Manual of Pediatric Balance Disorders

Second Edition

Manual of Pediatric Balance Disorders

Second Edition

Robert C. O'Reilly, MD, FACS
Thierry Morlet, PhD
Jacob R. Brodsky, MD, FACS, FAAP
Sharon L. Cushing, MD, MSc, FRCSC

Plural Publishing Inc.

PLURAL PUBLISHING INC.

5521 Ruffin Road
San Diego, CA 92123

e-mail: information@pluralpublishing.com
Website: https://www.pluralpublishing.com

Typeset in 11/13 Adobe Garamond Pro by Flanagan's Publishing Services, Inc.
Printed in the United States of America by Integrated Books International

Library of Congress Cataloging-in-Publication Data:

Names: O'Reilly, Robert (Robert Carlos), editor. | Morlet, Thierry, editor. | Brodsky, Jacob R., editor. | Cushing, Sharon L., editor.
Title: Manual of pediatric balance disorders / [edited by] Robert C. O'Reilly, Thierry Morlet, Jacob R. Brodsky, Sharon L. Cushing.
Description: Second edition. | San Diego, CA : Plural Publishing, Inc., [2020] | Includes bibliographical references and index.
Identifiers: LCCN 2019022621 | ISBN 9781635501469 (paperback) | ISBN 9781635501483 (ebook)
Subjects: MESH: Vestibular Diseases | Postural Balance | Movement Disorders | Nervous System Diseases—physiopathology | Child | Infant
Classification: LCC RF260 | NLM WV 255 | DDC 617.8/82083—dc23
LC record available at https://lccn.loc.gov/2019022621

Contents

Preface

The study of balance and vestibular disorders in adults has reached a degree of sophistication that parallels the study of auditory disorders. In contradistinction, our knowledge of balance problems in children is, so to speak, in its infancy but growing exponentially. The first edition of this book was born out of collaborations and discussions, with the editors recognizing that there was a paucity of materials available to the pediatric clinician and researcher regarding pediatric balance dysfunction. The limited information on this topic in other texts of vestibular and balance disorders has largely been a rehashing of adult topics without an in-depth analysis of what makes the pathophysiology and presentation of these problems so different in children. The genesis of this manual springs from an intention to rectify this deficit in knowledge. In the last 6 years, there has been tremendous growth in our knowledge about pediatric vestibular and balance disorders, leading to the revision of the first edition. This second edition has been thoroughly updated and is a testament to how far we have come in recognizing and managing this complex patient population.

This text is meant to be used by a broad array of clinicians and students. It has been intentionally named a "manual," reflecting its role in the classroom, clinic, bedside, and laboratory. Included with the text is a companion website with self-assessment questions, figures and videos, and suggested readings. We hope that the information contained within finds its way into the hands of physicians, audiologists, physical, occupational, and other therapists, as well as researchers.

The topics are broadly divided into four sections. The first chapters on basic mechanisms set the groundwork for understanding the anatomy and physiology of the vestibular and balance systems, with particular emphasis on maturation of these systems in children. These are followed by a series of chapters regarding the clinical evaluation of children with balance dysfunction. Tips and special techniques for testing in the young patient are emphasized and highlighted in the accompanying videos. Next, a series of chapters addresses the range of pathology encountered in this age group. The reader will find here a treasure trove of information directly applicable in the clinic and a spectrum of disease that is markedly different than what is encountered in adults. Finally, the book concludes with a careful review of treatment and a last chapter that looks to the future of this nascent field of study.

This second edition of the book is based on the foundation of the first and is the product of years of study, careful observation, fruitful collaborations with talented clinicians, and, most importantly, the byproduct of the desire and indeed necessity of helping those who cannot help themselves. We are deeply grateful to all participating authors for sharing their distinguished expertise. Last, none of this would have been possible without the willingness of our patients and their families to allow us to learn from them.

Robert C. O'Reilly
Thierry Morlet
Jacob R. Brodsky
Sharon L. Cushing

Acknowledgments

I would like to express my deepest gratitude to all the individuals who have given me opportunities throughout my career. I want to recognize the mentorship and friendship I received during my residency at Thomas Jefferson University and Neurotology fellowship at the University of Pittsburgh. I want to thank William Keane, Dale Lowry, Ed Pribitkin, Tom Willcox, Don Kamerer, Barry Hirsch, Steve Cass, Eugene Myers, Jonas Johnson, and my friends and colleagues at the Children's Hospital of Philadelphia. In particular, I want to thank my teacher and friend James S. Reilly, whose vision led me down this path.

For Maggie, Patrick, and Robby: life is a box of chocolates.

Robert C. O'Reilly

To Anaïs and Cylia

To L. Collet, J. D. Durrant, and C. I. Berlin for their remarkable mentorship over the years.

Thierry Morlet

Renée and Tobin, words cannot express my deep appreciation for your patience, love, and support.

Thank you to my parents and friends for your unwavering encouragement.

Thank you to my coeditors for your mentorship and for paving the way for this new field of pediatric vestibular medicine.

Thank you to my other mentors and colleagues, especially Dennis Poe, Daniel J. Lee, Margaret Kenna, Greg Licameli, Michael Cunningham, Richard Lewis, and Charles I. Woods.

Thank you to my patients and to the Balance and Vestibular Program team for your support and patience as we navigate a fledgling field where the best solutions are often ones that we learn together as we go along.

Jacob R. Brodsky

To Richard, Alicia, and Karen—You are my foundation and compass.

To Dr. Blake Papsin—You have provided me with mentorship and most importantly friendship that I will carry with me always.

To Drs. J. M. Filion, Ken Rose, and Karen Gordon—You have been the signposts along a career path that I didn't necessarily see coming.

To Dr. David Tomlinson—Your work and legacy remain a constant inspiration.

To my mentors, colleagues, and students—Thank you for your guidance and support throughout my residency at the University of Toronto, fellowship at Seattle Children's Hospital, and career at the Hospital for Sick Children.

Sharon L. Cushing

About the Editors

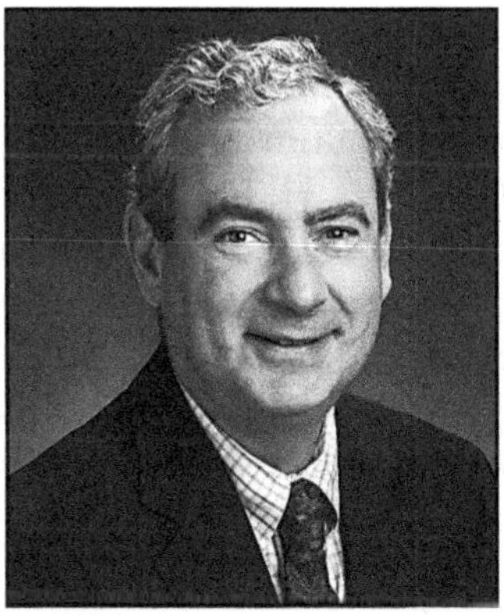

Robert C. O'Reilly, MD, FACS

Robert C. O'Reilly, MD, FACS, is director of the Balance and Vestibular Program at the Children's Hospital of Philadelphia. He is a professor of Otolaryngology-Head and Neck Surgery at the Children's Hospital of Philadelphia and the Perelman School of Medicine of the University of Pennsylvania. O'Reilly is a graduate of Thomas Jefferson University Medical School (1990) and completed residency in otolaryngology at the same institution. He completed a fellowship in neurotology at the University of Pittsburgh Medical Center and is board certified in otolaryngology-head and neck surgery. O'Reilly's basic science and research publications have included techniques of otologic surgery and disorders of the cochlea and vestibular systems. He has presented his work on pediatric balance disorders at national and international meetings. He is a winner of the Triological Society's Harris P. Mosher Award for clinical research. His current research includes assessment of static and dynamic balance in pediatric vestibulopathy, the genetics of vestibular disorders, and strategies for biofilm disruption.

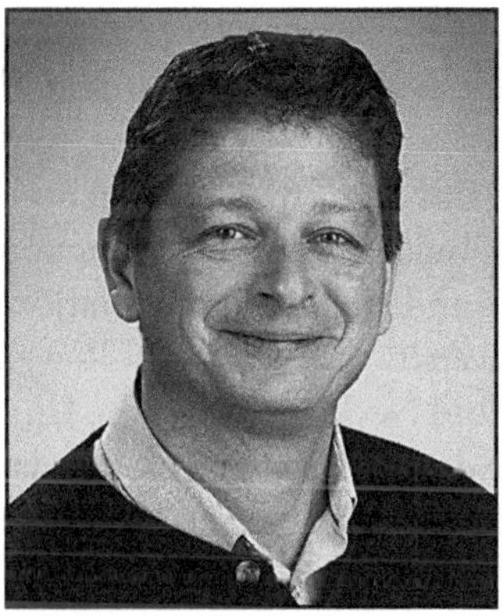

Thierry Morlet, PhD

Thierry Morlet, PhD, is a senior research scientist and head of the Auditory Physiology and Psychoacoustics Laboratory at the Nemours/Alfred I. duPont Hospital for Children, director of the Auditory Neuropathy program at Nemours, adjunct assistant professor in the Department of Linguistics and Cognitive Science, College of Arts and Science at the University of Delaware, adjunct professor in Communication Sciences and Disorders, College of Health Sciences at the University of Delaware, and adjunct faculty at the Georges Osborne College of Audiology, Salus University. With a PhD in Neuroscience from the University of Lyon (France), Morlet has a broad background in human auditory and vestibular physiology and has extensively studied otoacoustic emissions, efferent auditory pathways, and event-related potentials in the normally functioning and diseased auditory systems of children and adults. He is a member of the cochlear implant program, the "Hear We Go" 5K run/walk committee, and the auditory processing disorder program at Nemours, and is the chairperson of the Nemours Lectures on Pediatric Research. He has authored or coauthored more than 55 articles on the development of hearing, pediatric hearing loss, vestibular and balance disorders, auditory processing disorders, auditory neuropathy spectrum disorder, and inner ear malformations.

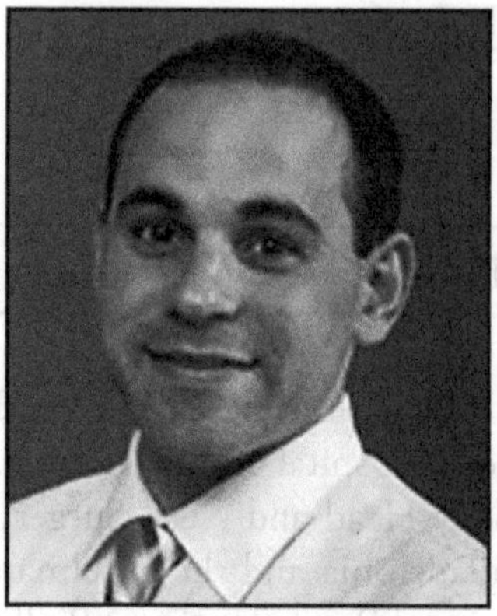

Jacob R. Brodsky, MD, FACS, FAAP

Brodsky's clinical and academic work focuses on disorders of the middle and inner ear, including the medical and surgical management of hearing loss and vestibular disorders. He has published widely on these topics and routinely presents his work at national and international meetings. He has a particular research interest in the effects of concussion and head trauma on the inner ear. He is the director of the Balance and Vestibular Program and co-coordinator of the Multidisciplinary Concussion Clinic at Boston Children's Hospital, Massachusetts. He is also an assistant professor of Otolaryngology at Harvard Medical School. Brodsky completed his otolaryngology residency at Upstate Medical University in 2011 and his pediatric otolaryngology fellowship at Boston Children's Hospital in 2012.

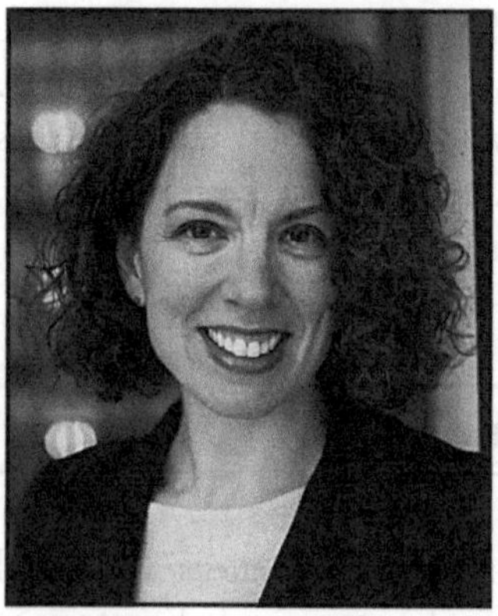

Sharon L. Cushing, MD, MSc, FRCSC

Sharon L. Cushing is a full-time pediatric otolaryngologist at the Hospital for Sick Children in Toronto, Canada, and an associate professor and clinician investigator in the Department of Otolaryngology-Head and Neck Surgery at the University of Toronto. She is the director of the Cochlear Implant Program at the the Hospital for Sick Children. Cushing has a clinical and surgical interest in disorders of the external, middle, and inner ear, including hearing loss and vestibular dysfunction. Her research interests include vestibular and balance function and dysfunction in children, and its association with hearing loss and cochlear implantation.

Cushing completed her undergraduate degree at Queen's University in Kingston, followed by medical school and residency training in Otolaryngology-Head and Neck Surgery at the University of Toronto. In addition, she completed a master's in science degree examining vestibular function and balance in children with hearing loss through the Surgeon Scientist Program at the University of Toronto. She completed her fellowship training in Pediatric Otolaryngology at Seattle Children's Hospital prior to returning to Sick Kids in Toronto.

Contributors

Jacob R. Brodsky, MD, FACS, FAAP
Assistant Professor of Otolaryngology
Harvard Medical School
Pediatric Otolaryngologist
Department of Otolaryngology and Communication Enhancement
Boston Children's Hospital
Director of the Balance and Vestibular Program
Boston Children's Hospital
Boston, Massachusetts
Chapters 15, 16, and 17

Jennifer L. Campos, PhD
Associate Director, Academic
Senior Scientist
Chief Scientist, Challenging Environments Assessment Laboratory
KITE, Toronto Rehabilitation Institute
University Health Network
Associate Professor
Department of Psychology
University of Toronto
Toronto, Ontario
Chapter 12

Nicole Captain, Msc (OT), BA, OT Reg (Ont)
Child Development Program
Holland Bloorview Kids Rehabilitation Hospital
Lecturer, Status Appointment
Department of Occupational Science and Occupational Therapy
University of Toronto
Toronto, Ontario
Chapter 27

Margaretha L. Casselbrant, MD, PhD
Professor Emerita of Otolaryngology
University of Pittsburgh School of Medicine
Pittsburgh, Pennsylvania
Chapter 16

Sharon L. Cushing, MD, MSc, FRCSC
Associate Professor
University of Toronto
Otolaryngologist, Director
Cochlear Implant Program
The Hospital for Sick Children
Toronto, Ontario
Chapters 4, 12, 14, 24, and 28

Wanda A. Dillon
Diploma in Nursing
Clinical Vestibular Nurse
The Hertz Multidisciplinary Neurotology Clinic
University Health Network–Toronto General Hospital
Toronto Ontario
Chapter 24

Philip Gerretsen, MD, PhD, FRCPC
Hertz Multidisciplinary Neurotology Clinic
Department of Otolaryngology-Head and Neck Surgery
Toronto General Hospital
Department of Psychiatry
Institute of Medical Science
University of Toronto
Toronto, Ontario
Chapter 24

Christina Y. Go, MD, DABPN-Neurology
Division of Neurology
The Hospital for Sick Children
Assistant Professor
Department of Pediatrics
University of Toronto
Toronto, Canada
Chapter 20

Karen A. Gordon, PhD, CCC-A, Reg. CASLPO
Archie's Cochlear Implant Laboratory
The Hospital for Sick Children, Toronto
Department of Otolaryngology-HNS
University of Toronto
Toronto, Ontario
Chapter 12

Nathalie Goulème, PhD
Lyon Neuroscience Research Center
Department of Audiology and Otoneurological Evaluation
Civil Hospitals of Lyon
Lyon, France
Chapter 9

Renée Haldenby, BSc, MSc PT
Physical Therapist
SickKids
University of Toronto
Toronto, Ontario
Chapter 10

John Henley, PhD
Senior Engineer
Gait Analysis Laboratory
Nemours/Alfred I. duPont Hospital for Children
Wilmington, Delaware
Chapter 11

George M. Ibrahim, MD, PhD, FRCSC, FAANS
Pediatric Neurosurgeon
The Hospital for Sick Children
Assistant Professor
IBBME
Institute of Medical Science
University of Toronto
Associate Scientist
Neurosciences and Mental Health
SickKids Research Institute
Toronto, Ontario
Chapter 18

Eugen Ionescu, MD
Otorhinolaryngologist
Senior Neurotologist
Department of Audiology and Neurotology
Civil Hospitals of Lyon
Lyon, France
Chapter 9

Huseyin Isildak, MD
Assistant Professor of Surgery
Director of Otology and Neurotology
Director of Cochlear Implant Program
Division of Otolaryngology-Head and Neck Surgery
The Pennsylvania State University
The Milton S. Hershey Medical Center
Hershey, Pennsylvania
Chapter 1

Michael Karl, PT, DPT, OCS, FAAOMPT
Physical Therapist
Balance and Vestibular Clinic
Sports Medicine and Performance Center
Children's Hospital of Philadelphia
Philadelphia, Pennsylvania
Chapter 26

Ana Marissa Lagman-Bartoleme, MD, FRCPC, Diplomate, UCNS (Headache)
Assistant Professor (Pediatrics)
Director, Pediatric and Adolescent Headache/Concussion Program
Centre for Headache
Women's College Hospital
The Hospital for Sick Children
University of Toronto
Toronto, Ontario
Chapter 21

Violette H. Lavender, AuD
Pediatric Audiologist
Division of Audiology
Cincinnati Children's Hospital
Cincinnati, Ohio
Chapter 7

Jane Lea, BSc, MD, FRCSC
Assistant Professor
Department of Surgery
Division of Otolaryngology-Head and Neck Surgery
The University of British Columbia
Director
BC Rotary Hearing and Balance Centre
St. Paul's Hospital, Providence Health Care
Vancouver, British Columbia
Chapter 14

Jessica R. Levi, MD
Director, Division of Pediatric Otolaryngology
Otolaryngology Clerkship Director
Department of Otolaryngology- Head and Neck Surgery and Department of Pediatrics
Boston University and Boston Medical Center
Boston, Massachusetts
Chapter 4

Gillian Liberman, MSW, RSW
Department of Otolaryngology-Head and Neck Surgery
Department of Social Work
The Hospital for Sick Children
University of Toronto
Toronto, Canada
Chapter 24

Sophie E. Lipson, BA
Research Assistant
Balance and Vestibular Program
Department of Otolaryngology and Communication Enhancement
Boston's Children Hospital
Boston, Massachusetts
Chapter 15

Abigail Lynch
Division of Neurology
Children's Hospital of Philadelphia
Philadelphia, Pennsylvania
Chapter 19

David R. Lynch, MD, PhD
Professor of Neurology and Pediatrics
University of Pennsylvania
Philadelphia, Pennsylvania
Chapter 19

Claire McSweeny, BA
The Hospital for Sick Children
University of Toronto
Toronto, Ontario
Chapter 12

Freeman Miller, MD
Pediatric Orthopedic Surgeon
Co-Director, Cerebral Palsy Program
Nemours/Alfred I. duPont Hospital for Children
Wilmington, Delaware
Chapter 11

Stephanie A. Moody Antonio, MD, FACS
Otology-Neurotology
Associate Professor
Eastern Virginia Medical School
Children's Hospital of the King's Daughters
Norfolk, Virginia
Chapter 23

Thierry Morlet, PhD
Head, Auditory Physiology and Psychoacoustics Laboratory
Center for Pediatric Auditory and Speech Sciences
Nemours/Alfred I. duPont Hospital for Children
Wilmington, Delaware
Adjunct Assistant Professor
Department of Linguistics and Cognitive Science
University of Delaware
Newark, Delaware
Chapter 2

Timothy A. Niiler, PhD
Associate Teaching Professor of Physics
Penn State Brandywine
Adjunct Biomechanist/Biostatistician
Nemours/Alfred I. duPont Hospital for Children
West Chester, Pennsylvania
Chapter 11

Robert C. O'Reilly, MD
Division Chief, Pediatric Otolaryngology
Nemours/Alfred I. duPont Hospital for Children
Wilmington, Delaware
Professor of Otolaryngology and Pediatrics
Jefferson Medical College of Thomas Jefferson University
Philadelphia, Pennsylvania
Chapters 4 and 28

Moira Pena, MOT, OT Reg (Ont)
Child Development Program
Holland Bloorview Kids Rehabilitation Hospital
Lecturer, Status Appointment
Department of Occupational Science and Occupational Therapy
University of Toronto
Toronto, Ontario
Chapter 27

James O. Phillips, PhD
Research Associate Professor
Department of Otolaryngology-Head and Neck Surgery
University of Washington
Seattle, Washington
Chapters 3 and 6

Melissa B. Ramocki, MD, PhD
Center for Vestibular and Balance Disorders, A Division of University Otolaryngology
East Greenwich, Rhode Island
Chapter 13

Y. Arun Reginald, MBBS, FRCSC
The Hospital for Sick Children
University of Toronto
Toronto, Ontario
Chapter 22

Pierre Reynard, MD
Department of Audiology and Otoneurological Evaluation
Civil Hospitals of Lyon
Claude Bernard University Lyon 1
Lyon, France
Chapter 9

Lance H. Rodan, MD
Division of Genetics and Genomics, Department of Pediatrics
Boston Children's Hospital
Department of Neurology
Harvard Medical School
Boston, Massachusetts
Chapter 13

Kim Schadt, MSN, CRNP
Children's Hospital of Philadelphia
Philadelphia, Pennsylvania
Chapter 19

Anne Scofich, BSc, PT, MSc
Clinical Director
Department of Rehabilitation
The Hospital for Sick Children
Toronto, Canada
Chapter 10

Teesta Soman, MD, MBA
Staff Neurologist
The Hospital for Sick Children
Assistant Professor of Pediatrics
University of Toronto
Toronto, Ontario
Chapter 21

Michael Teixido, MD
Assistant Clinical Professor

Department of Otolaryngology-Head and Neck Surgery
Jefferson Medical College of Thomas Jefferson University
Philadelphia, Pennsylvania
Chapter 1

Hung Thai-Van, MD, PhD
Head, Department of Audiology and Otoneurological Evaluation
Lyon University Hospital
Hearing Institute
Institut Pasteur, Inserm U1120
Lyon, France
Chapter 9

Henri Traboulsi, MD
Clinical Instructor
Pediatric Otolaryngology
Baylor College of Medicine
Texas Children's Hospital
Houston, Texas
Chapter 16

Joan Vertes, OT Reg (Ont)
Occupational Therapist
Department of Occupational Science and Occupational Therapy
University of Toronto
Department of Rehabilitation Services
The Hospital for Sick Children
Toronto, Ontario
Chapter 25

Richard Vincent, MD
ENT of Southeastern Connecticut
Old Saybrook, Connecticut
Chapter 1

Shelly Wang, MD, MPH, FRCSC
Pediatric Neurosurgery Fellow
Nicklaus Children's Hospital
Miami, Florida
Chapter 18

Vincent G. Wettstein, MD
Department of Otorhinolaryngology-Head and Neck Surgery
University Hospital Zürich
Zürich, Switzerland
Chapter 7

Sylvette Wiener-Vacher, MD
Vestibular and Oculomotor Evaluation Unit
ORL Department
Hopital Pédiatrique Robert Debré
Paris, France
Chapter 8

Janet Woodhouse, MEd, BSc OT, OT Reg (Ont)
Brain Injury Rehab Team
Holland Bloorview Kids Rehabilitation Hospital
Lecturer, Status Appointment
Department of Occupational Science and Occupational Therapy
University of Toronto
Toronto, Ontario
Chapter 27

Guangwei Zhou, ScD, CCC-A, FAAA
Balance and Vestibular Program
Department of Otolaryngology and Communication Enhancement
Boston Children's Hospital
Assistant Professor of Otolaryngology
Harvard Medical School
Waltham, Massachusetts
Chapters 7 and 8

Emily F. Zwicky, AuD, CCC-A
Senior Staff Audiologist
Virginia Commonwealth University
Audiology Department
Children's Hospital of Richmond
Richmond, Virginia
Chapter 5

SECTION I

Basic Mechanisms

CHAPTER 1

Anatomy and Embryology of the Vestibular Apparatus

Richard Vincent, Huseyin Isildak, Michael Teixido

Embryology

The vestibular apparatus is one of the systems of balance and equilibrium. Although balance and equilibrium depend on the interaction of multiple senses including vision and proprioception, it is primarily controlled by the vestibular apparatus. The vestibular apparatus consists of three semicircular canals, which are sensitive to angular accelerations, and two otolith organs, which are sensitive to linear accelerations. In this chapter, the anatomy and embryology of the vestibular apparatus are discussed in some detail. As an aid to understanding the complex three-dimensional anatomy of the vestibular apparatus, the reader is urged to use virtual models constructed from serial sections through the human temporal bone. They are available from the Eaton-Peabody Laboratory of Auditory Physiology/Massachusetts Eye and Ear Infirmary website (http://research.meei.harvard.edu/otopathology/3dmodels/).

While middle ear structures develop from mesoderm, external ear and inner ear develop from ectoderm. The Eustachian tube and middle ear cavity come from elongation of the endoderm-lined first pharyngeal pouch. The tympanic membrane (TM) develops from ectoderm, endoderm, and mesoderm.

The vestibular apparatus begins development around the third week of gestational age and is complete at 25 weeks of gestational age. When the human embryo reaches the third week of gestational age, surface ectoderm overlying the future site of the inner ear thickens to form the otic placode, which invaginates into the mesenchyme and forms an otic pit. During the fourth week, the otic pit becomes the otic vesicle. A portion of neural crest migrates to the forming otic vesicle and originates the acousticofacial ganglion. The ganglion differentiates into four distinguishable parts: geniculate, superior vestibular, inferior vestibular, and cochlear.

Within 1 or 2 days of formation of the otic vesicle, the otic vesicle elongates and differentiates to form a medial portion, the endolymphatic diverticulum, and a lateral portion, the utriculosaccular chamber. The endolymphatic diverticulum gives rise to the endolymphatic sac and duct. By a constriction of its middle, the utriculosaccular chamber divides into a utricular portion that later becomes the semicircular canals and the utricle, and a saccular portion destined to become the saccule and the cochlea (Figure 1–1).

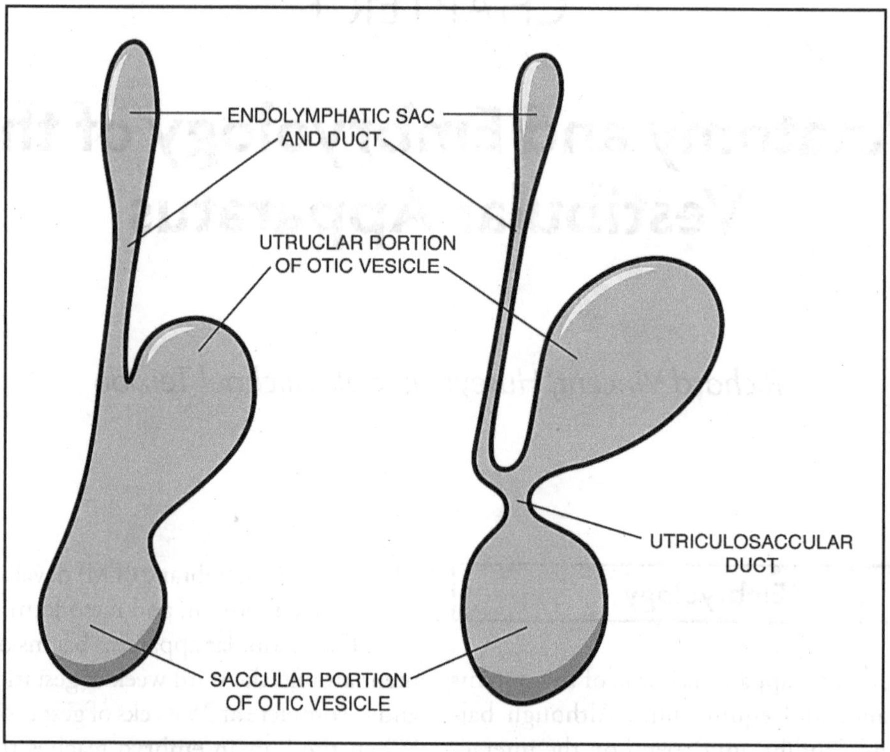

Figure 1–1. Morphogenesis of the vestibular system starts with partitioning of the otocyst into a utricular portion and a saccular portion. The two portions are separated by the utricolo-saccular duct. The semicircular canals will develop from the utricular portion of the otic vesicle. The future cochlear duct develops as a further partitioning of the saccular portion of the otic vesicle (not shown).

At about 6 weeks, the semicircular canals appear as flattened outpocketings of the utricular portion. The central portions of the walls of these outpocketings eventually approach and efface one another and finally disappear, leaving spaces around the perimeter that become the three semicircular canals (Figure 1–2). The superior semicircular canal forms first, followed by the posterior and lateral canals. Dilations of one end of each of the semicircular ducts become the ampullae. The opposite ends of the canals remain unwidened. The saccular portion of the utriculosaccular chamber gives rise to the saccule and the cochlea. The communication between the saccule and membranous cochlea narrows to form the ductus reuniens (Figure 1–3).

Parallel to the morphological changes within the otocyst, histological differentiations of the sensory epithelium are also occurring. The arrival of afferent endings in the epithelium precedes hair cell differentiation.[1,2] Around the third week, the vestibular sensory neuroepithelium develops from ectoderm. Its upper part gives rise to the utricular macula and crista ampullaris of the superior and lateral semicircular ducts, and its lower part gives rise to the saccular macula and crista ampullaris of the posterior semicircular duct.

The hair cells in the vestibular end organs reach adult form at about 9 weeks; the macu-

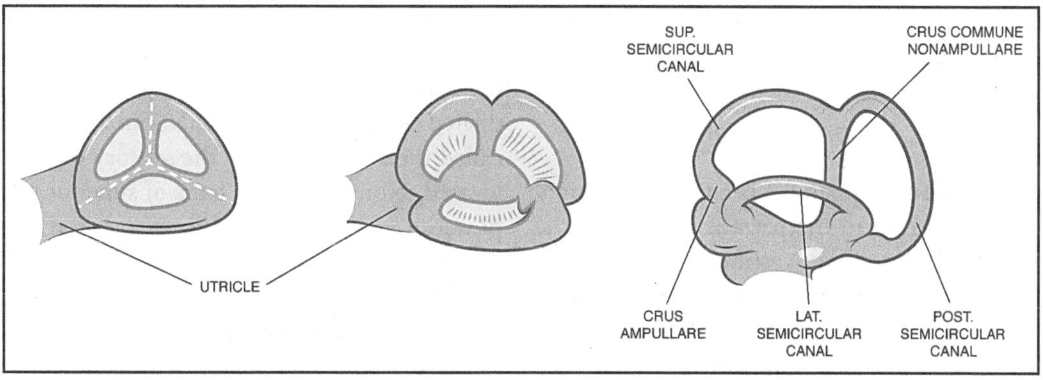

Figure 1–2. Morphogenesis of the labyrinth with formation of the semicircular canals from the utricular portion of the otic vesicle at 5, 6, and 8 weeks.

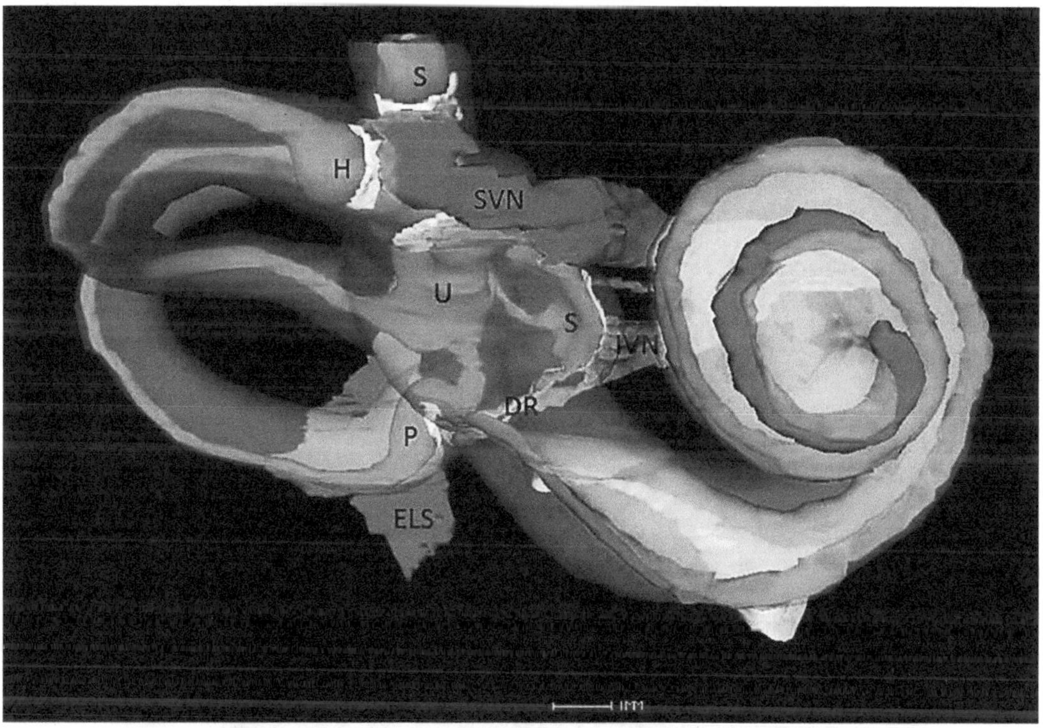

Figure 1–3. The human membranous labyrinth can be seen with its innervations and end organs within the larger perilymphatic space. (DR, ductus reuniens; ELS, endolymphatic sac; H, horizontal ampulla; IVN, inferior vestibular nerve; P, posterior ampulla; S, saccule; SA, superior ampulla; SVN, superior vestibular nerve; U, utricle.) http://research.meei.harvard.edu/otopathology/3dmodels/

lae at about 16 weeks; and the cristae, at about 23 weeks. The mesoderm surrounding the membranous labyrinth gives rise to the bony otic capsule. The membranous labyrinth is suspended in perilymph fluid within the bony labyrinth by loose connective tissue.

Anatomy

General Anatomy

The vestibular apparatus is enclosed within a bony labyrinth in the petrous portion of the temporal bone. The vestibular apparatus is contained within an endolymph-filled membranous labyrinth, which is itself contained in the perilymph-filled bony labyrinth. The vestibular apparatus consists of three semicircular canals (SCCs) and two otolith organs: utricle and saccule.

The three semicircular canals are formed like a bent torus. Within each bony and perilymph-filled semicircular canal lies the semicircular duct. Each semicircular duct rides along the outermost edge of its canal where it maintains an intermittent mesenteric attachment to the overlying endosteum. There is a dilated end of each semicircular canal and duct called the ampulla where the sensory organ is located. Nonampullated ends of superior and posterior canals unite and form a shared segment termed the common crus. The ampullated and nonampullated ends of the SCCs are connected to the utriculus.

Each SCC is oriented in a different plane: superior (or anterior), horizontal (or lateral), and posterior. Each canal is oriented at approximately right angles to the other two.[3] The superior and posterior canals are oriented roughly at 45° in relation to the sagittal plane, and the lateral canal angles 22° upward from the horizontal plane (Figure 1–4). Each semi-

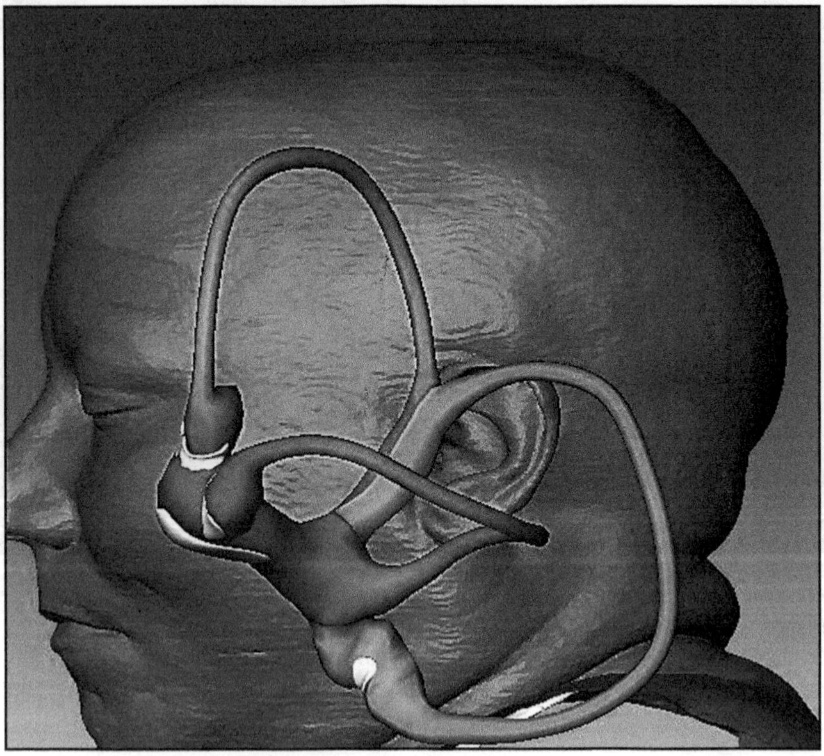

Figure 1–4. The utricle and semicircular ducts of the left membranous labyrinth can be seen in their anatomic position relative to the head. The horizontal canal plane is oriented 22° above the horizontal plane.

circular canal is maximally sensitive to motion in the plane of that canal. The result of this unique arrangement is that SCCs can specify the direction of any head rotation. The canals also act in functional pairs with one canal from each ear oriented in the same plane. Rotation in that plane will be excitatory to one canal and inhibitory to the other. The left and right lateral canals are one pair. The anterior canal on one side is paired with the posterior canal on the opposite side creating two functional planes commonly referred to as the RALP (right anterior-left posterior) and LARP (left anterior-right posterior) planes (Figure 1–5). One canal gives an excitatory response, and the other canal gives an inhibitory response for rotation in a given plane. This paired input is then integrated by the brainstem to control balance.

The structures of the utricle and saccule are different from the semicircular canals. They are irregular in shape; while the utricle is an oval shape tube, the saccule is a flattened shaped sac. The utricle lies mainly in the horizontal plane, and the saccule lies mainly in the vertical plane. The utricle and saccule fluid spaces communicate with one another via the utricular duct and saccular ducts that join the endolymphatic sinus. The utricle is connected to the endolymphatic duct via the utricular duct and endolymphatic sinus. The utricular duct originates from the inferior part of the utricle by a cleft-shaped opening and passes close to the utricle wall, and thus, the utriculo-endolymphatic valve is formed.[4,5] The utriculo-endolymphatic valve (UEV) was first described in a human fetus by Bast in 1928, and it is located in the posterior wall of the utricle at its junction with the utricular duct. The function of the UEV remains unclear, but some researchers suggest that the UEV may prevent loss of endolymph from the utricle and SCCs and preserve the anatomical features of the utricle and SCCs during developmental, disease-related, and traumatic events.[6,7] The saccule is connected to the endolymphatic duct via the saccular duct and to the cochlear duct via the ductus reuniens (Figure 1–6).

The anatomic orientations of the utricular and saccular maculae allow the utricle to sense motion in the horizontal plane (eg,

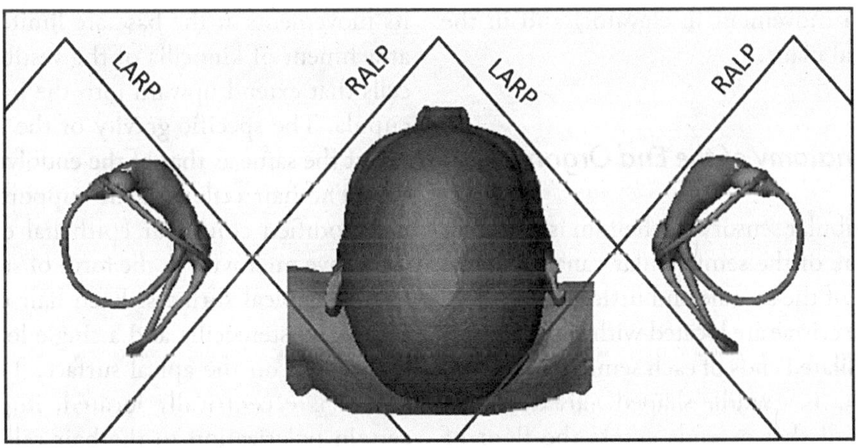

Figure 1–5. The RALP and LARP planes. The right anterior (RA) and left posterior (LP) canals are roughly coplanar and form the RALP plane in which excitation in one canal is associated with inhibition in the other. The left anterior (LA) and right posterior (RP) canals form another functional pair of canals in the LARP plane.

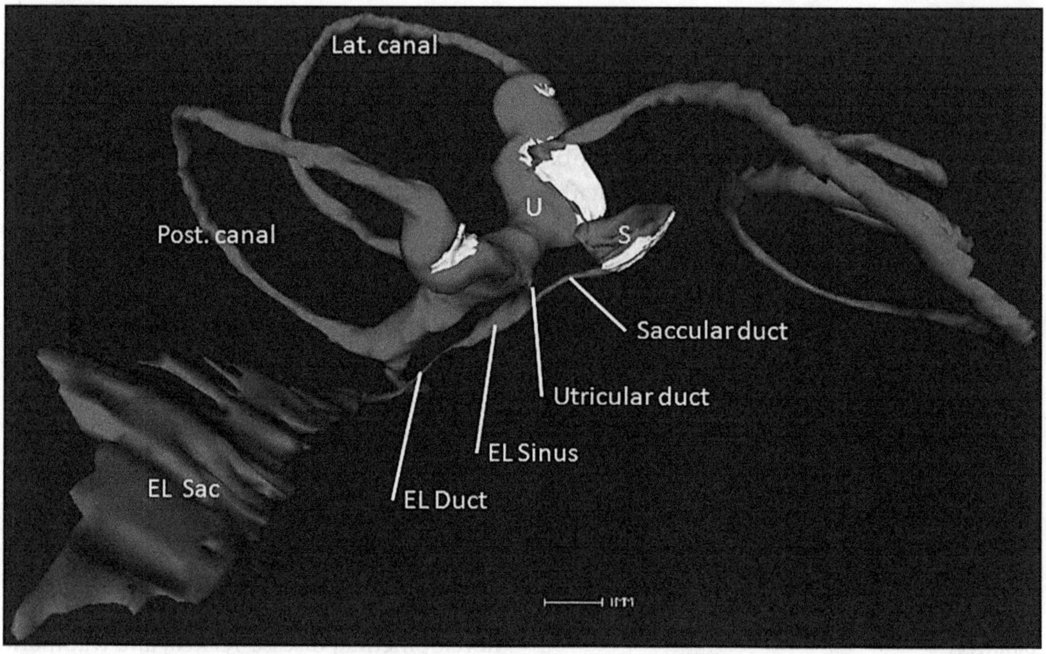

Figure 1–6. The human membranous labyrinth from below. Seen from below, the trifurcate connection of the utricle (U), saccule (S), and the endolymphatic sac (EL Sac) can be seen converging on the endolymphatic sinus (EL Sinus). From the endolymphatic sinus radiate the endolymphatic duct (EL Duct), the utricular duct, and the saccular duct. http://research.meei.harvard.edu/otopathology/3dmodels/

acceleration on forward-backward movement, left-right movement) and the saccule to sense accelerations in the vertical plane (eg, up-down movement in elevator) and in the horizontal plane.

Anatomy of the End Organs

The vestibular sensory epithelium is placed in the cristae of the semicircular canals and the maculae of the saccule and utricle.

The cristae are located within the ampullae, the dilated ends of each semicircular duct. The crista is a saddle-shaped, raised section of the wall that extends across the floor of the ampulla perpendicular to its long axis. It is surmounted by a bulbous, wedge-shaped, gelatinous mass called the cupula. The spinnaker-shaped cupula extends from the surface of the cristae to the roof and lateral walls of the membranous labyrinth, and forms a fluid-tight division. It is anchored at the roof and its movements at the base are limited by the attachment of kinocilia of the vestibular hair cells that extend upward into the base of the cupula. The specific gravity of the cupula is about the same as that of the endolymph.

The hair cells and the supporting cells are modified columnar epithelial cells, and they have microvilli in the form of stereocilia, on their apical surfaces. Each hair cell bears 50 to 100 stereocilia and a single long, thick kinocilium on the apical surface. This kinocilium is eccentrically located, imparting a certain polarization to the hair cell that has important functional implications. While in the superior and posterior semicircular canals, the kinocilia are located on the side of the hair cell away from the utriculus, in the lateral semicircular canals the kinocilium is located on the side nearest the utricle (Figure 1–7). The movement of the hair bundle toward the kinocilium causes an increase in the firing rate of the hair cell, while deflection away causes a decrease in the firing rate (see physiology section for more detail).

Hair cells are surrounded by supporting cells, and form tight junctions and desmosomes with the supporting cells that limit the endolymphatic space at the surface of the cristae. In this way, endolymph bathes the stereocilia above the cells, and perilymph is present below the apical surface.

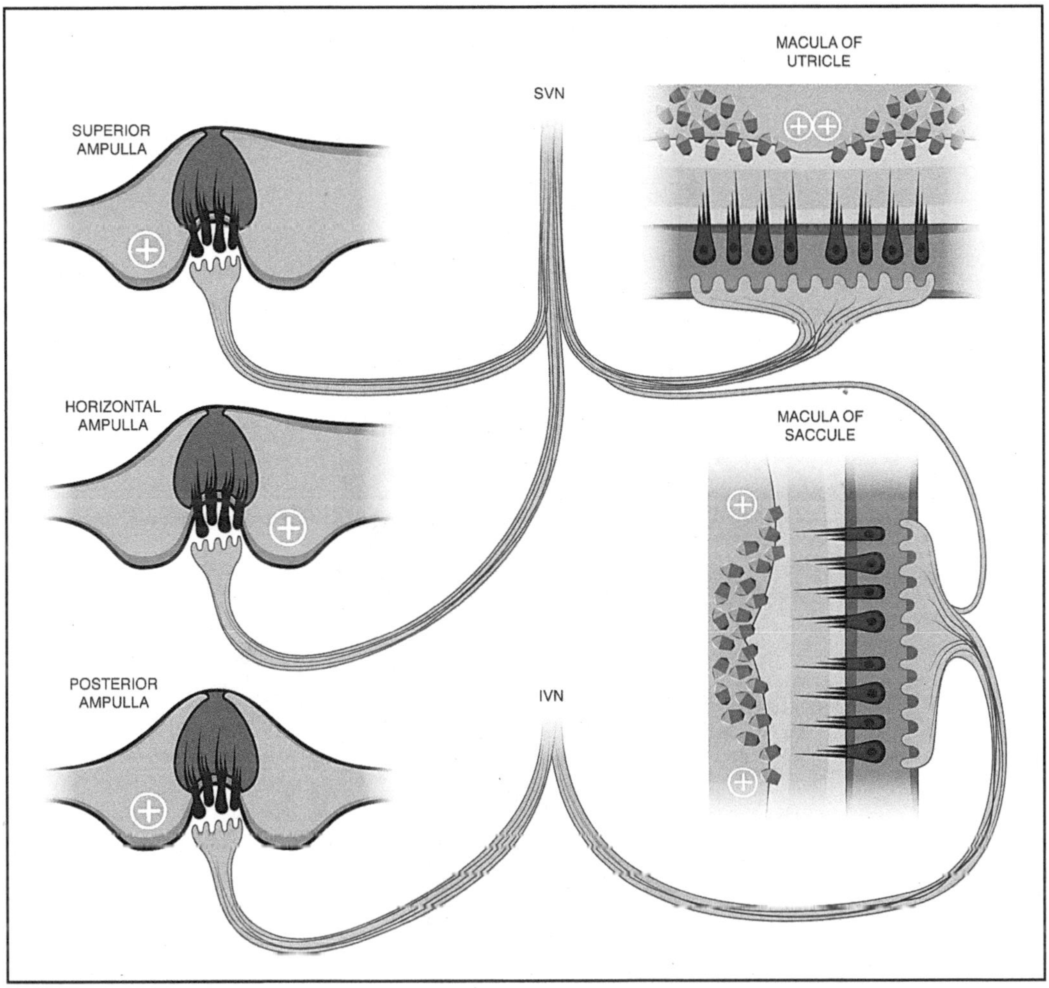

Figure 1–7. Polarization of the end organs. The relative positions of the three ampullae to the utricle and saccular maculae are shown. Deflection of the cupula of the superior and posterior ampullae away from the utricle is stimulatory, whereas deflection of the cupula of the horizontal ampulla toward the utricle is stimulatory. Note the orientation of the kinocilia of the utricular macula toward the striola and the orientation of the kinocilia of the saccular maculae away from the striola. The superior vestibular nerve (SVN) innervates the cristae of the superior and horizontal canals as well as the macula of the utricle and the superior portion of the macula of the saccule. The inferior vestibular nerve (IVN) innervates the crista of the posterior canal and the macula of the saccule.

Vestibular hair cells are of two types, type I and type II (Figure 1–8). The two hair cell types differ in several respects including their innervation characteristics and shapes. Type I hair cells are flask-shaped and are surrounded by a calyx ending. One calyx nerve ending can synapse with just one, or with two to four type I hair cells. Type II hair cells are cylinder-shaped cells that are contacted at their basal surfaces by numerous afferent and efferent synapses. Types I and II vestibular hair cells correspond morphologically to inner and outer hair cells of the organ of Corti.

Similar to the cristae ampullares, the maculae of the utriculus and sacculus consist of neuroepithelium, supporting cells, blood vessels, and nerve fibers. The maculae are covered with hair cells across their surface as well. The cilia of the hair cells protrude upward and are embedded in the otolithic membrane, a

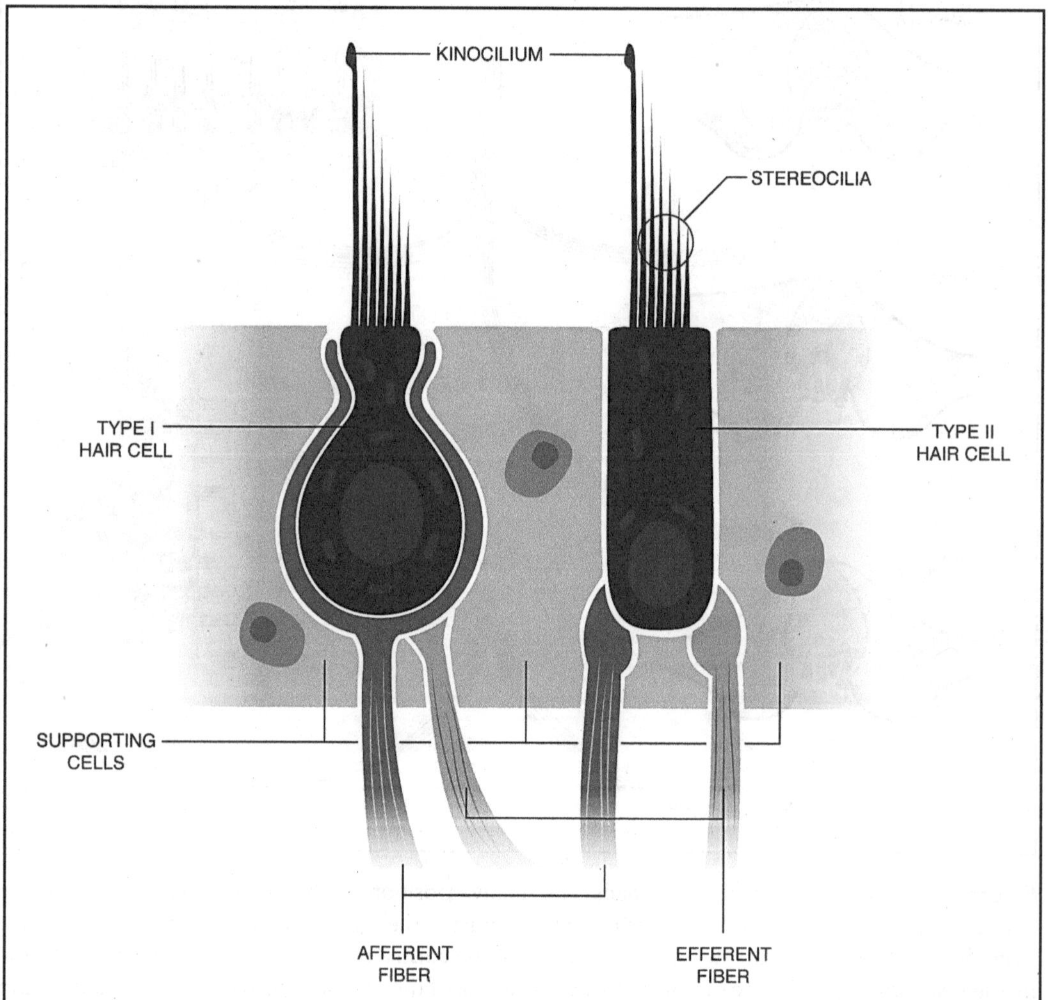

Figure 1–8. Type I and II hair cells. Type I hair cells are goblet shaped and are surrounded by a calyx-type afferent nerve ending. Type II hair cells are rod shaped and are contacted by bouton endings of afferent and efferent nerves. Both display similar arrangements of stereocilia and kinocilia and are surrounded by supporting cells.

gelatinous membrane analogous to the cupula but with no attachments to the utricular wall. Calcareous particles called otoconia (otoliths) are embedded in the otolithic membrane. Thus, the utriculus and sacculus are also referred to as the otolith organs. Otoconia are inorganic crystals composed of calcium carbonate.[8] They vary in size from 0.5 to 30 μm, with most being around 5 to 7 μm.[9] The otoconia have a slow turnover. They appear to be produced by the supporting cells of the sensory epithelium and to be resorbed by the dark cell region that surrounds the area of sensory cells. The dense embedded crystals make the specific gravity of the otolithic membrane much higher than that of the surrounding endolymph, around 2.71 to 2.94.[10] In the central portion of each otolithic membrane is a line called the striola. The striola is distinct as a thinning in the center of the otolithic membrane in the utricle and a thickening in that of the saccule. The striola divides the areas on the sensory epithelium with hair cells oriented in one direction from those oriented in the opposite direction. In the utricular macula, the hair cells are found to be polarized with the kinocilium facing the striola, whereas in the saccular macula, the kinocilium of each cell face away from the striola. Both the utricle and the saccule have a gently curved elliptical shape; thus, the striolae are curved lines. Because of the distributed orientation of the hair cell stereociliary bundles in all directions, static head tilts in any direction cause some hair cells to be excited and others to be inhibited in one or both of the otolithic organs.

Innervation of the Vestibular Apparatus

The basal portions of the hair cells synapse with afferent and efferent nerve fibers. According to more recent morphologic and physiologic work on vestibular afferents, three types of afferent endings are defined morphologically—pure calyx endings, bouton endings, and dimorphic endings (which may contain both calyx and bouton terminals).[11–13] Calyx endings are found in the central region of sensory epithelium, while bouton endings are found near the periphery. Dimorphic endings are found throughout the sensory epithelium. The classification of vestibular afferents correlates with numerous physiologic and morphologic features.[14,15] Calyx units innervate a few neighboring type I hair cells. Bouton units contact several type II hair cells. Dimorphic units innervate both kinds of receptors.

The primary vestibular neurons are bipolar neurons whose cell bodies make up the vestibular nerve ganglion called Scarpa's ganglion, located within the internal auditory meatus. Scarpa's ganglion consists of the bodies of the primary vestibular neurons, which are divided into a superior and an inferior group. The superior group innervates the cristae of the superior and lateral semicircular canals, the utricular macula, and the anterosuperior part of the saccular macula. The inferior group innervates the crista of the posterior semicircular canal and most of the saccular macula.

The fibers of the superior and inferior divisions of the vestibular nerve join the cochlear fibers to form the eighth nerve. In vivo magnetic resonance imaging (MRI) has shown the vestibulo-cochlear nerve is usually rectangular but sometimes round and rarely triangular in shape near the brainstem, and it becomes crescentic at the porus. The superior vestibular nerve keeps its posterosuperior position in the canal, and the inferior vestibular nerve and the cochlear nerve pass beneath the superior vestibular nerve. The vestibular fibers extend in a rostral-caudal direction in the internal auditory canal. These vestibular afferent fibers terminate in the vestibular nuclei in the floor of the fourth ventricle. The vestibular nuclei have been classified into four main regional subdivisions: superior, medial, lateral, and inferior vestibular nuclei.[16–18] The rostral branch projects to the superior and medial vestibular nuclei and sends a collateral branch to the cerebellum. The caudal branch projects to the inferior and medial vestibular nuclei and to the ventrolateral part of the lateral vestibular nucleus. Primary vestibular afferents do not cross the midline.

The projections from vestibular nucleus extend to the cerebellum, extraocular nuclei, and spinal cord. The projections of the superior vestibular nucleus go in an ascending direction to the nuclei of the extraocular muscles (III and IV) by way of the medial longitudinal fasciculus. The lateral vestibular nucleus has been shown to be the sole source of fibers to the vestibulospinal tract. These fibers terminate near the anterior horn cells of all the spinal cord levels and mediate trunk and limb muscle reflexes. The projections of the medial vestibular nucleus are ascending and descending in the medial longitudinal fasciculus. The ascending fibers course bilaterally to the extraocular muscles, and the descending fibers project to the cervical segment of the cord. The inferior vestibular nuclei integrate input from the vestibular system and the fastigial nucleus of the cerebellum. The vestibular cortex is in the temporal lobe near the auditory cortex. Functional MRI and positron emission tomography (PET) scanning studies implicate the insula as another possible cortical projection of the vestibular system.[19]

The Labyrinthine Fluids

The labyrinth contains two distinctly separate fluids: endolymph fills the membranous labyrinth, and perilymph fills the bony labyrinth. Thus, the endolymph-containing membranous labyrinth is surrounded by perilymph. Endolymph has ionic concentrations similar to intracellular fluid with high potassium and low sodium. It is produced by the marginal cells of the stria vascularis in the cochlea and by cells called dark cells in the maculae of the utricle and saccule. It is absorbed in the endolymphatic sac that is connected to the utricle and saccule via the endolymphatic, utricular, and saccular ducts.

Conversely, in perilymph the sodium content is high and the potassium content is low, which causes perilymph to resemble extracellular rather than intracellular fluid. The site of perilymph production is controversial. It may be formed from an ultrafiltrate of blood or cerebrospinal fluid as the perilymph compartment communicates with the cerebrospinal fluid containing subarachnoid space via the cochlear aqueduct.

Blood Supply of the Vestibular Apparatus

The main blood supply to the vestibular apparatus is the labyrinthine artery (internal auditory artery), which arises variably from the anterior inferior cerebellar artery (45%), superior cerebellar artery (24%), or from the basilar artery directly (16%).[20] After entering the inner ear, the labyrinthine artery splits into two branches: the anterior vestibular artery and the common cochlear artery. The anterior vestibular artery supplies the utricle, superior and lateral ampullae, and a small portion of the saccule, mirroring the distribution of fibers from the superior vestibular nerve. The common cochlear artery also splits in two divisions: the cochlear artery and the vestibulo-cochlear artery. The cochlear artery supplies the cochlea. The vestibulo-cochlear artery divides into a cochlear ramus and a vestibular ramus also known as the posterior vestibular artery. The cochlear ramus supplies the cochlea with the common cochlear artery. The posterior vestibular artery supplies the posterior ampulla, most of the saccule, part of the utricle, and part of the superior and lateral ampullae (Figure 1–9).

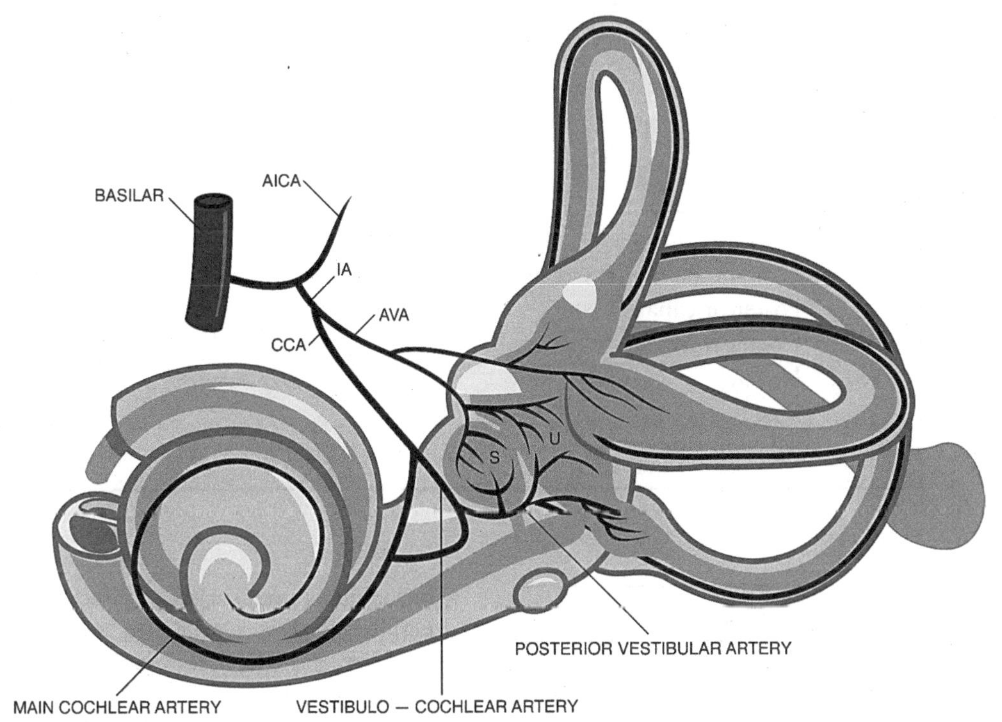

Figure 1–9. Blood supply of the cochlea. The internal auditory artery (IA) commonly arises from the anterior inferior cerebellar artery (AICA). The internal auditory artery divides into the common cochlear artery (CCA) and the anterior vestibular artery (AVA). The common cochlear artery gives rise to the cochlear artery, vestibulocochlear artery, and the posterior vestibular artery.

Self-Assessment Questions

1. Which canal is oriented in the same plane as the right anterior canal?
   a. Right horizontal
   b. Right anterior
   c. Left posterior
   d. Right posterior

2. The otolith organs sense:
   a. Head position in relation to gravity
   b. Angular acceleration
   c. Motion of the visual field
   d. Linear acceleration
   e. a and d

3. The inferior vestibular nerve innervates the:
    a. Posterior canal
    b. Saccule
    c. Anterior canal
    d. a and b
    e. All of the above

4. The saccule has connections to the:
    a. Posterior canal
    b. Cochlear duct
    c. Utricle
    d. b and c
    e. All of the above

References

1. Sans A, Deschesne CJ. Afferent nerve ending development and synaptogenesis in the vestibular epithelium of human fetuses. *Hear Res.* 1987;28:65–72.
2. Sans A, Deschesne CJ. Early development of vestibular receptors in human embryos: An electron microscopic study. *Acta Otolaryngol (Stockh) Suppl.*1985;423:51–58
3. Della Santina CC, Potyagaylo V, Migliaccio AA, Minor LB, Carey JP. Orientation of human semicircular canals measured by three-dimensional multiplanar CT reconstruction. *J Assoc Res Otolaryngol.* 2005 Sep;6(3):191–206.
4. Retzius G. *Das Gehorgan der Wirbelthiere.* Morphologische-histologische Studien II, 1884.
5. Werner CF. *Das Labyrinth.* Leipzig, Germany: Thieme; 1940:202–205.
6. Schuknecht HF, Belal AA. The utriculo-endolymphatic valve: Its functional significance. *J Laryngol Otol.* 1975;89(10):985–996.
7. Bachor E, Karmody CS. The utriculo-endolymphatic valve in pediatric temporal bones. *Eur Arch Otorhinolaryngol.* 1995;252(3): 167–171.
8. Ross MD, Pote KG, Perini F. Analytical studies of the organic material of otoconial complexes, including its amino acid and carbonate composition. In: Drescher DG, ed. *Auditory Biochemistry.* Springfield, IL: Charles C Thomas; 1985:500–514.
9. Lindemann HH. Studies on the morphology of the sensory regions of the vestibular apparatus. *Ergeb Anat Entwicklungsgesch.* 1969;42:1–113.
10. Money KE, Bonen L, Beatty JD, et al. Physical properties of fluids and structures of vestibular apparatus of the pigeon. *Am J Physiol.* 1971;220:140–147.
11. Baird RA, Desmadryl G, Fernández C, et al. The vestibular nerve of the chinchilla. II. Relation between afferent response properties and peripheral innervation patterns in the semicircular canals. *J Neurophysiol.* 1988;60: 182–203.
12. Fernández C, Baird RA, Goldberg JM. The vestibular nerve of the chinchilla. I. Peripheral innervation patterns in the horizontal and superior semicircular canals. *J Neurophysiol.* 1988;60:167–181.
13. Fernández C, Baird RA, Goldberg JM. The vestibular nerve of the chinchilla. III. Peripheral innervation patterns in the utricular macula. *J Neurophysiol.* 1990;63:767–780.
14. Goldberg JM, Brichta AM, Wackym PA. Efferent vestibular system: Anatomy, physiology and neurochemistry. In: Anderson JH, Beitz AJ, eds. *Neurochemistry of the Vestibular*

System. Boca Raton, FL: CRC Press; 2000: 61–94.

15. Lysakowski A, Goldberg JM. Morphophysiology of the vestibular sensory periphery. In: Highstein SM, Fay RR, Popper AN, eds. *The Vestibular System*. New York, NY: Springer-Verlag; 2004:57–152.
16. Brodal A, Pompeiano O. Thc vcstibular nuclei in cat. *J Anat.* 1957;91:438–454.
17. Brodal A, Pompeiano O, Walberg H. *The Vestibular Nuclei and Their Connections, Anatomy and Functional Correlations*. Edinburgh, Scotland: Oliver & Boyd; 1962.
18. Highstein SM, Holstein GR. The anatomy of the vestibular nuclei. *Prog Brain Res.* 2006; 151:157–203.
19. Dieterich M, Brandt T. Vestibular system: Anatomy and functional magnetic resonance imaging. *Neuroimaging Clin N Am.* 2001; 11(2):263–273.
20. Wende S, Nakayama N, Schwerdtfeger P. The internal auditory artery (embryology, anatomy, angiography, pathology). *J Neurol.* 1975;210: 21–31.

CHAPTER 2

Physiology and Maturation of Balance Mechanisms

Thierry Morlet

Introduction

The maintenance of balance relies on the complex peripheral and central interactions of three important senses: vision, vestibular function, and proprioception. The vestibular system, which functions to maintain equilibrium, direct the gaze of the eyes, and stabilize gaze in the presence of motion, is the first sensory system to develop in humans.[1] The vestibular nerve is the first cranial nerve to complete myelination, and the system itself becomes functional in the eighth to ninth month of gestation.[1] Morphologically, the sensory systems related to balance are fully developed at birth. Balance function continues to mature thereafter with sequential acquisition of general motor milestones (especially pertaining to posture) including head control, sitting, standing, and walking, followed by the ability to stabilize vision during head movements and finally, until adolescence, through experiential learning and adaptation. Changes in balance function are most rapid and pronounced during infancy and in preschool years when motor milestones needed for walking are realized and as postural control and coordinated movements are refined.

Embryology

Inner Ear

Ongoing research and technological advances have significantly improved our understanding of the morphogenesis and cellular differentiation of the human vestibular system.[2] As detailed in Chapter 1, the vestibular system is composed of two otolith organs (the saccule and utricle), which sense linear acceleration (ie, gravity and translational movements), and three semicircular canals, which lie orthogonal to each other and are responsive to angular acceleration. The development of the inner ear starts during the third week of gestation and is complete around 25 weeks. By that time, the vestibular apparatus has achieved adult form and size. The first stages of inner ear development begin as diffuse thickenings of surface ectoderm on either side of the embryonic (rhomboencephalon) hindbrain. Then the thickened surface ectoderm from either side of the embryonic hindbrain begins to invaginate forming the otic placodes.

During week 4 of gestation, the otic placodes are surrounded by proliferating embryonic mesoderm creating otic pits. The otic pits subsequently pinch off from the surface ectoderm to form the closed, rounded structures of the otic vesicles. The otic vesicles further differentiate into three subdivisions: (1) a small dorsal endolymphatic duct and sac, (2) an expanded central utricle, and (3) a ventral saccule. Different growth rates and timelines have been observed for the canals, vestibular aqueduct, oval window, round window, and cochlea, which suggests that each part of the inner ear follows a distinct developmental trajectory.[3] The vestibular apparatus, located superiorly in relation to the cochlea, develops earlier and grows at a faster rate than the cochlea. From the fourth to the seventh weeks, the utricle differentiates to form the three semicircular canals, and the ventral end of the saccule elongates and coils to form the cochlea. The superior semicircular canal forms first, followed by the posterior and lateral canals. A small expansion called the ampulla forms at one end of each semicircular duct. The communication between the saccule and membranous cochlea narrows to form the ductus reuniens. These otic vesicle derivatives collectively constitute the membranous labyrinth. The otic placode also gives rise to the sensory ganglia of the vestibulocochlear nerve.

The definitive membranous labyrinth is suspended in the fluid-filled perilymphatic space within the bony labyrinth of the petrous portion of the temporal bone. The bony capsule that encapsulates the membranous labyrinth forms rapidly from embryonic mesoderm over a period of approximately 5 weeks, between gestational weeks 19 and 23. Ossification of the otic capsule and encapsulation first occur in the area of the cochlea and anterior semicircular canal at approximately 19 weeks' gestation. Encapsulation then appears to progress in an outward fashion from the areas surrounding the vestibule to the canal vertices, with the last area of encapsulation being the posterolateral area of the horizontal semicircular canal at approximately 21 to 23 weeks of gestation.[4] The current consensus is that the vestibule is adult-like in form and size by 25 to 27 weeks of gestation, which coincides with the rotation of most fetuses into the birth position.[4] The superior semicircular canal is the first to attain adult size and to become fully ossified, followed by the lateral and then by the posterior semicircular canal, whereas the internal aperture of the vestibular aqueduct is still growing and smaller than adult size at 39 weeks.[3,4]

Maturation of Vestibular Receptors

Around the third week of gestation, the sensory epithelium develops from the ectoderm in the cristae of the forming semicircular canals and in the maculae of the forming otolithic organs. By 7 weeks of gestation, small quantities of otoconia are present in the utricle. Thereafter, development proceeds quite rapidly, and within 1 week, greater amounts of otoconia are present in both the utricle and saccule, and cellular differentiation of the macular neural substrate is readily evident. Observations during the period of 7 to 12 weeks of gestation show that the calcium content of the otoconia increases markedly in both the utricle and saccule; however, comparisons along the entire continuum of macular development reveal that the otoconia of the utricle appear to be more mature and varied in size and shape than the saccular otoconia.[5] During week 7 of gestation, some vestibular hair cells begin their differentiation. Even though the vestibular hair cells are not yet fully differentiated, synaptogenesis is observed in the human fetus at approximately 9 to 10 weeks' gestation. Differentiation of type I and type II hair cells begins between 11 and 13 weeks of gestation. In general, the morphological sequence is from apex to base in the cristae and from the center to the periphery in the maculae. Significant numbers of fully formed calyx nerve endings are observed at 20 weeks of gestation. The maturing ampullary cristae become active as early as the eighth or ninth week of fetal life,[6] and reflexogenically, vestibular receptors become fully active by the 32nd week, at which time a fully developed Moro reflex can be elicited.[7] These observations suggest that vestibular afferents are mature and functional in the early stages of human development.

Development of Vestibular Pathways

At approximately 4 weeks of gestation, a portion of the neural crest migrates to the vicinity of the otic vesicle and becomes the acousticofacial ganglion. Soon thereafter, the geniculate ganglion migrates away from this cluster of neurons, leaving the vestibulocochlear ganglion in close proximity to the otic vesicle. The arrival of afferent endings in the epithelium precedes hair cell differentiation. An increase in the number of synaptic bodies, which characterize the development of synapses between hair cells and afferent fibers, occurs between 9 and 10 weeks of gestation.[8] Vestibular ganglion cells are of various shapes until 21 weeks of gestation and become uniform in shape around 24 weeks of gestation when the development of the inner ear is nearly complete. Morphometric studies show that ganglion cells grow until the 39th week, reaching maturity around the time of birth.[9] Neuronal connections between the labyrinths and the oculomotor nuclei of the brainstem occur between 12 and 24 weeks of gestation. Myelination of the vestibular nerve begins around the 20th fetal week; it is the first cranial nerve to complete myelination and occurs even before the myelination of the acoustic fibers of the eighth nerve.[1] The vestibular nuclear complex is functional at 21 weeks of gestation.

Developmental Reflexes

With early development of anatomical structures and function, certain developmental reflexes can be elicited at birth or soon thereafter. They are primitive in nature, usually disappear as the child matures, and primarily reflect the integrity of the brainstem and spinal cord.[10] Their persistence beyond the normally expected age of dissipation indicates delayed maturation or impaired nervous system function. Their asymmetry suggests either a central or a peripheral nervous system disorder. The *Moro reflex*, which disappears by the age of 5 to 6 months, is elicited by holding the child supine and allowing his or her head to drop approximately 30° in relation to the trunk. Extension and abduction of the arms with fanning out of the fingers, followed by adduction of the arms at the shoulder, takes place as a normal response. The *tonic neck reflex* normally disappears by the age of 6 months and is tested by turning the head of the child to one side while he or she is lying supine with shoulders fixed. The arm and leg toward the side that the head is turned extend, while the arm and leg on the opposite side flex.

The *head righting reflex* develops by the age of 4 to 6 months. When the child's trunk is held 30° from the vertical plane, a normally responding infant will tilt the head so that it remains vertical. At about 5 months, the child will additionally move the lower limbs away from the side to which they have been tilted, thereby reflecting functional integration of visual, vestibular, and proprioceptive stimuli.[1] The *parachute reaction* is elicited after 5 months of age when a sudden downward movement of a vertically held child causes the lower limbs to extend and abduct. This reflex is considered to represent visual-vestibular interaction[1] with the otoliths presumably involved. The *doll's eye response* is normally found in full-term babies within 2 weeks of birth. When the baby (facing the examiner) is held at arm's length and rotated in one direction around the examiner, a deviation of the eyes and head opposite to the direction of the rotation is produced, representing vestibular activity. Due to an immature saccadic system at this stage, the fast component of a normal nystagmic response is not seen. During the following months, however, nystagmus is apparent with the fast component in the direction of rotation.[11]

Development of Vestibular-Induced Reflexes

Balance and equilibrium are maintained through a series of events triggered by sensory stimulation. Incoming sensory inputs received from the vestibular, visual, and somatosensory/proprioceptive systems are directed to the vestibular nuclei and cerebellum for processing and calibration. In response to afferent inputs, the vestibular nuclear complex creates direct and rapid efferent connections to the muscles controlling the eyes, neck, and spinal cord. These motor outputs stimulate three vestibular reflexes (vestibulo-ocular, vestibulospinal, and vestibulocollic) that allow for the maintenance of balance and equilibrium. Vestibular responses are gradually modulated by developing central inhibitory influences, cerebellar control, and central vestibular adaptation.[1,12] It is through examination of these reflexes that we are provided with a window for uncovering vestibular dysfunction.

Vestibulo-Ocular Reflex

Stability of vision in the presence of head or body movements is an important function of the vestibular system. The purpose of the vestibulo-ocular reflex (VOR) is to stabilize gaze and maintain clear vision when the body or head is in motion. Objects of visual interest are maintained on the fovea, the most sensitive part of the retina, through inputs from the semicircular canals and otoliths. The various types of eye movements have the important functions of projecting and maintaining this image of the object of interest onto the fovea. In general, fast eye movements called saccades bring the image of a target onto the fovea, and slow eye movements, including smooth-pursuit, vestibulo-ocular reflexes, and optokinetic nystagmus, help maintain the image there. A variety of techniques have been employed to explore and record the VOR in children. Despite previous technical difficulties inherent to achieving compliance and obtaining accurate recordings in addition to VOR alteration from a variety of nonvestibular influences (ie, subject attention and state of arousal, unintended ocular fixation due to light leaks, inadequate calibration, and insufficient head stabilization during testing), the VOR can be elicited and examined in the pediatric population. These techniques include caloric stimulation, per-rotatory (torsion swing) stimulation, as well as passive whole-body (en bloc) rotation techniques. Depending on the techniques employed, parameters such as speed of the slow component, amplitude of nystagmus beat, gain (ratio of peak eye velocity to peak head velocity), phase (timing difference between head and eye velocities), symmetry (comparison of rightward and leftward eye velocities), and time constant of decay (time for the slow-phase eye velocity to decline by two-thirds from its maximum value), as well as latency and duration of the response, have been recorded.[13]

The VOR is present at birth, although its time constants were found to be approximately one-half of normal adult values in neonates aged 24 to 120 hours. They appear to approach adult values by 2 months of age.[14]

These differences are likely a reflection of the immaturity of the visual pathways at birth, which suggests that maturation of the visual pathways is a necessary precursor for adequate calibration of the VOR and for competent function of the velocity storage mechanism necessary for stable vision. In response to angular acceleration, newborns show distinct nystagmus characterized by alternating slow and fast components. The reflexive slow-component nystagmus of the VOR generated by vestibular stimulation is routinely observed at birth; however, the centrally mediated fast component, which returns and maintains the eyes within the physical confines of the orbits, is variably present.[15]

Infants demonstrate inaccurate saccades, frequently requiring more than one saccade to reach the target. The saccadic system is immature at birth and continues to develop up to the age of 2 years.[16] The speed of the slow component as well as the frequency of beats were found to increase as a function of age until 6 to 12 months, after which values reached a plateau and stabilized.[13] Smooth pursuit is also only possible at very low frequencies in this age group due to foveal immaturity. In children, the canal-ocular reflex and otolith-ocular reflex, elicited by vertical-axis rotation and off-vertical-axis rotation, respectively, develop independently of each other. The canal-ocular reflex parameters remain unchanged after birth, whereas the otolith-ocular reflex parameters change with age, especially at the stage when children are learning to walk. Children present a higher gain of the VOR response to sinusoidal rotation than adults, and due to immature visual-vestibular interaction a poorer suppression of the VOR response is seen. Gain and time-constant parameters of the VOR in response to constant angular acceleration reveal that time constants increase, whereas VOR gains show small but significant decreases as a function of age from 2 months to 11 years of age.[16] In a large longitudinal study, Casselbrant et al[17] observed that in response to both sinusoidal and constant velocity rotations on an earth-vertical axis, VOR gain increases linearly as a function of age from 3 to 9 years, but that phase differences appeared to remain stable. These findings are in contrast to several other studies that have shown decreased or stable VOR gain as a function of a child's increasing age. As suggested by Casselbrandt,[17] changes in gain may be related to maturation of attentional mechanisms as part of the overall process of maturation of the vestibulo-ocular system because mental alertness plays a key role in VOR function. In a recent evaluation of the VOR using a video head impulse test, Wiener-Vacher and Wiener[18] observed a rapid change in VOR gain until about age 6 years, followed by slower growth after 6 years with adult values reached by age 16 years.

In summary, the VOR goes through several developmental stages, with a healthy response developing by several months beyond full term,[19] and absence of the VOR by the age of 10 months should be considered an abnormal finding.[19,20] It is evident that regardless of the parameters explored, the underlying constant prevailing across all studies of the pediatric VOR is that qualitative differences exist between the VOR function of children and adults,[21–25] and that these differences seem to persist until preadolescence.

Vestibulospinal Reflex

Whether the body is stationary or in motion, continuous afferent signals from the visual and vestibular systems detect the body's orientation and relationship to gravity. These inputs combine with touch receptors on the skin as well as proprioceptors on the soles of the feet, hands, and torso to detect the body's contact with the environment. The sum of these inputs provides the information needed to generate the vestibulospinal reflex (VSR), which stabilizes the body and helps to maintain postural control. Vestibulospinal reflex signals travel along three major pathways: the lateral, medial, and reticulospinal tracts. These tracts impact the anterior horn cells of the spinal cord and generate myotactic, deep tendon reflexes in the antigravity skeletal muscles of the limbs and trunk.

The VSR has more numerous and complex innervations than the VOR, but just as the VOR works to contract and relax paired ocular muscles, the VSR works similarly to create a push-pull arrangement of agonist and antagonist muscle firing across the neural axis. In general, when comparing the VSR function of children with that of adults, the postural control of these groups varies significantly.[26] As detailed later in this chapter, the vestibulospinal mechanism or effectiveness of the vestibular system in postural control continues to develop until at least 15 to 16 years of age.

Vestibulocollic Reflex

The vestibulocollic reflex (VCR) plays an important role in stabilizing vision by compensating for head movements when the body is in motion. Through patterned contractions of the neck muscles, the VCR stabilizes the bobbing of the head caused by vibrations transmitted from the heels as they strike the ground during walking and running; thus, the VCR assists in stabilizing the head on top of the neck, and in keeping the head still and level, especially during ambulation. During walking, vestibular signals caused by linear translations stimulate nerve receptors of the saccule. In response, the saccule transmits afferent signals along the inferior vestibular nerve and ganglion to the vestibular nuclear complex in the brainstem. From there, efferent signals are sent via the medial vestibulospinal tract and spinal accessory nerve to the neck muscles, including the sternocleidomastoid muscles, which are the long neck muscles extending from the thorax to the base of the skull behind the ear.

In the past decade, VCR function has become routinely explored through recordings of vestibular-evoked myogenic potentials (VEMPs; see Chapter 8). VEMPs have become an increasingly popular clinical technique because, unlike other tests of vestibular function, VEMPs provide information regarding saccular and inferior vestibular nerve function. Additionally, the VEMP test is an objective measure that can be reliably recorded from surface electrodes in a wide variety of patients, including infants and young children. Many recent studies recording VEMPs in preterm neonates, infants, and young children have confirmed the efficacy of VEMP recordings in the pediatric population. These studies have pointed out differences between the VEMP responses of children and adults, with a slightly shorter latency of the initial negative peak in children (3–11 years of age) than in adults,[27] suggesting again maturational effects from preschool age through adolescence.[25,27]

Development of Postural Control

With the development of postural control comes new motor behaviors, skills, and possibilities. Maintenance of postural balance requires an active sensorimotor control system. In adults, the sensory systems are well organized and act in a context-specific way.[28] Postural control involves sensory feedback,[29] and visual and proprioceptive inputs need to be integrated in order for the center of foot pressure to move in phase with the center of mass. In children, the sensory systems are not completely developed, although their anatomical structures mature early in life.[30] The proprioceptive, visual, and vestibular systems develop more slowly than the hierarchically lower automatic motor processes that mature early in childhood.[31] The importance of visual cues in maintaining static posture has been well demonstrated, particularly in children who are used to visually monitoring the body during posture.[32,33] As important are the cognitive functions for the organization and integration of available sensory information under both static and dynamic conditions, and this has also been well documented[34]; hence, the selection of the appropriate balance strategy not only depends on environmental demands but is also a function of neuromaturation and experience.

In typically developing children, the growth of postural stability proceeds in a cephalocaudal fashion, with the infant achieving first control of the head, then the trunk, and finally postural stability in standing.[35,36] The newborn infant when held ventrally with a hand under the abdomen cannot hold his or her head up. By 6 weeks of age the head is held in the plane of the body, and by 12 weeks it can be held above this level. Head control allowing the baby to look around in a horizontal plane is achieved by 16 weeks of age, and by the 36th week of life the infant is able to sit unsupported for a few minutes. In infants born preterm, however, there is a risk for decreased or delayed adaptability of the postural control system as their prematurity and medical factors may alter their experiences in the first year of life.[37] Head control in infants is usually considered as constituting the beginning of body equilibrium development and improves with the emergence of reaching. Articulated operation of the head–trunk unit associated with a descending temporal organization of postural control occurs during the first year of life. This is defined as the first period in the development of locomotor balance control that extends from birth to the acquisition of the upright stance.[38] By the age of 1 year, the typically developing child is able to crawl on hands and knees and is able to stand up holding onto furniture. At about 15 to 16 months of age, the child is normally able to start walking.[39] The second period in the development of locomotor balance control[38] takes place from the acquisition of upright stance up to approximately 6 years of age. This period is characterized by mastery of the effectors and development of coordination between the lower and upper parts of the body. During this period, with age, the ability to control several body segments during locomotion occurs with a caudocephalic progression. This chronological progression is consistent with an ascending temporal organization of balance control with hip movements occurring before shoulder movements and shoulder movements before head movements. Children from 3 to 6 years of age adopt a head-stabilization-in-space strategy only while walking on the flat ground without any equilibrium difficulty; however, when the level of equilibrium difficulty increases, these children show an increase in head-trunk stiffness. Children from 7 to 8 years of age become able to adopt the head-stabilization-in-space strategy even when balance difficulty increases. Last, in adulthood, the head-stabilization-in-space strategy is adopted most of the time.[40] The third period begins at around age 7 years and continues likely into adolescence. Adolescence might constitute a turning point in the development of balance control. This period is characterized by a return to an articulated mode of head-trunk operation, whereby the head stabilization necessary for the descending temporal organization of balance control is ensured. Adolescence is also marked by a period of accelerated increases in height and weight. This growth spurt affects variability smoothness and regularity of gait but not its stability.[41] The fourth period, which is reached during adulthood, combines the main features of the third period with a new skill involving the articulated operation of the head-trunk unit along with a selective control of the degrees of freedom at the neck level.

Under normal sensory conditions, the shorter the stature of children and the greater variability of their automatic postural adjustments combine to produce sway responses that are larger, more variable, and more oscillatory than those of adults. When deprived of support-surface inputs, visual input, or both, all young children performed within stable limits but, again, with larger and more variable oscillations than adults. When the control of postural stability does not require the resolution of conflicting sensory information, a significant increase in stability is observed between the fourth and fifth years of life.[42] Females show a greater rate of improvement in stability until the age of 11 to 12 years. Males younger than 10 years swayed more than females of the same age,[43–45] although gender differences were not observed in children 3 to 6 years of age when assessing the effect of altered sensory environment on postural stability.[42]

In balance control, somatosensory inputs are primary in adults, whereas children prefer visual inputs to vestibular information in achieving their postural equilibrium.[42] Infants and young children (aged 4 months to 2 years) are dependent on the visual system to maintain balance.[46,47] At 3 to 6 years of age, children begin to use somatosensory information appropriately,[31,42,45,48] although some studies indicate that development continues until the age of 9 to 11 years.[44] In the case of an intersensory conflict, the vestibular system acts as a referential function by suppressing input not congruent with vestibular information.[45] Due to presumed mature vestibular function, even with misleading visual information, adults can maintain their postural control. By 12 years of age, children are still not able to select and process misleading visual information.[49] Between the three sensory inputs in children, the vestibular system seems to be the least effective in postural control,[42,50–52] and functional efficiency of the vestibular system in children 10 to 15 years of age is still developing.[45,48,51] Visual function develops more slowly than somatosensory function, with adolescents aged 14 to 15 years displaying the same maturity as adults. Vestibular function develops more slowly than visual function, so even at the age of 14 to 15 years, tested subjects did not completely reach adult levels,[45] although a more recent study suggests that 11- to 13-year-old boys have the ability to select varying balance strategies as in adults.[53] The ultimate development of several visual functions, such as saccade latency and contrast or chromatic sensitivity, does not asymptote to adult level until approximately 12 years of age.[54] The visual influence on standing stability is reported to be established at adult levels around the age of 15 years.[45,48]

In summary, the coordination of postural responses develops until at least 10[28,31] to 16 years of age,[25,53,55-58] while the gait pattern reaches full maturity at around 7 to 10 years of age.[56] Adult-like postural stability resulting from complete maturation of the 3 sensory systems and the ability to solve an intersensory-conflict situation can thus be assumed in adolescents around 15 years of age.[25,45,48,51,55,57]

Conclusion

Examination and evaluation of balance and vestibular end-organ function in children require a thorough understanding of the developmental timeline and trajectory of the peripheral end organs and their neuronal pathways. Likewise, the weighting of various sensory inputs inherent to the maintenance of equilibrium are subject to maturation. Knowledge of this underlying developmental trajectory is imperative in identifying dysfunction of the vestibular system and determining its impact on balance in children.

Self-Assessment Questions

1. The development of the inner ear:
   a. Starts at around 10 weeks of gestation and is complete around 1 month after birth
   b. Starts at around 3 weeks of gestation and is complete around 1 month after birth
   c. Starts at around 3 weeks of gestation and is complete around 25 weeks of gestation

2. The vestibulo-ocular reflex is not present at birth:
   a. True
   b. False

3. Absence of the vestibulo-ocular reflex by the age of 10 months should be considered an abnormal finding:
   a. True
   b. False

4. The vestibular-evoked myogenic potentials are useful in testing the vestibulocollic reflex:
   a. True
   b. False

5. In balance control, visual inputs are primary in adults, whereas children prefer somatosensory inputs to vestibular information in achieving their postural equilibrium:
   a. True
   b. False

6. Children begin to use somatosensory information appropriately:
   a. At around 6 months of age
   b. Between 3 and 6 years of age
   c. After 12 years of age

7. Between the 3 sensory inputs in children, the vestibular system seems to be the most effective in postural control:
   a. True
   b. False

8. Synaptogenesis in the vestibular system is observed only when all vestibular hair cells are fully differentiated:
   a. True
   b. False

9. The persistence beyond the normally expected age of dissipation of the Moro and tonic neck reflexes indicates delayed maturation or impaired nervous system function:
   a. True
   b. False

References

1. Blayney AW. Vestibular disorders. In: Adams DA, Cinnamond MJ, eds. *Paediatric Otolaryngology, Scott-Brown's Otolaryngology*. Vol 6. 6th ed. Oxford, UK: Butterworth-Heinemann; 1997:1–29.
2. Jeffery N, Spoor F. Prenatal growth and development of the modern human labyrinth. *J Anat.* 2004;204:71–92.
3. Richard C, Laroche N, Malaval L, et al. New insight into the bony labyrinth: A microcomputed tomography study. *Auris Nasus Larynx.* 2010;37:155–161.
4. Richard C, Courbon G, Laroche N, Prades JM, Vico L, Malaval L. Inner ear ossification and mineralization kinetics in human embryonic development—microtomographic and histomorphological study. *Sci Rep.* 2017;7(1): 4825.
5. Wright CG, Hubbard DG. SEM observations on development of human otoconia during the first trimester of gestation. *Acta Otolaryngol.* 1982;94(1–2):7–18.
6. Holt K. Movement and child development. *Clin Dev Med.* 1975;55:1-182.
7. Schulte FJ, Linke I, Michaelis E. Excitation, inhibition and impulse conduction in spinal motoneurons of preterm, term and small-fordates newborn infants. In: Robinson RJ, ed. *Brain and Early Behavior Development in the Fetus and Infants.* CASDS Study Group on Brain Mechanisms or Early Behavioural Development. New York, NY: Academic Press; 1969.
8. Dechesne CJ. The development of vestibular sensory organs in human. In: Romand R, ed. *Development of Auditory and Vestibular Systems 2.* Amsterdam, Netherlands: Elsevier; 1992: 419–447.
9. Kaga K, Sakurai H, Ogawa Y, et al. Morphological changes of vestibular ganglion cells in human fetuses and in pediatric patients. *Int J Pediat Otorhinolaryngol.* 2001;60:11–20.
10. Swaiman KF, Ashwal S. *Pediatric Neurology: Principles and Practice.* 3rd ed. St. Louis, MO: Mosby; 1999:31–53.
11. Eviatar L, Eviatar A, Naray L. Maturation of neurovestibular responses in infants. *Dev Med Child Neurol.* 1974;16:435–446.
12. Ornitz EM, Atwell CW, Walter DO, Hartmann EE, Kaplan AR. The maturation of vestibular nystagmus in infancy and childhood. *Acta Otolaryngol.* 1979;88:244–256.
13. Eviatar L, Eviatar A. The normal nystagmic response of infants to caloric and perrotatory stimulation. *Laryngoscope.* 1979;89: 1036–1044.
14. Weissman BM, Di Seenna AO, Leigh RJ. Maturation of the vestibulo-ocular reflex in normal infants during the first 2 months of life. *Neurology.* 1989;39:534–538.
15. Cohen B. Origin of quick phases of nystagmus. In: Brodal A, Pompeiano O, eds. *Basic Aspects of Central Vestibular Mechanisms.* Amsterdam, Netherlands: Elsevier; 1972:1–649.
16. Ornitz EM, Kaplan AR, Westlake JR. Development of the vestibulo-ocular reflex from infancy to adulthood. *Acta Otolaryngol (Stockh).* 1985;100:180–183.
17. Casselbrant ML, Mandel EM, Sparto P, et al. Longitudinal posturography and rotational testing in children three to nine years of age: normative data. *Otol Head Neck Surg.* 2010; 142:708–714.

18. Wiener-Vacher SR, Wiener SI. Video head impulse tests with a remote camera system: Normative values of semicircular canal vestibule-ocular reflex gain in infants and children. *Front Neurol.* 2017;8:434
19. Donat JFG, Donat JR, Swe Lay K. Changing response to caloric stimulation with gestational age in infants. *Neurology.* 1980;30:776–778.
20. Fife TD, Tusa RJ, Furman JM, et al. Assessment: Vestibular testing techniques in adults and children. *Neurology.* 2000;55:1431–1441.
21. Van der Laan FL, Oosterveld WJ. Age and vestibular function. *Clin Aviat Aerosp Med.* 1974;45:540–547.
22. Mulch G, Petermann W. Influence of age on results of vestibular function tests. Review of literature and presentation of caloric test results. *Ann Otol Rhinol Laryngol Suppl.* 1979; 88:1–17.
23. Andrieu-Guitrancourt JA, Peron JM, Dehesdin D, Aubet J, Courtin P. Normal vestibular responses to air caloric tests in children. *Int J Pediatr Otolaryngol.* 1981;3:245–250.
24. Staller SJ, Goin DW, Hildebrandt M. Pediatric vestibular evaluation with harmonic acceleration. *J Otolaryngol Head Neck Surg.* 1986; 95:471–476.
25. Valente M. Maturational effects of the vestibular system: A study of rotary chair, computerized dynamic posturography, and vestibular evoked myogenic potentials with children. *J Am Acad Audiol.* 2007;18:461–481.
26. Rine RM. Management of the pediatric patient with vestibular hypofunction. In: Herdman S, ed. *Vestibular Rehabilitation.* 3rd ed. Philadelphia, PA: F.A. Davis; 2007:360–375.
27. Kelsch TA, Schaefer LA, Esquivel CR. Vestibular evoked myogenic potentials in young children: Test parameters and normative data. *Laryngoscope.* 2006;116:895–900.
28. Shumway-Cook A, Woollacott MH. The growth of stability: Postural control from a development perspective. *J Motor Behav.* 1985;17:131–147.
29. Nashner LM, Stupert CL, Horak FB, Black FO. Organization of postural controls: An analysis of sensory and mechanical constraints. *Prog Brain Res.* 1989;80:411–418.
30. Ornitz EM. Normal and pathological maturation of vestibular function in the human child. In: Romand R, ed. *Development of Auditory and Vestibular Systems.* New York, NY: Academic Press; 1983:479–536.
31. Forssberg H, Nashner LM. Ontogenetic development of postural control in man: Adaptation to altered support and visual conditions during stance. *J Neurosci.* 1982;2:545–552.
32. Wiener-Vacher SR, Toupet F, Narcy P. Canal and otolith vestibule-ocular reflexes to vertical and off vertical axis rotation in children learning to walk. *Acta Otolaryngol.* 1996;116: 657–665.
33. Bucci MP, Kapoula Z, Yang Q, Brémond-Gignac D, Wiener-Vacher S. Speed-accuracy of saccades, vergence and combined eye movements in children with vertigo. *Exp Brain Res.* 2004;157:286–295.
34. Shumway-Cook A, Woollacott M. Attentional demands and postural control: The effect of sensory context. *J Gerontol A Biol Sci Med Sci.* 2000;55:M10–M16.
35. Bradley NS. Motor control: Developmental aspects of motor control in skill acquisition. In: Campbell SK, ed. *Physical Therapy for Children.* Philadelphia, PA: Saunders; 1997: 39–77.
36. Burleigh AL, Horak FB, Malouin F. Modification of postural responses and step initiation: Evidence for goal-directed postural interactions. *J Neurophysiol.* 1994;72:2892–2902.
37. Dusing SC, Thacker LR, Galloway JC. Infant born preterm have delayed development of adaptive postural control in the first 5 months of life. *Infant Behav Dev.* 2016;44:49–58.
38. Assaiante C. Development of locomotor balance control in healthy children. *Neurosci Biobehavior Rev.* 1998;22:527–532.
39. Illingworth RS. *The Normal Child.* 8th ed. Edinburgh, Scotland: Churchill Livingstone; 1983.
40. Assaiante C, Amblard B. Ontogenesis of head stabilization in space during locomotion in children: Influence of visual cues. *Exp Brain Res.* 1993;93:499–515.
41. Bisi MC, Stagni R. Development of gait motor control: What happens after a sudden

increase in height during adolescence? *BioMed Eng OnLine.* 2016;15:47.

42. Foudriat BA, Di Fabio RP, Anderson JH. Sensory organization of balance responses in children 3–6 years of age: A normative study with diagnosis implication. *Int J Pediatr Otorhinolaryngol.* 1993;27:255–271.
43. Odenrick P, Sandstedt P. Development of postural sway in the normal child. *Hum Neurobiol.* 1984;3:241–244.
44. Riach CI, Hayes KC. Maturation of postural sway in young children. *Dev Med Child Neurol.* 1987;29:650–658.
45. Hirabayashi S, Iwasaki Y. Developmental perspective of sensory organization on postural control. *Brain Dev.* 1995;17:111–113.
46. Starkes J, Riach CL. The role of vision in the postural control of children. *Clin Kinesiol.* 1990;44:72–77.
47. Woollacott MH, Debu B, Mowatt M. Neuromuscular control of posture in the infant and child: Is vision dominant? *J Motor Behav.* 1987;19:167–186.
48. Steindl R, Kunz K, Schrott-Fischer A, Scholtz AW. Effect of age and sex on maturation of sensory systems and balance control. *Dev Med Child Neurol.* 2006;48:477–482.
49. Ionescu E, Morlet T, Froehlich P, Ferber-Viart C. Vestibular assessment with Balance Quest: Normative data for children and young adults. *Int J Pediatr Otorhinolaryngol.* 2006; 70:1457–1465.
50. Ferber-Viart C, Ionescu E, Morlet T, Froehlich P, Dubreuil C. Balance in healthy individuals assessed with Equitest: Maturation and normative data for children and young adults. *Int J Pediatr Otorhinolaryngol.* 2007; 71:1041–1046.
51. Cherng RJ, Chen JJ, Su FC. Vestibular system in performance of standing balance of children and young adults under altering sensory conditions. *Percep Motor Skills.* 2001;92: 1167–1179.
52. Charpiot A, Tringali S, Ionescu E, Vital-Durand F, Ferber-Viart C. Vestibulo-ocular reflex and balance maturation in healthy children aged from six to twelve years. *Audiol Neurotol.* 2010;15:201–210.
53. Hatzitaki V, Zisi V, Kollias I, Kioumourtzoglou E. Perceptual-motor contributions to static and dynamic balance control in children. *J Motor Behav.* 2002;34(2):161–170.
54. Yang Q, Bucci MP, Kapoula Z. The latency of saccades, vergence, and combined eye movements in children and in adults. *Invest Ophthalmol Vis Sci.* 2002;43:2939–2949.
55. Shinjo Y, Jin Y, Kaga K. Assessment of vestibular function of infants and children with congenital and acquired deafness using ice-water caloric test, rotational chair test and vestibular-evoked myogenic potential recording. *Acta Oto-Laryngol.* 2007;127:736–747.
56. Hsu YS, Kuan CC, Young YH. Assessing the development of balance function in children using stabilometry. *Int J Pediatr Otorhinolaryngol.* 2009;73:737–740.
57. Mallau S, Vaugoyeau M, Assaiante C. Postural strategies and sensory integration: No turning point between childhood and adolescence. *PLOS ONE.* 2010;5(9):e13078.
58. Gouleme N, Debue M, Spruyt K, Vanderveken C, De Siati RD, Ortega-Solis J, Petrossi J, Wiener-Vacher S, Bucci MP, Ionescu E, Thai-Van H, Deggouj N. Changes of spatial and temporal characteristics of dynamic postural control in children with typical neurodevelopment with age: Results of a multicenter pediatric study. *Int J Ped Otorhinolaryngol.* 2018; 113:272–280.

CHAPTER 3

Vestibular Adaptation and Compensation

James O. Phillips

Pediatric vestibular disorders are often difficult to diagnose, and when they are identified they often go untreated. There is an implicit assumption among many pediatricians and primary care physicians that the extraordinary plasticity of the developing nervous system can "solve" the problem of vestibular dysfunction without any intervention from a health care provider. While it is arguably true that the nervous system in young patients is highly plastic, and indeed that the vestibular system is very capable of compensation and adaptive change in response to injury throughout life, there is strong evidence to suggest that there are many limitations to vestibular compensation and adaptation, and that medical treatment or vestibular rehabilitation may be critical for full functional recovery in pediatric vestibular patients. This chapter explores the characteristics of vestibular adaptive change and the natural process of vestibular compensation to acute loss of function, and also briefly touches on the literature evaluating the benefits of vestibular rehabilitation, in general, and specifically with regard to recovery in pediatric patients.

Normal Central Vestibular Processing of Motion and Static Orientation Inputs

The central nervous system is constructed to make active comparisons between the inputs from the vestibular end organs in the inner ear. Individual neurons in the vestibular nucleus receive convergent inputs from afferents from multiple canals and from both canal and otolith end organs. In addition, the vestibular system utilizes the bilateral symmetry of the vestibular end organs of both ears to its advantage. To sense rotation, the inputs from complementary canals in either ear, which are aligned in the same rotational plane but have opposite signs, are compared. Since the input from each ear projects ipsilaterally in the brain, this means that there is a direct comparison of the inputs to each side of the brain. When the canal inputs are balanced, the brain calculates that the head is not rotating. When the otolith inputs are balanced, the brain calculates that the head is in its normal upright orientation and is not translating. Together, balanced input from both systems produces the sensation of a stationary head. This information is then immediately combined with nuchal afferent information, visual information, and kinesthetic information from the trunk and limbs to define the position of the head on the trunk, in the world, and relative to the various parts of the body.

During head rotation the canal inputs are naturally unbalanced, due to increased frequency of afferent discharge from the end organ and ear that the head is turning toward, and decreased frequency of afferent discharge from the end organ and ear that the head is turning away from. The imbalance indicates head rotation, and the degree of the difference in inputs is a direct indication of the velocity or acceleration of the head. Similarly, linear acceleration or tilt of the head changes the relative depolarization of individual receptors, and the frequency of firing of afferents with different tuning within the otolith organs of each ear. However, in this system, complementary inputs within individual end organs must be reconciled, since the direction of tuning of hair cells within these organs systematically varies with location within the end organ relative to the striola. The central nervous system reinforces the comparison between complementary inputs from the right and left ear with powerful commissural connections between the right and left side of the brainstem. These connections aid the detection of movement by facilitating inhibitory networks that accentuate differences in firing rate between the neurons with complementary sensitivity in the right and left vestibular nuclei, thereby increasing the depth of modulation of firing rate of vestibular nuclear neurons in response to head motion.

Acute Consequences of Vestibular Loss

The proper functioning of the ear is predicated on the presentation of adequate and balanced excitatory input from each ear to nuclei on both sides of the brainstem in the resting state. When the input from one ear fails, the neurons of the vestibular nuclei initially respond as though there is a very rapid sustained motion away from the affected ear. The patient experiences a sensation of whirling vertigo, with rotation toward the intact ear, from unbalanced canal input. The patient may also misperceive vertical orientation due to unbalanced otolith system input. These changes also induce a host of reflex responses aimed at stabilizing the body and the eyes in space. Patients may experience an ocular (utricular) tilt reaction to an inaccurately sensed head tilt. Unilateral loss of utricular afferent input produces rotation of the top of the eye toward the lesioned ear, elevation of the eye on the side of the intact ear, and tilt of the head toward the lesioned ear. All of these are consistent with a compensatory reflex response to sensation of tilt toward the intact ear. Patients with unilateral lesions often fall, or feel pushed, toward the lesioned ear, reflecting the effect of descending vestibulospinal reflexes that maintain posture and balance. Unbalanced canal input produces robust nystagmus with slow phase eye movement toward the side of the lesion, as the vestibulo-ocular reflex (VOR) attempts to stabilize the eye in response to an inaccurately sensed head rotation. Basically, these changes reflect the fact that the secondary vestibular neurons ipsilateral to the lesion dramatically decrease their resting discharge rate or fall silent, and the vestibular neurons contralateral to the lesion actually increase their resting discharge rate. In response to actual head rotation, the vestibular nuclei in a patient with unilateral vestibular loss respond with decreased modulation of the resting rate bilaterally, with modulation being virtually eliminated in the ipsilateral vestibular nuclei. Therefore, acutely, this system is designed to fail catastrophically in response to failure of input from one ear.[1]

Peripheral Changes After Inner Ear Vestibular Loss

Following the loss of vestibular input due to the death or injury of vestibular hair cells, there are numerous changes that take place in the periphery. Some of these changes may aid in the later compensation for loss. Unlike cochlear hair cells, there is evidence in mammalian vestibular end organs that hair cells do, in fact, regenerate.[2–11] In some cases, this regeneration is robust. For example, Stone and colleagues have shown that after targeted ablation of inner ear hair cells with diphtheria toxin, which eliminates 98% of vestibular hair cells, approximately 17% of all utricular hair cells are regenerated in lesioned mouse ears.[12] Such cells have basolateral processes typical of type II hair cells, form ribbon synapses, and show proper alignment toward the striola.[12] Type I hair cells show little if any regeneration. Preliminary observations suggest that this regeneration does not restore compensatory eye movement reflexes, which is consistent with the observation that loss of type I input reduces stimulus-driven responses, but inconsistent with the fact that regular afferent input alone is thought to be sufficient to drive eye movement responses in the mid to lower frequencies.[13–15] However, such changes may provide critical inputs that allow central mechanisms to drive recovery after loss.

Central Compensation for Peripheral Vestibular Loss

In response to the previously described significant changes, the central nervous system begins to implement systematic modifications in the weighting of various sources of sensory information immediately after a loss of function. This global response is the first line of defense in response to an acute catastrophic central misinterpretation of sensory input because the mechanisms are already in place and can act quickly. Sensory cues provided by other intact sensory systems can assist in the process of suppressing the consequences of abnormal vestibular afferent input. Kinesthetic and tactile cues are still reliably available in this situation, as are a variety of enteroceptive sensory inputs that can detect changes in the forces exerted on the body's tissues in response to motion.[16] Auditory information can also provide important orientation cues during this period. It has been demonstrated that sound stimuli can aid standing balance and postural stability during gait.[17–22] All of these inputs can theoretically be used to reduce the symptoms of an acute attack. Unfortunately, visual sensation, which contributes significantly to normal vestibular function, is compromised in response to acute unilateral loss by the action of the VOR, which drives a nystagmus beating toward the intact ear. If the loss of function is complete in the lesioned ear, the nystagmus is largely horizontal and torsional because the vertical canals have offsetting vertical vestibular sensitivity; therefore, the loss of both vertical canals produces no net vertical sensation. However, the retinal slip generated by the pathologic nystagmus in the light does help to engage cerebellar and brainstem circuits that normally modulate the VOR gain in response to contextual cues, in this case, by partially suppressing the pathological nystagmus. In response to actual motion, these mechanisms produce a modulation of the gain of the VOR in the vestibular nuclei by combining inhibitory inputs from vestibular and eye movement sensitive cells in the cerebellum with excitatory inputs from the vestibular end organ. The net result, depending on the phase and depth of modulation of the cerebellar neurons, can be either a cancellation or suppression of the VOR, or enhancement of VOR gain. In the pathologic case, this mechanism can suppress the aberrant VOR to produce a suppression of the pathological nystagmus.

It is tempting to speculate that the central nervous system uses efferent modulation of peripheral input during this process of recovery. Vestibular efferent input can influence vestibular afferents through synaptic inputs to hair cells and to afferent fibers.[23–24] Vestibular efferents, which exist in relatively small numbers, have been shown to primarily inhibit but also may excite vestibular hair cells.[25–28] It would make sense that such interactions could reduce the initial imbalance in peripheral vestibular input following injury, and perhaps participate in the later restoration of function, by modulating the specific firing characteristics and overall contribution of vestibular input from intact peripheral hair cells and afferents. Indeed, it has been shown that vestibular efferents can produce weak modulation of type I vestibular afferents in nonhuman primates,[29] and there are systematic changes in the regularity of background firing in vestibular afferents during recovery from unilateral vestibular loss.[30] When efferent inputs are compromised by mutation of the receptors in efferent vestibular neuron synapses, functional recovery of the VOR after unilateral lesion is significantly compromised.[31] However, since changes in afferent modulation do not appear to play a significant role in VOR adaptation or vestibular compensation from injury,[30,32] the mechanism by which the benefits of efferent contributions are derived is not clear. Perhaps changes in the patterning of peripheral input primarily facilitate central adaptive processes.

The next step in the recovery of vestibular function following an acute unilateral peripheral lesion is the reweighting of inputs to the neurons in the vestibular nucleus. This complex process reestablishes the resting background activity in vestibular nuclear neurons ipsilateral to the affected ear and reduces the resting discharge of contralateral vestibular nuclear neurons. Animal experiments have shown a restoration of resting vestibular neuron discharge in cells ipsilateral to a peripheral lesion within 12 hours after a unilateral lesion that initially eliminates all ipsilateral activity. Within 1 week, the resting discharge returns to the prelesion levels.[33] These changes are heavily dependent on synaptic inputs from other neurons, and presumably also reflect changes in neuromodulatory inputs from other structures.[34] For example, there is an immediate downregulation of γ-aminobutyric acid (GABA) receptors in ipsilesional vestibular nucleus neurons, which reduces their inhibition from the contralesional nucleus.[35] As a result of these changes, a balanced discharge of ipsilateral and contralateral vestibular nuclear neurons is restored, and the vestibular system no longer interprets a stationary head as moving. In addition, a slower process of changes to vestibular neuron intrinsic membrane properties is initiated at the same time, so that the compensation produced initially by changes in network properties is sustained by changes in the neurons themselves. For example, animal experiments show that compensation to unilateral loss produces increases in membrane input resistance, depolarization of resting membrane potential, decrease in the threshold for firing of many ipsilesional vestibular neurons, and complementary changes in the intrinsic properties of contralesional neurons.[36–38] These changes in intrinsic cellular properties may also be accompanied by changes in the number and type of vestibular neurons and supporting cells, since both neurogenesis and gliosis have been observed after unilateral peripheral loss in animal experiments.[39,40]

As the process of rebalancing the resting discharge of vestibular nuclear neurons proceeds, there is also a progressive change in the response to motion stimuli. Initially, when there is no resting activity in ipsilesional vestibular neurons, they are also largely, although not entirely, unresponsive to rotational inputs. Contralateral vestibular neurons remain responsive to head rotation, but the depth of their modulation is reduced by a lack of appropriate commissural input from the ipsilateral side. Over time, the imbalance in rate modulation is reduced, although it is never completely eliminated. Therefore, there is a trend toward a modulation of both ipsilesional and contralesional vestibular neurons with head rotation as compensation progresses. The modulation of ipsilesional neurons is presumably primarily through inhibition from the contralesional side. The response is also not perfect in terms of its timing or its dynamic range. Since the signals are virtually all derived from afferent input from a single ear, the push-pull symmetry of the normal vestibular system is compromised. Inputs from the intact ear reach the ipsilateral brainstem first, and then must take more time to traverse the commissural pathways to the side ipsilateral to the lesioned ear. The brain cannot perfectly resolve these timing delays, and the result is a change in the phase of the VOR with respect to the head movement. Also, the brain normally performs an integration and storage of vestibular velocity information. One consequence of this is that the normal phase of the VOR is compensatory over a greater dynamic range than would be achieved by the vestibular afferent discharge itself. Following central compensation, this storage of velocity information is compromised, resulting in a more dramatic shift in phase (phase lead) with decreasing rotational frequency. Finally, since the input to the adapted system is dependent on afferent input from one ear, and increase of afferent discharge above resting discharge has a larger dynamic range than decrease of afferent discharge below resting discharge, there is a residual deficit in dynamic range of rotational inputs to which the system can now adequately respond. Put simply, following a unilateral peripheral loss, the vestibular afferents cannot accurately indicate the velocity of rotations that completely suppress their discharge, even if the head velocities toward the lesioned ear dramatically differ.

Cerebellar Contributions to Compensation and Adaptation

The cerebellum also plays a critical role in all stages of vestibular compensation, although this role is less well defined than the role it plays in normal adaptation and calibration of vestibular reflexes. It is known that the vestibulo-cerebellum is necessary for the increase in resting firing rate in ipsilesional vestibular neurons after a unilateral loss.[41] Also, in animals the behavioral recovery of VOR gain seems to involve both early cerebellum independent and later cerebellum dependent processes.[42] The cerebellum is surely heavily involved in the final recalibration of vestibular reflexes, including the angular VOR. A massive literature supports the involvement of the cerebellum in motor learning in general and VOR adaptation specifically. These experiments have shown adaptive changes in the vestibulo-cerebellum and the vestibular nucleus following experimental manipulation of visual feedback with prisms, magnifying or minifying lenses, or moving visual stimuli during head rotation. The motor learning that results can change the gain and phase (even the direction) of the VOR, matching the motion of the eyes to the motion of the visual world elicited in association with the head movement.[43–45] The visual signals for this learning are relayed via mossy fiber and climbing fiber input to the vestibulocerebellum, the latter fibers providing a presumed error signal for the detection of abnormal retinal image motion. The neurons in the inferior olive of the brainstem, which give rise to these climbing fibers, receive massive inputs from neurons in the nucleus of the optic tract, which are exquisitely sensitive to small slip of the visual image across the retina. The adapted signals from the cerebellum then converge with vestibular inputs, either directly from the end organs of the ear or indirectly via commissural pathways, onto flocculus target neurons within the vestibular nuclei, where neurons also undergo long-lasting adaptive changes.[46–49] This learning is true adaptation, in that the adapted VOR response is sustained in the absence of new visual input over long periods of time. Animals and humans placed in dark environments largely retain their learning of an experimentally altered VOR gain until they have an opportunity to experience normal image motion resulting from head motion.

Why Does This System Sometimes Fail?

Ultimately, the vestibular system has the capacity for dramatic recovery, such that the brain accurately interprets stationary head and body position, and accurately reports active motion over a range of frequencies and velocities of movement even after complete unilateral vestibular loss. However, this recovery is not perfect and is subject to many limitations. For example, VOR adaptation experiments suggest that adaptation of the VOR to different combinations of head and visual motion is limited to the frequencies of stimulation that are experienced during the adaptation period. This suggests that there are limitations to the generalization of the motor learning that restores natural vestibular function. In patients, a similar phenomenon occurs in which those patients who restrict head and body motion during the period of their recovery tend to have poorer outcomes than those who force themselves to safely and progressively experience destabilizing and challenging visual, vestibular, and support surface environments. Furthermore, the adaptive mechanisms that generally restore function can seek local solutions to the global challenge of restoring balance and orientation. Since patients generally employ both substitution of alternate sensory inputs and adaptation of altered vestibular inputs to solve the challenges presented by a loss of peripheral vestibular function, partial recovery can be achieved through a wide variety of sensory strategies. The result, however, is often suboptimal for the wide range of environments and contexts in which vestibular information is normally utilized. For example, a patient who recovered at home in an environment with minimal head on trunk movement, lots of stationary vertical visual cues, and flat hardwood floors might unknowingly choose to utilize visual and proprioceptive cues to maintain balance and orientation. However, this strategy would be likely to betray that same patient when she moves into the chaotic outside world of moving visual stimuli and uneven and compliant support surfaces. A globally appropriate strategy that strikes a compromise between visual, proprioceptive, and residual adapted vestibular inputs would be far more appropriate for the full restoration of the normal activities of daily living.

Of course, it is not always the case that a single strategy will be appropriate for all environments. Even an optimal compromise is still a compromise. Fortunately, the vestibular system is capable of context-dependent adaptive change as well. Vestibular gain can be adapted to multiple adaptation states such that a single, one-size-fits-all adaptation state is not an absolute requirement for compensation. The classic example of this is the anecdotal observation of Gauthier that the gain of the VOR experienced by divers in aquatic and terrestrial environments must increase when diving due to the magnification produced by wearing a diving mask in the water, and must return to normal gain when the diver returns to daily activity on dry land. The vestibular system in these individuals must rapidly assume different gain states when the divers don their diving masks. The mask would serve as a context cue for the change in adaptation state.[50] Training in such context-dependent adaptation is being investigated as a countermeasure for the challenges of rapid adaptation during transitions from 1 g to near 0 g environments in astronauts who are often disoriented for sustained periods during and following spaceflight.[51] The key to successful transitions in adaptation state is learning to associate certain specific cues with the context-appropriate adaptation state. This is a natural process, which may be facilitated by preexposure training in comparable environments with highly salient cues.

Vestibular Rehabilitation Aids Optimal Adaptation

Vestibular rehabilitation encompasses a range of treatment strategies to facilitate effective calibration of vestibular reflexes and optimal utilization of altered vestibular inputs. Therefore, vestibular rehabilitation does more than just augment natural vestibular compensation, by aiding both optimal adaptive change and habituation to the ongoing symptoms that result from imperfect or incomplete compensation for vestibular loss. The activities of vestibular adaptation are derived in part from exercises developed by Cawthorne and Cooksey to encourage physical activity in patients with vestibular loss.[52,53] These exercises challenge the vestibular system by forcing patients recovering from a static vestibular insult to safely engage in activities that progressively produce uncompensated disequilibrium or incompletely compensatory reflex behavior. The nervous system responds to this adaptive demand by adjusting the gain of vestibular reflexes, engaging other sensory inputs to substitute for inadequate vestibular information, and habituating to stimuli that are produced by the mismatch between the expected and actual responses generated by the recovering vestibular system. In controlled trials in adults, specific forms of vestibular rehabilitation have been shown to be effective in facilitating recovery of gaze stabilization after acoustic neuroma surgery.[54–55] Other exercises have been shown to have a positive effect on balance.[56] Simple admonitions to maintain physical activity but without instructions for the specific directed exercises and activities of vestibular rehabilitation do not appear to be as effective in producing recovery of function.

Vestibular rehabilitation exercises tend to fall into two distinct categories: gaze stabilization exercises and balance exercises. Together they represent a program of exercises that is tailored to the unique challenges faced by an individual patient. Gaze stabilization exercises are designed to reduce the retinal slip and oscillopsia produced by inadequate VOR function. The exercises are performed with and without ongoing visual feedback, visual distracters, or other task demands such as standing on foam. The idea of the task is to maintain stable gaze on a visual target while the head is moving in a variety of contexts. The adaptive strategies that are most effective in compensating for loss of vestibular function appear to be substitution of visually elicited eye movements, such as smooth pursuit for the reduced VOR, and increases in the gain of the reduced VOR itself. Often, moving visual targets are employed, which force the patient to maintain gaze on objects that move with or against their own head movement. The idea behind these specific exercises is to force the patient to use various context-dependent gain states to maintain gaze. Occasionally, multiple targets are used and the head movement is actually part of a coordinated gaze shift to realign the eyes and head on the new visual target. Under normal conditions, the VOR is naturally modulated throughout the gaze shift (ie, it is turned off to allow the eye to be carried toward the target by the head, and then turned on to stabilize gaze on the target while the head is completing its deceleration to rest).[57] In patients with vestibular disorders, this complex situation produces demands that are not present during normal combinations of volitional head movement and stable fixation. Often, compensation and recovery in this context require use of (1) both substitution and VOR gain changes, and (2) the use of efference copy of the commanded head movement or preprogrammed compensatory eye counter-rotation to compensate for head movement while the eye is fixating on the newly acquired target.[58] This demanding situation is highly relevant because we naturally employ eye and head movement in this coordinated fashion to look at visual objects, and this is one of the most commonly avoided natural behaviors after a loss of vestibular function.

Balance and gait retraining exercises comprise the other large group of vestibular rehabilitation exercises. The exercises are performed either alone or in combination with the gaze stabilization exercises described previously. To adapt and optimize standing posture, the patient is asked to maintain stable stance in a variety of situations that challenge postural stability. These include standing with a reduced base of support, standing on a compliant surface, and standing during head or upper body and hip motion (eg, in a circle). To adapt and optimize gait, patients are asked to walk in a straight line and turn 180°, walk around obstacles, step over obstacles, and walk while moving the head in a repetitive pitch or yaw motion, or in different head postures. Often, cognitive tasks such as counting are superimposed on the exercises to limit the attention that can be devoted to the motor task, further stressing the balance control system.

There have been numerous controlled trials demonstrating the efficacy of vestibular rehabilitation against control procedures for the treatment of unilateral peripheral vestibular loss.[54,56,59–82] These studies examined both subjective assessment of vestibular or balance function and quantitative measures such as dynamic visual acuity, posturography scores, and sway path. The results of these studies clearly support the use of vestibular rehabilitation in adult patients. It is reasonable to assume that these procedures could be successfully adapted to pediatric vestibular patients, but there is still very little evidence from controlled studies to demonstrate this conclusively. In one placebo-controlled study, however, Rine and colleagues demonstrated a significant difference in motor development score (Peabody Developmental Motor Scales [PDMS]) improvement following vestibular rehabilitation versus a control procedure of auditory rehabilitation.[83] There is much work still to be done to confirm the efficacy of vestibular rehabilitation in children who face many of the same challenges as adult patients. This leaves the door open for other treatment alternatives, which share some characteristics with those of adult vestibular rehabilitation but are dramatically different in terms of their underlying theory and are totally unproven in this patient population (eg, sensory integration therapy,[84] see Zimmer and Deschel[85]).

Summary

The fields of rehabilitation medicine and vestibular neuroscience have produced parallel observations on the natural history of and progressive compensation to unilateral vestibular loss. The observations of neuroscientists clearly demonstrate that the vestibular system is capable of significant recovery from a peripheral vestibular loss if some peripheral function is preserved. These compensatory and adaptive changes occur naturally and progressively as the system adjusts to the loss of its basic functional strategy of bilateral comparison of vestibular inputs. The new, adapted system can solve many problems but at the cost of the precise timing and symmetry of vestibular responses. Augmentation of vestibular inputs with increased reliance on other sensory cues can further compensate for a loss, but it can also produce adaptive solutions that are limited to certain contexts. Ultimately, the central nervous system must learn to use this new combination of sensory inputs effectively in a wide variety of situations. This requires effort and exposure to challenging environmental contexts that provide the full range of challenges encountered in normal activities. Vestibular rehabilitation provides a valuable adjunct to this natural process by defining, through structured activities, the appropriate contexts required for maximal recovery from a vestibular loss.

Self-Assessment Questions

1. List the clinical features of a unilateral loss of utricular afferent input.
2. What complaints might a patient with unilateral utricular lesion complain of?
3. What are the findings in the setting of unbalanced canal input?
4. Which sensory cues provided by other intact sensory systems can assist in the process of suppressing the consequences of abnormal vestibular afferent input? Choose all that apply.
   - Kinesthetic cues
   - Tactile cues
   - Enteroceptive sensory inputs
   - Visual sensation
5. Outline the steps involved in central compensation of a peripheral vestibular loss.
6. List one patient factor that can lead to a poor functional outcome following a peripheral vestibular loss.
7. What are the two main categories of vestibular rehabilitation exercises?

References

1. Precht W, Shimazu H, Markham CH. A mechanism of central compensation of vestibular function following hemilabyrinthectomy. *J Neurophysiol.* 1966; 29(6):996–1010.
2. Warchol ME, Lambert PR, Goldstein BJ, Forge A, Corwin JT. Regenerative proliferation in inner ear sensory epithelia from adult guinea pigs and humans. *Science.* 1993; 259: 1619–1622.
3. Forge A, Li L, Corwin JT, Nevill G. Ultrastructural evidence for hair cell regeneration in the mammalian inner ear. *Science.* 1993; 259: 1616–1619.
4. Rubel EW, Dew LA, Roberson DW. Mammalian vestibular hair cell regeneration. *Science.* 1995;267:701–707.
5. Forge A, Li L, Nevill G. Hair cell recovery in the vestibular sensory epithelia of mature guinea pigs. *J Comp Neurol.* 1998;397:69–88.
6. Walsh RM, Hackney CM, Furness DN. Regeneration of the mammalian vestibular sensory epithelium following gentamicin-induced damage. *J Otolaryngol.* 2000;29:351–360.
7. Oesterle EC, Cunningham DE, Westrum LE, Rubel EW. Ultrastructural analysis of [3H] thymidine-labeled cells in the rat utricular macula. *J Comp Neurol.* 2003;463:177–195.
8. Kawamoto K, Izumikawa M, Beyer LA, Atkin GM, Raphael Y. Spontaneous hair cell regeneration in the mouse utricle following gentamicin ototoxicity. *Hear Res.* 2009; 247: 17–26.
9. Wang GP, Chatterjee I, Batts SA, et al. Notch signaling and Atoh1 expression during hair cell regeneration in the mouse utricle. *Hear Res.* 2010;267:61–70.
10. Lin V, Golub JS, Nguyen TB, Hume CR, Oesterle EC, Stone JS. Inhibition of notch activity promotes nonmitotic regeneration of hair cells in the adult mouse utricles. *J Neurosci.* 2011;31:15329–15339.
11. Golub JS, Tong L, Ngyuen TB, et al. Hair cell replacement in adult mouse utricles after targeted ablation of hair cells with diphtheria toxin. *J Neurosci.* 2012;32(43):15093–15105.
12. Stone J, Pujol R, Schlobohm L, Finkbeiner C, Gonzalez-Garrido A, Eatock RA. Anatomical observations of sensorineural degeneration and regeneration after destruction of hair cells in adult mouse utricles. *ARO Abstracts.* 2017; 40:126
13. Hirvonen TP, Minor LB, Hullar TE, Carey JP. Effects of intratympanic gentamicin on vestibular afferents and hair cells in the chinchilla. *J Neurophysiol.* 2005;93(2):643–655.
14. Stone J, Phillips J, Nguyen T, et al. Morphological and functional analyses of vestibular hair cell loss and replacement in adult Pou4f3-DTR mice after treatment with two different doses of diphtheria toxin *ARO Abstracts.* 2015; 38:4.
15. Minor LB, Goldberg JM. Vestibular-nerve inputs to the vestibulo-ocular reflex: A functional-ablation study in the squirrel monkey. *J Neurosci.* 1991;11(6):1636–1648.
16. Yates BJ, Miller DM. Integration of nonlabyrinthine inputs by the vestibular system: Role in compensation following bilateral damage to the inner ear. *J Vestib Res.* 2009;19(5–6): 183–189.
17. Buchman C, Joy J, Hodges A, Telischi FF, Balkany TJ. Vestibular effects of cochlear implantation. *Laryngoscope.* 2004;114:1–22.
18. Zhong X, Yost WA. Relationship between postural stability and spatial hearing. *J Am Acad Audiol.* 2013;24:782–788.
19. Stevens MN, Barbour DL, Gronski MP, Hullar TE. Auditory contributions to maintaining balance. *J Vestib Res.* 2016;26:433–438.
20. Hallemans A, Mertens G, Van de Heyning P, Van Rompaey V. Playing music may improve the gait pattern in patients with bilateral caloric areflexia wearing a cochlear implant: Results from a pilot study. *Front Neurol.* 2017; 8:404.
21. Weaver TS, Shayman CS, Hullar TE. The effect of hearing aids and cochlear implants on balance during gait. *Otol Neurotol.* 2017;38: 1327–1332.
22. Shayman CS, Earhart GM, Hullar TE. Improvements in gait with hearing aids and cochlear implants. *Otol Neurotol.* 2017;38: 484–486.

23. Goldberg JM, Lysakowski A, Fernàndez C. Morphophysiological and ultrastructural studies in the mammalian cristae ampullares. *Hear Res.* 1990;49:89–102.
24. Lysakowski A, Goldberg JM. A regional ultrastructural analysis of the cellular and synaptic architecture in the chinchilla cristae ampullares. *J Comp Neurol.* 1997;389:419–443.
25. Sugai T, Yano J, Sugitani M, Ooyama H. Actions of cholinergic agonists and antagonists on the efferent synapse in the frog sacculus. *Hear Res.* 1992;61:56–64.
26. Boyle R, Rabbitt RD, Highstein SM. Efferent control of hair cell and afferent responses in the semicircular canals. *J Neurophysiol.* 2009; 102:1513–1525.
27. Castellano-Munoz M, Israel SH, Hudspeth AJ. Efferent control of the electrical and mechanical properties of hair cells in the bullfrog's sacculus. *PLOS ONE.* 2010;5:e13777.
28. Rabbitt RD, Boyle R, Highstein SM. Mechanical amplification by hair cells in the semicircular canals. *Proc Natl Acad Sci USA.* 2010; 107:3864–3869.
29. Sadeghi SG, Goldberg JM, Minor LB, Cullen KE. Efferent-mediated responses in vestibular nerve afferents of the alert macaque. *J Neurophysiol.* 2009;101:988–1001.
30. Sadeghi SG, Minor LB, Cullen KE. Response of vestibular-nerve afferents to active and passive rotations under normal conditions and after unilateral labyrinthectomy. *J Neurophysiol.* 2007;97:1503–1514.
31. Hübner PP, Khan SI, Migliaccio AA. The mammalian efferent vestibular system plays a crucial role in vestibulo-ocular reflex compensation after unilateral labyrinthectomy. *J Neurophysiol.* 2017;117:1553–1568.
32. Miles FA, Braitman DJ. Long-term adaptive changes in primate vestibuloocular reflex. II. Electrophysiological observations on semicircular canal primary afferents. *J Neurophysiol.* 1980;43:1426–1436.
33. Ris L, Capron B, de Waele C, Vidal PP, Godaux E. Dissociations between behavioural recovery and restoration of vestibular activity in the unilabyrinthectomized guinea-pig. *J Physiol.* 1997;500(pt 2):509–522.
34. Guilding C, Dutia MB. Early and late changes in vestibular neuronal excitability after deafferentation. *Neuroreport.* 2005;16(13):1415–1418.
35. Yamanaka T, Him A, Cameron SA, et al. Rapid compensatory changes in GABA receptor efficacy in rat vestibular neurones after unilateral labyrinthectomy. *J Physiol-Lond.* 2000;523:413–424.
36. Him A, Dutia MB. Intrinsic excitability changes in vestibular nucleus neurons after unilateral deafferentation. *Brain Res.* 2001; 908:58–66.
37. Beraneck M, Hachemaoui M, Idoux E, et al. Long-term plasticity of ipsilesional medial vestibular nucleus neurons after unilateral labyrinthectomy. *J Neurophysiol.* 2003;90(1): 184–203.
38. Beraneck M, Idoux E, Uno A, Vidal PP, Moore LE, Vibert N. Unilateral labyrinthectomy modifies the membrane properties of contralesional vestibular neurons. *J Neurophysiol.* 2004;92(3):1668–1684.
39. Tighilet B, Brezun JM, Sylvie GD, Gaubert, C, Lacour, M. New neurons in the vestibular nuclei complex after unilateral vestibular neurectomy in the adult cat. *Eur J Neurosci.* 2007; 25:47–58.
40. Dutheil S, Brezun JM, Leonard J, Lacour M, Tighilet B. Neurogenesis and astrogenesis contribution to recovery of vestibular functions in the adult cat following unilateral vestibular neurectomy: Cellular and behavioral evidence. *Neuroscience.* 2009;164(4):1444–1456.
41. Johnston AR, Seckl JR, Dutia MB. Role of the flocculus in mediating vestibular nucleus neuron plasticity during vestibular compensation in the rat. *J Physiol.* 2002;545(Pt 3):903–911.
42. Beraneck M, McKee JL, Aleisa M, Cullen KE. Asymmetric recovery in cerebellar-deficient mice following unilateral labyrinthectomy. *J Neurophysiol.* 2008;100(2):945–958.
43. Melville Jones G. Plasticity in the adult vestibulo-ocular reflex arc. *Philos Trans Roy Soc Lond Biol.* 1977;278:319–334.
44. Miles FA, Fuller JH. Adaptive plasticity in the vestibulo-ocular responses of the rhesus monkey. *Brain Res.* 1974;80:512–516.

45. Robinson DA. Adaptive gain control of vestibuloocular reflex by the cerebellum. *J Neurophysiol.* 1976;39:954–969.
46. Lisberger SG. Neural basis for motor learning in the vestibuloocular reflex of primates. III. Computational and behavioral analysis of the sites of learning. *J Neurophysiol.* 1994;72: 974–998.
47. Lisberger SG, Pavelko TA, Bronte-Stewart HM, Stone LS. Neural basis for motor learning in the vestibuloocular reflex of primates. II. Changes in the responses of horizontal gaze velocity Purkinje cells in the cerebellar flocculus and ventral paraflocculus. *J Neurophysiol.* 1994;72:954–973.
48. Lisberger SG, Pavelko TA, Broussard DM. Neural basis for motor learning in the vestibuloocular reflex of primates. I. Changes in the responses of brain stem neurons. *J Neurophysiol.* 1994;72:928–953.
49. Hirata Y, Highstein SM. Plasticity of the vertical VOR: A system identification approach to localizing the adaptive sites. *Ann NY Acad Sci.* 2002;978:480–495.
50. Gauthier GM, Robinson DA. Adaptation of the human vestibuloocular reflex to magnifying lenses. *Brain Res.* 1975;92(2):331–335.
51. Shelhamer M, Zee DS. Context-specific adaptation and its significance for neurovestibular problems of space flight. *J Vestib Res.* 2003; 13(4–6):345–362.
52. Cawthorne T. Vestibular injuries. *Proc R Soc Med.* 1946;39:270–273.
53. Cooksey FS. Rehabilitation in vestibular injuries. *Proc R Soc Med.* 1946;39:273–278.
54. Herdman SJ, Clendaniel RA, Mattox DE, Holliday MJ, Niparko JK. Vestibular adaptation exercises and recovery: Acute stage after acoustic neuroma resection. *Otolaryngol Head Neck Surg.* 1995;113:77–87.
55. Enticott JC, O'Leary SJ, Briggs RJ. Effects of vestibulo-ocular reflex exercises on vestibular compensation after vestibular schwannoma surgery. *Otol Neurotol.* 2005;26(2):265–269.
56. Vereeck L, Wuyts F, Truijen S, De Valck C, Van de Heyning P. The effect of early customised vestibular rehabilitation on balance after acoustic neuroma resection. *Clin Rehab.* 2008; 22:698–713.
57. Fuchs AF, Ling L, Phillips JO. Behavior of the position vestibular pause (PVP) interneurons of the vestibuloocular reflex during head-free gaze shifts in the monkey. *J Neurophysiol.* 2005;94(6):4481–4490.
58. Newlands SD, Ling L, Phillips JO, Siebold C, Duckert L, Fuchs AF. Short- and long-term consequences of canal plugging on gaze shifts in the rhesus monkey. I. Effects on gaze stabilization. *J Neurophysiol.* 1999;81(5):2119–2130.
59. Horak FB, Jones-Rycewicz C, Black FO, Shumway-Cook A. Effects of vestibular rehabilitation on dizziness and imbalance. *Otolaryngol Head Neck Surg.* 1992;106(2):175–180.
60. Scott B, Larsen H-C, Lyttkens L, Melin L. An experimental evaluation of the effects of transcutaneous nerve stimulation and applied relaxation on hearing ability, tinnitus and dizziness in patients with Ménières disease. *Br J Audiol.* 1994;28:131–140.
61. Szturm T, Ireland DJ, Lessing-Turner M. Comparison of different exercise programs in the rehabilitation of patients with chronic peripheral vestibular dysfunction. *J Vestib Res.* 1994;4:461–479.
62. Mruzek 1995, Long-term plasticity of ipsilesional medial vestibular nucleus neurons after unilateral labyrinthectomy. *J Neurophysiol.* 2003;90(1):184–203.
63. Yardley L, Beech S, Zander L, Evans T, Weinman J. A randomised controlled trial of exercise therapy for dizziness and vertigo in primary care. *Br J Gen Pract.* 1998;48:1136–1140.
64. Strupp M, Arbusow V, Maag KP, Gall C, Brandt T. Vestibular exercises improve central vestibulospinal compensation after vestibular neuritis. *Neurology.* 1998;51:838–844.
65. Zimbelman JE, Stoecker J, Haberkamp TJ. Outcomes in vestibular rehabilitation. *Physical Therapy Case Reports.* 1999;2:232–240.
66. Toledo H, Cortés ML, Pane C, Trujillo V. Semont maneuver and vestibular rehabilitation exercises in the treatment of benign paroxysmal postural vertigo. A comparative study. *Neurologia.* 2000;15(4):152–157.
67. Cohen HS, Kimball KT, Jenkins HA. Factors affecting recovery after acoustic neuroma resection. *Acta Otolaryngologica.* 2002;122: 841–850.

68. Cohen HS, Kimball KT. Increased independence and decreased vertigo after vestibular rehabilitation. *Otolaryngol Head Neck Surg.* 2003;128:60–70.
69. Herdman SJ, Schubert MC, Das VE, Tusa RJ. Recovery of dynamic visual acuity in unilateral vestibular hypofunction. *Arch Otolaryngol Head Neck Surg.* 2003;129:819–824.
70. Krebs DE, Gill-Body KM, Parker SW, Ramirez JV, Wernick-Robinson M. Vestibular rehabilitation: Useful but not universally so. *Otolaryngol Head Neck Surg.* 2003;128:240–250.
71. Resende CR, Taguchi CK, de Almeida JG, Fujita RR. Vestibular rehabilitation in elderly patients with benign paroxysmal positional vertigo. *Brazilian J Otorhinolaryngol.* 2003; 69:online.
72. Pavlou M, Lingeswaran A, Davies RA, Gresty MA, Bronstein AM. Simulator based rehabilitation in refractory dizziness. *J Neurol.* 2004; 251:983–995.
73. Yardley L, Donovan-Hall M, Smith HE, Walsh BM, Mullee M, Bronstein AM. Effectiveness of primary care-based vestibular rehabilitation for chronic dizziness. *Ann Intern Med.* 2004;141:598–605.
74. Kammerlind AC, Ledin TEA, Odkvist LM, Skargren EIB. Effects of home training and additional physical therapy on recovery after acute unilateral vestibular loss—A randomized study. *Clin Rehab.* 2005;19:54–62.
75. Barozzi S, Berardino F, Arisi E, Cesarini A. A comparison between oculomotor rehabilitation and vestibular electrical stimulation in unilateral peripheral vestibular deficit. *Int Tinnitus J.* 2006;12:45–49.
76. Yardley L, Kirby S. Evaluation of booklet-based self-management of symptoms in Ménière disease: A randomised controlled trial. *Psychosom Med.* 2006;68:762–769.
77. Venosa A, Bittar R. Vestibular rehabilitation exercises in acute vertigo. *Laryngoscope.* 2007; 117:1482–1487.
78. Kulcu D, Yanik B, Boynukalin S, Kurtais Y. Efficacy of a home-based exercise program on benign paroxysmal positional vertigo compared with betahistine. *J Otolaryngol Head Neck Surg.* 2008;37(3):373–379.
79. Giray M, Kirazli Y, Karapolat H, Celebisoy N, Bilgen C, Kirazli T. Short-term effects of vestibular rehabilitation in patients with chronic unilateral vestibular dysfunction: A randomised controlled study. *Arch Phys Med Rehab.* 2009;90(8):1325–1331.
80. Teggi R, Caldirola D, Fabiano B, Pecanati P, Bussi M. Rehabilitation after acute vestibular disorders. *J Laryngol Otol.* 2009;123:397–402.
81. Hall CD, Heusel-Gillig L, Tusa RJ, Herdman SJ Efficacy of gaze stability exercises in older adults with dizziness. *J Neurol Phys Ther.* 2010;34(2):64–69.
82. Yardley L, Barker F, Muller I, et al. Clinical and cost effectiveness of booklet based vestibular rehabilitation for chronic dizziness in primary care: Single blind, parallel group, pragmatic, randomised controlled trial. *BMJ.* 2012;344:e2237.
83. Rine RM, Braswell J, Fisher D, Joyce K, Kalar K, Shaffer M. Improvement of motor development and postural control following intervention in children with sensorineural hearing loss and vestibular impairment. *Int J Pediatr Otorhinolaryngol.* 2004;68(9):1141–1148.
84. Ayres A. Sensory integration and the child. Torrance, CA: Western Psychological Services; 1979.
85. Zimmer M, Desch L. Section on Complementary and Integrative Medicine; Council on Children with Disabilities; American Academy of Pediatrics, Sensory integration therapies for children with developmental and behavioral disorders. *Pediatrics.* 2012;129(6): 1186–1189.

SECTION II

Clinical Evaluation

CHAPTER 4

History and Physical Examination of the Child With a Balance Disorder

Sharon L. Cushing, Jessica R. Levi, and Robert C. O'Reilly

Introduction

Children typically do not complain about vestibular dysfunction or vertigo (the sensation of movement) and therefore the diagnosis can be difficult. The diagnosis relies on questioning of the child and parents, physical examination, and an astute clinician to make the diagnosis. It is important to distinguish whether the problem resides within the vestibular system, within the vestibular pathways, or with abnormalities in the visual, motor, or proprioceptive systems or ultimately with their integration.

Patient History

Many children do not have the vocabulary or understanding to articulate the feeling or sense of "vertigo." In addition, the central vestibular projections to the cerebral cortex are diffuse. As such, vestibular disorders in children can be difficult to recognize and diagnose appropriately. Children with vestibular disorders are often initially thought to be clumsy and uncoordinated, or are diagnosed with a behavioral abnormality. Their presentation is variable, including ataxia, headache, visual disturbances, hearing loss, otalgia, and otorrhea, and at times their symptoms can go unrecognized or misdiagnosed for years. Other symptoms that are important in diagnosing vestibular disorders include vertigo, oscillopsia, drop attacks without loss of consciousness, lateropulsion (sensation of being pushed to one side), and vegetative symptoms (nausea, emesis, malaise). It is also important to determine if there is any history of delayed motor development (Table 4–1) or frequent falls. Learning disabilities can sometimes be a presenting complaint due to poor dynamic visual acuity secondary to deficiency of the vestibulo-ocular reflex (VOR). Beyond their reports of poor balance and incoordination, parents of children with severe vestibular dysfunction will often report that the child seems to perform all activities at very high speed, preferring to run than walk, for example.

Table 4–1. Gross Motor Milestones by Age

Age (months)	*Gross Motor Skills*
0–1	Prone: knees to abdomen Prone: rotates head side to side Ventral suspension: head held down Supine: head usually to side, tonic neck reflex position predominates
2	Prone: knees no longer under abdomen Prone: lifts head to 45° briefly Ventral suspension: head held erect briefly (bobbing) Supine: head kept in mid position briefly
3	Prone: lifts head to 45° for sustained period Ventral suspension: head up above level of body Sitting: head mostly steady, occasional bob only Supine: head in mid position predominantly
4	Prone: head up 90° on extended arms Bears weight briefly on extended legs Rolls front to back Downward parachute response emerges Ventral suspension: head and legs held up Sitting: head steady but slightly forward
5	Supine: lifts legs high Sitting: head erect and steady When pulled to sit no head lag May roll back to front
6	When pulled to sit, assists by lifting head Pivots in prone position Sits leaning forward on arms Bears full weight on legs if held standing Anterior propping response emerges Asymmetric tonic neck reflex fully inhibited
7	Bounces when held standing Sits erect for brief periods Assumes crawling position
8	Sits steadily on hard surface for 10 minutes In sitting, leans forward to reach and re-erects Lateral protection response in sitting emerges Stands holding rail if placed in position
9	Sits indefinitely on hard surface Gets to sitting position Pulls to stand Reciprocal crawl Forward parachute response present
10	Cruises using two hands on rail or furniture Lets self down from stand with partial control Posterior propping response present
11	Stands momentarily Walks with one hand held

Table 4–1. *continued*

Age (months)	*Gross Motor Skills*	*Age (months)*	*Gross Motor Skills*
12	Walks a few steps Stands independently well Creeps upstairs Climbs into small chair and sits	24	Jumps with both feet from floor Jumps off step Kicks a ball on request Throws the ball overhand
15	Walks well Creeps downstairs Climbs onto furniture to reach things Throws the ball while standing without falling Walks up steps with one hand held Gets to standing without support	30	Alternates feet going up stairs Stands briefly on one foot (1 second)
		36	Pedals tricycle Broad jump Stands on one foot (2 seconds) Alternates feet going down stairs
18	Walks pulling toys or carrying object Walks downstairs when hand is held Runs stiffly	48	Balances on one foot (5 seconds) Hops on one foot
21	Runs well Walks up- and downstairs holding rail Kicks a large ball with demonstration	School-Aged Child	Age 5 years: stands on one foot (10 seconds) Skips alternating feet Age 6: smooth heel–toe gait

Source: Shea S. Developmental Assessment. In: Goldbloom RB, ed. *Pediatric Clinical Skills*. 2nd ed. Philadelphia, PA: Churchill Livingstone; 1997:419.

Sometimes patients are asymptomatic; in a study of 62 children with basilar skull fracture, 34% of whom had sensorineural hearing loss (SNHL) and often vestibular injury, "few" of the children had vestibular complaints[1] despite the high likelihood that many of them suffered a concurrent vestibular injury. In addition, children with congenital deficits of vestibular function may not experience vertigo but rather have balance deficits that go unrecognized. With such variable presentation, diagnosis can be a challenge; however, a series of focused questions, based on the work by G. Michael Halmagyi,[1] can differentiate the pathology in most children.

Question 1: "Can You Tell Me How It Feels?"

This question can differentiate vertigo (an illusion of movement that is indicative of an abnormality in the vestibular end organ) from other sensations such as lightheadedness or presyncope. For example, anxiety with hyperventilation can produce a light-headed feeling and orthostatic hypotension that is particularly common in teenage females, and results in a presyncopal sensation. Peripheral vestibular disorders typically produce a true sense of whirling or spinning vertigo that is always exacerbated by movement. In contradistinction, the vertigo resulting from disorders of the central vestibular pathways typically are not exacerbated by movement. Central disorders are also characterized by fewer vegetative symptoms than peripheral disorders. Any change in sensorium related to the vertigo (particularly in the setting of a previously diagnosed seizure disorder) should prompt investigation into temporal lobe seizures.

Question 2: "Is There Anything That Makes Your Symptoms Better or Worse or Brings Your Symptoms On?"

Precipitating, aggravating, and alleviating factors can also be clues to the etiology of the vestibulopathy. Vertigo that worsens with straining or Valsalva can indicate perilymph fistula (especially if these symptoms are seen in conjunction with head trauma or in children with known inner ear dysplasias). Vertigo associated with benign paroxysmal positional vertigo (BPPV) is often worse or begins with rolling over, bending over, or looking up.

Question 3: "How Many Episodes Have You Had and How Long Do Your Symptoms Last?"

The duration of the vertigo and if it is recurrent may be the most helpful distinguishing factors. Brief episodes (seconds to minutes) of vertigo may indicate BPPV or benign paroxysmal vertigo of childhood (BPVC) (also called benign recurrent vertigo of childhood [BRVC]). Vertigo lasting hours may indicate endolymphatic hydrops, migraine, or, significantly less likely in children, posterior circulation compromise. A single longer episode usually indicates an insult to the vestibular system such as vestibular neuritis or labyrinthitis. Vertigo that is of a peripheral vestibular cause should always be episodic with variable duration of the episodes as previously described. Constant unrelenting vertigo that never subsides and is present for long durations of time is unlikely to be peripheral in nature. While it often takes adults weeks to months to compensate for such disorders, otherwise normal children will develop central compensation very rapidly, typically within a period of several days.

Question 4: "Do You Feel Anything Else With It and What Other Medical Problems Do You Have?"

Vestibular disorders are variable in terms of etiology, but sometimes it is possible to determine a specific cause or preceding event such as exposure to ototoxic medications or head/ear trauma. Autoimmune diseases can also have vestibular manifestations. A personal history of otologic disease, hearing loss, or any otologic surgery (eg, cholesteatoma or cochlear implantation) is also important. One should also elicit a history of seizures, ophthalmologic disease, and vascular or cardiac disease. Family history is important for malignancy, hearing loss, and migraine.

Concurrent symptoms can also help differentiate vestibulopathies and therefore should be examined. Many vestibulopathies have associated hearing loss or aural fullness. A history of headache or history of paroxysmal torticollis may help one differentiate migraine or BPVC. Other neurologic symptoms or symptoms of palpitations or anxiety should also be noted.

Physical Examination

A comprehensive head and neck exam should be performed including a full neurotologic and cranial nerve exam. The clinician should investigate static and dynamic imbalance. Vision should also be tested, and one should consider dynamic visual acuity testing (Video 4–1). For young children who do not as yet know their alphabet, an eye chart with symbols can be used (ie, LEA symbols chart). Complete age-appropriate audiometric evaluation including stapedius reflex testing should be performed. Specific tests of vestibular end-organ function (vestibular-evoked myogenic potentials [VEMPs], caloric testing, etc) should be performed when feasible (see Chapters 5, videonystagmography [VNG]/electronystagmography [ENG]; 6, rotational testing; 7, video head impulse testing [vHIT]; and 8, VEMP) for specific tests of vestibular end-organ function).

Developmental Reflexes

Developmental reflexes should be tested when examining infants. Failure of these reflexes to appear and more importantly disappear along an appropriate timeline can indicate an underlying neurologic abnormality. The timeline for these developmental reflexes is outlined in Table 4–2, and a full description of these reflexes can be found in Chapter 2.

Static Imbalance

Older children, who are able to cooperate with the exam, are instructed to stare at a finger or some other interesting object in order to determine the presence of spontaneous or gaze-evoked nystagmus (Figure 4–1). When evaluating for spontaneous nystagmus, it is important that the patient not look beyond 30° (extremes of gaze) where physiologic nystagmus occurs.

All cardinal gazes should be evaluated. Sometimes it is necessary to remove fixation with Frenzel glasses (Figure 4–2) in order to appreciate spontaneous nystagmus. If seen, spontaneous nystagmus indicates an active asymmetry in vestibular function; gaze-evoked nystagmus will indicate a central nervous system disorder.

In infants and young children who are unable to cooperate with most of the exam, one can still evaluate for a functional VOR by evaluating the presence and characteristics of per-rotatory and post-rotatory nystagmus. The child, with or without a parent depending on age, sits on a rotating stool. The clinician then accelerates the child in a circle and then comes to a stop. This is then repeated in the alternating direction. With an intact VOR,

Table 4–2. Timeline of Developmental Reflexes

Age at Appearance	*Age at Disappearance*	*Reflex*
Birth	5 to 6 months	Moro reflex
Birth	6 months	Tonic neck reflex
4–6 months	N/A	Head righting reflex
5 months	N/A	Parachute reaction
Birth	2 to 3 weeks	Doll's eye response

Source: Lehman R, Schor N. Neurologic Evaluation. In: Kliegman R, Behrman R, Jenson H, Stanton B, eds. *Nelson Textbook of Pediatrics*. 19th ed. Philadelphia, PA: Saunders Elsevier; 2011.

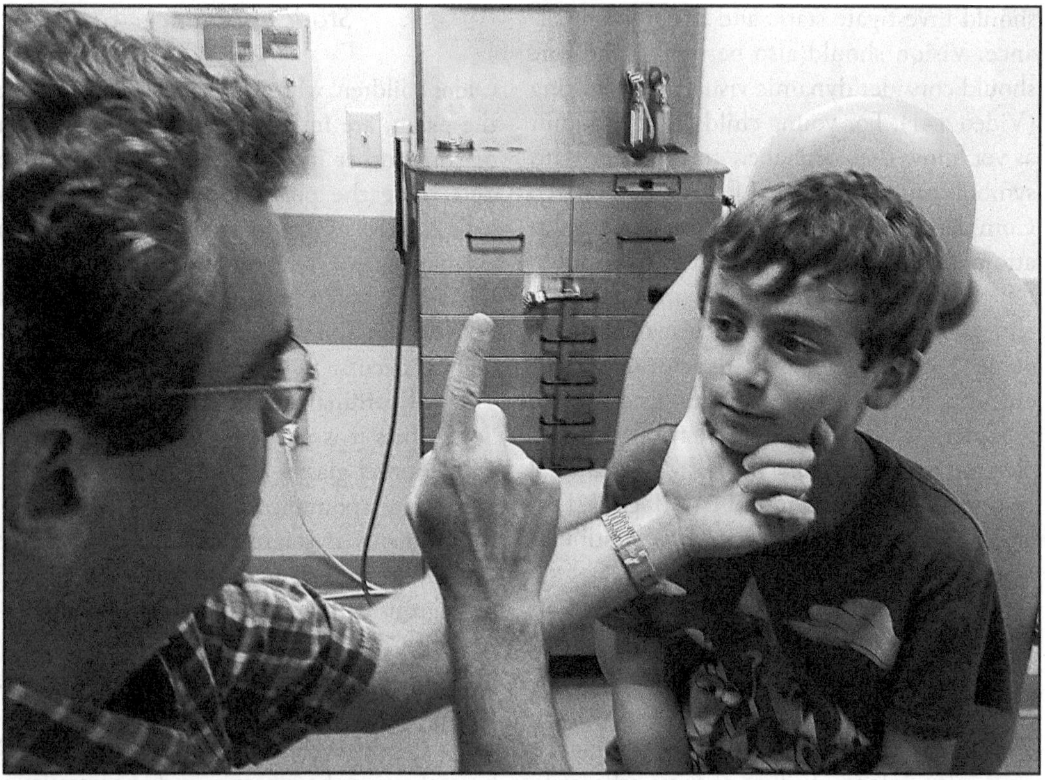

Figure 4–1. Search for spontaneous and gaze-evoked nystagmus.

fast phase nystagmus toward the direction of acceleration can be observed throughout rotation (per-rotatory nystagmus). Once the acceleration is halted, reversal of the nystagmus will be observed with the fast phase directed away from the direction of the acceleration (post-rotatory nystagmus) (Video 4–2). The nystagmus is best seen using Frenzel lenses or in the dark (ie, wearing occlusive goggles). However, young infants (<6 months of age) have an inability to suppress their VOR; therefore, their horizontal canal function can be examined in this way without the removal of visual fixation (Video 4–3).

A perilymph fistula may produce horizontal nystagmus and symptomatic vertigo that is worse with tragal compression, impedance testing (Hennebert's sign), or loud sound (Tullio phenomenon). Vertical nystagmus can indicate either a cranial cervical junction lesion that will have down-beating nystagmus or a pontine lesion with up-beating nystagmus. A child with a large Chiari malformation, for example, would likely have down-beating nystagmus with worsening upon Valsalva. "Cervical vertigo" can lead to nystagmus upon neck rotation, and hyperventilation can elicit nystagmus produced by demyelinating lesions of the brain or eighth nerve compression.

Patients recovering from an acute peripheral vestibular injury will progress through the different degrees of nystagmus as they develop central compensation. They will initially experience third-degree nystagmus (nystagmus is seen in the primary and both lateral positions of gaze) and then progress to second-degree

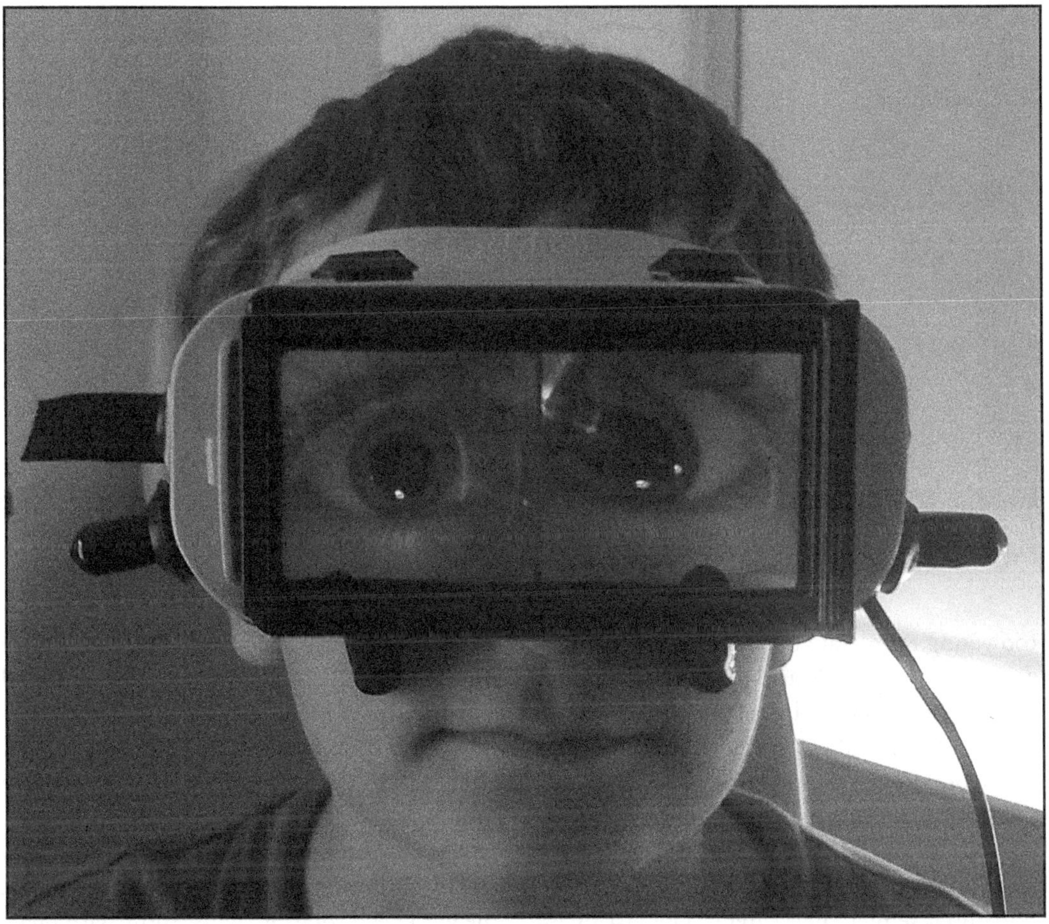

Figure 4–2. Frenzel glasses (high diopter lenses) prevent fixation and aid in identification of nystagmus.

nystagmus (nystagmus is seen in the primary and one lateral position). Finally, they will experience first-degree nystagmus (nystagmus is seen in only one position of lateral gaze), and then will have no spontaneous nystagmus. An extended discussion of static imbalance can be found in Chapter 9.

Dynamic Imbalance

Tests of dynamic imbalance are important for evaluating the VOR and include the "head thrust maneuver," "Halmagyi maneuver," or "head impulse test." The patient fixates on a stationary target and the head is rapidly moved up, down, left, or right (Figure 4–3). In patients with a deficient VOR, stationary gaze cannot be maintained, and one can appreciate corrective saccades (Videos 4–4, 4–5, and 4–6).

Deficiency of the VOR can also be examined with the head shake maneuver, looking for post head shake nystagmus. Fixation must be prevented during this test, as it will lead to visual suppression of the nystagmus, and this can be achieved using Frenzel glasses. If Frenzel glasses are unavailable or the child is

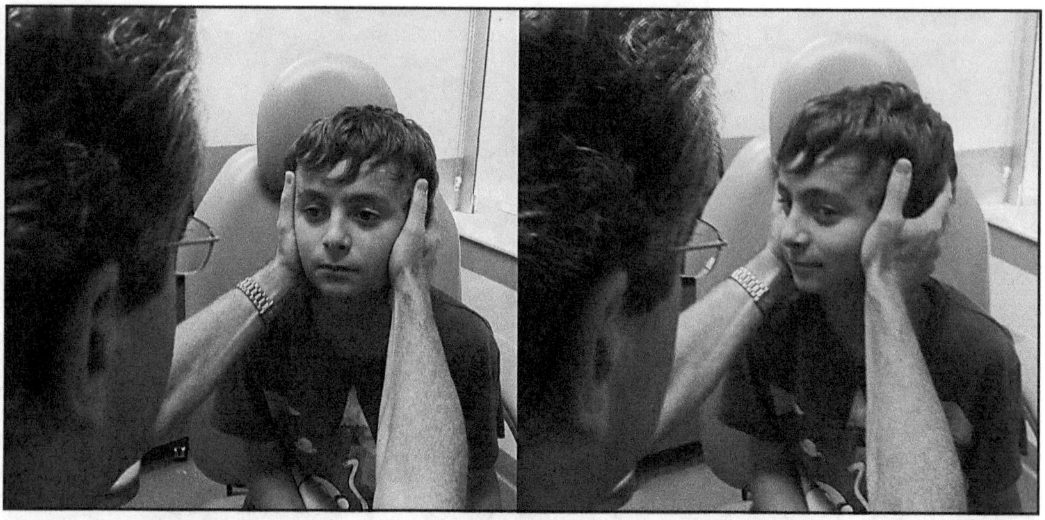

Figure 4–3. Head thrust maneuver tests the vestibulo-ocular reflex (VOR).

too young to tolerate them, a dark room with a video camera with a night vision function can be used instead. In this test, the head is oscillated from side to side symmetrically at a frequency greater than 2 Hz and then stopped (Video 4–7). Several beats of nystagmus will be observed in patients with vestibular imbalance or asymmetry of function between the horizontal semicircular canals. The fast phase will be directed to the side of the intact horizontal semicircular canal. Suppression of the VOR should also be examined and can be performed with the child seated alone or in the caregiver's lap with a target for fixation at approximately arm's length away. The child is then rotated from side to side and maintenance of fixation suggests intact ability to suppress the VOR (Video 4–8). Inability to visually suppress nystagmus during head rotations suggests a defect at the level of the vestibulocerebellum. The Dix-Hallpike maneuver with right, left and center head hanging positions as well as bilateral supine head roll maneuvers should also be performed to search for evidence of BPPV (Figure 4–4). If necessary, this can be followed with a particle repositioning maneuver. Dynamic visual acuity testing is useful for detecting bilateral VOR deficiency due to bilateral areflexia. Following standard visual acuity testing, repeat visual acuity testing is performed while the head is oscillated from side to side symmetrically a frequency greater than 2 Hz at an amplitude of approximately 20°. Adults with intact vestibular function often show no more than a loss of a single line with head rotation, while those with bilateral loss may show up to a five-line decline in visual acuity with head rotation (Video 4–1).[2] An extended discussion of dynamic imbalance can be found in Chapter 10.

Vestibulospinal Testing

In order to test the vestibulospinal tract, the clinician should test the Romberg, sharpened Romberg (patient stands heel to toe), past pointing, and the Fukuda stepping test (where the child marches in place with eyes closed for 30 seconds). Abnormal responses for the Romberg and sharpened Romberg and dyskinesia in the past pointing test should be recorded. Any rotation during the Fukuda step test may indicate a unilateral vestibular loss, with the

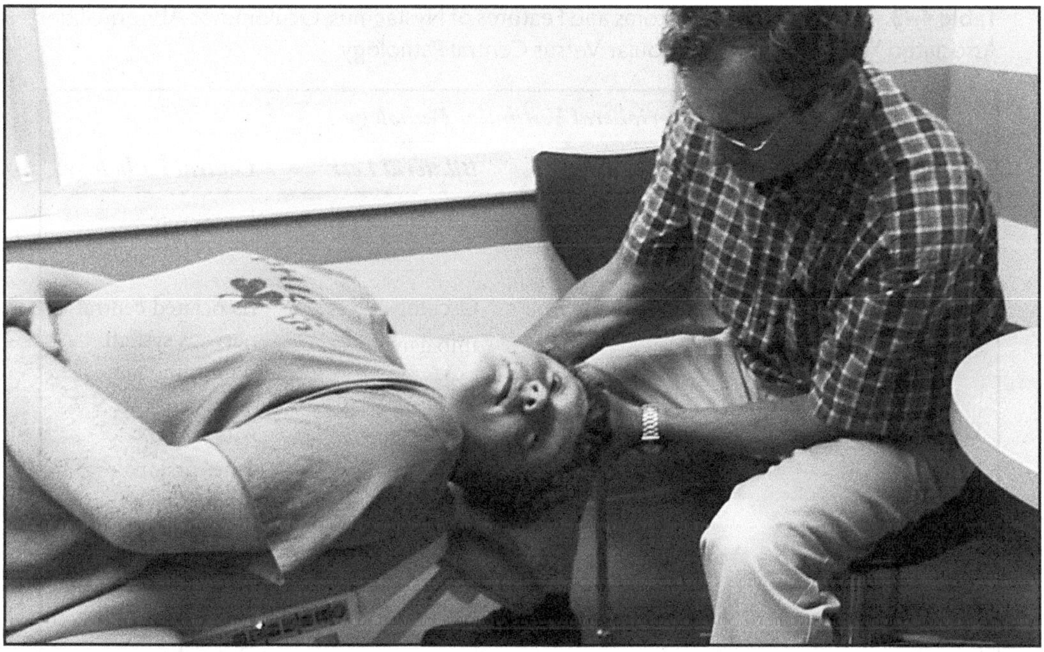

Figure 4–4. Dix-Hallpike maneuver.

patient rotating more than 45° toward the side of weakness (Figure 4–5, Video 4–9). For the Fukuda stepping test, it is important to observe for a minimum of 30 seconds as deviation in children can often occur late in the assessment and would be missed if only a short duration was observed. Gait and gross motor skills must be assessed as well. An in-depth review of gait assessment can be found in Chapter 11.

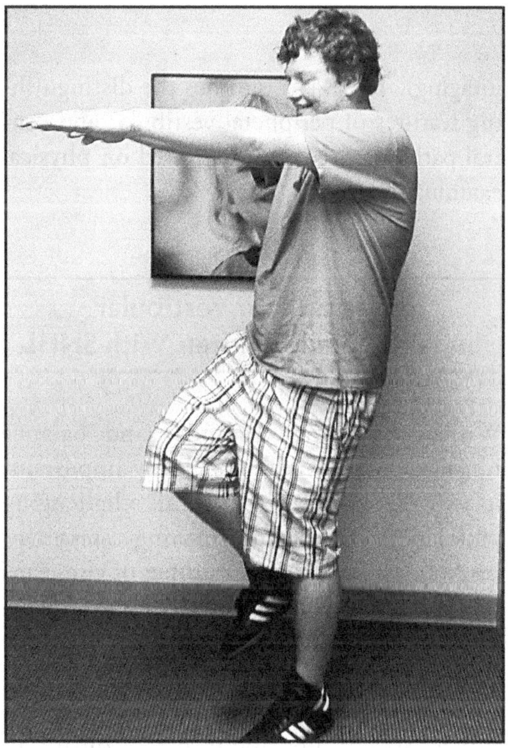

Figure 4–5. Fukuda stepping test.

Characteristics of Peripheral Vestibular and Central Pathology

While history and physical examination alone may not be sufficient to characterize the underlying disorder in all cases, it should provide the means to distinguish between peripheral vestibular versus central pathology. This ability is key in directing further evaluation of the child who will not tolerate exhaustive testing or who may require anaesthesia for certain investigations (eg, magnetic resonance

Table 4–3. Characteristic Symptoms and Features of Nystagmus, Oculomotor Abnormalities Associated With Peripheral Vestibular Versus Central Pathology

	Peripheral Vestibular Pathology		
	Acute Unilateral Loss	*Bilateral Loss*	*Central Pathology*
Characteristics of vertigo	Severe Motion aggravated	No vertigo	Less severe
Other symptoms	Vegetative symptoms	Oscillopsia Imbalance Gait ataxia	Associated central nervous system symptoms
Direction of nystagmus	Mixed horizontal torsional	No vertigo	Mixed Pure torsional Pure vertical
Fixation/suppression	Yes	Yes	No
Smooth pursuit	Normal	Normal	Typically saccadic
Saccades	Normal	Normal	Often dysmetric

Source: Rutka JA. Physiology of the Vestibular System. In: Roland PS, Rutka JA, eds. *Ototoxicity*. Hamilton: BC Decker; 2004.

imaging). Table 4–3 outlines the distinguishing features of peripheral vestibular and central pathology that can be noted on physical examination.

Screening for Vestibular Impairment in Children With SNHL

While identifying vestibular and balance impairment in children is clearly important, it may be impractical in this challenging population. The ideal screening assessment could be applied by any number of clinicians to identify those at risk of vestibular impairment who should be referred for more thorough testing.

Asking caregivers about motor milestones, specifically about neck control in infancy and age at sitting and walking, can identify risk of vestibular impairment (see Table 4–1). Second, one-foot standing eyes open and eyes closed is an effective screening tool for balance dysfunction in children (Table 4–4).[3] Finally a measure of horizontal canal function can be obtained without specialized equipment in the form of a clinical head impulse test or as outlined previously, by looking for post-rotary nystagmus following rotation of an infant younger than 6 months.[4] While completing all three parts of the screen is ideal, however, completion of any one assessment is useful in the identification of children at risk of vestibular impairment. At times, findings across these screening tests may be discordant; they may be abnormal not only in peripheral vestibular dysfunction but also in central and combined dysfunction. More thorough evaluation will better define the presence and contribution of any peripheral vestibular deficit.

Table 4–4. Expected and Red Flag One-Foot Standing Times by Age[9,10]

Age	*Duration (second), One Foot Standing*
30 months	1 (briefly)
36 months	2
4 years	5
5 years	10
≥5 years	Red flag for vestibular impairment
Eyes open	<8 seconds
Eyes closed	<4 seconds

Conclusions

In 1974, Rapin eloquently expressed that "The testing of children rarely fulfills all the conditions for an ideal vestibular study."[5] This quote certainly reflects the sentiment that surrounds testing of any kind in a pediatric clinical setting and a number of modifications to adult neuro-otologic testing techniques have been suggested in the literature.[6–8] Ultimately, complete evaluation of the child with a balance disorder may not be possible; however, results can be optimized through good preparation of the family, time, patience, and creativity and may require breaks in testing and, at times, several visits to the clinic.

Self-Assessment Questions

1. If the vertiginous episodes last seconds to minutes, which causes of vertigo are in your differential diagnosis?
2. Is vertigo of a peripheral origin episodic or continuous?
3. Children with BPVC are at risk of developing which condition later in life?
4. What is the utility of using Frenzel glasses or testing in darkness when examining for nystagmus?
5. What tests may be abnormal in the setting of a complete bilateral vestibular loss (horizontal canal)?
6. Which clinical tests may be abnormal in the setting of asymmetric horizontal canal function?
7. At what age should a child be able to stand on one foot for 10 seconds?
8. What oculomotor features suggest an underlying central cause for the symptoms?

9. What does vertical nystagmus indicate?
10. What is the progression of nystagmus that occurs following an acute vestibular injury?

References

1. Halmagyi G, ed. History II. Patient with Vertigo. In: Baloh RW, Halmagyi GM, eds. *Disorders of the Vestibular System*. New York, NY: Oxford University Press; 1996:171–177.
2. Kasai T, Zee DS. Eye-head coordination in labyrinthine-defective human beings. *Brain Res*. 1978;144(1):123–141.
3. Oyewumi M, Wolter NE, Heon E, Gordon KA, Papsin BC, Cushing SL. Using balance function to screen for vestibular impairment in children with sensorineural hearing loss and cochlear implants. *Otol Neurotol*. 2016;37:926–932.
4. Cohen B. Erasmus Darwin's observations on rotation and vertigo. *Hum Neurobiol*. 1984;3(3):121–128.
5. Rapin I. Hypoactive labyrinths and motor development. *Clin Pediatr (Phila)*. 1974;13(11):922–923, 926–929, 934–937.
6. Cyr DG, Brookhouser PE, Valente M, Grossman A. Vestibular evaluation of infants and preschool children. *Otolaryngol Head Neck Surg*. 1985;93(4):463–468.
7. Eviatar L, Eviatar A. Neurovestibular examination of infants and children. *Adv Otorhinolaryngol*. 1978;23:169–191.
8. Snashall SE. Vestibular function tests in children. *J R Soc Med*. 1983;76(7):555–559.
9. Shea S. *Developmental Assessment*. 2nd ed. Philadelphia, PA: Churchill Livingstone; 1997.
10. Oyewumi M, Wolter NE, Heon E, Gordon KA, Papsin BC, Cushing SL. Using balance function to screen for vestibular impairment in children with sensorineural hearing loss and cochlear implants. *Otol Neurotol*. 2016;37(7):926–932.

CHAPTER 5

Videonystagmography/ Electronystagmography Testing With Children

Emily F. Zwicky

Introduction

Why Test Children?

The recent focus on identifying and treating balance and vestibular pathology in children stems in large part from mandates for universal newborn hearing screening and genetic advances resulting in increased awareness among professionals that auditory and vestibular pathology frequently co-occur.[1] There is also mounting evidence that vestibular pathology can result in significant negative impacts on a child's development and well-being.

Vestibular pathology can lead to a cascade of interrelated problems, potentially reducing a child's quality of life. For example, delays in motor development secondary to vestibular pathology may prompt decreased participation in physical activity resulting in deconditioning, and reduced peer interaction. Subsequent feelings of isolation may compromise psychological well-being. Further symptoms of vestibular pathology such as malaise, gait instability, loss of postural control, nausea, and fatigue may lead to missed school days, difficulty with attention and focus in class, and deficits in reading secondary to reduced dynamic visual acuity. These scenarios support prompt identification and treatment of vestibular pathology to minimize the impacts on children and their families.[2]

Preparing the Family for Testing

It is important to adequately prepare the family for videonystagmography (VNG)/electronystagmography (ENG) testing. When possible, it is best to set an appointment with the parents and child prior to their scheduled testing to establish rapport, review case history, and complete a comprehensive diagnostic hearing evaluation, which is an integral preliminary component of any vestibular test battery. Issues such as excessive cerumen, which may interfere with caloric testing, can also be addressed during this visit, and if a significant hearing loss exists, other strategies for testing can be discussed. A description of upcoming test procedures and a brief tour of the test facility can often help to put the child and parents at ease, especially if care has been taken to utilize child-friendly furnishings and decor in your vestibular laboratory. Parents should be coached on how to best assist during the actual evaluation and should be questioned regarding any motivators that are particularly effective for their child. A discussion of medications to avoid prior to testing as well as eating and change-of-clothing instructions should also be reviewed. If the family is traveling some distance, a face-to-face meeting prior to testing may not be possible. In these cases, it is helpful to conduct a phone interview to discuss the child's case history and to review test instructions and answer any questions. For traveling families, it may also be helpful to arrange overnight accommodations close to the test facility so that the child will be well rested on the date of testing. Literature or brochures describing test procedures and clear pretest instructions should always be provided well in advance.

Normative Data

The VNG/ENG battery is largely composed of tests derived from common bedside examinations of vestibular function. Electro-oculography (EOG) techniques used to make objective recordings of the corneoretinal potential were first introduced by researchers including Schott in 1922, Meyers in 1929, and Jacobsen in 1930.[3] Jung in 1939[4] was the first to use EOG for exploration and recording of eye movements in patients with dizziness complaints. Since these earliest EOG recordings, technological advances providing computerized control of stimuli and analysis of recordings have increased the accuracy and diagnostic utility of the VNG/ENG by allowing the recording of objective data that can be precisely measured and compared among patients. For many clinics, this has facilitated the gathering of normative data, and has thereby enhanced test sensitivity and specificity. As a result, VNG/ENG is widely considered the cornerstone of diagnostic testing in assessing adult vestibular function. Before engaging children in any vestibular testing, especially tests that are difficult and challenging, it is important to consider whether the selected tests will generate meaningful data to assist in diagnosis and treatment planning. The vestibular system is the first of the body's organ systems to complete development, and although it appears structurally complete at birth, it is well documented that the vestibular and balance systems continue to develop and undergo sequential maturational changes well into adolescence.[5] To this end, it is vitally important to collect and utilize clinic-specific normative data obtained from a variety of representative age groups, and to use the same test techniques and equipment used in collecting norms when applying tests to patients.

Central Versus Peripheral Vestibular Function

The eyes provide our most accessible window for exploring vestibular function. The typical VNG/ENG test battery takes advantage of this fact by combining a series of tests to capture both the centrally mediated eye movements of the central vestibulo-ocular pathways and the peripherally mediated reflexive eye movements of the vestibular ocular reflex (VOR). By combining tests that explore both central and peripheral vestibular function, the VNG/ENG battery may provide information to assist in distinguishing between central versus peripheral pathology. Peripheral vestibular pathology is characterized by dysfunction of any of the 5 motion sensors of the vestibular labyrinth (the semicircular canals [SCCs] and the otolith organs) or within the afferent pathways of the superior and inferior vestibular nerves carrying signals to the level of the root entry zone in the brainstem. Central pathology involves abnormalities beginning at the level of the root entry zone of the brainstem, the central vestibular nuclei, or ascending neural connections in the brainstem, cerebellum, and cortex.[6] In general, VNG/ENG testing allows only generalized statements regarding site of lesion and typically findings fall into one of the following categories, for example, peripheral pathology, central pathology, mixed peripheral and central pathology, or nonlocalizing.

VNG/ENG Limitations

It is important to recognize the limitations of the VNG/ENG test battery. It assesses the function of the superior vestibular nerve with its ascending connections to the extraocular muscles controlling eye movement by stimulating the horizontal semicircular canals. However, the stimulation used in caloric testing is nonphysiologic in that it mimics only very low frequency rotational stimulation and, therefore, does not replicate the stimuli that occur during normal active head or body movements. Important contributions made by other vestibular receptors serving the vestibulospinal reflex, vestibulocolic reflexes, and gravity sensitive otoliths (saccule and utricle), as well as the superior and posterior SCCs are not assessed in VNG/ENG testing. Fortunately, other clinical tests—that is, rotary chair (Chapter 6), vestibular-evoked myogenic potential (Chapter 7), and platform posturography (Chapter 9) supplement the VNG/ENG battery and have been successfully adapted for use in children.

Videonystagmography Versus Electronystagmography

VNG uses goggle-mounted infrared cameras to capture eye movements (Figure 5–1A) and because of the advantages of high resolution and playback of video recordings, VNG has surpassed ENG in popularity for adult testing. VNG is also preferred when testing children; however, ENG techniques with application of electrodes for recording both horizontal and vertical eye movements (Figure 5–1B) are very useful for children who are unable to wear VNG goggles due to limited tolerance or poor fit related to small head size or craniofacial anomalies.

Keys to Success

When testing children, numerous patient-related factors including the child's age, size, cognitive abilities, and limits of compliance will interact to determine whether or not the VNG/ENG test battery can be successfully completed. Non-patient-related factors also come into play. These factors include the skill of the clinician conducting the test in appropriately modifying test protocols and establishing rapport, thereby maintaining the child's compliance. The clinician must be skillful in putting both the child and parents at ease and must make the entire experience as engaging and nonthreatening as possible in order to record useful and valid data from the child. This requires creativity, patience, flexibility, and a warm personality.

Modifying the Adult Test Battery for Pediatric Testing

In general, furnishings and decor in the pediatric vestibular lab should be child friendly, yet not infantile, so as to appeal to children of varying ages. Children with vestibular complaints may be unsteady, and issues of inattention and fidgety behavior can arise during testing. To assure safety, testing on an exam table or bed with retractable side rails is recommended. Often short breaks between subtests

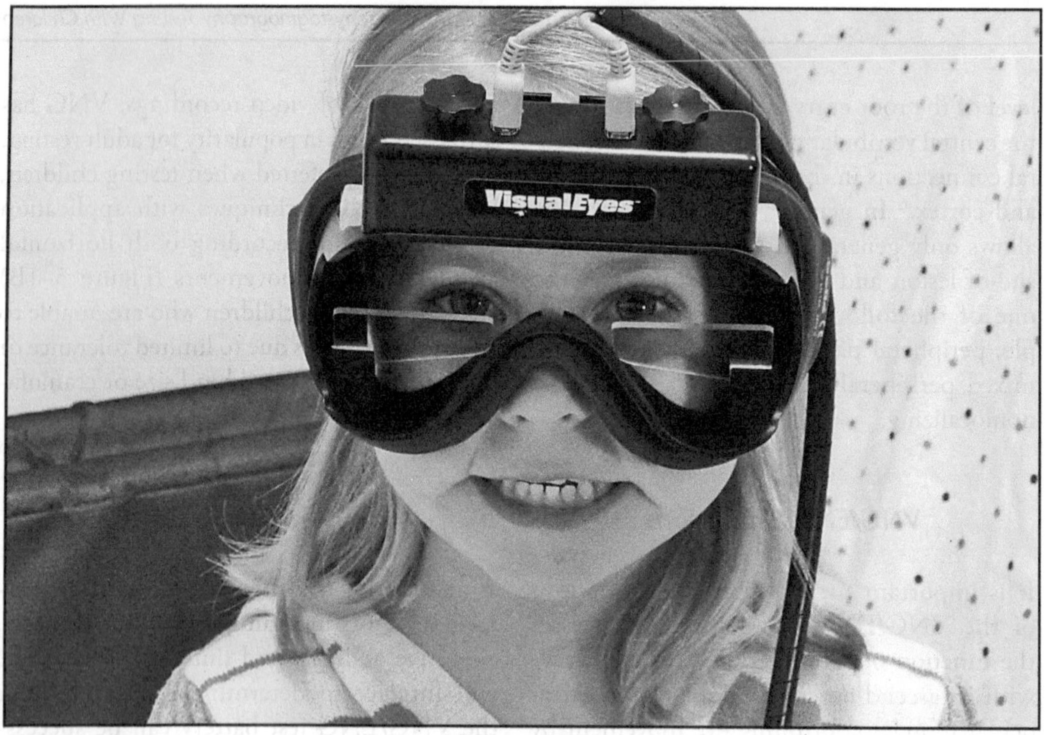

A

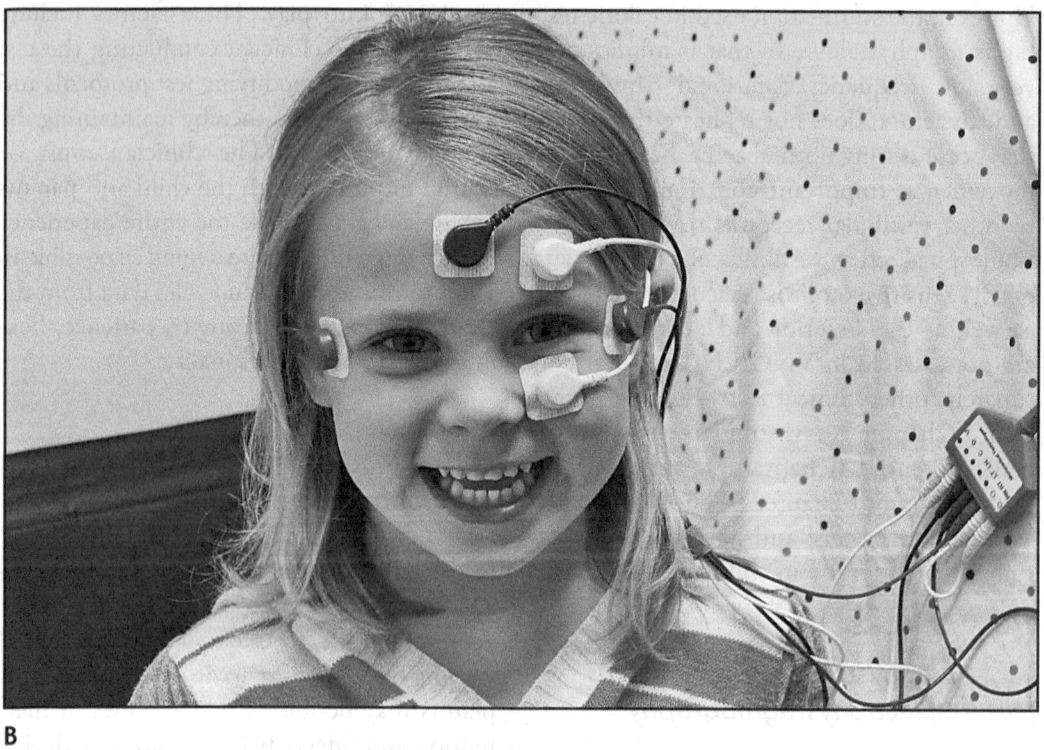

B

Figure 5–1. A. VNG goggles worn by pediatric patient. **B.** ENG electrode montage—Braiding electrode wires and securing away from the face helps reduce issues with intentional removal of electrodes by pediatric patients.

are needed to promote compliance; therefore, appointment times required for VNG/ENG testing with children are typically longer than with adults. If VNG goggles or electrodes are removed or lighting is altered, it is important to recalibrate eye movements before proceeding (Video 5–1). See Table 5–1 for a list of typical subtests of the pediatric VNG/ENG test battery.

Eye Movement Exam

Prior to VNG/ENG recording, a bedside examination of eye movements should be conducted. To engage a child, finger puppets, small toys, or lighted spinners can be used as targets and will help facilitate bedside assessment of ocular alignment, range of motion, vergence, saccades, and pursuit. The eye movement exam provides information for accurate interpretation of recorded tests by revealing such issues as disconjugate eye movements, ocular misalignment, or other abnormalities, which impact findings or require modification of test recording techniques.[7–9] See Video 4–2 for an example of a pediatric bedside eye movement exam.

Oculomotor Testing

The oculomotor test battery serves to explore the function of the central oculomotor control systems located in the brainstem and cerebellum. VNG/ENG recordings generally include tests of gaze stability, saccades, pursuit tracking, and optokinetic nystagmus. See Videos 5–3, 5–4, 5–5, and 5–6, for additional details regarding oculomotor testing, interpretation, and discussion of ocular-motor development in children.

Oculomotor Test Modifications

When performing oculomotor testing with children, teasing out true abnormalities from poor performance related to inattention or lack of effort can sometimes be challenging. Ensuring that you have achieved an accurate calibration of eye movements is a fundamental prerequisite to making accurate judgments of recordings. Strategies for successful recording include making the test fun by turning it into a game. For example, allowing a child to "score points" during testing and awarding carnival tickets that can later be redeemed for a "prize" can be highly motivating and enhance performance for some children. Use of colorful,

Table 5–1. Typical Subtests of the Pediatric VNG/ENG Test Battery

Spontaneous	*Oculomotor*	*Positioning*	*Static Positional*	*Caloric*
Sitting; Head Center (without fixation)	Gaze stability; center and eccentric gaze with and without fixation Random saccades Pursuit Tracking Optokinetic nystagmus	Dix-Hallpike maneuver	Supine; head at 30° Head left, (body left, if indicated) Head right, (body right, if indicated)	Bithermal warm and cool calorics Fixation Suppression

interesting, and relatively large visual targets such as cartoon characters, or a "smiley" face will also help sustain attention to task. Providing clear and simple directions and checking for understanding of tasks are also critical factors to obtaining reliable recordings. To facilitate understanding, it is often helpful to begin with a brief practice run demonstrating the visual target and to use a laser pointer to simulate and demonstrate the eye movements required during the task. A child's fatigue and tolerance can be unpredictable; therefore, it is important to strategize the order of tests and to prioritize and record the most meaningful information first. If it becomes apparent that a child's compliance is waning, it may be useful to record certain oculomotor subtests first. It is important to record a sufficient amount of data in order to adequately judge recordings and to repeat any tests that show abnormal results. When abnormalities appear, a review of directions and additional motivation to assure the child's best effort are helpful prior to re-recording. Table 5–2 provides suggestions for oculomotor test modifications.

Spontaneous Nystagmus Testing

Spontaneous nystagmus testing is performed to look for the presence of any nystagmus in the neutral (typically sitting) position in the absence of vestibular stimulation. Spontaneous nystagmus testing is done without fixation; therefore, as in all tests done without fixation, mental tasking should be applied. Examples include involving the child in conversation regarding the child's family, pets, or any particular interests. See Table 5–3 for a list of suggestions for tasking with children.

Table 5–2. Oculomotor Test Modifications

Make it fun; turn it into a game.
Use interesting child-friendly targets.
Use a practice run to demonstrate the task.
Check for understanding of the task.
Prioritize and record the most important information first.
Record sufficient data.
Repeat tests with abnormal results to ensure reliability.

Positioning Tests

The purpose of positioning testing is to search for evidence of benign paroxysmal positioning vertigo (BPPV). Recent evidence suggests that BPPV may be more common in children than previously thought.[9] When present, BPPV fatigues during repeated movement of the head with respect to gravity; therefore, positioning testing with Dix-Hallpike or other provocative maneuvers should be done *prior* to static position testing. Use of VNG recordings for capturing video evidence of rotary nystagmus is preferred to ENG since ENG cannot

Table 5–3. Suggestions for Tasking With Children

Favorite TV shows
Kids in your class; who sits in front of you, behind you, left and right of you
Foods (alphabetically)
Three-letter words or any words (alphabetically)
Baseball/football teams
Types of candy
Types of Halloween costumes
Geography (cities, states, countries; alphabetically)
Simple addition, subtraction, or multiplication
Spelling tests
Colors

capture pure rotary nystagmus (Video 5–7). To assist the examiner in interpretation of complex eye movements, use of Frenzel lenses may be helpful by magnifying eye movements for inspection.

Children do not frequently have issues with arthritis or restricted range of motion and are usually able to tolerate this test quite well with limited modifications. It is always best to support a child's head and neck throughout the test and to stabilize VNG goggles with light pressure to prevent slippage while the head is reclined. Tasking is not necessary during this test.

Static Position Tests

The rationale for performing static position testing is to seek evidence of nystagmus or other abnormal eye movements when the vestibular labyrinths are statically altered with respect to gravity. Explanations for the mechanisms responsible for positional nystagmus of *peripheral origin* relate to the keen sensitivity of the otoliths to gravity. When the head and body are gravitationally altered from the neutral sitting position, an otolithic lesion, usually in the undermost ear, may cause disruption of the VOR due to a tonic asymmetry between the paired otoliths, which in turn impacts neural firing of the SCCs resulting in nystagmus. Lesions of the central vestibular nuclei located within the brainstem may also cause asymmetries resulting in positional nystagmus of *central origin.* Whether positional nystagmus is abnormal or whether it is due to central or peripheral pathology is determined by examining characteristics of the recorded nystagmus including its *intensity, beat direction,* and any *impacts of fixation* on the nystagmus. Several axioms do exist for identifying positional nystagmus of central origin. These include the *presence of nystagmus with fixation* (which does not increase in intensity with fixation removed) and the observation of *direction changing nystagmus* in a single head position.[10]

When testing children, the strategy should always be to acquire useful information in a time-efficient manner; therefore, recommended positions to include during testing include *supine with head at 30°, head left,* and *head right.* If the history reveals positions that trigger symptoms, these should be added when feasible. Tasking should routinely be applied during testing and should be geared to the child's age, interests, and capabilities. If nystagmus is present, the child should be questioned regarding any subjective sensation of vertigo or dizziness. Unless nystagmus is evident, positional testing with fixation is not considered necessary. In addition, to save time, lateral positions should only be added if nystagmus is present in the supine or head left/right positions.[10]

Caloric Testing: Air Versus Water?

Opinions regarding preference for air versus water irrigators do exist; however, research does not conclusively support the use of either technique as more effective and, therefore, the choice is largely one of clinician preference.[11] Some clinicians prefer open- or closed-loop water irrigators and have excellent success using these techniques with children. Children who enjoy water play sometimes find the sensation of water in the ear pleasing or soothing. Air caloric irrigation also has its advantages when testing children. For example, when needed, air stimulation can be rapidly ceased by simply moving the irrigator away from the ear canal, whereas (closed-loop) water systems typically require a momentary wait for balloon deflation prior to removal from the ear canal. This added time, although only a few seconds, can be highly stressful for a child who has already lost composure and is crying or upset. Open-loop water irrigators can also be problematic if a child moves suddenly and may result in accidentally wetting the patient if the head is jerked quickly away from the irrigator. Another advantage of air irrigators is that unlike open-loop water irrigators, they are not contraindicated in the presence of pressure-equalizing (PE) tubes, which are more common in the pediatric population. A variety of factors should be considered and the choice of irrigator should be made based on clinician experience and preference.

Directions for Caloric Testing

Caloric testing is not usually tolerated by children less than 5 years of age; however, precocious 4-year-olds may sometimes be successfully tested. Motivators such as allowing the child to select one prize from the prize box for each irrigation completed can be helpful. Before caloric testing, it is important to prepare the child with an accurate, nonthreatening description of what to expect. Allowing a child to feel the air from the irrigator on the hand and describing the air as "cool and breezy" or as "warm and windy" can reduce apprehension. When using water, you may allow the child to feel the warm/cool tubing "hose" of water before the irrigation. A sample narrative of directions for pediatric caloric testing follows (Video 5–8):

> *I'm going to blow a little cool breeze into your ear. It might sound a little bit noisy, but it won't hurt. The air will only be in your ear for exactly 60 seconds. You can help me count to 60 if you like. Afterward, you might start to feel a little bit like you're spinning or floating and that will only last a minute, too. If you do feel a little "floaty" that's good because it means that your inner ear is working well. I'll be right here next to you the whole time, and you can hold onto me or onto mom's hand if you want to. After we are finished with the air, we are going to play a game. I'll call out letters of the alphabet and you tell me any word you can think of that starts with that letter. During the game, I need you to keep your eyes* (open *for VNG)* (closed *for ENG) for me. Don't worry, I'll keep reminding you, if you forget.*

For younger children, singing familiar songs such as, "Old MacDonald's Farm," "Five Little Monkeys," "The Wheels on the Bus," "Bingo," "The Itsy-Bitsy Spider," or "Twinkle, Twinkle Little Star," can be used for tasking. For older middle and high school age children, tasks such as reviewing their class schedule (ie, your first period teacher/subject/who sits in front, behind, to the left, to the right) are often engaging. When performing ENG it may help to put a soft eye mask, such as a sleeping mask over the child's eyes to remind the child to keep the eyes closed and to prevent fixation. Use of a small night light or lamp with a red light bulb can be used to bring minimal light into the test suite and minimize impact of light changes on calibration of eye movements.

Despite best efforts to alleviate fears (Table 5–4), some children will not be able to tolerate a full battery of caloric testing or to tolerate any at all. Although not ideal, in some instances, it may be necessary to attempt only 2 caloric irrigations, and in those cases, research suggests that warm calorics may in general provide slightly higher sensitivity and specificity than cool calorics.[12,13] Reducing the irrigation time to 40/45/50 seconds may also assist in maintaining compliance during calorics and if applied, times must be held constant for all irrigations.[14] The use of age- and

Table 5–4. VNG/ENG Adaptations

Perform monothermal warm irrigations when necessary.
Reduce irrigation time, if needed.
Award a prize for each irrigation completed.
Make tasking fun and gear it to the child's interests.

clinic-specific norms for evaluating responses is also vital. The caloric subtest of the VNG/ENG battery is often performed last. Upon completion of the VNG/ENG test battery, the child should be required to rest briefly before leaving the exam table and should be monitored for gait stability to prevent falls. A light snack may be offered by the parents if desired.

Conclusions

For children with vestibular and balance complaints, the primary goal of VNG/ENG assessment is to provide information to assist in achieving an accurate differential diagnosis. The underlying etiology of the vestibular problems will often dictate specific treatments from a variety of available options; therefore, an accurate diagnosis is prerequisite to applying timely and appropriate intervention. At times, the goals of testing may be to simply assist in treatment planning, for example, when performing VNG/ENG on children being considered for cochlear implantation, the diagnosis of a unilateral vestibular weakness may support selection of the weaker side for implantation in order to reduce the possibility of bilateral vestibular weakness. Ultimately, the overriding goal of testing is to help the child to avoid, overcome, or minimize any limitations imposed by pathology and to maximize the child's ability to participate fully in activities of daily living.

Acknowledgments. Many thanks to Miss Sophia Szymkowski, and to Master Ryan and Miss Sarah Cox for kindly agreeing to serve as subjects for videotaping. Much appreciation goes to Drs. Stacy Szymkowski, AuD, CCC-A, and Dr. Annemarie Cox for kindly allowing and assisting with videotaping. Sincere thanks also go to Dr. Annemarie Cox, AuD, CCC-A, and Dr. Robert O'Reilly for reading the initial manuscript and providing valuable remarks. To Dr. James Reilly, thank you for your invaluable assistance and for doing "whatever it takes." Finally, thanks also to Jessica Godovin, MS, for her assistance with videography.

Self-Assessment Questions

1. All peripheral vestibular pathology may be detected by VNG/ENG.
   a. True
   b. False

2. When performing positional subtests of the VNG test battery, if eye movement recordings without fixation show no evidence of abnormality, testing with fixation is not necessary.
   a. True
   b. False

3. Monothermal caloric testing is a preferred method when testing children due to advantages of reduced patient discomfort and decreased test time.
   a. True
   b. False

4. The following test adaptations are useful with children:
   a. Examination table with side rails
   b. Rewards for completing subtests
   c. Extra examination time to allow for breaks when needed
   d. Use of interesting child-friendly targets for ocular motor testing
   e. All of the above

5. A physical examination of eye movements should be performed before initiating VNG/ENG testing.
   a. True
   b. False

6. Prior to VNG/ENG testing, a bedside exam of eye movements should be performed and should include:
   a. Check of gross eye movements in an H pattern, 30° left, right, up, and down
   b. Tests of vergence
   c. Saccade and smooth pursuit testing
   d. All of the above

7. Calibration of eye movements must be repeated if a child removes the infrared goggles during testing or if goggles are removed during a break in testing.
   a. True
   b. False

8. Tasking is unnecessary during tests performed without fixation.
   a. True
   b. False

9. Oculomotor test results can be impacted by:
   a. Central vestibular pathology
   b. Patient effort and attention
   c. Medications
   d. All of the above

10. A thorough case history and diagnostic audiological testing are important prerequisites to any vestibular testing.
   a. True
   b. False

References

1. Iwasaki S, Egami N, Fujimoto C, et al. The mitochondrial A3243G mutation involves the peripheral vestibule as well as the cochlea. *Laryngoscope*, 2011;121(8):1821–1824.
2. Rine RM, Management of the pediatric patient with vestibular hypofunction. In: Wolf SL, Herdman SJ, eds. *Vestibular Rehabilitation*, 3rd ed. Philadelphia, PA: F. A. Davis; 2000:360–375.
3. Yarbus AL. *Eye Movements and Vision*, New York, NY: Plenum Press; 1967. Haigh B, Translator, Riggs L. Translation ed. Original Russian text published by Nauka Press, Moscow, 1965.
4. Cyr DG, Harker LA. Vestibular function tests. In: Cummings C, Fredrickson J, Harker LA, et al., eds: *Otolaryngology: Head and Neck Surgery*. St Louis, MO: Mosby, 1993.
5. Mulch G, Petermann W. Influence of age on results of vestibular function tests. Review of literature and presentation of caloric test results. *Ann Otol Rhinol Laryngol Suppl.* 1979;88:1–17.
6. Baloh RW, Hornrubia V. *Clinical Neurophysiology of the Vestibular System.* New York, NY: Oxford University Press; 2001.
7. McCaslin DL, Dundas JA, Jacobson GP. The bedside assessment of the vestibular system. In Jacobson GP, Shephard NT, eds. *Balance Function Assessment and Management.* San Diego, CA: Plural Publishing; 2008:63–97.
8. Nandi R, Luxon LM. Development and assessment of the vestibular system. *Int J Audiol.* 2008;48:566–577.
9. Brodsky JR, Lipson S, Wilber J, Zhou G. Benign paroxysmal positional vertigo (BPPV) in children and adolescents: clinical features and response to therapy in 110 pediatric patients. *Otol Neurotol.* 2018;39(3):344–350.
10. Roberts RA, Gans RE. Background, technique, interpretation, and usefulness of positional/positioning testing. In: Jacobson GP, Shephard NT, eds. *Balance Function Assessment and Management.* San Diego, CA: Plural Publishing; 2008:171–196.
11. Zapala DA, Olsholt KF, Lundy LB. A comparison of water and air caloric responses and their ability to distinguish between patients with normal and impaired ears. *Ear Hear.* 2008;29(4):585–600.
12. Murnane OD, Akin FW, Lynn SG, Cyr DG. Monothermal caloric screening test performance: A relative operating characteristic curve analysis. *Ear Hear.* 2009;30(3):313–319.
13. Keith RW, Pensak ML, Katbamna B. Prediction of bithermal caloric response from monothermal stimulation. *Otolaryngol Head Neck Surg.* 1991;104 (4):499–502.
14. Fife TD, Tusa RJ, Furman JM, et al. Assessment: Vestibular testing techniques in adults and children: Report of the therapeutics and technology assessment subcommittee of the American Academy of Neurology. *Neurology.* 2000;55:1431–1441.

APPENDIX 5–1

Sample Case History

Following is a sample case history for pediatric patients:

A. I. duPont Hospital for Children

Audiology Division—Vestibular Case History

Name: ______________________ MR#: ______________________

Age: ________ Date of Birth: ______________ Today's Date: ______________

1. Main complaints/complications and characterizations:
2. Observations by the parent(s):
3. Patients complaints (ear pain, headaches, tinnitus, fullness, hearing loss, nausea, spinning, lightheadedness):
4. When did it start?
5. Possible participating factors (head trauma, new meds, stressors, etc):
6. How long does the problem last? (Seconds, minutes, hours, days, continuous):
7. Frequency (times/day, days, week, month):
8. How does it manifest?
9. Exacerbating or relieving factors?
10. Developmental motor milestones met?
11. Past medical history:
12. Enrolled in other rehabilitation programs?
13. Current medications:

Comments: ____

____

CHAPTER 6

Rotary Chair Testing

James O. Phillips

Introduction: Relative Advantages and Disadvantages of Rotary Chair Testing

Rotary chair testing has been an important diagnostic tool for vestibular assessment since the turn of the 20th century when Robert Barany pioneered the application of both rotational testing and caloric testing for the investigation of vestibular function in humans. These are two of the most commonly used testing modalities in the vestibular laboratory today. The relative advantages and disadvantages of rotary chair testing can best be understood through a comparison of it with Barany's caloric test, and with a modern test of vestibular function called the video head impulse test (vHIT).

Perhaps one of the best ways to compare rotary chair testing with caloric testing and vHIT in children is to examine the sensitivity and specificity of each test using another test as a reference. Children with hearing loss and potential vestibulopathy have been examined with batteries of these assessment tools, allowing such an analysis to be performed.[1] Compared to caloric tests, rotary chair tests have a sensitivity of 80% to 61%, and a specificity of 80% to 21% in determining loss of vestibular function.[2–5] Compared to rotary chair testing, lateral canal vHIT has been shown in a single study to have a sensitivity and specificity of 100%.[6] It is tempting to conclude, therefore, that caloric testing is superior to the other forms of testing, and that vHIT and rotary chair are lesser tests but equivalent. This conclusion would be incorrect. These results simply show that there are differences in the findings of such tests when evaluating children with potential vestibular dysfunction. Each test has significant limitations and advantages, as later discussed.

For adult testing, the caloric test was for many years the gold standard for the assessment of vestibular function. It has several advantages for the diagnosis of most common forms of unilateral peripheral vestibular loss. The caloric test requires simple and relatively inexpensive equipment. It is easy to perform. It assesses a simple reflex behavior, the angular vestibulo-ocular reflex (aVOR), which is easy to quantify and, in its simplest incarnation, involves only three neurons from input to out put. This means that the complications of central processing of peripheral inputs to produce the dependent measure of eye movement are reduced but not eliminated. Caloric testing can be used to assess each ear independently. Most importantly, there is a very robust set of normative data on which to base a diagnosis, and clinicians are widely knowledgeable about the interpretation of such tests.

vHIT is a relatively new alternative to traditional caloric testing. It is a modern laboratory implementation of a well-established clinical tool called the head thrust test, which was developed and popularized by Michael Halmagyi, Ian Curthoys, and colleagues. vHIT shares many of the same advantages of caloric testing. First, it is simple, and the equipment required today is relatively inexpensive. It is conceptually straightforward. It too assesses the VOR. It can do so in multiple canal planes, although assessment of the vertical canals is challenging and generally less reliable. It can be used as a unilateral test of function, since it relies heavily on excitatory responses from the vestibular end organ and therefore can differentiate between the functions of coplanar semicircular canals in opposite ears by the direction of the head thrust that is applied.

Unfortunately, these tests also have several weaknesses. First, each test primarily assesses vestibular function across a small portion of the vestibular system's dynamic frequency range. Caloric testing is focused on the lower-frequency responses due to the slow transmission of a thermal stimulus and its conversion into the adequate stimulus for activation of hair cells in the lateral semicircular canal. vHIT relies on a high acceleration head impulse and cannot be performed primarily at low or intermediate frequencies. Since different afferent populations have different frequency response characteristics, each test emphasizes only part of normal vestibular afferent sensation.

In standard assessment protocols, the caloric test assesses only the activity of one of the five vestibular end organs of the inner ear. This is not a limitation of vHIT. While the caloric test is easy to perform, it is not always easy to get reliable results. Small external ear canals, middle and inner ear structural abnormalities, otitis media, tympanic membrane perforation, or pressure equalization tubes are among the issues that can compromise or invalidate assessment with this tool. Determination of bilateral vestibular hypofunction is notoriously difficult with the caloric test, and assessment of central compensation to a vestibular insult is virtually impossible. Reliable responses are also difficult to obtain with vHIT. Any slippage of the recording mask produces artifact that is difficult to disambiguate from the high-velocity eye movement that is elicited transiently by the impulsive head movement. Neck stiffness, inattention, and inconsistent fixation behavior all compromise the reliability of vHIT. Similar to caloric assessment, vHIT is currently primarily a tool to assess peripheral vestibular function.

More importantly, the caloric test is aphysiologic. It provides the healthy vestibular system with an isolated unilateral change in input that it never processes during normal behavior. While vHIT measures the function of the vestibular system under physiologic conditions, it does so with a trunk fixed head rotation. Since neck afferents provide a robust input to secondary vestibular neurons, and can contribute heavily to the modulation of VOR interneurons in the face of compensated vestibular loss, the interpretation of this test is potentially clouded by convergent neck afferent input during the head thrust. Therefore, neither test provides an evaluation of the physiological response of the vestibular end organ in isolation.

Finally, and most critically for the assessment of pediatric function, the caloric test and vHIT are often poorly tolerated by many patients, especially young children. This means that there is limited normative data available for pediatric testing, and the tests can be quite challenging in this patient population. Fluid calorics provide a strong aversive stimulus that must be maintained for many seconds while the patient remains motionless. Air calorics produce more variable results and are very loud for young patients with intact hearing. vHIT demands consistent fixation of a point target by a young child wearing a tightly fitting mask during manual head thrusts by the clinician. Such movements must be rapid, consistent, and precisely aligned with the tested canal planes. These techniques can and do produce valuable results in pediatric testing, but they require patience and often repeat evaluation, and they must be interpreted in the context of their limitations.

Rotary chair assessment overcomes many of the weaknesses of caloric testing and vHIT. Because it is very well tolerated in children, many clinicians have considered it to be the gold standard for pediatric vestibular assessment.[7] The testing can be performed successfully using either sophisticated servo-controlled motorized chairs, or manual rotation. It is easy to perform and can be complemented with direct clinical rotational assessments such as the Halmagyi head thrust test. It assesses the same simple reflex behavior as the caloric test and vHIT (aVOR) but does so with a physiologically relevant stimulus that spans much or all of the dynamic frequency range of the vestibular system, depending on the protocol that is used. Because it uses a stimulus that is comparable to the natural rotation that the vestibular system senses in normal activity, rotational testing can be used to assess compensation and central adaptive change of vestibular function in response to peripheral vestibular dysfunction. It has been the consensus test for the assessment of bilateral vestibular hypofunction in adults and children.[7] For adult testing, there is a large set of normative data to rely on in the determination of clinical abnormalities, and for pediatric testing there is a small but growing set of normative data that generally suggest the pediatric responses are similar to those of adults, and perhaps even more robust in infants and very young children.[8–26] The validity of rotary chair testing is unaffected by inner and middle ear structural abnormalities and disease, and small external ear canals, because it does not rely on these structures to transmit the test stimulus. Unlike vHIT, rotary chair testing does not require a volitional behavior from the patient; however, the patient must be either head restrained, or the head must be monitored, to ensure that there is a consistent relationship between the rotation of the chair and the rotational stimulus that is applied to the vestibular end organs in the head. The rotary chair test directly assesses the function of the inner ear when it processes rotational or linear acceleration stimuli, which are adequate stimuli for the natural response.

The standard rotary chair is constructed to produce vertical axis rotation, which can be used to directly assess horizontal (lateral) semicircular canal function; however, many chairs also have the capability of performing off-vertical axis rotation (OVAR) and unilateral centrifugation, which can be used to assess specifically the function of the otolith organs. In addition, simple head motion in association with rotational testing can be used to assess both otolith organ and cerebellar function with a rotary chair. Many devices also accommodate visual stimulus projection, so that the rotary chair and enclosure can perform the oculomotor subtests of basic vestibular assessment. Some devices can even accommodate performance of the positional and positioning subtests of basic vestibular testing as well.

Rotary chairs also have significant limitations, which are important to consider. For example, these devices can be very costly and often require a large amount of space. Unlike the vHIT, the rotations of a standard rotary chair are restricted to a single horizontal canal plane. The physiological stimulus that they deliver is delivered to both ears simultaneously, so that pure stimulation of a single ear is not possible. The chairs are designed to deliver a very pure rotational stimulus, but at higher intermediate frequencies of 0.32 to 1 Hz, there are additional stimuli, such as tactile and kinesthetic cues, from which an eye movement response not dependent on VOR can be generated, compromising the test at those frequencies. In young patients, good head stabilization may be difficult to achieve for the sustained periods of time required for data collection. Alertness can affect the angular VOR response, and young children may fall asleep in the dark and quiet environment typical of the rotary chair enclosure. Conversely, older children may find the small, darkened environment of the enclosure stressful and anxiety provoking. Finally, clinicians generally have less exposure to the results and interpretation of rotary chair testing than to those of caloric tests, which makes adoption of this tool problematic in an external, referral-based practice.

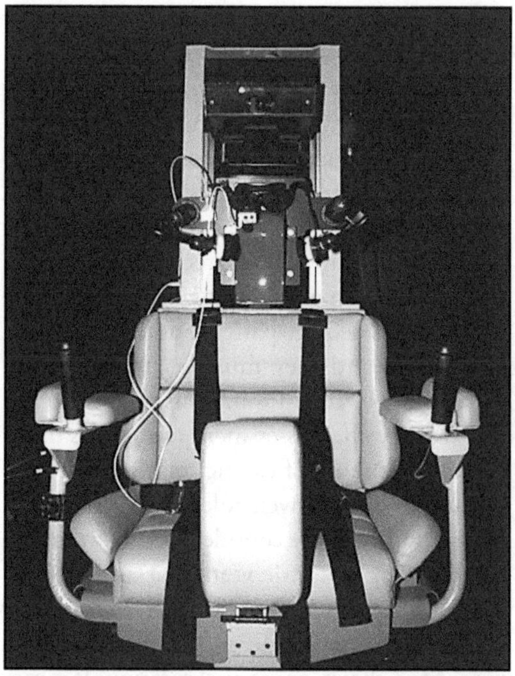

Figure 6–1. A typical vertical axis rotary chair inside a light tight enclosure configured for testing of a 10-year-old child. This direct drive chair (Neurokinetics) is capable of high accelerations and velocities and is equipped with a laser projection system, optokinetic drum, manual anterior-posterior translation, and motorized lateral translation for unilateral centrifugation. Three-dimensional binocular videonystagmography (VNG) and electronystagmography (ENG) are utilized for eye position monitoring. In addition, the device has a positionable head restraint for high acceleration and velocity stimulation.

Rotary Chair Testing Equipment

There are many types of rotary chairs that are currently available for clinical testing. Several manufacturers make clinical devices that differ in the range of frequencies that they can deliver, the type of drive system that they employ, the type of head restraint that they utilize, the axes of rotation about which the patient can rotate, and the total load that they can accommodate. The typical rotary chair is a vertical-axis rotator with a chair located at a single position above the rotational axis as shown in Figure 6–1. Some laboratories have adapted chairs to hold child and infant car seats with padded head restraints, while others simply have a parent or technician hold the child facing forward in their lap or in a soft infant carrier on their chest.[27,28] The mode of restraint is a critical variable in the performance of rotary testing because most rotary chair systems do not monitor the actual position or velocity of the child's head. While manual stabilization is widely used, the ability to deliver consistent high-frequency rotational stimuli with this method is limited. Some laboratories utilize independent monitoring of head position for rotational testing to overcome this limitation. The position of the head and body is typically optimized for lateral canal stimulation using en bloc yaw rotation about a vertical axis at the midline of the interaural axis. The main reason for this is that such yaw rotation is easily achieved with relatively low inertia, whereas pitch and roll en bloc rotation require generating large torques to move the mass of the body off axis.

There are many modifications of the standard rotary chair to achieve specialized testing goals. For example, if the pediatric patient is to be seated with a parent or technician, the chair may be able to be translated to allow the axis of rotation to pass through the patient in this seating arrangement. In addition, chairs from multiple manufacturers allow for controlled chair displacement laterally to accommodate unilateral centrifugation testing of the utricular end organ. Also, many chairs are capable of changing the rotation axis from an earth vertical orientation to an off-vertical orientation to allow for assessment of otolith organ function using OVAR. Some devices, such as the Epley Omniax or the manually operated Thomas Richard-Vitton (TRV) chair, which are displayed in Figure 6–2, are uniquely designed to provide multiaxis rotation and static orientation testing. Such testing is very useful in the diagnosis and treatment of complex positional vertigo. Because rotary chairs are large and clinical space utilization is at a premium, many chairs are designed with adjustable backs to allow the chair to be used as an examination chair or for caloric, positional, or positioning tests.

Data Collection for Rotary Chair Testing

The recording of eye position is a key to data collection using the rotary chair. The timing, amplitude, and symmetry of slow-phase eye velocity in response to changing chair velocity are the dependent measures used in most rotary chair tests. In pediatric rotary chair testing, all of the available tools for acquiring reliable eye position in adults can be used, although with age-appropriate modification.

Electronystagmography (ENG) provides a reliable if inexact measure of horizontal eye position in pediatric and adult rotary chair testing. The electrodes are relatively well tolerated in infants and young children, and bitemporal placement of electrodes can be performed in very young infants to obtain a fairly robust signal average of the horizontal position of both eyes. Of course, the conjugacy of eye movements must be clinically assessed in young patients before utilizing bitemporal recordings. ENG must be carefully calibrated in young patients, and this can be challenging. In our laboratory, we use manual placement of a bright red target light and direct observation of the corneal reflection of the target when calibrating the ENG with infants and very young children in a darkened environment.[16] Other laboratories use low-amplitude mid-frequency chair rotation while infants are fixating a large, interesting target in either a darkened or red light illuminated room as a means of calibrating the ENG. This method is based on the assumption that eye and target motion will be equal and opposite under these conditions even with significant vestibular dysfunction. Older children can use a simple adult calibration requiring them to track stepped or ramped point targets. All calibration must be performed after a period of dark adaptation, since the corneoretinal potential is strongly affected by adaptation state. Well-calibrated ENG will provide a horizontal resolution of about a degree over a range of up to about ±40°, with a temporal resolution of 40 Hz. The calibrated accuracy of vertical ENG is very low due to the contamination of the corneoretinal potential by electrical signals associated with movement of the lid. The absolute position accuracy of the ENG is poor even for horizontal eye movements, since the

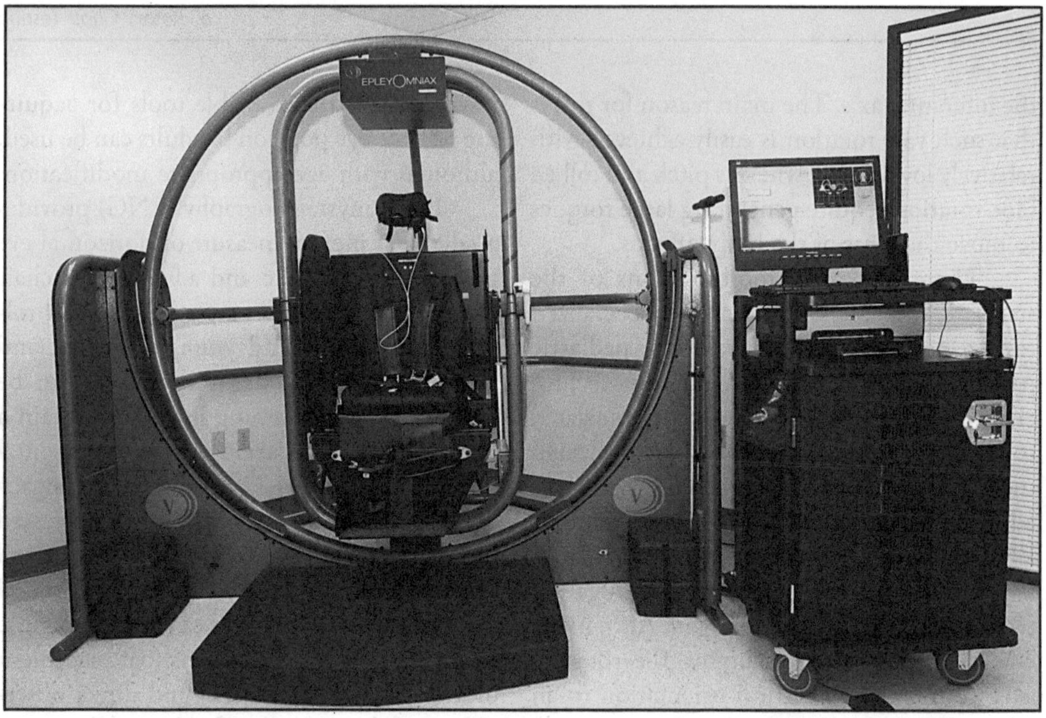

A

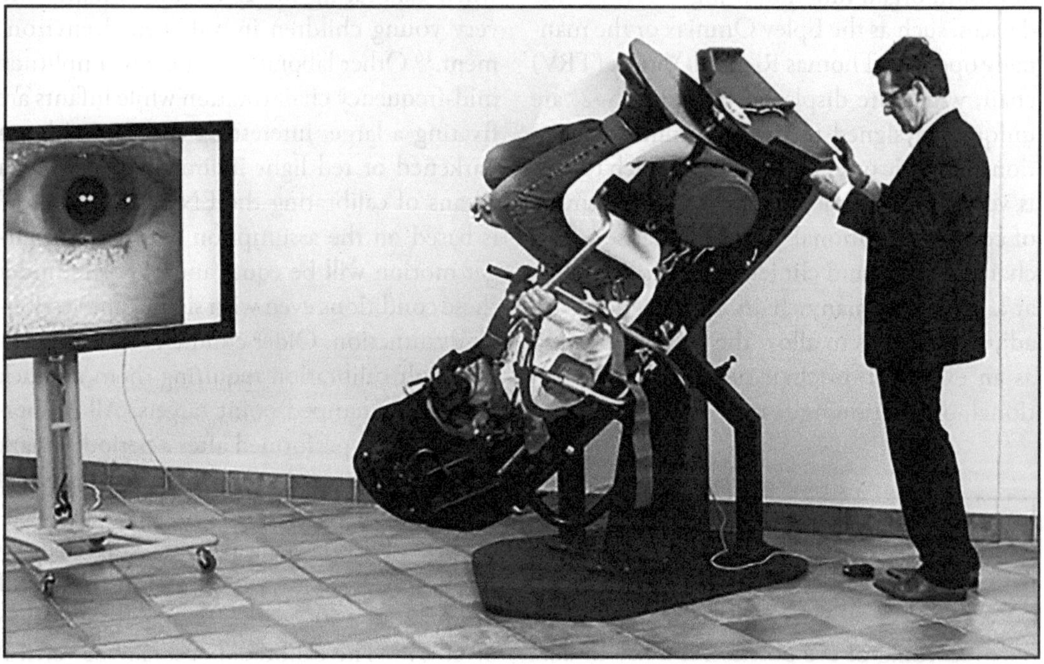

B

Figure 6–2. Two clinical multiaxis rotators. **A.** The Epley Omniax is capable of slow rotation in canal planes and static orientation in multiple positions. **B.** The Thomas Richard-Vitton (TRV) chair is a manually operated device capable of three-dimensional canal plane rotations at higher velocity and impulsive decelerations to static orientation. Both devices use three-dimensional VNG for eye position monitoring.

recorded potentials tend to drift and are noisy due to muscle, 60 Hz, changing impedance, and other artifacts.

In adults, the most commonly used new eye movement monitoring technique is videonystagmography (VNG). VNG relies on the recording of reflected infrared light to track the pupil or limbus of the eye. Various systems are available for the recording of eye position, and each of these has advantages and disadvantages. Depending on the reflections that are tracked, some of these systems are more or less challenged by artifact created by differential motion of the camera and the eye, differential oblique positioning of the camera, transillumination of the iris, dilation of the pupil, drying of the eye, and ptosis, to name a few. The standard clinical VNG has resolution of about 0.25° to 0.5°, and calibrated absolute position accuracy of less than 1°. Modern clinical VNG systems have a relatively high sampling rate of ≥100 Hz. VNG requires calibration, and this can be tricky in children, although the techniques described earlier for ENG can be used successfully here. In addition, camera systems with fixed geometry can employ a geometric calibration by making assumptions about the size and location of the eye relative to the camera, although the accuracy of this calibration is reduced. Some VNG systems are capable of limited three-dimensional eye position recording, by tracking fiducial marks on the iris to acquire torsional records. However, two-dimensional eye position recording is adequate for most clinical assessments. In addition, binocular recording is an option for most systems. In adults, the most common VNG camera configuration is a mask or goggle. Most manufacturers do not make a pediatric goggle currently, but these can be constructed by using children's swim masks with a fitting to house the camera. In addition, a fixed head rest, camera, and IR reflective mirror can be mounted to the chair to obtain stable recordings, or a remote camera can be used if the head is adequately stabilized. The main limitation with all of these approaches except the remote camera is that very young children tolerate objects in contact with the face very poorly. This can limit the duration and accuracy of testing.

A third technique for monitoring eye movements is to use a scleral coil. This technology can be used successfully to record eye movements even in very young infants. The scleral coil consists of several turns of very fine wire embedded in a Silastic annulus that is placed on the eye following application of local anesthetic. This technique, which is used primarily in research applications, produces high-quality recording of eye position in three dimensions, with a resolution of 0.01°, virtually no noise or drift, and a temporal resolution of 500 Hz. The scleral coil can be precalibrated on a gimble, which slightly reduces the accuracy of the recording but greatly simplifies its use in patients. The main limitations to this technology are that the coil is invasive, it requires a skilled clinician to insert it into a child's eye, and it is only practical to use the coil for relatively short recording sessions, typically less than 30 minutes. Furthermore, the coil system itself is bulky, requiring the construction of large driver coils that are either freestanding in the clinic or can be incorporated into an enclosure for the rotary chair as shown in Figure 6–3. Still, the scleral coil is remarkably well tolerated in young infants and older children, who largely forget that the Silastic annulus is present after it has been placed in the eye.

Standard Rotary Chair Test Protocols

The most common tests of pediatric vestibular function using rotary chair involve either sinusoidal rotation of the chair about a vertical

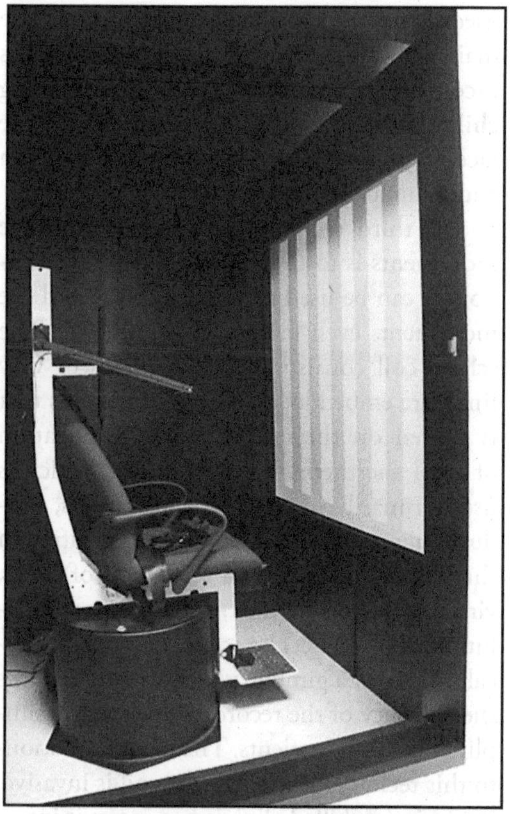

Figure 6–3. A belt-driven servo-controlled rotary chair (Micromedical) located within a light-resistant enclosure with a back projection tangent screen. The enclosure is designed to incorporate 1.83 meter (6-foot) driver coils for a three-dimensional scleral and head coil monitoring system. This high torque device is capable rotating pediatric patients and a parent or technician holder. Scleral coil, two-dimensional binocular VNG, or ENG are used for eye position monitoring.

axis, or rapid acceleration or deceleration of the chair to and from a sustained angular velocity. The resulting eye movements are recorded, as is the movement of the chair, and the status of the stimulated vestibular end organs can be assessed by a quantitative comparison of the slow phase of the recorded eye movements and the recorded chair motion.

Sinusoidal harmonic acceleration (SHA) testing involves sinusoidally accelerating the rotary chair to a standard peak velocity of 50 to 100°/s across several frequencies of rotation from 0.01 to 0.64 Hz or higher.[3,29] Typically, rotations are presented in sets of fixed frequency, with higher frequencies of rotation obtained over a higher number of cycles due to practical time limitations. However, some laboratories have employed pseudorandom rotation across a broad frequency range. In adults, lower frequencies of rotation are associated with disorientation and nausea, but in children these frequencies are well tolerated. The main limitation of SHA is that children need to be stabilized in a dark and unfamiliar environment for long periods of time to complete the test protocol across all tested frequencies. In some laboratories, the use of video games and the presentation of images between sets of chair rotation can be used to increase patient compliance with the protocol. This may require the construction of special enclosures with video projection systems or rear projection screens, see Figure 6–3, which can be used for oculomotor testing with interesting stimuli as well. An alternative in some labs is the use of a dedicated tablet computing device or portable game system to occupy young subjects between trials.

SHA generates three primary measures of vestibular function: gain, phase, and symmetry. These are predicated on sinusoidal fits to the instantaneous eye and chair velocity through several cycles of sinusoidal rotation. Figure 6–4 shows multiple cycles of chair rotation at 0.16 Hz and 60°/s peak velocity, and the eye movements that result in a 9-year-old female patient. The traces in the upper panel represent the eye position recorded during rotation with VNG (see curve) and the gray sections/circles are fast-phase eye movements that are extracted from the record automatically based on velocity and acceleration cri-

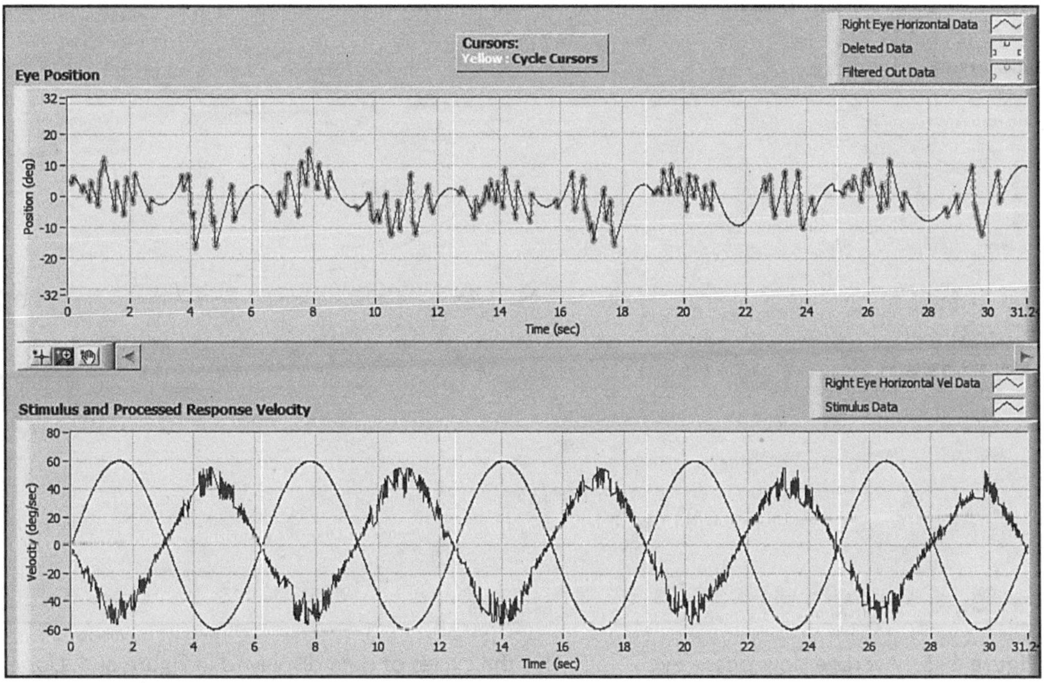

Figure 6–4. Eye position and velocity resulting from 0.16-Hz sinusoidal rotation of a 9-year-old patient with normal caloric function. *Upper panel:* gray line represents horizontal eye position; gray circles indicate fast phases eliminated from the analysis. *Lower panel:* gray trace indicates slow-phase horizontal eye velocity, and black trace indicates horizontal chair velocity. Vertical white lines indicate the beginning and end of each rotation cycle.

teria. The resulting slow-phase eye velocity is displayed as a gray trace in the lower panel, which is superimposed on the velocity of the rotary chair. Figure 6–5 shows the subsequent analysis of the averaged accumulated slow-phase eye velocity. The average eye velocity in the upper panel is superimposed on a calculated sine wave (white line) derived from the data and compared to the average chair rotation to extract gain, phase angle, and symmetry data. The lower panel shows that the calculated sine wave represents virtually all of the power in the response.

The gain of the response is the ratio of the slow-phase eye velocity to the chair velocity. The phase angle of the response is a representation of the timing difference between the eye and chair velocity fits. Typically, the phase difference is shifted by 180° in the report, so that perfectly compensatory eye movement has a phase angle of 0°. The symmetry of the response is the ratio of the rightward and leftward slow-phase eye velocities. Each of these values must be compared to age-appropriate normative data to determine if the patient's response falls within two standard deviations of the mean response for that group. In Figure 6–6, the gain, phase, and symmetry results are shown for the patient whose 0.16 Hz data are displayed in Figures 6–4 and 6–5. The adult norms for the same data ranges are displayed for comparison. It is clear from the data that the response of this child, who had normal caloric responses, is largely comparable

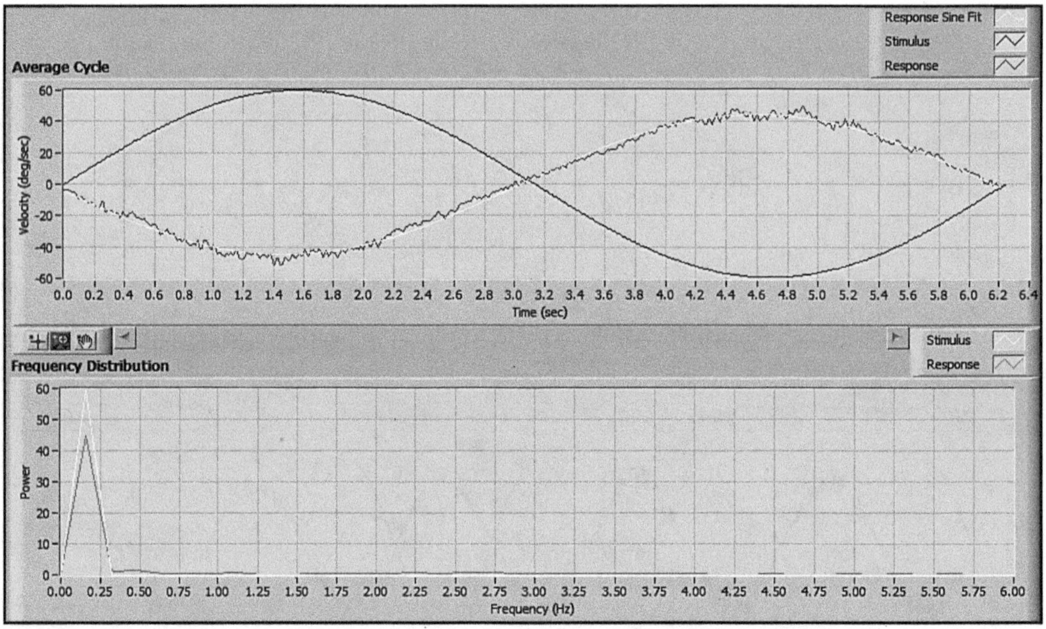

Figure 6–5. Average slow-phase eye velocity for the cycles of data displayed in Figure 6–4. *Upper panel:* Jagged curve represents average horizontal eye velocity; black curve represents the average chair velocity; white curve indicates a sinusoidal fit (by fast Fourier transform [FFT]) to the average horizontal eye velocity. *Lower panel:* Frequency distribution of the power in various harmonics of the FFT, indicating that the fundamental harmonic (0.16 Hz) captures most of the data.

to the response of an adult. The phase of the response at low frequency shows a significant phase lead relative to the adult norms but is borderline normal for this age group.

Most manufacturers provide normative data for adult patients only, and these can be used as a guide for pediatric testing, but to evaluate children most laboratories develop their own set of control data for the unique testing paradigms that they employ. Generally speaking, mean pediatric gains decrease with increasing age, with infants having near unity gain even at lower frequencies of rotation.[9,16] Pediatric gains are also generally higher than adult gains.[9,11–13,16] Practically speaking, this means that consistent below-normal gains across frequency compared to published adult norms are a reliable indication of vestibular hypofunction in a pediatric patient. Low-frequency phase angle in infants and young children is often phase advanced with respect to adult norms, due to the progressive development of velocity storage in children.[23,30] In adults, symmetry during SHA testing is not a strong indication of the presence or absence of a unilateral loss, since the symmetry of the response tends to normalize with compensation following a loss of peripheral function. In young children, the range of normal symmetry values is much greater than in adult patients due to the high variability of the measure across control subjects. Despite this fact, abnormal symmetry compared to pediatric norms is often present long after a unilateral vestibular loss in pediatric patients.

The second widely used test of pediatric vestibular function is the velocity step test. In this test, slow-phase eye velocity resulting

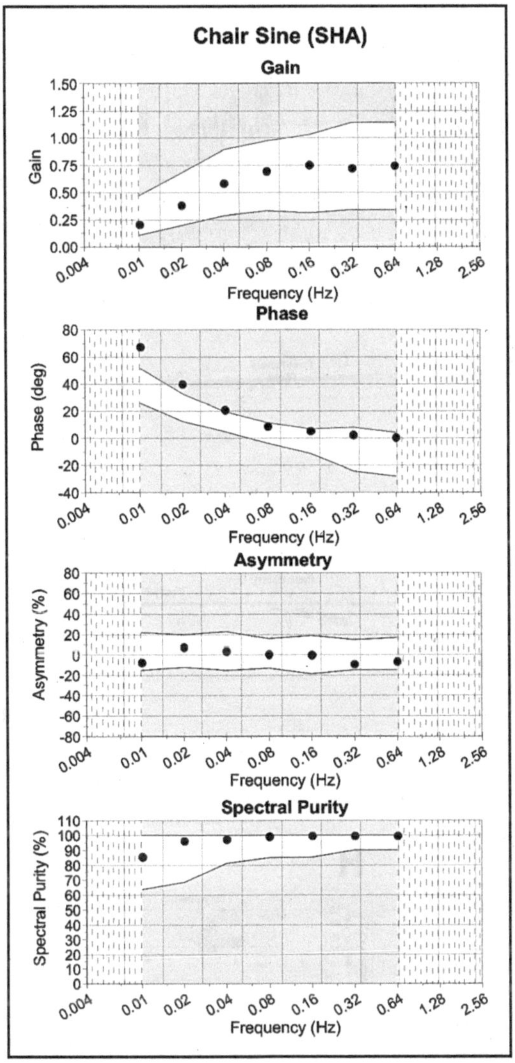

Figure 6–6. Results of SHA rotary chair testing across frequency for the patient whose 0.16 Hz data are displayed in Figures 6–4 and 6–5. Gain, phase, symmetry, and spectral purity are displayed. The dots indicate the response of the patient, and the lines and shading indicate the normal range (*white*) and abnormal range (*gray shading*) of data for adult control subjects performing the same tests. For descriptions of gain, phase, and symmetry, see the text. Spectral purity is an indication of how much of the power of the FFT is captured by the fundamental harmonic at each frequency (ie, how good is the fit on which the other calculations are based).

from symmetric presentations of a rapid acceleration of the chair to a constant rotational velocity, and subsequent deceleration of the chair to rest, is used to assess the state of the vestibular end organ and the central processing of vestibular information. The test produces three primary measures of vestibular function: gain, time constant, and symmetry. The gain of the response is the ratio of the slow-phase velocity of the fastest, typically the first, beat of nystagmus in response to the rapid step in chair velocity, to the amplitude of the velocity step (ie, the change in velocity of the step). Although a pure velocity step is not possible, relatively high acceleration velocity trapezoids are typically used. However, some laboratories use low-acceleration trapezoids in a reduced protocol for pediatric testing presumably because they are well tolerated and can be delivered reliably.[31] The time constant of the response is the time constant of a single exponential decay function that is fit to the slowly decaying eye velocity that results from this stimulus. The symmetry of the response is the ratio of the rightward and leftward peak slow-phase eye velocity in response to symmetric steps of velocity in each direction. Figure 6–7 displays the velocity step responses of the young patient whose data are displayed in Figure 6–6. Figure 6–7A displays the eye position traces that result from repeated presentation of 100°/s steps: right, left, left, right at 45-second intervals. The slow-phase velocity extracted from those position traces is displayed in Figure 6–7 B–E, with the sequence of steps being B, C, D, E. From those slow-phase velocity values, the gain, time constant, and symmetry values are calculated. The exponential fits are displayed as light gray lines in Figure 6–7 B–E, and the calculated values for peak slow-phase eye velocity, time constant, and symmetry are displayed in Figure 6–7 F–H. The adult norms for this test are displayed for comparison.

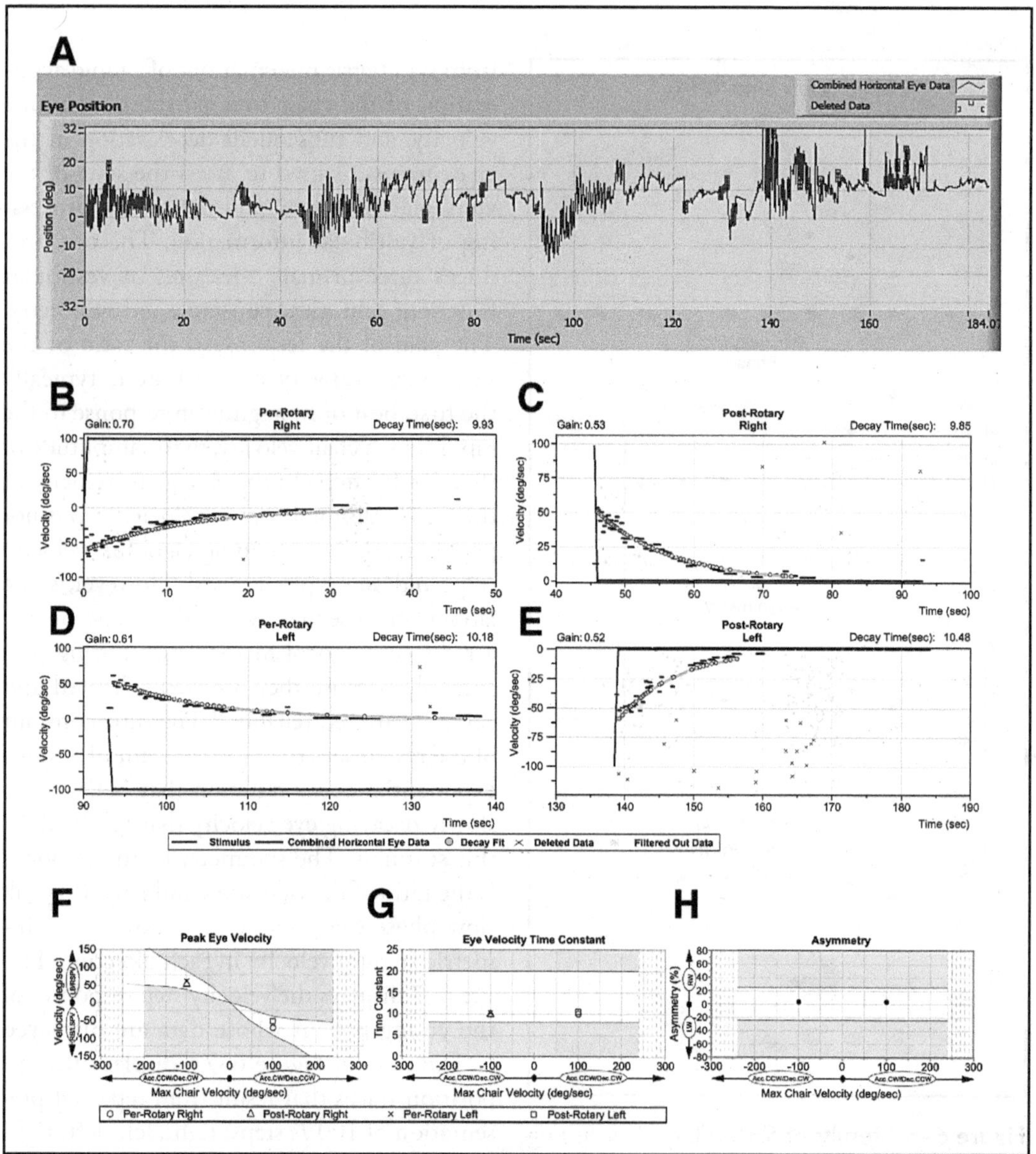

Figure 6–7. Results of velocity step testing for the patient whose SHA test data are displayed in Figure 6–6. *Panel A:* Jagged trace indicates horizontal eye velocity resulting from serial velocity steps of 100°/s. Black vertical lines indicate the timing of the steps. Dark gray rectangles that appear at the tips of the signal indicates artifact that was removed from consideration in the analysis. *Panels B, C, D, E:* The velocity of each slow phase (*short black lines*) resulting from a step and an exponential fit to the velocity data (*light gray curve with open circles*) are superimposed on the velocity of the chair (*long black line*). The calculated gain and time constant (decay time) for each step are displayed above each panel. *Panels F, G, H:* The subject data are displayed using open shapes (F, G) and solid circles (H), and the lines and shading indicate the normal range (*white*) and abnormal range (*gray shading*) of data for adult control subjects performing the same tests. The direction of the rotation is indicated by the arrows below each panel. Panels F, G, and H display the peak slow-phase horizontal eye velocity, the time constant of the exponential fit, and the gain symmetry of the response, respectively.

Since pediatric patients have a robust response to rapid chair acceleration, this is an effective tool for the evaluation of such patients. The gain of the response is typically high in pediatric patients, and the symmetry, although more variable than that of adults, also provides a reliable measure. Unfortunately, because the neural networks that are responsible for the central storage of velocity information are relatively slow to develop, the time constant is not always an effective measure of vestibular loss in very young infants who have time constants close to the time constant of the normally functioning end organ, ≈6 seconds.[30,32–34] However, in older children, this test can be interpreted in the same manner as with adult patients. Unilateral vestibular loss produces a reduction of the time constant for rotations toward the affected ear, which accompanies a reduction in the gain of the response in the same direction, producing an overall gain asymmetry.

Common Additions to the Standard Protocols

Several modifications of the two basic rotational tests are also frequently used in the assessment of pediatric vestibular function. These tests, which are also widely used in adults, superimpose additional stimuli on the two basic rotational test paradigms to obtain additional data about central or otolith organ function.

In the visually enhanced VOR test, the vestibular test environment is illuminated with a high-contrast large-field stationary visual stimulus, such as a random dot or grating stimulus used with optokinetic nystagmus testing. The stimulus remains stationary while the chair is rotated sinusoidally at relatively high frequency, such as 0.8 Hz. The purpose of this test is to evaluate the visually enhanced VOR. In children and adults, this test should produce a symmetric response with a gain approaching 1.0, and a phase of 0.0. Low gain responses indicate vestibular hypofunction, whereas gains above 1.0 are associated with central vestibular dysfunction (eg, cerebellar lesions).

The fixation suppression test is performed with a similar combination of rotational and visual stimuli. This test is performed in adults with a fixation spot that moves with the subject as the chair rotates at a moderate frequency, such as 0.5 Hz. Since smooth pursuit is not fully mature in young children, and they are unlikely to follow verbal instructions to track visual targets, the pediatric version of this test is performed with combined point and optokinetic stimuli, producing a naturally stable visual environment that rotates with the chair. The purpose of this test is to evaluate the ability of the brain to suppress the VOR in a context-appropriate manner. While this test is not appropriate for infants, who naturally lack both high gain smooth pursuit and the ability to suppress the VOR, the test produces a significant reduction in VOR gain in older children and adults (ie, reduction to a gain below 0.20).

Finally, in the canal and otolith organ interaction test, patients are rotated to a constant velocity for at least 45 seconds, and then the chair is rapidly decelerated to rest. This would ordinarily evoke a robust post-rotary nystagmus that would decay relatively slowly in children and adults. However, when the deceleration of the chair is followed with a quick pitch down rotation of the head, the resulting nystagmus is cut short. This phenomenon is called dumping of stored velocity, and it reflects both the function of the vestibulocerebellum and input from the otolith organs. Therefore, it is a quick and easy evaluation of both peripheral and central processes and can be performed with older children. The resulting tumbling sensation is relatively brief and not aversive to most pediatric patients.

Evaluations Requiring Specialized Rotary Chairs

There are many modifications to the test protocols described above, and most of these do not require significant modifications to the rotational chair. However, there are a few important tests that demand chairs with specialized capabilities such as a tilting rotation axis, lateral displacement of the rotation axis, or multiple rotation axes. These tests extend the capability of rotary chair testing to the evaluation of otolith organ function and the function of multiple semicircular canals.

Assessment of otolith organ function can be accomplished with the use of a chair that rotates the patient about a nonvertical or tipped rotation axis. This test, which is called off-vertical axis rotation (OVAR), testing, stimulates the otolith organs by using constant velocity yaw rotation about an axis that is tilted off of earth vertical.[15] A sinusoidal yaw oscillation about a tipped axis is also used in adult clinical testing, but this has not been applied to pediatric testing. For clinical testing, the tilt of the axis is typically 10° to 14°, since patients poorly tolerate greater tilt angles. The observed eye movement response is primarily produced by the constantly changing gravito-inertial vector resulting from the tilted yaw rotation and transduced by the otolith organs. The resulting eye movements have both a steady-state slow-phase eye velocity that is directed opposite to the direction of yaw rotation, known as the bias component, and oscillations in eye position and velocity in all directions of eye movements, known as the modulation component. This test is very sensitive to loss of otolith function and will report changes in the central storage of vestibular velocity information. The test has been used regularly in young pediatric patients, employing a tilt angle of 14° and a constant velocity rotation of 60°/s.

Another assessment of otolith organ function is the unilateral centrifugation test. This test, which primarily evaluates the function of the utricle, requires a rotary chair with a laterally positionable seat. In some versions of this test, the seat is manually positioned before rotation, whereas in other versions, the chair is controlled by a motor that laterally offsets the chair to the right and left after the rotator has reached a constant velocity of rotation, typically 300°/s or higher. The offset of the chair turns the rotator into a centrifuge that activates the utricular end organ on the side to which the chair is displaced. The other utricle is aligned with the rotation axis and is therefore minimally activated. The result of this action is a compelling sensation of roll tilt. In addition, there is a torsional rotation of the eye in response to this fictive tilt stimulus. The eye movements can be recorded directly with three-dimensional eye position measurement, or the patient can attempt to vertically align a projected or positionable line during rotation. This is called subjective visual vertical testing. The absence of an otolith response in the stimulated canal produces a reduction in the observed eye torsion or line tilt. Subjective visual vertical testing can, of course, be performed without chair rotation, with acute loss of utricular function producing a tilted subjective vertical of 2° or more in pediatric subjects. However, compensated chronic loss of utricular function typically produces a restoration of accurate alignment of static subjective vertical. Unilateral centrifugation is well tolerated in older pediatric patients but is not appropriate for younger children. The test requires precise alignment and stabilization of the head of the patient to ensure that the proper positioning of the head occurs during translation of the chair relative to the rotational axis.

Finally, rotational chair testing can be used to align or rotate subjects in multiple axes. A number of institutions have either specially constructed rotators or commercially available systems that allow for controlled rotation in all canal planes and also static alignment of the patient in virtually any orientation. These devices tend to be relatively large, but they have the advantage of being able to test for and treat vestibular dysfunction by performing both multiple canal diagnostic procedures and carefully controlled therapeutic maneuvers such as the canalith-repositioning maneuver.

Summary

Rotary chair testing is performed in many pediatric clinical laboratories and has high value as a diagnostic tool. The devices vary widely as do the various tests that can be performed. The primary utility of rotary chair testing is that it produces robust measures of the function of multiple end organs within the ear, and of the central processing of vestibular signals within the brain. Although this chapter has described many of the most commonly applied pediatric tests and tools available for rotary chair testing, it has omitted the clinical tests of manual head and chair rotation assessment that are performed in the general otology clinic. Such tests contribute to the first line of assessment for abnormal vestibular function and may trigger referral to the vestibular laboratory for extensive testing including the rotary chair tests described here.

Self-Assessment Questions

1. List the advantages of rotary chair testing in children.
2. List the limitations/challenges of rotary chair testing in children.
3. Which rotary chair tests can be used to evaluate the otolith organs (saccule and utricle)?
4. What means can be used to record eye movements during rotary chair testing?
5. What are the three primary measures that are generated using sinusoidal harmonic acceleration?
6. How is the gain of the response calculated?
7. How is the symmetry of the response calculated?
8. What are the three primary measures that are generated using the velocity step test?
9. What caveat is required during the interpretation of the time constants generated during velocity step testing in the pediatric population?

10. What are the features of a unilateral vestibular loss on velocity step testing?

References

1. Verbecque E, Marijnissen T, De Belder N, et al. Vestibular dysfunction in children with sensorineural hearing loss: A systematic review. *Int J Audiol.* 2017;56(6):361–381.
2. Inoue A, Iwasaki S, Ushio M, et al. Effect of vestibular dysfunction on the development of gross motor function in children with profound hearing loss. *Audiol Neurootol.* 2013; 18(3):143–151.
3. Cushing SL, Papsin BC, Rutka JA, James AL, Gordon KA. Evidence of vestibular and balance dysfunction in children with profound sensorineural hearing loss using cochlear implants. *Laryngoscope.* 2008;118(10):1814–1823.
4. Kaga K, Shinjo Y, Jin Y, Takegoshi H. Vestibular failure in children with congenital deafness. *Int J Audiol.* 2008;47:590–599.
5. Shinjo Y, Jin Y, Kaga K. Assessment of vestibular function of infants and children with congenital and acquired deafness using the ice-water caloric test, rotational chair test and vestibular-evoked myogenic potential recording. *Acta Oto-Laryngol.* 2007;127:736–747.
6. Janky K, Givens D. Vestibular, visual acuity, and balance outcomes in children with cochlear implants: A preliminary report. *Ear Hear.* 2015;36,E364–E372.
7. Fife TD, Tusa RJ, Furman JM, et al. Assessment: Vestibular testing techniques in adults and children: Report of the Therapeutics and Technology Assessment Subcommittee of the American Academy of Neurology. *Neurology.* 2000;55(10):1431–1441.
8. Lotfi Y, Rezazadeh N, Moossavi A, et al. Rotational and collic vestibular-evoked myogenic potential testing in normal developing children and children with combined attention deficit/hyperactivity disorder. *Ear Hear.* 2017; 38(6):E352–E358.
9. Chan FM, Galatioto J, Amato M, Kim AH. Normative data for rotational chair stratified by age. *Laryngoscope.* 2015;126(2):460–463.
10. Maes L, De Kegel A, Van Waelvelde H, Dhooge I. Rotatory and collic vestibular evoked myogenic potential testing in normal-hearing and hearing-impaired children. *Ear Hear.* 2014; 35:E21–E32.
11. Casselbrant ML, Mandel EM, Sparto PJ, Perera S. Longitudinal posturography and rotational testing in children 3–9 years of age: Normative data. *Otolaryngol Head Neck Surg.* 2010;142:708–714.
12. Charpiot A, Tringali S, Ionescu E, Vital-Durand F, Ferber-Viart C. Vestibulo-ocular reflex and balance maturation in healthy children aged from six to twelve years. *Audiol Neurootol.* 2010;15:203–210.
13. Valente M. Maturational effects of the vestibular system: A study of rotary chair, computerized dynamic posturography, and vestibular evoked myogenic potentials with children. *J Am Acad Audiol.* 2007;18(6):461–481.
14. Selz PA, Girardi M, Konrad HR, Hughes LF. Vestibular deficits in deaf children. *Otolaryngol Head Neck Surg.* 1996;115:70–77.
15. Wiener-Vacher SR, Toupet F, Narcy P. Canal and otolith vestibulo-ocular reflexes to vertical and off vertical axis rotations in children learning to walk. *Acta Otolaryngol (Stockh).* 1996; 116:657–665.
16. Finocchio DV, Preston KL, Fuchs AF. Infant eye movements: Quantification of the vestibulo-ocular reflex and visual-vestibular interactions. *Vision Res.* 1991;31(10):1717–1730.
17. Goodkin F. The development of mature patterns of head-eye coordination in the human infant. *Early Human Develop.* 1980;4(4): 373–386.
18. Ornitz EM, Kaplan AR, Westlake JR. Development of the vestibulo-ocular reflex from

infancy to adulthood. *Acta Otolaryngol.* 1985; 100(3–4):180–193.
19. Regal DM, Ashmead DH, Salapatek P. The coordination of eye and head movements during early infancy: A selective review. *Behav Brain Research.* 1983;10:125–132.
20. Reisman JE, Anderson JH. Compensatory eye movements during head and body rotation in infants. *Brain Res.* 1989;484:119–129.
21. Staller SJ, Goin DW, Hildebrandt M. Pediatric vestibular evaluation with harmonic acceleration. *Otolaryngol Head Neck Surg.* 1986;95: 471–476.
22. Cyr D, Brookhauser P, Valente M, Grossman A. Vestibular evaluation of infants and preschool children. *Otolaryngol Head Neck Surg.* 1985;93:463–468.
23. Cioni G, Favilla M, Ghelarducci B, LaNoce A. Development of the dynamic characteristics of the horizontal vestibulo-ocular reflex in infancy. *Neuropediatrics.* 1984;15:125–130.
24. Ornitz E, Atwell C, Walter D, Hartmann E, Kaplan A. The maturation of vestibular nystagmus in infancy and childhood. *Acta Otolaryngol.* 1979;88:244–256.
25. Eviatar L, Eviatar A. The normal nystagmic response of infants to caloric and per-rotary stimulation. *Laryngoscope.* 1979;89:1036–1044.
26. Eviatar L, Miranda S, Eviatar A, Freeman K, Borkowski M. Development of nystagmus in response to vestibular stimulation. *Ann Neuro.* 1979;5:508–514.
27. Cyr DG. Vestibular testing in children. *Ann Otol Rhinol Laryngol.* 1980;89(5 pt 2):63–69.
28. Phillips JO, Backous DD. Evaluation of vestibular function in young children. *Otolaryngol Clin North Am.* 2002;35(4):765–790.
29. O'Reilly RC, Greywoode J, Morlet T, et al. Comprehensive vestibular and balance testing in the dizzy pediatric population. *Otolaryngol Head Neck Surg.* 2011;144(2):142–148.
30. Weissman BM, DiScenna AO, Leigh RJ. Maturation of the vestibuloocular reflex in normal infants during the first 2 months of life. *Neurology.* 1989;39:534–538.
31. Wiener-Vacher SR, Mazda K. Asymmetric otolith vestibulo-ocular responses in children with idiopathic scoliosis. *J Pediatr.* 1998; 132(6):1028–1032.
32. Clark DL, Cordero L, Bates J. Development of postrotatory nystagmus time constants. *Acta Otolaryngol.* 1984;98:287–291.
33. Cordero L, Clark DL, Urrutia JG. Post-rotational nystagmus in full term and premature infants. *Int J Pediatr Otorhinolaryngol.* 1983; 5:47–57.
34. Kaga K, Suzuki JI, Marsh R, Tanaka V. Influence of labyrinthine hypoactivity on gross motor development of infants. *Ann NY Acad Sci.* 1981:374:412–420.

CHAPTER 7

Video Head Impulse Testing (vHIT)

Guangwei Zhou, Violette H. Lavender, and Vincent G. Wettstein

Vestibular laboratory testing on pediatric patients can be technically challenging with conventional procedures (eg, caloric and rotary chair test) since they may elicit fear or anxiety in young children.[1,2] In recent years, noninvasive and child-friendly vestibular tests such as vestibular-evoked myogenic potential (VEMP) and video head impulse test (vHIT) have been developed and become valuable tools in the vestibular evaluation of pediatric patients.[3–7] Based on the head impulse/thrust test introduced by Halmagyi and Curthoys, vHIT incorporates a high-speed camera, usually fixed on lightweight video goggles, to measure eye velocity and record corrective saccades in patients with vestibulo-ocular reflex (VOR) impairment.[8–10] Along with quantitative analysis by accompanying computer software, vHIT can precisely calculate the VOR gain of all 6 semicircular canals. Also, vHIT is capable of differentiating between overt and covert saccades, as the latter are difficult to identify with the naked eye. Clinical studies have shown that vHIT is tolerated well among pediatric patients since it does not evoke vertigo or nausea, and the test does not require the child to be confined in a dark enclosed space.[4,5,11–13] Also, the video goggles are relatively comfortable to wear, and the testing can be completed in a short amount of time.

Overview of vHIT Technology and Equipment

The first vHIT system was approved by the U.S. Food and Drug Administration (FDA) in 2013, and many manufacturers have since developed their own version of the product for clinical use. Although differences in design exist among available vHIT systems, the key component of any VHIT system is a high-speed video camera (usually with a minimum of 250 frames per second), which is required to record clear images of a patient's eyes during fast head motion. The software then processes each image to determine the center position of the pupil, calculating the eye velocity and VOR gain. Here, an overview of available vHIT products that can be used for pediatric patients is provided, with a brief discussion.

ICS Impulse

In collaboration with Otometrics, now a division of Natus (Pleasanton, California), a group of Australian researchers developed the first vHIT system based on many years of research.[10,14] The current product features lightweight goggles (weighing about

60 grams) with built-in sensors and calibration lasers. The frame is similar to regular glasses and connects to a laptop computer via a USB cable. The high-speed camera is located on the right side of the frame. Coupled with a face cushion, the goggles can be adjusted to fit the head of most children age 3 or older. Results of vHIT from this well-designed system have been clinically validated against scleral search coils. The software is user friendly, and the interface is easy to navigate. One useful feature in the software is autodetection of eye blinks, which enables exclusion of trials where eye blinks affect the calculation of average VOR gain. Nonetheless, clinicians should pay attention when using this product in small children for a few reasons: (1) The mirror, a thin glass sticking out of the frame, is very fragile, as seen in Figure 7–1. Therefore, patients should be told specifically not to grab or touch it. (2) Slippage may happen when the headband is not properly tightened and secured, especially for girls with straight hair. (3) For children with a smaller head or under the age of 3 years, fitting these goggles can be problematic, and results may be invalid. Other details in using the ICS Impulse system for pediatric patients are discussed further in the section on testing procedures.

Interacoustics EyeSeeCam

The EyeSeeCam vHIT system is another portable product that features lightweight goggles. A high-speed camera is incorporated, as well, which can be snapped on either the left or the right side of the frame, as seen in Figure 7–2. Immediately after collecting data, the software conducts a velocity regression to calculate VOR gain at 40, 60, and 80 milliseconds post-impulse onset and gain asymmetry. Covert and overt saccades can be easily identified in tracings. According to recent studies,[5,15] this system can be used for younger children, including infants; however, some children may feel that the goggles are too tight and less comfortable to wear. Notably, data

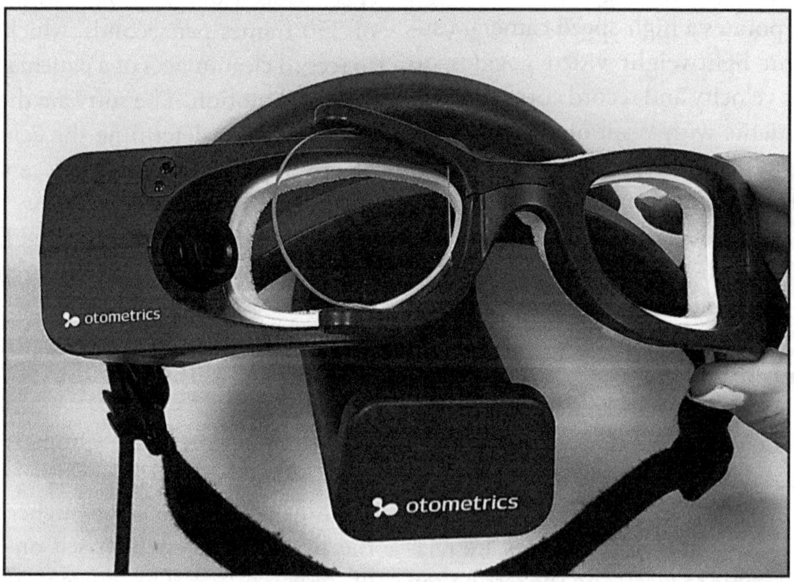

Figure 7–1. ICS Impulse vHIT goggles.

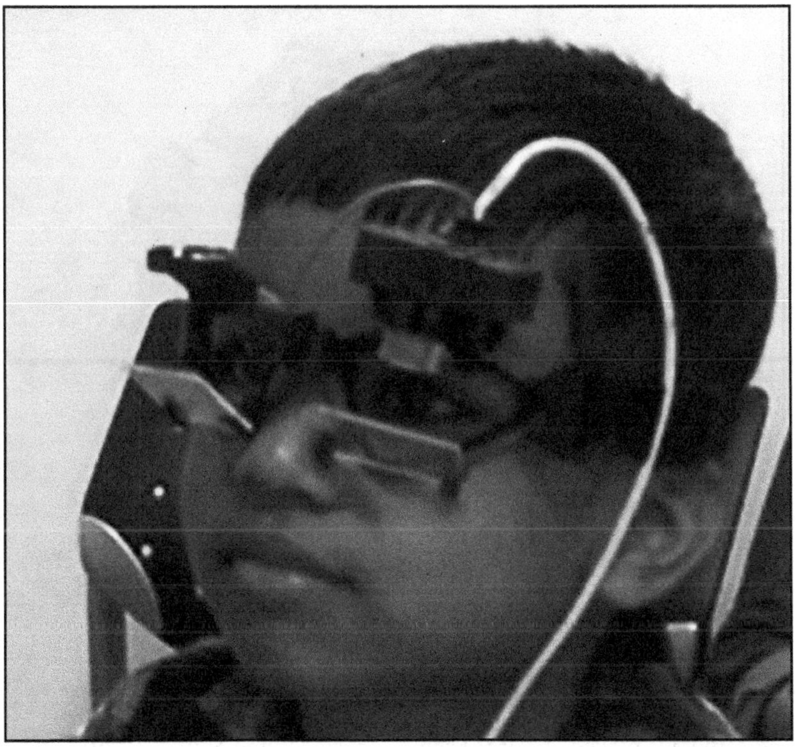

Figure 7–2. Interacoustics EyeSeeCam goggles (Courtesy of Sharon Cushing, MD).

may be contaminated by eye blinks, which can impact the automatic calculation of VOR gain when children are not able to control their eye blinks effectively.

Micromedical vHIT (A Subtest of VORTEQ)

Micromedical Technologies (Chatham, Illinois) employs their VisualEyes binocular high-speed camera in their vHIT product. With two separate cameras tracking eye motions on each side, binocular recording limits errors due to disconjugate eye movements, strabismus, or poor eye tracking, which can occur more often in pediatric patients. Customized criteria can be set in the software, and video playback provides crystal clear images. While this product works well for older children, the goggles are large and heavy (Figure 7–3) and may not fit well on small heads/faces.

Synapsys vHIT Ulmer

In contrast to vHIT systems with a goggle-mounted video camera that requires tight fitting, the Synapsys (Marseilles, France) vHIT Ulmer device records eye and head movements from a remote position with a space-fixed camera in front of the patient.[16] Without goggles or other devices attached to the patient, the examination is tolerated well even by children under the age of 3 years.[17]

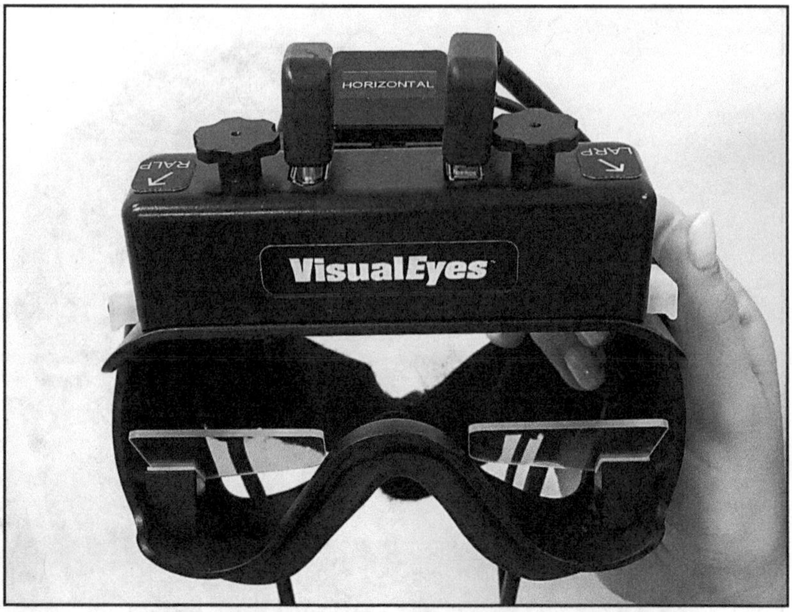

Figure 7–3. Micromedical VisualEyes goggles, with vHIT option.

The recording camera is placed about 90 centimeters in front of the child and a fixation target is positioned about 1 meter farther away. A screen displaying a cartoon can be used to attract the child's attention. The child can sit sideways on the lap of a parent or caregiver, as demonstrated in Figure 7–4.

The software allows flexible shifting between horizontal, LARP (left anterior-right posterior), and RALP (right anterior-left posterior) acquisition within the same session since it automatically detects the plane in which the head impulse is delivered. The system also has unique algorithms that allow elimination of invalid trials before VOR gain calculation and detection of covert and overt saccades. The software interface exhibits VOR gain in the "canalogram," individual vHIT tracings, and head velocity, as seen in Figure 7–5 (an example of normal lateral canal findings from a child of 7 weeks of age).

While this system is commercially available and a good option to conduct valid vHIT for infants, it is not approved yet for clinical use in the United States. Additional pediatric studies on this system may be warranted, as well.

Testing Procedures

To conduct vHIT, the testing room should be well lit to prevent pupil dilation, which can degrade video data collection. Typically, the patient sits in a chair about 3 feet (or 1 m) away from a visual target. The target should contrast with the background, which can be a wall or a screen. The height of the target should be at the patient's eye level. Corrective glasses should be removed from the patient before fitting the vHIT goggles, but contact lenses do not need to be removed. Any eye makeup, especially mascara, must be cleaned off completely because it can interfere with recording the eyes. Here, the testing steps using the ICS Impulse are discussed. A similar approach may be applied to other vHIT systems, as well.

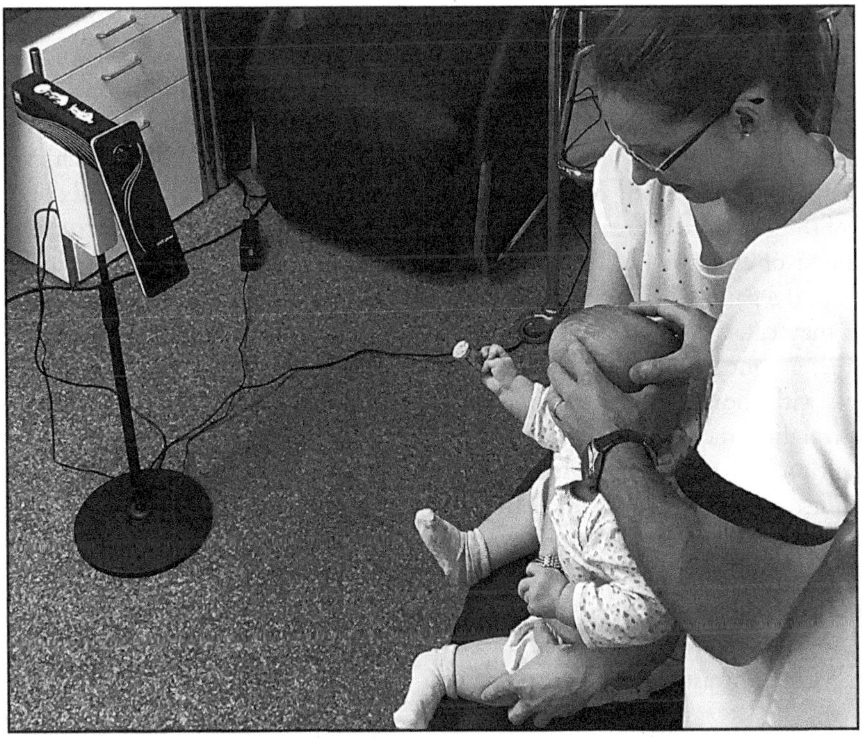

Figure 7–4. The setup of SYNAPSYS vHIT Ulmer system for testing an infant.

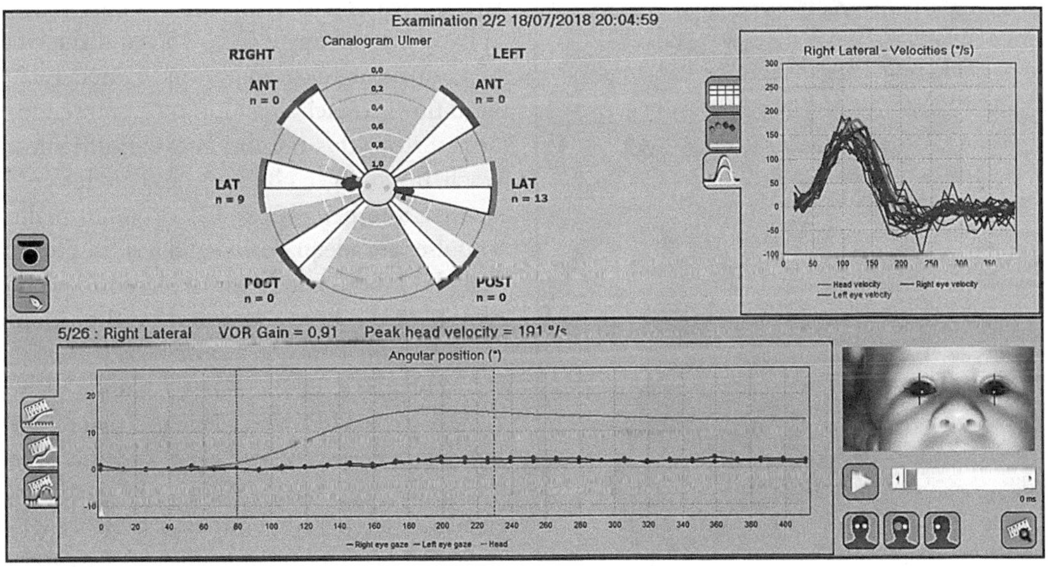

Figure 7–5. The software interface of SYNAPSYS vHIT Ulmer system, which displayed the "canalgram" (*top-left*), vHIT tracings (*top-right*), head velocity (*bottom-left*), and patient's face/eyes (a 7-week-old infant).

Goggle Fitting and Calibration

Proper fitting of vHIT goggles is the first important step to obtain valid results. The head strap on the goggles should be tightly fitted on the patient's head; otherwise, any slippage of the goggles will create errors in the measurement of eye motion. This should be explained to the patient beforehand, since the tightness may cause some discomfort. Most of the time, a tight fit can be easily achieved in patients with short hair. For children with long or straight hair, it is important to pay extra attention to avoid slippage during head motion. Putting the hair in a low ponytail below the strap can be helpful to prevent the strap from sliding down the back of the head during testing (Figure 7–6).

In order to measure eye velocity accurately, a precise contrast threshold setting and *in vivo* calibration are necessary. The software allows for the adjustment of the contrast threshold, so that the image of the pupil becomes a sharp white circle against a black background. Calibration is achieved using a built-in laser that projects a red dot on the wall or screen. The patient is instructed to follow the motion of the laser dot visually until the software acquires enough information about the pupil displacement. Younger children have the tendency to move their head during calibration, so the clinician may have to hold their head gently and ask them to "count the dots" with their eyes. If the calibration process is unsuccessful for any reason or cannot be finished in a short time, then default calibration can be adopted to proceed with testing.

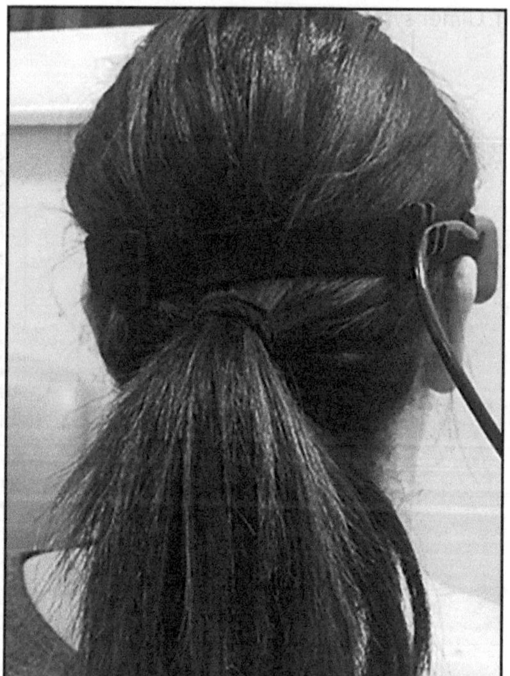

Figure 7–6. Patient's hair in a low ponytail to prevent the strap from sliding down. (Cited from Bachmann, Sipos, Lavender, and Hunter.[11])

Performing vHIT in the Horizontal and Vertical Planes

To conduct vHIT, the clinician stands behind the patient with his or her hands on the patient's head without touching the head strap. The clinician turns the head unpredictably by a small angle (eg, ~15°) and the stop of head turns must be abrupt. Generally, 20 head turns to each direction is recommended; nonetheless, this number may be difficult to reach in younger children, and therefore, a smaller number (10 to 12) of good-quality impulses are adequate for valid results. For lateral vHIT, both hands can be placed above the temple of the head to control head motions, see a demonstration in Figure 7–7.

For vHIT in the vertical planes, either LARP or RALP, the clinician places one hand on the top of the head and the other one under the chin, as shown in Figure 7–8. Before delivering head impulses in the vertical planes, the patient turns the head 30° to 40° to one side (ie, to the right for LARP and to the left for RALP) while keeping his or her eyes on the target.

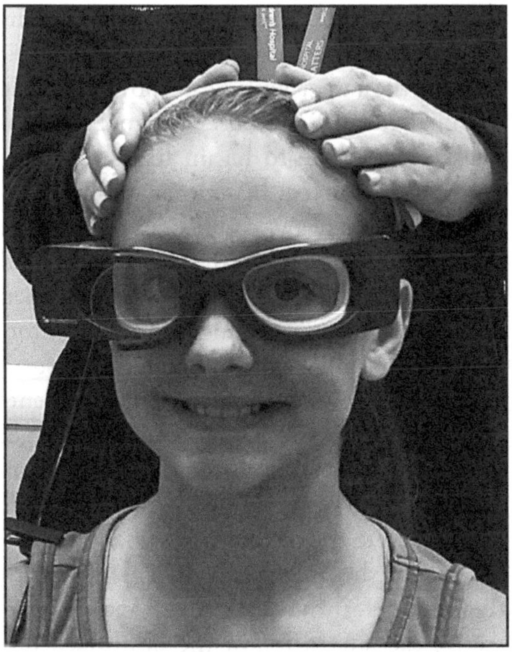

Figure 7–7. Examiner's hands position for lateral canal vHIT.

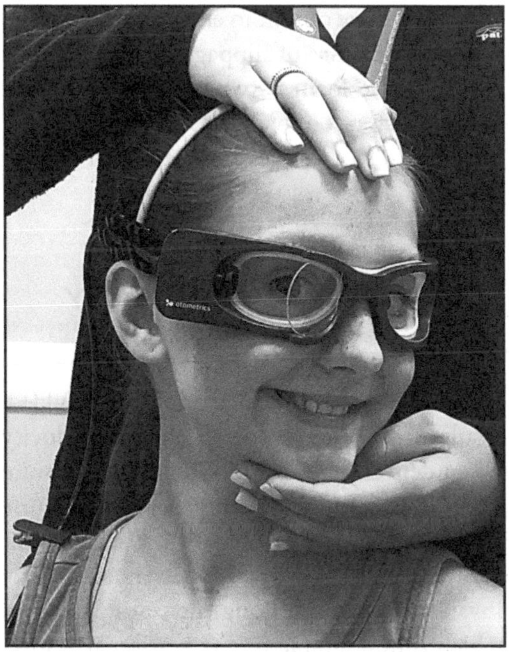

Figure 7–8. Examiner's hands position for vertical canal vHIT.

It is imperative to instruct patients to fix their eyes on the visual target during testing, regardless of how their head is moved around. Frequent eye blinks should be avoided with the patient's best efforts, and it may be necessary to encourage them to finish the session without a break.

Accommodations for Successful Testing on Young Children

To achieve valid and reliable vHIT results, modifications are often necessary to ensure young children are fully engaged during testing. Although the time needed to finish vHIT in all three planes is not very long, usually around 10 to 15 minutes, some children may have a very short attention span and get bored quickly looking at a fixed target.[11] Instead of using the default visual target, a colorful sticker containing a child-friendly image or character can be adopted. Asking questions about the sticker (eg, what color sprinkles do you see on the cupcake?) can also help children maintain their gaze on the target.

For young children unable or unwilling to sit alone, one solution is to have them sit on their parent's lap and perform head impulses with the clinician's arms around the adult. A booster seat or high chair can be used if the child can sit alone but the height of the head is too low compared to the target. Alternatively, an attractive target with adjustable height (eg, sticker on a Velcro strip) can be mounted on the wall or screen. Also, it may be beneficial to have an assistant who can help to maintain continued gaze on the target when testing a child with a short attention span.

As mentioned previously, tight fitting of vHIT goggles is required for valid outcomes. Although the head strap is adjustable, it may still be difficult to achieve the desired fit when facing a young child or a child with smaller head/face. One option to ensure a snug fit and reduce the chance of slippage is to add a piece of disposable foam between the hair and the strap, which not only increases the bulk of the head but also provides some friction against the hair.

Required Peak Head Velocity of Head Impulses

Another key requirement for valid vHIT results is to reach proper peak head velocity when delivering head impulses. The software of an ICS impulse system can reject impulse trials with low velocity from the calculation of average VOR gain. However, too many invalid trials will prolong the testing session, which is undesirable in any vestibular testing of pediatric patients. Clinicians who plan to regularly conduct vHIT on children should have extensive training in delivering effective head impulses. Practice of head thrusts with the aid of software that can provide feedback about the velocity of each head impulse is highly recommended.

Peak head velocity of 150°/s or higher for vHIT is usually recommended because head impulses with low peak head velocities (eg, below 100°/s) are not adequate to reveal a loss in semicircular canal function.[18–21] Although such high peak head velocities can be easily achieved in adults, it is not practical for all pediatric patients, especially for the young ones, due to the physical characteristics (ie, stiffness and flexibility) of their cervical spines. A recent study suggested that a head velocity of 100° to 150°/s is more feasible and sufficient for pediatric patients.[22]

New Paradigm in ICS Impulse: SHIMP

For the conventional paradigm of vHIT (now also called HIMP), patients are instructed to maintain eye fixation on a preset target in front of them during head motion. Patients with vestibular loss are unable to keep their eyes on the target with head movement due to impaired VOR, and they will make a compensatory saccade to regain fixation on the target, as instructed. In contrast, healthy subjects barely make any compensatory saccades. Complementing HIMP, the suppression head impulse paradigm (SHIMP) was developed with the aim of providing additional information regarding VOR function.[9,23] Instead of using a preset/earth-fixed target, patients are instructed to follow a head-fixed target (projected from a head-mounted laser) during head motion. Patients with impaired VOR can complete the testing without any corrective saccade because their eyes will move with the head. Healthy subjects will make a corrective saccade to follow the head-fixed target. Therefore, corrective saccades indicate a functioning VOR system. While patients with vestibular loss may still show a reduced VOR gain in SHIMP, the pattern of corrective saccades is completely different from HIMP. It seems that the SHIMP test is more intuitive for the patients, where lack of corrective saccades indicates a vestibular loss. Clinical studies demonstrating the utility of SHIMP have been reported in adults, but studies on this approach have not yet been reported in children.[23,24]

Interpretation of vHIT Results

The goal of vHIT is to assess the functional status of the individual semicircular canals and/or the two branches of the vestibular nerves, and to aid in the clinical diagnosis of vestibular disorders. High-velocity head accelerations in vHIT primarily produce an excitation to the semicircular canal on one side and limit the contribution from the corresponding canal on the other side, resulting in an ear-/canal-specific assessment.

Outcome Measures of vHIT

The results of vHIT have both qualitative and quantitative components. Qualitative measures of vHIT refer to whether the tracings of eye velocity match the tracings of head velocity. If mismatches occur, the terms overt and covert saccades are used to define the tracings (Figure 7–9). Overt saccades can be easily detected since they occur after the head turns have stopped. In contrast, covert saccades occur during head turns, which are almost impossible to detect visually but are clearly indicated in vHIT tracings.

Quantitative measures of vHIT refer to the average VOR gain for each semicircular canal, which is shown in a graph when vHIT is completed for the paired-semicircular canals (Figure 7–10). Manufacturers usually define their own normal VOR gain ranges and asymmetry ratios, which are generally based on adult data and should be used with caution for pediatric patients.

Normative Data

There are only a handful of studies evaluating normative vHIT findings in children.[4,5,20] These studies suggest that there is no significant maturational trend among most age groups. For the horizontal canals, the average VOR gain in vHIT was close to 1, which is similar to adults. In contrast, the cutoff value for VOR gain in the vertical canals dipped as low as 0.6, and more variability was observed. Recently, a group of researchers from Cincinnati Children's Hospital published a study on 30 healthy children ages 4 to 12 years using the ICS Impulse, along with a small control group of adults.[11] These children did not have any hearing loss or vestibular symptoms. Normative vHIT values of VOR gain are summarized in Table 7–1. The authors also evaluated the amount of time needed to complete vHIT testing for all six semicircular canals, as shown

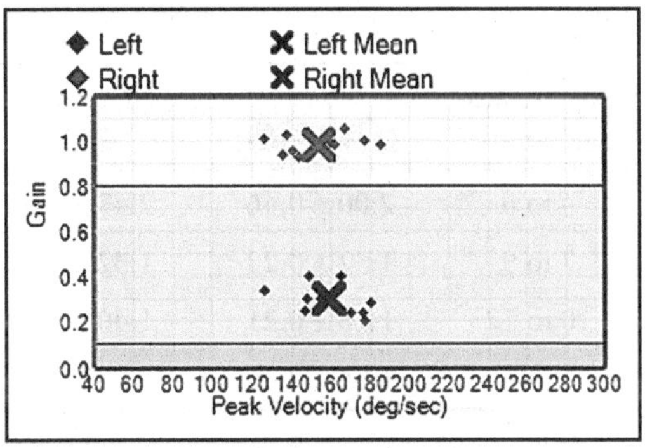

Figure 7–10. A graph of VOR gain in vHIT for each individual canal, as average gain marked with "X". Here, the gain for the right canal is normal while the gain for the left is reduced (*falling in the shaded area*). Corresponding head velocity also indicated.

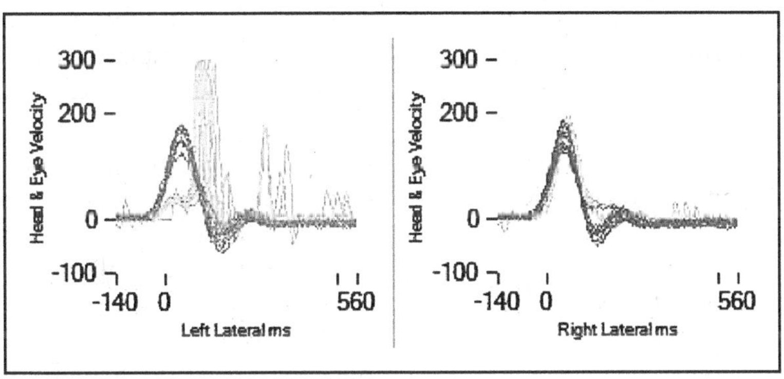

Figure 7–9. Examples of covert and overt saccades in left horizontal canal vHIT. Normal right horizontal canal vHIT tracing.

Table 7–1. VOR Gain (mean ± standard deviation) in vHIT in Children, Comparing to That in Adults[a]

		Children (4 to 12 years)	*Adults*
Lateral canal	Left	0.96 ± 0.09 (0.79–1.14)	0.91 ± 0.06 (0.79–1.04)
	Right	1.04 ± 0.09 (0.87–1.23)	1.03 ± 0.06 (0.91–1.14)
Anterior canal	Left	0.80 ± 0.11 (0.58–1.02)	0.93 ± 0.07 (0.78–1.07)
	Right	0.90 ± 0.19 (0.53–1.27)	0.95 ± 0.18 (0.60–1.30)
Posterior canal	Left	0.91 ± 0.14 (0.65–1.18)	0.95 ± 0.09 (0.77–1.12)
	Right	0.83 ± 0.09 (0.65–1.01)	0.89 ± 0.08 (0.73–1.05)

[a]Numbers in parentheses are 5th to 95th percentile confidence intervals. Data cited from Bachmann, Sipos, Lavender, and Hunter.[11]

Table 7–2. The Amount of Time Needed to Complete vHIT Testing for All Six Semicircular Canals[a]

Age Group (Years)	*Lateral*	*RALP*	*LARP*	*Maximum Total Test Time (Mean ±2 SD)*
4 to 6	2:00 ± 0:46	2:47 ± 1:40	3:23 ± 2:18	17:38
7 to 9	1:32 ± 0:22	1:32 ± 0:40	2:01 ± 0:47	8:43
10 to 12	1:18 ± 0:21	1:40 ± 0:43	2:02 ± 1:27	10:18
Adults	1:24 ± 0:30	1:26 ± 0:46	1:49 ± 1:00	9:10

[a]Maximum total test time includes the mean ±2 standard deviation for each age group to complete lateral, LARP, and RALP tests but does not include time used for patient setup, calibration, breaks, or instruction.

in Table 7–2. Specifically, all of the children were able to complete the testing in less than 18 minutes (not including calibration and setup). However, there was a noticeable increase in test time as age decreased. It should be noted that normative values may not be universally equivalent across all manufacturers' devices and all testing facilities, so each testing center is encouraged to determine their own normative ranges, whenever feasible.

Importance of Clean Data

Data contamination can be seen more often when conducting vHIT in pediatric patients than in adults. Before giving an interpretation of vHIT outcomes, the clinician must ensure that contaminated trials are not counted in the calculation of the average VOR gain. As mentioned previously, goggle slippage and eye blinks can cause data contamination, even though the ICS Impulse software has built-in features to minimize the effects of these problems. If young children blink too frequently throughout the testing session, the acquired data are most likely invalid. Another source of vHIT tracing contamination seen in young children is the eyelid "flick."[9,11] Compared to adults, children often have a bigger pupil diameter but smaller eyelid opening. This may alter the detection of the pupil center when conducting vHIT in the vertical planes, especially for the anterior canal, as shown in Figure 7–11.

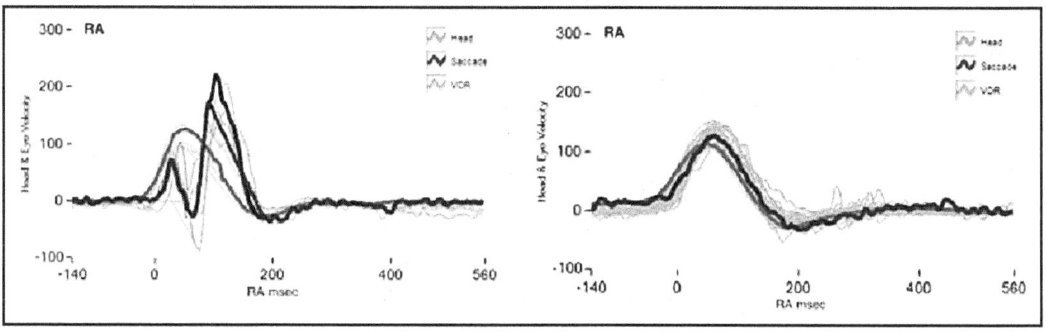

Figure 7–11. Example of a normal right anterior canal vHIT tracing (*on the right*), and a right anterior canal vHIT tracing with eyelid artifact (*on the left*) which has a "V"-shaped dip in the tracing. (Cited from Bachmann, Sipos, Lavender, and Hunter.[11])

Clinical Applications

Unilateral Peripheral Vestibular Loss

Traditionally, caloric testing has been considered the "gold standard" for diagnosing unilateral, peripheral vestibular loss.[25–27] vHIT is a much easier test than calorics to perform in children for confirmation of unilateral loss in suspected acute peripheral vestibular disorders such as acute vestibular neuritis or labyrinthitis. Typical vHIT findings in these disorders include reduced VOR gain of the canal(s) involved and the presence of overt/covert saccades.[28] In cases of vestibular neuritis, VOR gain reduction and saccades are found in the lateral and anterior semicircular canals if the superior branch of the vestibular nerve is involved (more common) and in the posterior semicircular canal if the posterior branch of the vestibular nerve is involved (rare).[29–31] In contrast, reduced VOR gain and corrective saccades are most likely found in all three semicircular canals on the affected side with labyrinthitis, typically in conjunction with hearing loss on audiometric testing.[32] While overt saccades can often be seen in acute vestibular loss, clinical vHIT studies have shown that the presence of covert saccades after the acute stage may indicate some degree of vestibular compensation. Some studies have suggested that vHIT may not be sensitive enough to determine the side of lesion in chronic, unilateral losses.[33–35]

Although vHIT may show reduced VOR gain in patients with benign paroxysmal positional vertigo (BPPV), a recent study did not find a consistent pattern to identify which semicircular canal is involved, and vHIT may often be normal in cases of BPPV.[36] Other peripheral disorders that are relatively common in adults, such as Ménière's disease and vestibular schwannoma, are very uncommon among pediatric patients, and vHIT is not the optimal tool for clinical evaluation of these disorders.

Bilateral Peripheral Vestibular Loss

Bilateral vestibular loss in adult patients is often suspected if postural imbalance and/or oscillopsia are present.[37] In contrast, the diagnosis of bilateral vestibular loss in children is often missed or delayed, because the signs may be less obvious and may present as a gross motor delay in conjunction with other associated developmental delays.[38–41] Bilateral vestibular loss in children may be due to structural congenital anomalies of the inner ear, acquired from perinatal infections, or genetic, particularly in conjunction with congenital hearing loss. Another potential cause of bilateral peripheral vestibular loss is the use of ototoxic drugs,[42] which include chemotherapy agents and high doses of aminoglycoside antibiotics (eg, gentamycin). Clinically, hearing loss is the most watched-for side effect while possible vestibular loss is rarely on the radar.[43] Not only can vHIT provide objective and quantitative assessment of the ototoxic effect from these drugs, but it can also be used to monitor the progress of the vestibular loss, if necessary.

Vestibular Impairment in Children With Hearing Loss

With the implementation of newborn hearing screening over the past 20 years, a diagnosis of hearing impairment can be achieved at a very young age. In contrast, assessment of vestibular function is often neglected in these children. Clinical studies have shown substantial vestibular impairment in children with hearing loss.[41,44–46] vHIT has many advantages over other vestibular testing, such as rotational or caloric testing, in screening children with hearing loss for vestibular impairment.[12] The presence of corrective saccades or reduction of VOR gain in vHIT will confirm suspected peripheral vestibular loss in young children.

Central Vestibular Loss

Lesions in the vestibular pathway, which includes the brainstem, medial longitudinal fasciculus (MLF), and vestibulocerebellum, may affect VOR and vHIT outcomes.[47–49] Although strokes and degenerative diseases are unlikely in pediatric patients, other diseases such as metabolic diseases or neuropathies may exist in children. The possibility of central involvement should be raised if unusual vHIT outcomes are found.

Nonspecific Vestibular Loss

A small percentage of patients with vestibular migraine or postconcussive syndrome were found to have reduced VOR gain in vHIT and/or minor saccades. Currently, it is not entirely clear whether this abnormal vHIT reflects impaired canal function or issues with the VOR pathway without confirmation from other vestibular testing.[12,50,51] It is argued that such isolated vHIT findings may be coincidental if there are no other abnormal vestibular findings. Otherwise, comorbid conditions such as persistent postural-perceptual dizziness (PPPD) should be considered (see Chapter 24).[52]

Potential Pitfalls of vHIT in Clinical Use

Although vHIT is a valid clinical tool that assesses the dynamic function of all six semicircular canals and has particular benefits in evaluating children, clinicians must be aware of its limitations in clinical use. First, vHIT should not be performed on any patients with a neck injury, pain, or stiffness that may make head impulses ineffective. Second, vHIT software usually enables automatic calculation of the average VOR gain based on the vHIT trials acquired; however, the quality of data acquisition is not automatically guaranteed. Without inspecting the quality of vHIT traces before ending the test, mistakes can occur in interpretation. For accurate interpretation, any recording artifacts or data outliers should be deleted from the calculation of the average VOR gain. If not, the test should be repeated before a final conclusion is made. Last, clinical applications of vHIT have expanded to a variety of vestibular disorders as the popularity of vHIT grows. As with any new test, it is essential to understand what vHIT is actually assessing. It is not appropriate to make a clinical diagnosis purely based on vHIT results since a normal vHIT outcome cannot rule out certain vestibular losses, and similarly abnormal vHIT outcomes do not always indicate a definite vestibular loss. While the sensitivity and specificity of vHIT are still under debate and currently being investigated in clinical studies, vHIT should not be treated as the single "gold standard" of vestibular evaluation.

Conclusion

vHIT is still a relatively new tool in vestibular laboratory testing, particularly for pediatric patients. Nonetheless, vHIT is a reliable clinical test to quantify individual semicircular canal function. It offers a noninvasive procedure as part of a vestibular test battery. Appreciating the challenges of working with young children will help in the collection of accurate vHIT results.

Self-Assessment Questions

1. Calibration is not needed for vHIT.
   a. True
   b. False

2. All six semicircular canals can be tested by vHIT individually.
   a. True
   b. False

3. Abnormal vHIT findings include:
   a. Reduced VOR gain
   b. Covert and overt saccades
   c. Both a and b

4. Trials of vHIT with peak head velocities below 100°/s are acceptable.
   a. True
   b. False

5. Only peripheral vestibular lesions influence vHIT responses.
   a. True
   b. False

6. Normal VOR gain of lateral canal vHIT in children is usually higher than:
   a. 0.6
   b. 0.7
   c. 0.8

References

1. Cyr DG, Brookhouser PE, Valente M, Grossman A. Vestibular evaluation of infants and preschool children. *Otolaryngol Head Neck Surg*. 1985;93(4):463–468.
2. Valente LM. Assessment techniques for vestibular evaluation in pediatric patients. *Otolaryngol Clin North Am*. 2011;44(2):273–290, vii.
3. Zhou G, Dargie J, Dornan B, Whittemore K. Clinical uses of cervical vestibular-evoked myogenic potential testing in pediatric patients. *Medicine*. 2014;93(4):e37.
4. Hamilton SS, Zhou G, Brodsky JR. Video head impulse testing (VHIT) in the pediatric population. *Int J Pediatr Otorhinolaryngol*. 2015;79(8):1283–1287.
5. Hulse R, Hormann K, Servais JJ, Hulse M, Wenzel A. Clinical experience with video head impulse test in children. *Int J Pediatr Otorhinolaryngol*. 2015;79(8):1288–1293.
6. Shinjo Y, Jin Y, Kaga K. Assessment of vestibular function of infants and children with congenital and acquired deafness using the ice-water caloric test, rotational chair test and vestibular-evoked myogenic potential recording. *Acta Oto-Laryngol*. 2007;127(7):736–747.
7. Singh S, Gupta RK, Kumar P. Vestibular evoked myogenic potentials in children with sensorineural hearing loss. *Int J Pediatr Otorhinolaryngol*. 2012;76(9):1308–1311.
8. Halmagyi GM, Curthoys IS. A clinical sign of canal paresis. *Arch Neurol*. 1988;45(7):737–739.
9. Halmagyi GM, Chen L, MacDougall HG, Weber KP, McGarvie LA, Curthoys IS. The video head impulse test. *Front Neurol*. 2017;8:258.
10. MacDougall HG, Weber KP, McGarvie LA, Halmagyi GM, Curthoys IS. The video head impulse test: Diagnostic accuracy in peripheral vestibulopathy. *Neurology*. 2009;73(14):1134–1141.
11. Bachmann K, Sipos K, Lavender V, Hunter LL. Video head impulse testing in a pediatric population: Normative findings. *J Am Acad Audiol*. 2018;29(5):417–426.
12. Sommerfleck PA, Gonzalez Macchi ME, Weinschelbaum R, De Bagge MD, Bernaldez P, Carmona S. Balance disorders in childhood: Main etiologies according to age. Usefulness of the video head impulse test. *Int J Pediatr Otorhinolaryngol*. 2016;87:148–153.
13. Ross LM, Helminski JO. Test-retest and interrater reliability of the video head impulse test in the pediatric population. *Otol Neurotol*. 2016;37(5):558–563.
14. MacDougall HG, McGarvie LA, Halmagyi GM, Curthoys IS, Weber KP. Application of the video head impulse test to detect vertical semicircular canal dysfunction. *Otol Neurotol*. 2013;34(6):974–979.
15. Wenzel A, Eck S, Hulse K, et al. Development of a new software and test setup for analyzing hVOR in very young children by vHIT. *J Vestib Res*. 2017;27(2–3):155–162.
16. Murnane O, Mabrey H, Pearson A, Byrd S, Akin F. Normative data and test-retest reliability of the SYNAPSYS video head impulse test. *J Am Acad Audiol*. 2014;25(3):244–252.
17. Wiener-Vacher SR, Wiener SI. Video head impulse tests with a remote camera system: Normative values of semicircular canal vestibulo-ocular reflex gain in infants and children. *Front Neurol*. 2017;8:434.
18. Seo YJ, Park YA, Kong TH, Bae MR, Kim SH. Head position and increased head velocity to optimize video head impulse test sensitivity. *Eur Arch Otorhinolaryngol*. 2016;273(11):3595–3602.
19. Patterson JN, Bassett AM, Mollak CM, Honaker JA. Effects of hand placement technique on the video head impulse test (vHIT) in younger and older adults. *Otol Neurotol*. 2015;36(6):1061–1068.
20. McGarvie LA, MacDougall HG, Halmagyi GM, Burgess AM, Weber KP, Curthoys IS. The video head impulse test (vHIT) of semicircular canal function—Age-dependent normative values of VOR gain in healthy subjects. *Front Neurol*. 2015;6:154.
21. Weber KP, Aw ST, Todd MJ, McGarvie LA, Curthoys IS, Halmagyi GM. Head impulse

test in unilateral vestibular loss: Vestibulo-ocular reflex and catch-up saccades. *Neurology*. 2008;70(6):454–463.

22. Zhou G, Goutos C, Lipson S, Brodsky J. Range of peak head velocity in video head impulse testing for pediatric patients. *Otol Neurotol.* 2018;39(5):e357–e361.
23. MacDougall HG, McGarvie LA, Halmagyi GM, et al. A new saccadic indicator of peripheral vestibular function based on the video head impulse test. *Neurology*. 2016;87(4):410–418.
24. Du Y, Liu XJ, Ren LL, Zhang SZ, Yang SM, Wu ZM. [The application value of suppression head pulse paradigm (SHIMP) in vestibular examination]. *J Clin Otolaryngol Head Neck Surg.* 2018;32(10):728–732.
25. Redondo-Martinez J, Becares-Martinez C, Orts-Alborch M, Garcia-Callejo FJ, Perez-Carbonell T, Marco-Algarra J. Relationship between video head impulse test (vHIT) and caloric test in patients with vestibular neuritis. *Acta Otorrinolaringol Espanola.* 2016;67(3): 156–161.
26. McCaslin DL, Jacobson GP, Bennett ML, Gruenwald JM, Green AP. Predictive properties of the video head impulse test: Measures of caloric symmetry and self-report dizziness handicap. *Ear Hear.* 2014;35(5):e185–191.
27. van Esch BF, Nobel-Hoff GE, van Benthem PP, van der Zaag-Loonen HJ, Bruintjes TD. Determining vestibular hypofunction: Start with the video-head impulse test. *Eur Arch Otorhinolaryngol.* 2016;273(11):3733–3739.
28. Brodsky JR, Cusick BA, Zhou G. Vestibular neuritis in children and adolescents: Clinical features and recovery. *Int J Pediatr Otorhinolaryngol.* 2016;83:104–108.
29. Rambold HA. Prediction of short-term outcome in acute superior vestibular nerve failure: Three-dimensional video-head-impulse test and caloric irrigation. *Int J Otolaryngol.* 2015; 2015:639024.
30. Guan Q, Zhang L, Hong W, et al. Video head impulse test for early diagnosis of vestibular neuritis among acute vertigo. *Can J Neurol Sci.* 2017;44(5):556–561.
31. Hou L, Chen T, Xu K, et al. [Evaluation of the injured range of vestibular superior and inferior nerves in sudden deafness patients with vertigo using video head impulse test]. Zhonghua er bi yan hou tou jing wai ke za zhi/ *Chinese J Otorhinolaryngol Head Neck Surg.* 2015;50(9):718–723.
32. Magliulo G, Gagliardi S, Ciniglio Appiani M, Iannella G, Re M. Vestibular neurolabyrinthitis: A follow-up study with cervical and ocular vestibular evoked myogenic potentials and the video head impulse test. *Ann Otol Rhinol Laryngol.* 2014;123(3):162–173.
33. Mezzalira R, Bittar RSM, do Carmo Bilecki-Stipsky MM, Brugnera C, Grasel SS. Sensitivity of caloric test and video head impulse as screening test for chronic vestibular complaints. *Clinics*. 2017;72(8):469–473.
34. Park P, Park JH, Kim JS, Koo JW. Role of video-head impulse test in lateralization of vestibulopathy: Comparative study with caloric test. *Auris Nasus Larynx.* 2017;44(6):648–654.
35. Burston A, Mossman S, Mossman B, Weatherall M. Comparison of the video head impulse test with the caloric test in patients with sub-acute and chronic vestibular disorders. *J Clin Neurol.* 2018;47:294–298.
36. Guan Q, Zhang L, Hong W, et al. [Video head impulse test for evaluation of vestibular function in patients with vestibular neuritis and benign paroxysmal positional vertigo]. Zhejiang da xue xue bao. Yi xue ban/*J Zhejiang Univ Med Sci.* 25 2017;46(1):52–58.
37. Strupp M, Kim JS, Murofushi T, et al. Bilateral vestibulopathy: Diagnostic criteria Consensus document of the Classification Committee of the Barany Society. *J Vestib Res.* 2017;27(4):177–189.
38. Inoue A, Iwasaki S, Ushio M, et al. Effect of vestibular dysfunction on the development of gross motor function in children with profound hearing loss. *Audiol Neurootol.* 2013; 18(3):143–151.
39. Masuda T, Kaga K. Relationship between acquisition of motor function and vestibular function in children with bilateral severe hearing loss. *Acta Otolaryngol.* 2014;134(7): 672–678.
40. Oyewumi M, Wolter NE, Heon E, Gordon KA, Papsin BC, Cushing SL. Using balance function

to screen for vestibular impairment in children with sensorineural hearing loss and cochlear implants. *Otol Neurol.* 2016;37(7):926–932.

41. Kimura Y, Masuda T, Kaga K. Vestibular function and gross motor development in 195 children with congenital hearing loss—Assessment of inner ear malformations. *Otol Neurol.* 2018;39(2):196–205.
42. Chen KS, Bach A, Shoup A, Winick NJ. Hearing loss and vestibular dysfunction among children with cancer after receiving aminoglycosides. *Pediatr Blood Cancer.* 2013;60(11): 1772–1777.
43. Agrawal Y, Bremova T, Kremmyda O, Strupp M. Semicircular canal, saccular and utricular function in patients with bilateral vestibulopathy: Analysis based on etiology. *J Neurol.* 2013;260(3):876–883.
44. Cushing SL, Gordon KA, Rutka JA, James AL, Papsin BC. Vestibular end-organ dysfunction in children with sensorineural hearing loss and cochlear implants: An expanded cohort and etiologic assessment. *Otol Neurol.* 2013;34(3):422–428.
45. Sokolov M, Gordon KA, Polonenko M, Blaser SI, Papsin BC, Cushing SL. Vestibular and balance function is often impaired in children with profound unilateral sensorineural hearing loss. *Hear Res.* 2019;372:52–61.
46. Verbecque E, Marijnissen T, De Belder N, et al. Vestibular (dys)function in children with sensorineural hearing loss: A systematic review. *Int J Audiol.* 2017;56(6):361–381.
47. Pavlovic I, Ruska B, Pavicic T, et al. Video head impulse test can detect brainstem dysfunction in multiple sclerosis. *Mult Scler Relat Disord.* 2017;14:68–71.
48. Guler A, Karbek Akarca F, Eraslan C, et al. Clinical and video head impulse test in the diagnosis of posterior circulation stroke presenting as acute vestibular syndrome in the emergency department. *J Vestib Res.* 2017; 27(4):233–242.
49. Armato E, Ferri E, Pinzani A, Ulmer E. Cerebellar haemorrhage mimicking acute peripheral vestibulopathy: The role of the video head impulse test in differential diagnosis. *Acta Otorhinolaryngol Ital.* 2014;34(4):288–291.
50. Zhou G, Brodsky JR. Objective vestibular testing of children with dizziness and balance complaints following sports-related concussions. *Otolaryngol Head Neck Surg.* 2015; 152(6):1133–1139.
51. Brodsky JR, Cusick BA, Zhou G. Evaluation and management of vestibular migraine in children: Experience from a pediatric vestibular clinic. *Eur J Paediatr Neurol.* 2016;20(1): 85–92.
52. Staab JP, Eckhardt-Henn A, Horii A, et al. Diagnostic criteria for persistent postural-perceptual dizziness (PPPD): Consensus document of the committee for the Classification of Vestibular Disorders of the Barany Society. *J Vestib Res.* 2017;27(4):191–208.

CHAPTER 8

Vestibular-Evoked Myogenic Potential (VEMP) Testing

Sylvette Wiener-Vacher and Guangwei Zhou

The vestibular-evoked myogenic potential (VEMP) test was first described by Colebatch and Halmagyi and involves the activation of otolith receptors by acoustic stimuli (loud clicks or tone bursts by air or bone conduction) causing stimulation of a tonically contracted muscle, which can then be recorded as an electrical response.[1–3] The original version of the VEMP test is the cervical VEMP (cVEMP), in which the tonically active muscle is the sternocleidomastoid (SCM) muscle. More recently, a version was developed where the response is recorded near eye muscles (inferior rectus/oblique muscles) and is called ocular VEMP (oVEMP).[4] The cVEMP tests the ipsilateral descending vestibulospinal pathway (via the saccule and the utricle), while the oVEMP tests the contralateral ascending vestibulo-ocular pathway (mostly from the utricle).[5]

Cervical VEMP

The potentials recorded from the SCM muscle correspond to a biphasic change in tonic electromyogram (EMG) activity labeled P13 and N23, according to their polarities and latencies. These responses are ipsilateral to the stimulation and depend on vestibulospinal pathway activation. The cVEMP is a reliable method for evaluating the function of the otolith vestibulospinal pathway in adults as well as in children. The stimuli can be delivered by air conduction (AC) or bone conduction (BC).[6,7] In animal studies, AC stimulates mostly the saccule, while bone conduction stimulates both the saccule and the utricle.[8] In contrast to AC, BC can bypass the problem of conductive hearing loss, which prevents sufficient high levels of stimulation for cVEMP to be detected. This is very useful for young children in whom middle ear effusion and Eustachian tube dysfunction are frequent. The amplitude of the cVEMP is proportional to the level of tonic muscle activity.[9,10] Because sufficient muscle contraction is not always easy to obtain in children, it is critical to generate a sufficient intensity and stable intensity of neck muscle contraction to avoid false negative results.

Stimulation and Recording Methodology

Because cVEMP measurement is a useful approach for otolith evaluation, it has been a part of our vestibular test battery (with bone and air conduction) for patients with hearing loss and prior to cochlear implantation.[11] Many recording systems currently available for cVEMP testing in a clinical setting do not accurately monitor the EMG level and, hence, require a high number of stimuli to compensate for the variability in active muscle contraction. The test can become tiresome and even more difficult to administer in fatigued patients or children.

Stimulus

Otolith stimulation is achieved with tone bursts (750 Hz, 6.6-ms duration) delivered at a rate of 4 Hz through headphones for AC. For BC, a vibrating bone stimulator provides the same stimulus on the mastoid. An additive amplifier can produce tone bursts up to 110 dB HL. Stimulus intensities usually vary between 75 and 100 dB. Stimuli of 100 to 110 dB HL are used in cases of profound hearing loss and when no response was obtained at 100 dB HL. Stimuli lower than 75 dB that produce a response can be seen in the setting of third window anomalies, such as superior semicircular canal dehiscence.

The neck EMG activity is recorded with contact electrodes. In young children, these electrodes are placed higher than those in adults (at the superior third of the anterior border of the SCM muscles), the manubrium arch, and the forehead. Our stimulation and analysis program permits recording in real time with simultaneous screen visualization of the amplitude of the EMG and the responses consist of a positive peak at a latency of 13 ms (P13) followed by a negative deflection at a latency of 23 ms (N23). EMG sampling is done every 150 ms. The P13-N23 responses obtained with the same level of EMG recording are selected to be averaged. The P13-N23 amplitude obtained with the same EMG can then be compared between sides. The responses are averaged at several stimuli intensities, selecting the same EMG in order to determine and compare cVEMP thresholds.

Muscle Contraction

To obtain a good neck-muscle contraction in children, the head is turned toward the side opposite the sound stimulation. In adults, the patient usually lies on a bed and is asked to lift and rotate his or her head toward the side opposite the stimulated ear. This position is too tiring for young children and infants. In our experience, we have found two positions to be efficient to obtain a good EMG with regard to age as shown in Figures 8–1 and 8–2. In the case of very young children, this feedback will be used by the technician to adjust the position or the amount of neck muscle contraction of the child accordingly during the trial. The postanalysis after the trials allows selection of all responses obtained with an identical and sufficient EMG level. Older children (>6 years) can lie down on a bed in a half-sitting position propped up on their elbows. They are asked to lift and turn their head toward the side opposite the ear stimulation.

Increasing Test Efficiency and Reliability

With proper techniques and experience, cVEMP testing can be applied as part of a pediatric vestibular evaluation as soon as a child can support his or her head, which is typically at about 2 to 3 months of age. To reduce the duration of the test, our recording system requires only 25 to 50 stimulations per trial and level of stimulation (performed with 5 dB HL steps starting at 100 dB HL). Two to three trials are performed at threshold. In our opinion, the Difra Neurosoft system

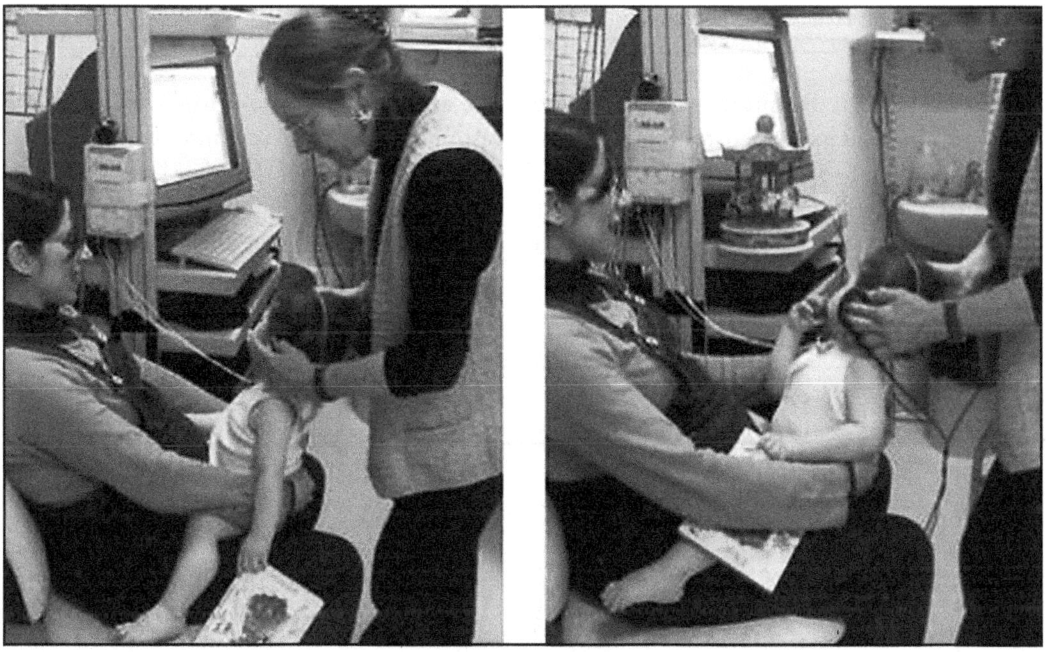

A B

Figure 8–1. A and **B.** Air conduction (AC) and bone conduction (BC) cVEMP recording procedure for children younger than 6 years. The child is seated on a parent's lap, face to face, while the parent supports the lowest part of the child's back. During stimulation the examiner tilts the child's trunk slightly backward. The child is encouraged to make an effort to straighten up, look at, and reach for a toy. To obtain a more efficient neck-muscle contraction, the toy is presented on the opposite side of the stimulus. Encouraging the child to reach the toy with the hands, unlock the head and shoulders (a reflex strategy that the child uses to minimize tiring neck-muscle contraction). The stimulation is applied with AC by placing one speaker on the pinna (**B**) or with BC by placing a vibrator Radio ear B71 on the parietal flat area just above the pinna (**A**). Speaker as well as vibrator are maintained by hand without any headband to control the position of the stimulator and be less restrictive for the child.

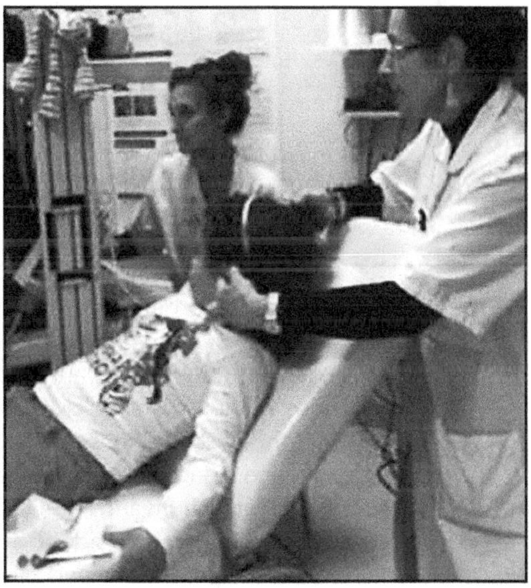

Figure 8–2. Bone-conduction cVEMP recording procedure for children older than 6 years. The child lies partially upright on an examination table and is asked to lift and rotate the head toward the side opposite from the stimulus. With one hand, the assistant holds the vibrating probe against the mastoid and closes the external meatus. With the other hand, the assistant helps the child to keep his or her head lifted. The amplitude of the EMG displayed simultaneously on the computer screen is efficient feedback for the assistant (and if possible, the subject) to maintain an intense and regular neck-muscle contraction.

(Difra Neurosoft, Belgium) provides some important advantages when testing pediatric patients (Figure 8–3), and greatly increases the tolerance of the test by young children. For each tone burst, the EMG is recorded in real time during the 150 ms following the stimulus, averaged, and then stored with the corresponding cVEMP response that is recorded on the first 50 ms of the recording. Then after each trial all individual evoked responses with the same best EMG levels can be selected and averaged together making possible a compari-

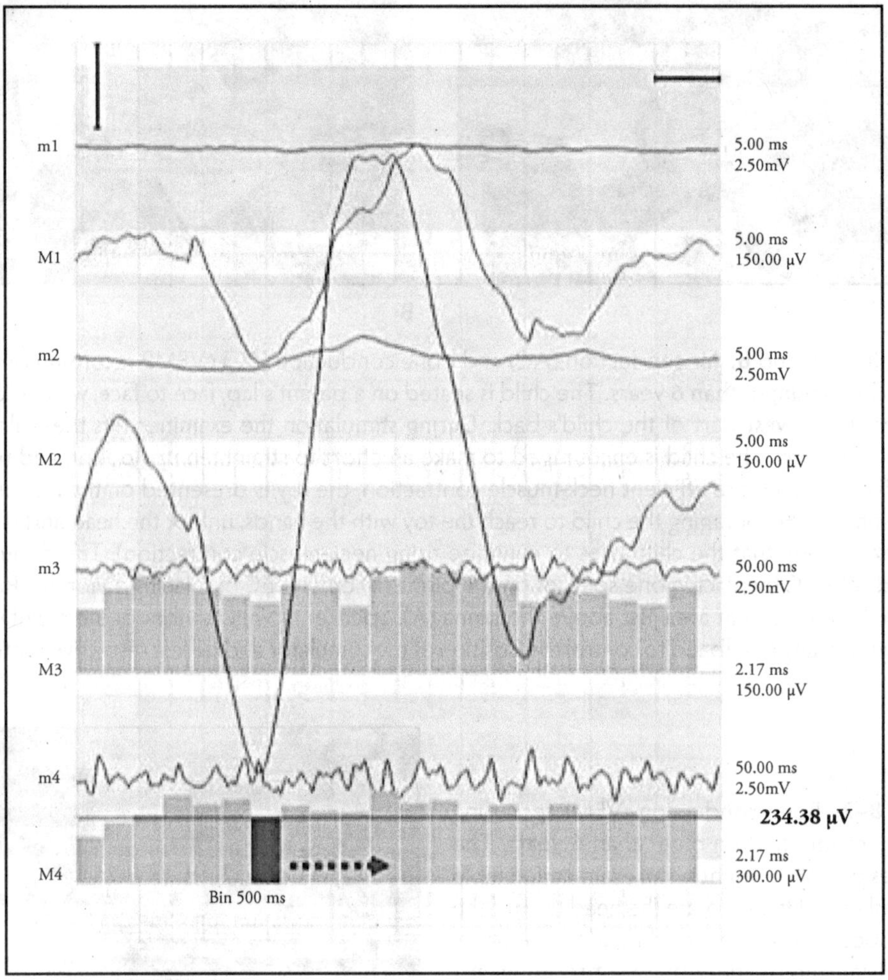

Figure 8–3. Post-recording analysis. c-VEMP analysis is performed after each trial (here 25 stimulations per trial and per level of stimulation). From top to bottom: traces 1 and 2, respectively, represent right- and left-muscle EMG; **m**, non-averaged trace; **M**, averaged trace; **M3**, left-averaged EMG; **M4**, right-averaged EMG. Histogram of the averaged EMG for the 21 stimulations (averaged over a 250-ms period per stimulation). The dotted lines (a and b) indicate the EMG levels (the higher value a and the lower value b) between which stimulations and P13-N23 responses are selected for further averaging. From one trial to another, one side to another, and one session to another, the same selection of EMG range is maintained, making comparison feasible and reliable.

son between sides for amplitudes, thresholds, and latencies (Figure 8–4). This EMG level control also allows for comparison of the cVEMP for the same subject at various times (eg, before and after surgery, after an initial vestibular impairment).

Normal cVEMP Characteristics in Children

The characteristics of vestibulospinal responses vary by age.[12] In our experience, children's cVEMP characteristics differ slightly from those of adults (Figure 8–5). The variability between individuals is slightly greater for N23 latencies than P13 latencies. Latencies increase slightly with age from childhood to adulthood (increase of <2 ms over 65 years). In children P13 mean latency is 12.8 ± 1 ms, and for N23 mean latency is 19 ± 2 ms. The P13-N23 amplitude is higher in children between the ages of 6 months and 12 years than in adults, while it is lower in children before the age of 6 months. Air conduction cVEMPs and BC cVEMPs have the same latencies. The amplitude is often slightly greater for BC cVEMP than for AC cVEMP. Thresholds for AC cVEMPs and BC cVEMPs slightly increase during childhood with an average of 90 ± 5 dB. After the age of 12 years, thresholds increase as a function of age only for BC

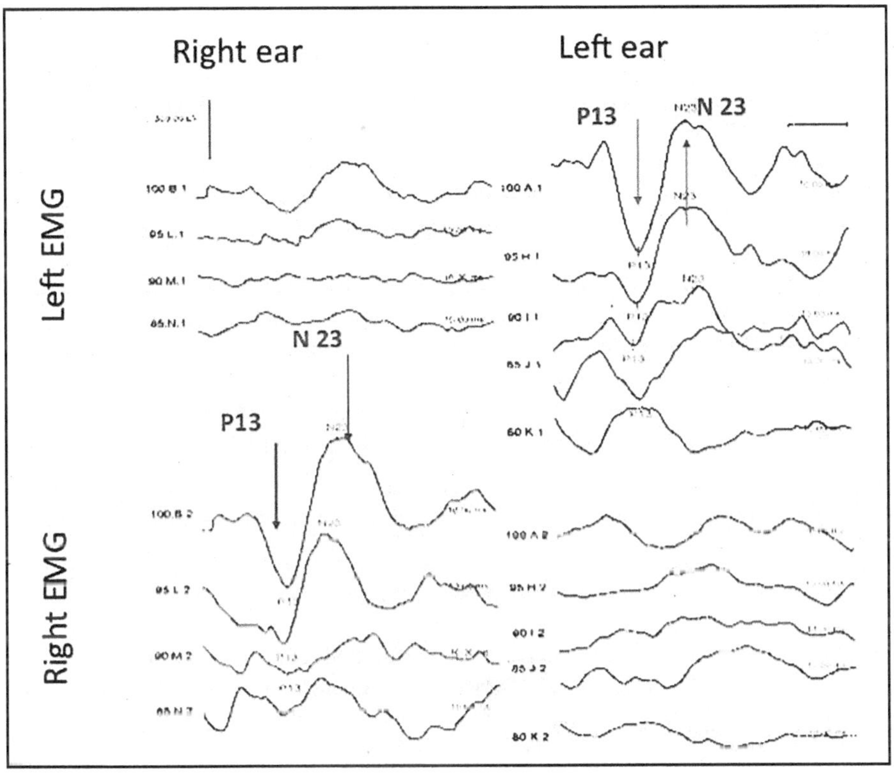

Figure 8–4. Latencies, amplitudes, and thresholds can be compared between sides. The two top traces correspond to the left neck-muscle recordings, the bottom two traces to the right neck muscle recordings. The left column corresponds to the recordings when the stimulus is applied to the right ear, and the right column corresponds to the recordings when the stimulus is applied to the left ear.

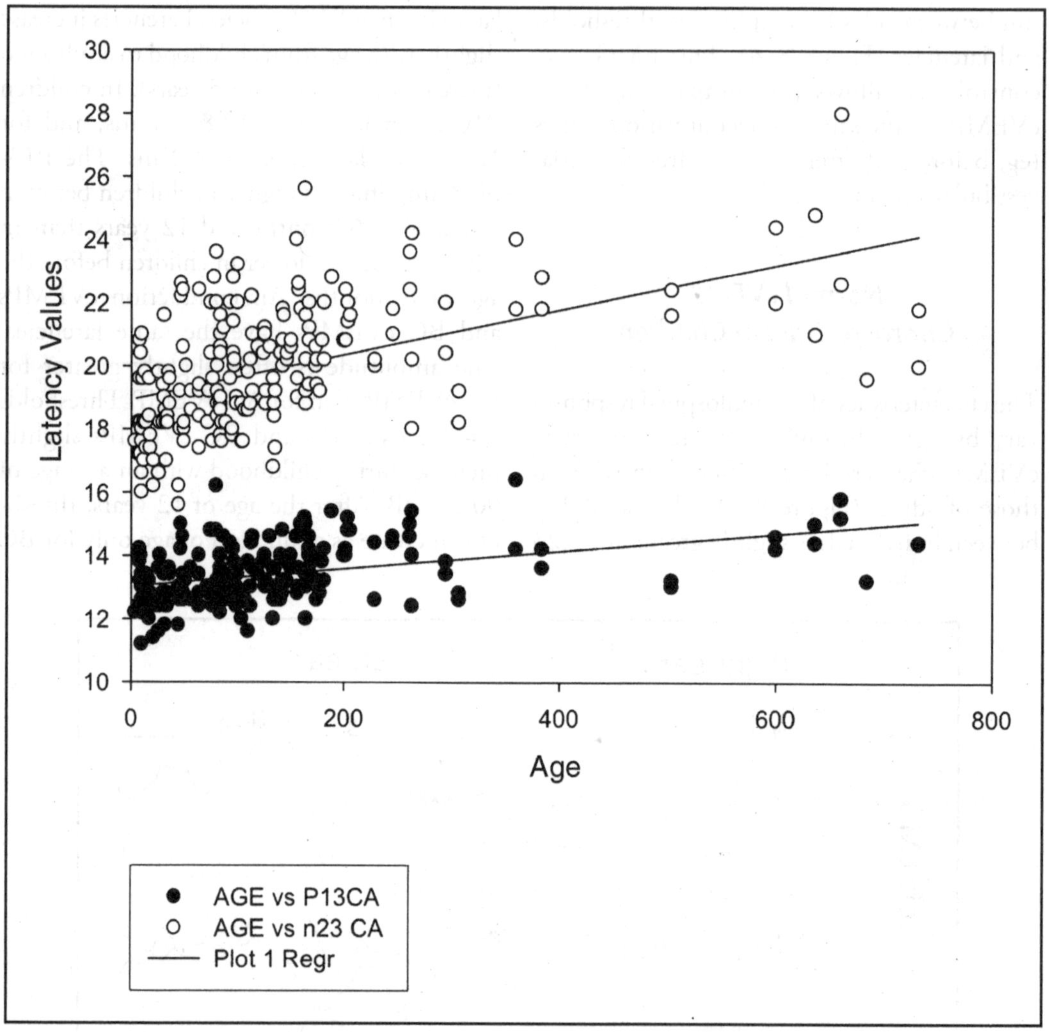

Figure 8–5. The cVEMP P13 and N23 latencies: normal values with regard to age. The latencies of P13 and N23 increase slightly with age. The latency values (*y*-axis) of P13 (solid circles) and N23 (open circles), obtained with BC stimulation, as a function of age (*x*-axis in months) are represented. P13 latencies are less variable than N23 latencies.

cVEMP. Sixty percent of adult subjects above the age of 40 years do not have BC cVEMPs at 110 dB HL but show remaining recordable AC cVEMPs usually with a slightly higher threshold than in children (thresholds mean values in adult: 100 ± 5 dB). This may be due to changes in mechanical properties of the skull with age that may lead to less efficient transmission of vibration to the vestibule than in children. The amplitude, latencies, and threshold of cVEMPs are usually symmetric in children without inner ear or middle ear pathology.

cVEMP in Children With Middle Ear Effusion

Eustachian tube dysfunction is very common in young children and can cause a middle ear effusion with an associated decrease in sound transmission. Air conduction cVEMPs are often absent in the setting of a middle ear effusion or other conductive hearing loss. When present, they have very high thresholds and small amplitudes. Bone conduction cVEMPs remain normal, however, because BC bypasses the transmission problem. In ears with tympanostomy tubes or negative middle ear pressure without effusion, AC cVEMPs can be normal or slightly modified (small amplitude and higher thresholds compared with BC cVEMP). Therefore, BC stimuli should be preferred for cVEMP in cases of young children with middle ear dysfunction.

cVEMP in Children With Sensorineural Hearing Loss

Normal AC and BC cVEMPs can be found in children with sensorineural hearing loss (SNHL). Such a result indicates that there is no otolithic impairment associated with the hearing loss. In the presence of hearing loss, abnormal BC cVEMPs indicate an impairment of the vestibular otolith receptors. The vestibular impairment can be symmetric or asymmetric and may not be correlated to the degree of hearing loss. A total absence of cVEMPs (either with BC or AC) is found in only 20% of children with profound bilateral hearing loss, while in candidates for cochlear implantation, 40% show normal AC or BC cVEMPs, and 40% have unilateral or bilateral abnormal cVEMPs.

cVEMP and Neuropathy

Latencies for cVEMP can be delayed in peripheral neuropathies. This is rare but has been described in adults and children.[13] All neuropathies (eg, multiple sclerosis, Guillain-Barré syndrome, mitochondrial cytopathy) can potentially impair the vestibulospinal pathway. For example, cVEMP latencies increased in the acute phase of Guillain-Barré syndrome in a young girl and normalized gradually over 6 months of follow-up in parallel to the clinical motor recovery.[13]

Conclusion on cVEMP in Children

The cVEMP is a practical test to evaluate vestibulospinal function for children (>2–3 months of age, capable of supporting their head). While AC cVEMP (testing predominantly saccule) can be absent in the presence of middle ear effusion, BC cVEMP (testing saccule and utricle) can overcome the frequent conduction problem in children. Latencies can be useful for the diagnosis of neuropathy impairing vestibulospinal pathways. The cVEMP test supplements the canal vestibular evaluation and should be included in vestibular testing for SNHL and preimplant vestibular testing in children.

Ocular VEMP

Studies on oVEMP have demonstrated that oVEMP testing can be used for assessing utricular function.[14–18] Therefore, oVEMP testing will complement cVEMP testing in the clinical evaluation of dynamic otolith function. Although both cVEMP and oVEMP are vestibular reflexes and may share many similarities, there are significant differences between them. For example, the cVEMP is an inhibitory response that can be recorded on the ipsilateral SCM muscle, whereas the oVEMP is an excitatory response that is best recorded near the extraocular muscle on the side contralateral to stimulation.

The neuropathway of oVEMP starts with the ipsilateral utricle, routes through the superior vestibular nerve to the vestibular nuclei, crosses the midline via the medial longitudinal fasciculus, reaches the contralateral oculomotor nucleus (ie, the third cranial nerve nucleus), and ends at extraocular muscles (primarily the inferior oblique muscle).[19,20] A typical oVEMP recorded with surface EMG electrodes features a series of biphasic waves: the first negative peak (n1) around 10 milliseconds (ms), followed by a positive peak (p1), as seen in Figure 8–6. Measurements of n1/p1 latencies, peak-to-peak (n1-p1) amplitude and threshold are the key values in the interpretation of oVEMP testing outcomes.

Stimulation and Recording Methodology

Historically, there has been a debate about the origins of oVEMP, and these debates are most likely associated with the type of stimulus used to elicit the oVEMP. Although oVEMP can be elicited by multiple modes of stimulation, including vibration and tapping on the forehead or mastoid using a mini shaker, acoustic stimuli are preferred to evoke oVEMP in a clinical setting, especially in young children. With acoustic stimulation, current evidence suggests that oVEMP predominately reflects utricular function. To simplify the use of oVEMP testing for clinical patients, we only discuss oVEMP testing via acoustic stimulation in this chapter, with a focus on air-conducted stimuli.

Acoustic Stimuli

Clicks can be used to elicit oVEMP responses; however, research on oVEMP in animal and human studies has concluded that the best acoustic stimuli are tone-bursts, specifically 500 Hz tone-bursts.[5,8,21,22] For pediatric patients, insert phones are preferred over headphones to deliver the stimuli since insert phones are much lighter in weight and more comfortable to wear. The intensity of the stimuli needs to be calibrated in decibel (dB) sound pressure level (SPL), or peak SPL (pSPL) before oVEMP testing on patients. For clinical convenience, the intensity can be described in normal hearing level (nHL) with proper biocalibration for any given recording system. The correction factor between SPL/pSPL and nHL may vary with the characteristics of the tone-bursts used, usually it is about

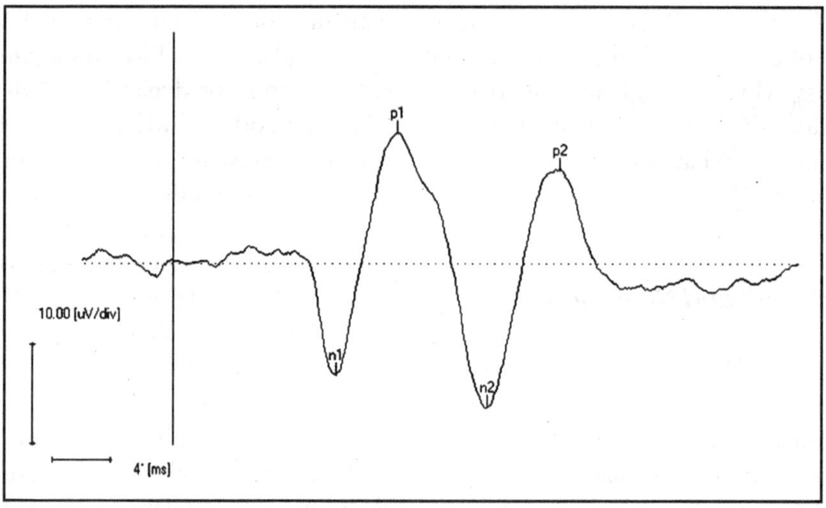

Figure 8–6. Typical oVEMP waveform.

25 to 35 dB. Generally, stimuli of Blackman-gated 500 Hz tone-bursts (8-ms duration) are presented at a slower rate of 5 to 7 per second via insert phones. In cases of children with conductive hearing loss due to known middle ear pathology (eg, otitis media with effusion), air-conducted stimuli delivered through insert phones may not produce oVEMP responses since the stimuli are attenuated. Instead, bone-conducted stimuli via the B71 bone oscillator may be used to elicit the oVEMP.

Electrode Montage

To record oVEMP responses, disposable surface EMG electrodes are often used in pediatric patients. These electrodes need to be good quality and smaller in size (eg, 1 cm in diameter) to avoid falling off, with snap lead on preferred. Typically, the ground (common) electrode should be on the forehead for easy access and retaining. The active (noninverting) electrode is positioned beneath each lower eyelid, while the reference (inverting) electrode is placed about 1 cm below the active electrode. For younger children with a small face, the placement of 2 individual electrodes risks contamination of oVEMP responses, since they are so close together. Therefore, pregelled dual electrodes, as seen in Figure 8–7, are recommended. Ideally, the impedance of individual electrodes should be under 5000 ohms to produce high-quality oVEMP tracings. While other types of electrode montage have been reported in the literature, the one previously described will produce the most reliable oVEMP responses.

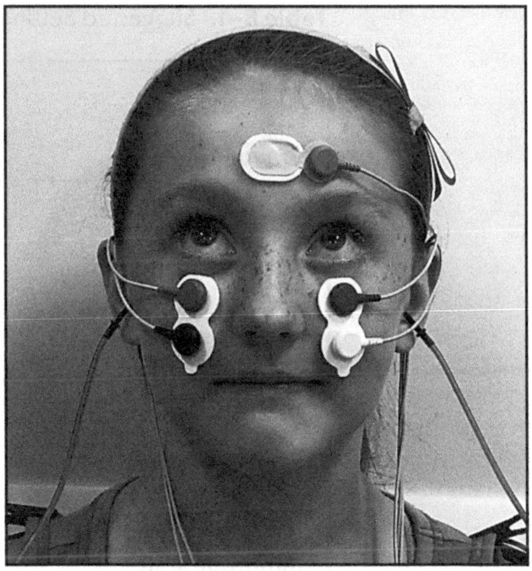

Figure 8–7. Electrode placement for oVEMP.

Recording Protocol of Pediatric oVEMP

Currently, oVEMP recording protocols vary from clinic to clinic. Although no formal consensus is reached at this time regarding the optimal protocol, published studies have produced sufficient data to establish a general approach on this topic.[23–27] Since oVEMP is mostly a contralateral response, a single-channel evoked potential system is capable of recording oVEMP responses; however, a true two-channel recording system is preferred because oVEMP responses can be seen on the ipsilateral side as well, although the waves may look a little different. The setups of pediatric oVEMP recording parameters are summarized in Table 8–1.

To elicit oVEMP responses with acoustic stimulation, patients are instructed to look up (eg, up gaze 30° to 45°) while they are in a sitting position with the head fixed. An attractive visual target may be employed to ensure the patient's best effort to the task. The intensity of the stimuli initially can be set at a level to ensure producing a clear and reliable oVEMP response, such as 125 dB SPL or 90 dB nHL. If no oVEMP response emerges at this level, stimulus intensity can go up to the maximal output level of the recording system used. If oVEMP response is present, the intensity can be dropped by 5 or 10 dB until

Table 8–1. Suggested Settings of oVEMP Testing for Children

Stimuli	***500 Hz Tone-Bursts (duration = 8 ms, eg, 2 cycles rise/fall, no plateau)***
Rate of stimulation	5.1 or 7.1/second
Starting intensity	125 dB SPL or 90 dB nHL
Minimal gain setting	× 5000
Band-pass filter	10 to 1000 Hz
Minimal recording epoch	50 milliseconds (ms)
Number of sweeps	100 to 150
Minimal accepted run	2
Amplitude scale	5 to 10 microvolt (μV)

oVEMP responses disappear. To have a replicable oVEMP, at least two averaging runs are required at a specific intensity.

Measurements of oVEMP

When no clear and repeatable oVEMP responses can be identified with the maximal intensity of stimulation, the oVEMP outcome is generally stated as absent. When oVEMP is present, oVEMP recordings should be described by these parameters: threshold, latency, and amplitude. Threshold of oVEMP is defined as the lowest intensity of stimulus at which oVEMP responses can be identified. For latency, n1 and p1 peaks are marked, and the corresponding time is measured. The amplitude of oVEMP is calculated from peak to peak (eg, n1 to p1). Of note, the amplitude of oVEMP is much lower (eg, 10 to 20 times smaller) than that in cVEMP. Other amplitude measurements (eg, asymmetry ratio) have been reported in the literature to define the oVEMP amplitude difference between the two sides. Each of the parameters has certain diagnostic value in evaluating vestibular disorders, and this topic is addressed in the section on clinical applications.

Feasibility of oVEMP Testing in Children

oVEMP responses usually start to emerge after age 2 years, which differs from cVEMP responses, which can be obtained in patients as early as infancy.[23,28] While older children are capable of following instructions to achieve an up-gaze position during oVEMP testing, younger children (eg, under the age of 5 years) may not maintain the appropriate gaze throughout a session. In our practice, we use attractive toys or videos on a smartphone to get patients' visual attention, ensuring proper gaze during testing. Normally, the patient can be sitting upright with head still for oVEMP testing. To make oVEMP testing more comfortable for younger children, they may choose the supine position, lying on a table. When facing uncooperative children, an assistant is helpful in either controlling the patients or operating the recording system.

Because middle ear issues (such as Eustachian tube dysfunction and otitis media with effusion) are quite common in pediatric patients, otoscopic examination and/or tympanometry are necessary to determine if a child has a healthy middle ear prior to oVEMP testing. Abnormal oVEMP findings (either absent or reduced response to air-conducted stimuli) are common in children with middle ear pathology. Additional testing with bone-conducted stimuli or retesting after the middle ear pathology has resolved is necessary to determine the true status of utricular function in patients with middle ear dysfunction.

Normal oVEMP Characteristics in Children

As mentioned previously, oVEMP responses may be absent in infants but can be recorded in a certain percentage of young children ages 2 to 3 years. Also, oVEMP responses recorded from children aged 3 years or older are very much like those from adults.[23] For oVEMP responses elicited by air-conducted stimuli, the variability of oVEMP threshold, latency, and amplitude is relatively small in healthy children. For example, the n1 latency is normally around 11 to 12 ms, and the p1 latency is about 15 to 16 ms, when Blackman-gated 500 Hz tone-bursts are used as stimuli via insert phones. Normal oVEMP thresholds in children are usually near 80 to 90 dB nHL. The amplitude of oVEMP responses may have some degree of variation depending on the intensity level of the stimulus and patients' effort of maintaining eyes in the upgaze position[29]; nonetheless, it is typically in the range of several to tens of microvolts (μV). Most importantly, these oVEMP measurements are not significantly different between the left side and right side, and gender difference is negligible, as well.[30–33] Unlike in adults, bone-conducted stimuli are also effective in eliciting oVEMP responses in pediatric patients; however, the waveforms may differ to some extent.[34]

oVEMP in Children With Vestibular Disorders

Accurate diagnosis of pediatric vestibular disorders can be challenging, since standard vestibular evaluations such as caloric and rotational tests are difficult for young children to do. Contemporary vestibular tests such as cVEMP and oVEMP are proven to be effective and more feasible to conduct in young children with suspected vestibular disorders.

In patients with vestibular neuritis, oVEMP testing, along with cVEMP testing, can be helpful in determining which branch of the vestibular nerve is involved.[35–37] Specifically, oVEMP is usually absent or abnormal, while the cVEMP is intact in cases of superior vestibular neuritis. In contrast, both oVEMP and cVEMP responses are most likely absent in children with labyrinthitis. Vestibular migraine (VM) can be frequently seen in pediatric patients, especially in teenagers. Benign paroxysmal vertigo of childhood (BPVC) is another common cause of episodic vertigo in young children. It is commonly believed that children with VM or BPVC should have normal vestibular function. Recent studies, however, have shown a certain degree of vestibular loss in some children with VM or BPVC. When compared to healthy children, abnormal cVEMP and oVEMP responses were reported in children with VM and BPVC, including amplitude asymmetry and delayed latency.[19,38,39]

oVEMP in Children With Hearing Loss

About 60% of children with hearing loss also have some degree of vestibular loss.[40] Absent cVEMP and oVEMP responses were found in hearing-impaired children, especially in children with syndromic hearing loss (eg, Usher syndrome), hearing loss associated with viral infection (eg, cytomegalovirus) or use of ototoxic drugs.[41–46] Although oVEMP results may not correlate with the degree of a child's hearing loss, the absence of oVEMP responses is most likely a result of malformed vestibules or postinfection utricular dysfunction. The loss of peripheral vestibular function in early life can lead to delays in a child's motor development and balance function.[47,48] Therefore, hearing-impaired children with balance problems or delayed motor development should be referred for a full vestibular evaluation, including oVEMP testing.

It should be noted that abnormal cVEMP and oVEMP responses can also be found in children with hearing loss associated with neuropathies (eg, Charcot-Marie-Tooth disease[49] and Guillain-Barré syndrome[13]). Typical oVEMP findings in this setting may include the absence of oVEMP responses or delays in oVEMP latencies.

oVEMP Testing and Cochlear Implantation

A number of studies in the last few years have published on vestibular outcomes in children with cochlear implants (CIs), and subsequently, pre- and post-CI vestibular testing has been recommended as a required evaluation for all CI candidates.[11,36,50–53] Since limited tools are available to assess vestibular function in young children, oVEMP along with cVEMP testing can provide valuable information on children's peripheral vestibular function. As previously stated, peripheral vestibular loss can be found in children with SNHL; therefore, pre-CI vestibular testing will establish a baseline. If abnormal oVEMP is found, it should be explained to the parents and reported to the surgeon who can make a better decision about CI surgery. Post-CI oVEMP testing is also valuable, either confirming stable utricular function after the surgery or identifying a functional change.

oVEMP in Children With Third Window Conditions

The most common third window conditions in pediatric patients are superior semicircular canal dehiscence (SSCD) and enlarged vestibular aqueduct (EVA). First described by Minor et al in 1998,[54] patients with SSCD may have auditory and/or vestibular symptoms.[55,56] While symptomatic SSCD is found primarily in adults, a few studies have demonstrated SSCD in the pediatric population. In fact, many believe SSCD is a developmental failure, and there may be a higher incidence of SSCD in young children compared to adults.[57,58] Although diagnosis of SSCD usually requires imaging confirmation, cVEMP and oVEMP testing has proved to be a valuable tool (with high sensitivity and specificity) in the clinical evaluation of SSCD.[19,56,59] Recently, oVEMP testing is reported to be more effective in diagnosing SSCD.[60–62] Similar to adults with SSCD, oVEMP responses with high amplitude can be found in pediatric patients with SSCD. If tested, a lower threshold is also noticeable.

The association between hearing loss and EVA has been well established clinically since the initial report by Valvassori and Clemis in 1978.[63] EVA is reported to be the most common structural inner ear anomaly in children with permanent hearing loss.[64,65] Hearing loss associated with EVA varies greatly and can be sensorineural, conductive, or mixed. Clinical studies of cVEMP and oVEMP responses in patients with EVA have demonstrated similar

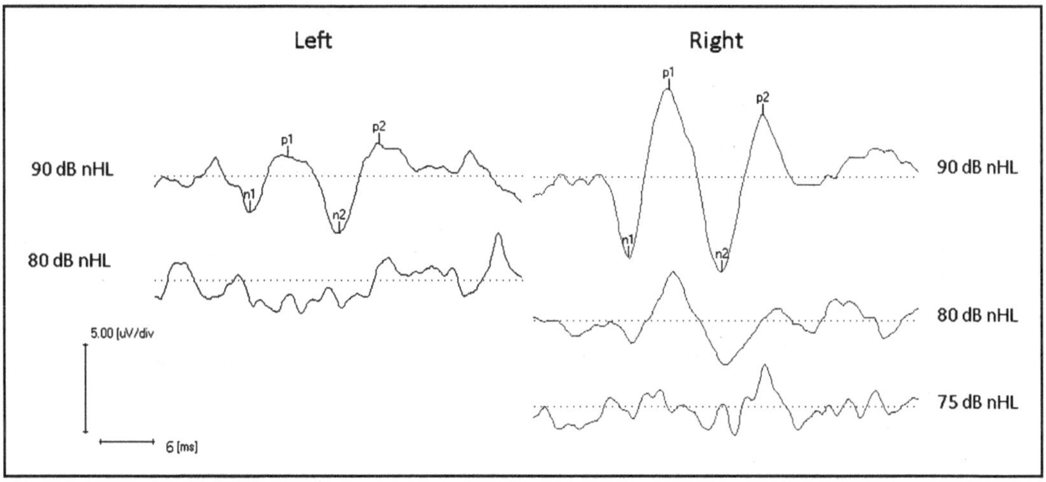

Figure 8–8. Waveforms of oVEMP from a child with right EVA.

features (ie, extremely high amplitudes and low thresholds, see Figure 8–8) to SSCD.[66–69] It is also common to see air-bone gaps in the hearing loss associated with EVA, especially at lower frequencies, such as 250 and 500 Hz.[66] Unlike the conductive hearing loss caused by middle ear pathologies, the air-bone gaps in cases of EVA are not middle ear related. Therefore, oVEMP responses can still be present regardless of the presence of air-bone gaps. In a small percentage of pediatric patients with bilateral EVA and Pendred syndrome, oVEMP responses can be absent, suggesting a peripheral vestibular loss.

Conclusion on oVEMP Testing in Children

Complementary to cVEMP testing for saccular function, oVEMP testing can assess the vestibular function of the utricle. Clinically, it can be used to evaluate pediatric patients (age >2 years) with suspected vestibular impairment. Abnormal oVEMP findings can be seen in children with several disorders, including vestibular neuritis, labyrinthitis, malformation of the inner ear (eg, SSCD and EVA), and neuropathies. Other clinical applications of oVEMP are still evolving.

Self-Assessment Questions

1. VEMPs are always absent in patients with SNHL:
   a. False
   b. True
2. BC cVEMPs can be recorded in the presence of a conductive hearing loss:
   a. True
   b. False

3. cVEMPs can be recorded in:
   a. Adults only
   b. Adults and children 5 years and older
   c. Adults, children, and infants

4. There is no difference in cVEMP characteristics between children and adults:
   a. True
   b. False

5. Peripheral neuropathies do not influence VEMP responses:
   a. False
   b. True

6. What otolith structure is tested by cVEMP by BC?
   a. The saccule
   b. Both saccule and utricle
   c. The utricle

7. oVEMPs can be recorded in infants:
   a. False
   b. True

8. Which otolith organ is tested by oVEMP?
   a. The saccule
   b. Both saccule and utricle
   c. The utricle

References

1. Colebatch JG, Halmagyi GM. Vestibular evoked potentials in human neck muscles before and after unilateral vestibular deafferentation. *Neurology*. 1992;42(8):1635–1636.
2. Colebatch JG, Halmagyi GM, Skuse NF. Myogenic potentials generated by a click-evoked vestibulocollic reflex. *J Neurol Neurosurg Psychiatry*. 1994;57(2):190–197.
3. Halmagyi GM, Colebatch JG, Curthoys IS. New tests of vestibular function. *Baillieres Clin Neurol.* 1994;3(3):485–500.
4. Rosengren SM, McAngus Todd NP, Colebatch JG. Vestibular-evoked extraocular potentials produced by stimulation with bone-conducted sound. *Clin Neurophysiol.* 2005;116(8):1938–1948.
5. Curthoys IS, Iwasaki S, Chihara Y, Ushio M, McGarvie LA, Burgess AM. The ocular vestibular-evoked myogenic potential to air-conducted sound; probable superior vestibular nerve origin. *Clin Neurophysiol.* 2011;122(3):611–616.
6. Welgampola MS, Rosengren SM, Halmagyi GM, Colebatch JG. Vestibular activation by bone conducted sound. *J Neurol Neurosurg Psychiatry.* 2003;74(6):771–778.

7. Sheykholeslami K, Murofushi T, Kermany MH, Kaga K. Bone-conducted evoked myogenic potentials from the sternocleidomastoid muscle. *Acta Otolaryngol.* 2000;120(6):731–734.
8. Curthoys IS, Kim J, McPhedran SK, Camp AJ. Bone conducted vibration selectively activates irregular primary otolithic vestibular neurons in the guinea pig. *Exp Brain Res.* 2006;175(2):256–267.
9. Lim CL, Clouston P, Sheean G, Yiannikas C. The influence of voluntary EMG activity and click intensity on the vestibular click evoked myogenic potential. *Muscle Nerve.* 1995;18(10):1210–1213.
10. Colebatch JG, Rothwell JC. Motor unit excitability changes mediating vestibulocollic reflexes in the sternocleidomastoid muscle. *Clin Neurophysiol.* 2004;115(11):2567–2573.
11. Jacot E, Van Den Abbeele T, Debre HR, Wiener-Vacher SR. Vestibular impairments pre- and post-cochlear implant in children. *Int J Pediatr Otorhinolaryngol.* 2009;73(2):209–217.
12. Welgampola MS, Colebatch JG. Vestibulocollic reflexes: Normal values and the effect of age. *Clin Neurophysiol.* 2001;112(11):1971–1979.
13. Jacot E, Wiener-Vacher S. Potential value of vestibular evoked myogenic potentials in paediatric neuropathies. *J Vestib Res.* 2008;18(4):231–237.
14. Todd NP, Rosengren SM, Aw ST, Colebatch JG. Ocular vestibular evoked myogenic potentials (OVEMPs) produced by air- and bone-conducted sound. *Clin Neurophysiol.* 2007;118(2):381–390.
15. Iwasaki S, McGarvie LA, Halmagyi GM, et al. Head taps evoke a crossed vestibulo ocular reflex. *Neurology.* 2007;68(15):1227–1229.
16. Iwasaki S, Chihara Y, Smulders YE, et al. The role of the superior vestibular nerve in generating ocular vestibular-evoked myogenic potentials to bone conducted vibration at Fz. *Clin Neurophysiol.* 2009;120(3):588–593.
17. Curthoys IS, Vulovic V, Manzari L. Ocular vestibular-evoked myogenic potential (oVEMP) to test utricular function: Neural and oculomotor evidence. *Acta Otorhinolaryngol Ital.* 2012;32(1):41–45.
18. Curthoys IS, Burgess AM, McGarvie LA. What is the adequate stimulus for the oVEMP n10 to bone-conducted vibration? A reply to the letter by Todd and Colebatch (2014). *Ear Hear.* 2014;35(4):487–489.
19. Fife TD, Colebatch JG, Kerber KA, et al. Practice guideline: Cervical and ocular vestibular evoked myogenic potential testing: Report of the Guideline Development, Dissemination, and Implementation Subcommittee of the American Academy of Neurology. *Neurology.* 2017;89(22):2288–2296.
20. Dlugaiczyk J. Ocular vestibular evoked myogenic potentials: Where are we now? *Otol Neurotol.* 2017;38(10):e513–e521.
21. Curthoys IS, Vulovic V. Vestibular primary afferent responses to sound and vibration in the guinea pig. *Exp Brain Res.* 2011;210(3–4):347–352.
22. Curthoys IS, Vulovic V, Burgess AM, et al. The basis for using bone-conducted vibration or air-conducted sound to test otolithic function. *Ann NY Acad Sci.* 2011;1233:231–241.
23. Wang SJ, Hsieh WS, Young YH. Development of ocular vestibular-evoked myogenic potentials in small children. *Laryngoscope.* 2013;123(2):512–517.
24. Young YH, Chen CN, Hsieh WS, Wang SJ. Development of vestibular evoked myogenic potentials in early life. *Eur J Paediatr Neurol.* 2009;13(3):235–239.
25. Wang SJ, Jaw FS, Young YH. Ocular vestibular-evoked myogenic potentials elicited from monaural versus binaural acoustic stimulations. *Clin Neurophysiol.* 2009;120(2):420–423.
26. Piker EG, Jacobson GP, McCaslin DL, Hood LJ. Normal characteristics of the ocular vestibular evoked myogenic potential. *J Am Acad Audiol.* 2011;22(4):222–230.
27. Mallinson A, Kuijpers A, Longridge N. Optimum number of sweeps in clinical OVEMP recording; How many sweeps are necessary? *J Int Adv Otol.* 2018;14(1):72–76.
28. Young YH. Assessment of functional development of the otolithic system in growing children: A review. *Int J Pediatr Otorhinolaryngol.* 2015;79(4):435–442.
29. Rosengren SM, Colebatch JG, Straumann D, Weber KP. Why do oVEMPs become larger

when you look up? Explaining the effect of gaze elevation on the ocular vestibular evoked myogenic potential. *Clin Neurophysiol.* 2013; 124(4):785–791.

30. Rosengren SM, Govender S, Colebatch JG. Ocular and cervical vestibular evoked myogenic potentials produced by air- and bone-conducted stimuli: Comparative properties and effects of age. *Clin Neurophysiol.* 2011; 122(11):2282–2289.
31. Walther LE, Schaaf H, Sommer D, Hormann K. [Air conducted ocular VEMP: I. Determination of a method and application in normal patients]. *Laryngo- rhino- otologie.* 2011; 90(7):410–415.
32. Hsu YS, Wang SJ, Young YH. Ocular vestibular-evoked myogenic potentials in children using air conducted sound stimulation. *Clin Neurophysiol.* 2009;120(7):1381–1385.
33. Kastanioudakis I, Saravakos P, Leontis T, Balatsouras DG, Ziavra N. Ocular vestibular-evoked myogenic potentials using air-conducted sound: Test parameters and normative data in healthy children; effect of body position on threshold. *Eur Arch Otorhinolaryngol.* 2016;273(9):2385–2394.
34. Chou CH, Hsu WC, Young YH. Ocular vestibular-evoked myogenic potentials via bone-conducted vibration in children. *Clin Neurophysiol.* 2012;123(9):1880–1885.
35. Govender S, Colebatch JG. Ocular vestibular evoked myogenic potential (oVEMP) responses in acute vestibular neuritis. *Clin Neurophysiol.* 2012;123(5):1054–1055; author reply 1055–1056; discussion 1056–1057.
36. Kantner C, Gurkov R. Characteristics and clinical applications of ocular vestibular evoked myogenic potentials. *Hear Res.* 2012; 294(1–2):55–63.
37. Govender S, Rosengren SM, Colebatch JG. Vestibular neuritis has selective effects on air- and bone-conducted cervical and ocular vestibular evoked myogenic potentials. *Clin Neurophysiol.* 2011;122(6):1246–1255.
38. Brodsky J, Kaur K, Shoshany T, Lipson S, Zhou G. Benign paroxysmal migraine variants of infancy and childhood: Transitions and clinical features. *Eur J Paediatr Neurol.* 2018; 22(4):667–673.
39. Brodsky JR, Cusick BA, Zhou G. Evaluation and management of vestibular migraine in children: Experience from a pediatric vestibular clinic. *Eur J Paediatr Neurol.* 2016;20(1): 85–92.
40. Wiener-Vacher SR, Quarez J, Priol AL. Epidemiology of vestibular impairments in a pediatric population. *Semin Hear.* 2018;39(3): 229–242.
41. Zagolski O. Vestibular system in infants after systemic therapy with amikacin. *J Otolaryngol Head Neck Surg.* 2008;37(4):534–539.
42. Zagolski O. Vestibular-evoked myogenic potentials and caloric stimulation in infants with congenital cytomegalovirus infection. *J Laryngol Otol.* 2008;122(6):574–579.
43. Magliulo G, Iannella G, Gagliardi S, et al. Usher's syndrome: Evaluation of the vestibular system with cervical and ocular vestibular evoked myogenic potentials and the video head impulse test. *Otol Neurotol.* 2015;36(8): 1421–1427.
44. Magliulo G, Gagliardi S, Ciniglio Appiani M, Iannella G, Re M. Vestibular neurolabyrinthitis: A follow-up study with cervical and ocular vestibular evoked myogenic potentials and the video head impulse test. *Ann Otol Rhinol Laryngol.* 2014;123(3):162–173.
45. Zagolski O. Vestibular-evoked myogenic potentials and caloric tests in infants with congenital rubella. *B-ENT.* 2009;5(1):7–12.
46. Wiener-Vacher SR, Obeid R, Abou-Elew M. Vestibular impairment after bacterial meningitis delays infant posturomotor development. *J Pediatr.* Aug 2012;161(2):246–251 e241.
47. Inoue A, Iwasaki S, Ushio M, et al. Effect of vestibular dysfunction on the development of gross motor function in children with profound hearing loss. *Audiol Neurootol.* 2013; 18(3):143–151.
48. Shall MS. The importance of saccular function to motor development in children with hearing impairments. *Int J Otolaryngol.* 2009; 2009:972565.
49. Sinha SK, Shankar K, Sharanya R. Cervical and ocular vestibular evoked myogenic potentials test results in individuals with auditory neuropathy spectrum disorders. *Audiol Res.* 2013;3(1):e4.

50. Cushing SL, Papsin BC, Rutka JA, James AL, Blaser SL, Gordon KA. Vestibular end-organ and balance deficits after meningitis and cochlear implantation in children correlate poorly with functional outcome. *Otol Neurotol.* 2009;30(4):488–495.
51. Licameli G, Zhou G, Kenna MA. Disturbance of vestibular function attributable to cochlear implantation in children. *Laryngoscope.* 2009; 119(4):740–745.
52. Cushing SL, Gordon KA, Rutka JA, James AL, Papsin BC. Vestibular end-organ dysfunction in children with sensorineural hearing loss and cochlear implants: An expanded cohort and etiologic assessment. *Otol Neurotol.* 2013; 34(3):422–428.
53. Janky KL, Givens D. Vestibular, visual acuity, and balance outcomes in children with cochlear implants: A preliminary report. *Ear Hear.* 2015;36(6):e364–e372.
54. Minor LB, Solomon D, Zinreich JS, Zee DS. Sound- and/or pressure-induced vertigo due to bone dehiscence of the superior semicircular canal. *Arch Otolaryngol Head Neck Surg.* 1998;124(3):249–258.
55. Minor LB. Clinical manifestations of superior semicircular canal dehiscence. *Laryngoscope.* Oct 2005;115(10):1717–1727.
56. Zhou G, Gopen Q, Poe DS. Clinical and diagnostic characterization of canal dehiscence syndrome: A great otologic mimicker. *Otol Neurotol.* 2007;28(7):920–926.
57. Carey JP, Minor LB, Nager GT. Dehiscence or thinning of bone overlying the superior semicircular canal in a temporal bone survey. *Arch Otolaryngol Head Neck Surg.* 2000;126(2):137–147.
58. Zhou G, Ohlms L, Liberman J, Amin M. Superior semicircular canal dehiscence in a young child: Implication of developmental defect. *Int J Pediatr Otorhinolaryngol.* 2007; 71(12):1925–1928.
59. Hunter JB, Patel NS, O'Connell BP, et al. Cervical and ocular VEMP testing in diagnosing superior semicircular canal dehiscence. *Otolaryngol Head Neck Surg.* 2017;156(5):917–923.
60. Zuniga MG, Davalos-Bichara M, Schubert MC, Carey JP, Janky KL. Optimizing ocular vestibular evoked myogenic potential testing for superior semicircular canal dehiscence syndrome: Electrode placement. *Audiol Neurootol.* 2014;19(4):239–247.
61. Janky KL, Zuniga MG, Schubert MC, Carey JP. The effect of increased intracranial pressure on vestibular evoked myogenic potentials in superior canal dehiscence syndrome. *Clin Neurophysiol.* 2015;126(4):780–786.
62. Janky KL, Nguyen KD, Welgampola M, Zuniga MG, Carey JP. Air-conducted oVEMPs provide the best separation between intact and superior canal dehiscent labyrinths. *Otol Neurotol.* 2013;34(1):127–134.
63. Valvassori GE, Clemis JD. The large vestibular aqueduct syndrome. *Laryngoscope.* 1978;88(5):723–728.
64. Madden C, Halsted M, Benton C, Greinwald J, Choo D. Enlarged vestibular aqueduct syndrome in the pediatric population. *Otol Neurotol.* 2003;24(4):625–632.
65. Berrettini S, Forli F, Bogazzi F, et al. Large vestibular aqueduct syndrome: Audiological, radiological, clinical, and genetic features. *Am J Otolaryngol.* 2005;26(6):363–371.
66. Zhou G, Gopen Q, Kenna MA. Delineating the hearing loss in children with enlarged vestibular aqueduct. *Laryngoscope.* 2008;118(11): 2062–2066.
67. Taylor RL, Bradshaw AP, Magnussen JS, Gibson WP, Halmagyi GM, Welgampola MS. Augmented ocular vestibular evoked myogenic potentials to air-conducted sound in large vestibular aqueduct syndrome. *Ear Hear.* 2012;33(6):768–771.
68. Sheykholeslami K, Schmerber S, Habiby Kermany M, Kaga K. Vestibular-evoked myogenic potentials in three patients with large vestibular aqueduct. *Hear Res.* 2004;190(1–2):161–168.
69. Zhou G, Gopen Q. Characteristics of vestibular evoked myogenic potentials in children with enlarged vestibular aqueduct. *Laryngoscope.* 2011;121(1):220–225.

CHAPTER 9

Static Balance: Computerized Dynamic Posturography

Eugen Ionescu, Pierre Reynard, Nathalie Goulème, and Hung Thai-Van

History of Static Balance Testing

In physics, an object is said to be in a state of equilibrium when the forces that act on it are balanced. In proper standing position, the center of gravity (COG) of the human body is a hypothetical point around which the force of gravity acts. Static balance control implies to keep strictly the projection at ground of the COG called center of pressure (COP) in the interior of the supporting polygon (SP), which is the area beneath the body, between the feet (Figure 9–1). If the COP falls outside the SP, in order to stay balanced, a motor reaction is needed. This task is coordinated by sensorimotor strategies that stabilize the COP during both self-initiated or externally triggered stimuli, which constitutes postural control (PC).[1]

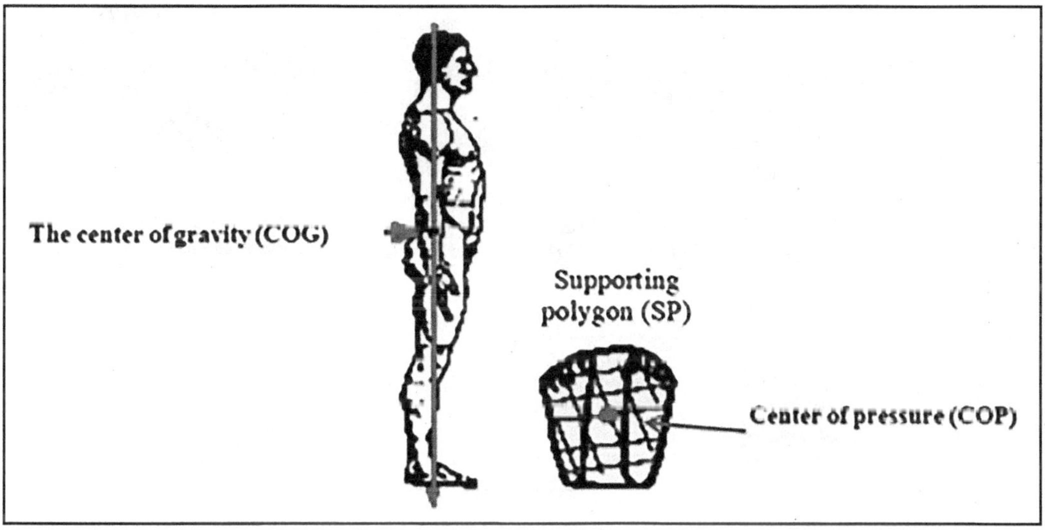

Figure 9–1. Static equilibrium condition: projection of the center of gravity (COG) in the interior of the supporting polygon (SP).

Static balance evaluation provides a functional measurement of the contribution to PC of the sensory systems. At the advent of the development of neurologic evaluation, the Romberg test (RT) or Romberg maneuver was the first tool to assess balance. The RT was described in 1846 by Khasnis and Gokula,[2] then by another clinician who understood the great value of this sign that became one of the cornerstones of the neurologic examination.[3] Optimal PC requires accurate information from three peripheral sensorial systems: visual, vestibular, and proprioceptive (somatosensory). Although disturbance in any of these sensorial modalities can be completely or partially substituted by input from the other two systems, loss and distortion of inputs as well as difficulties with regard to integrating information, is often associated with disequilibrium. Patients with significant somatosensory impairment or with vestibular dysfunction may fall when vision is suppressed.

The RT is positive when the patient shows important disequilibrium laterally or backward while keeping his or her eyes closed (Figure 9–2). Early in its history, the Rom-

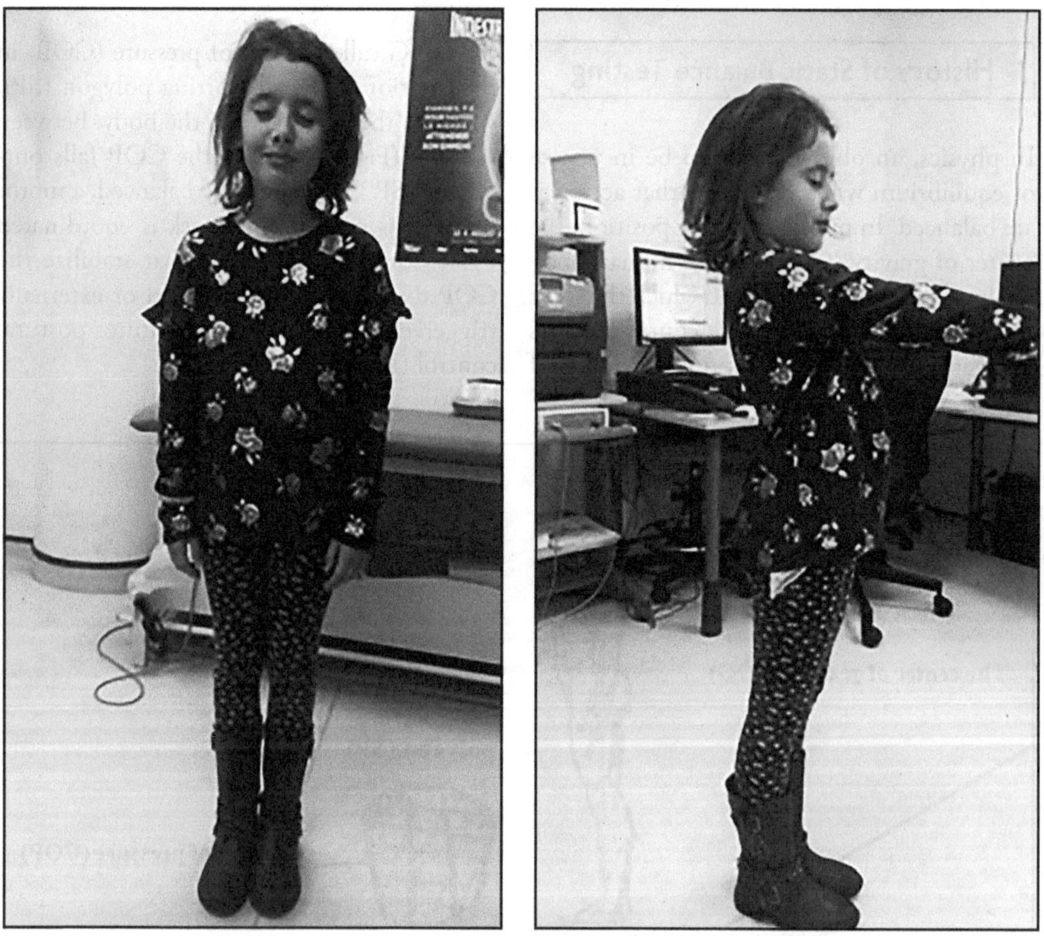

A B

Figure 9–2. Romberg Test. **A.** The feet are in contact, eyes closed, neutral head, teeth without contact, the arms along the body, we observe the spontaneous inclination of the body. **B.** Then, we ask the child to stretch the arms in front of her, the index in contact, we observe the oscillation.

berg sign was described as specific to the diagnosis of tabes dorsalis. Presently, it is widely accepted that a positive RT indicates proprioceptive loss. Positive RT can also be present in labyrinthine impairment (eg. vestibular Romberg sign). In acute labyrinthine disorders, it has been described that the imbalance appears shortly after closing the eyes and consists of a slow lateral inclination of the body toward the affected side.[4] This deviation is reproducible and may vary with the position of the head. Generally, this condition is attributed to a positive index test. Lateral deviation of the index is noted toward the side of labyrinthine impairment.

Clinical evaluation of the peripheral vestibular system continued to improve and expand as well it became more specific with the Fukuda test or stepping test.[5] This test is derived from a variation on the "Tretversuch test," initially described in 1938.[6] The stepping test evaluates motor reactions of the head and neck, which rely on vestibulospinal reflexes. Patients are required to step in place for 50 to 100 steps with both arms extended. Normal subjects generally show slight or no deviation or axial rotation (spin), whereas patients with acute peripheral vestibular dysfunction rotate progressively toward the side of their lesion. A spin greater than 30° suggests labyrinthine impairment, the weaker side being identified by the direction of rotation.

Lanska has reported use of a quantitative computer-calculated RT and concluded that it is a reasonable way of measuring postural stability.[3] As a result, RT has contributed significantly to the development of mechanical devices for evaluating balance control.

Posturographic Evaluation

Posturography is an approach to assess static balance using force platforms. In this way, posturography provides various objectives measures such as quantification of body sway. Two types of platforms have been developed to evaluate postural control: static and dynamic.

Static Platforms

On this type of platform, subjects are evaluated while they stand still on a flat, horizontal, unperturbed surface with eyes open initially and then with the eyes closed generally for 30 seconds in each condition. The spontaneous movements called postural sway are recorded through the trajectory of the COP, which is proportional to the ground-reaction torque and coincides with the vertical projection of the body's center of mass.[7] The result represents the body sway named statokinesigram (Figure 9–3). This first evaluation condition uses the RT and the outcome is quantified with respect to changes in COP displacement amplitude, distance, and/or velocity, the subject being in still stance in order to measure the influence of vision on postural stability. The ratio of surface of the COP with eyes

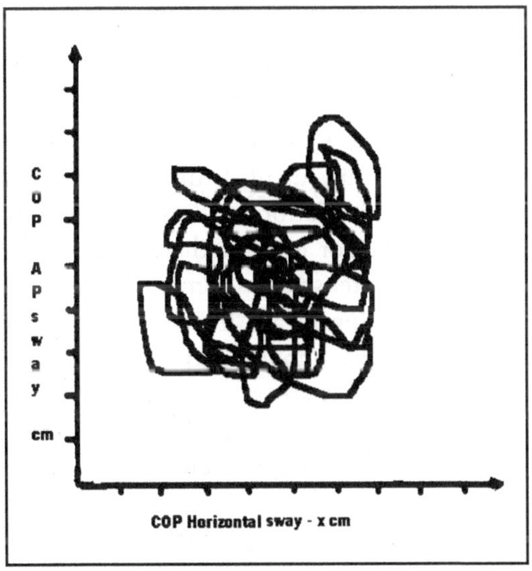

Figure 9–3. Oscillation of center of pressure (statokinesogram).

closed and eyes open is called the Romberg quotient (RQ) and reflects the influence of vision on the postural sway. An RQ >2.5 is considered to be pathologic.

Dynamic Platforms

This method principally consists of the intentional perturbation of the subject's equilibrium is in order to observe its ability to appropriately use visual, vestibular, and/or somatosensory inputs for regaining stability by diminishing postural sway.

There are many commercially available devices developed by manufacturers around the world. The most sophisticated but also more expensive are the "computerized platforms." The advantage of these machines are that somatosensory, visual, and vestibular input may be alternatively attenuated or suppressed while evaluating the subject's sway. Each sensory condition provides a specific vestibular score that is sway dependent. The limitation of these methods are that normative data (for children and/or adults) may not be available when purchasing one or another system. Therefore, before using a computerized dynamic platform, each center needs to produce their own normative data in their target clinical or research population.

Since 1999, we have had the experience of the daily us of 2 different dynamic posturographic platforms (EquiTest and Balance Quest). For each of these systems, we performed extensive assessments in normal subjects ranging in age from 3 to 80 years. The results were published previously and are revisited in this chapter.

We developed some basic aspects of posturology and used our technique to assess young subjects on both devices. Some insights about dynamic posturography based on nearly 20 years of experience will be summarized in this chapter.

Physiologic Concept and Basis of the Dynamic Posturography

The PC concept evolved in the 1970s through several groups.[8,9] The authors hypothesized that the brain uses vestibular inputs as an internal reference system for orientation about which adaptive changes in proprioceptive and visual inputs are made. Several studies were designed to confirm this hypothesis in returning astronauts.[10] All of them demonstrated transient vestibular-dependent deterioration of postural control upon return to normal gravity. One of the major conclusions of these studies was that the postural impairment observed on landing was caused by a temporary inability to use vestibular information. These and other results[11] support the hypothesis, documenting the effects of gravitational vector on the otolith system, and point out the prominent gravity-dependent role of the vestibular system on PC.[8]

The EquiTest Platform

At the time he postulated his theory, Nashner developed computerized dynamic posturography (CDP) (EquiTest, NeuroCom International, Clackamas, Oregon).[9] The EquiTest system consists of a motor-driven footplate capable of translations in the anterior-posterior directions and rotations about the ankle joint. The computer processes signals from the force-sensing support surface to quantify the subject's postural stability under modified sensory conditions and the motor reactions to unexpected perturbations. Subsequently, and despite some criticisms,[12] CDP has become the standard for balance-control assessment in medical and scientific institutions worldwide.

A key test in the dynamic posturography system is the Sensory Organization Test

(SOT). It provides information about the integration of the visual, proprioceptive, and vestibular components of balance, which leads to an outcome measure called the equilibrium score (ES). The ES is calculated from the maximum anterior and posterior angle sway compared with the theoretical limits of stability, anteriorly and posteriorly, as shown in the following equation:

$$ES = \{12.5 - [\theta max\ (ant) - \theta max\ (post)]\}/12.5$$

where θmax (ant) is the maximum anterior sway angle in degrees (8.25°) during a trial, and θmax (post) is the maximum posterior sway angle in degrees (4.25°) measured during the same trial.[12,13] That score is expressed as a percentage. The higher the ES, the less the subject swayed. The sensory analysis (SA) measures the patient's ability to make effective use of visual, vestibular, and proprioceptive information, or to suppress it if inappropriate. Scores represent the influence of each sensory system on the individual's stability (Table 9–1).

SOT Assessment in Children With EquiTest

The SOT is performed in standing position for 6 conditions as described in Figure 9–4.

The standard protocol as described by NeuroCom includes three trials of 20 seconds for each condition. When a trial ends by a fall (injury being prevented by the safety harness) or by stepping off of the platform marks, it is scored zero. The EquiTest software automatically calculates the results of ES and SA. Recorded data for each EquiTest condition as well as SA ratios must be compared with normative data. There are two ways to display the results: graphically and numerically. The graphic result is easy to use and comprehensive

Table 9–1. The Algorithm to Obtain Sensory Analysis Using Equilibrium Score Produced Through the Six Conditions[a]

Ratio	*Comparison*	*Functional Relevance*
Somatosensory	C2 C1	Patient's ability to use input from the somatosensory system to maintain balance
Visual	C4 C1	Patient's ability to use input from the visual system to maintain balance
Vestibular	C5 C1	Patient's ability to use input from the vestibular system to maintain balance
Preference	C3 + C6 C2 + C5	The degree to which a patient relies on visual information to maintain balance, even when the information is incorrect

Abbreviations: *C1* eyes open, visual surround, stable platform (SP); *C2* eyes closed, SP; *C3* eyes open, sway-referenced visual surround, SP; *C4* eyes open, fixed visual surround, unstable platform (UP) (sway-referenced surface); *C5* eyes closed, UP (sway-referenced surface); *C6* eyes open, UP (sway-referenced visual surround).

[a]Data from NeuroCom (Clackamas, Oregon). Sensory analysis was calculated through equilibrium score ratios.

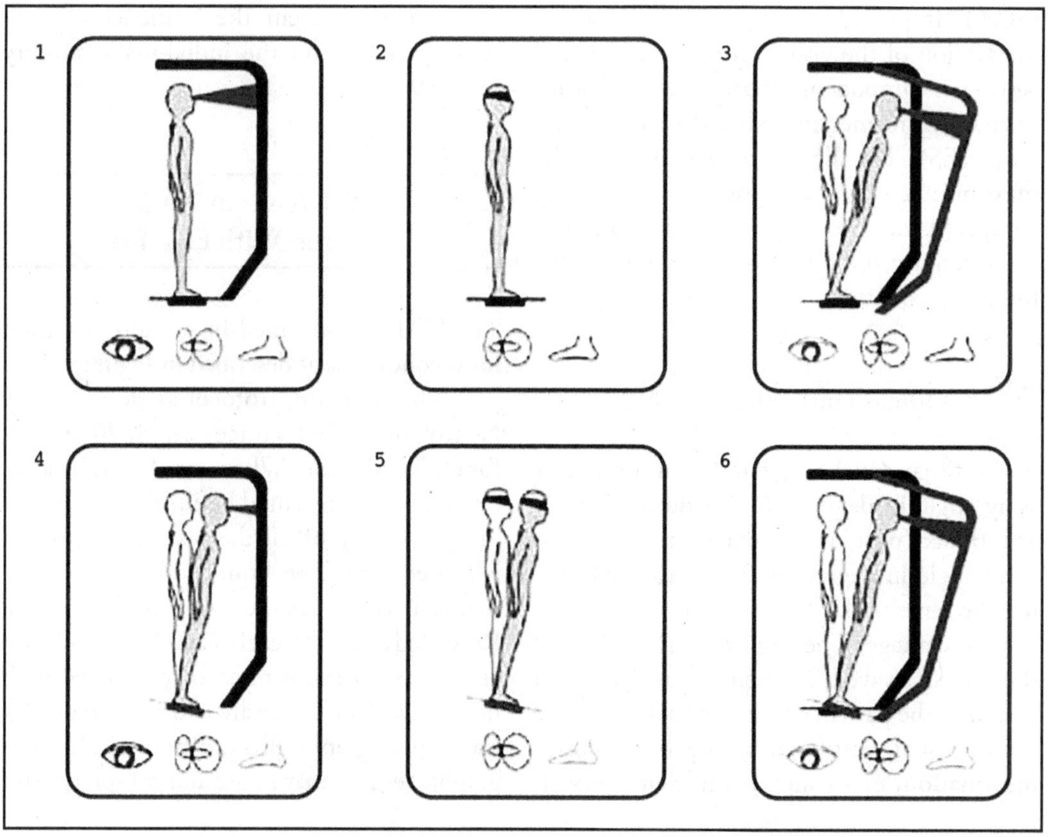

Figure 9–4. Equitest: Sensory Organization Test. The six sensorial conditions. (Reproduced with permission of Neurocom, Clackamas, Oregon.)

because the scores for each trial are displayed as a green or red bar while comparing with the available normative data (gray bar). The lack of reliable normative data calculated according to age and anthropologic characteristics (eg, weight, height, or gender) has been reported by several authors.[14–19] Some studies have focused on normative data for SOT in children, but only a few of them were performed on the EquiTest platform.[20–22]

Our method to produce normative data including SOT was slightly modified by adapting it for young subjects as follows: in order to keep the children's visual attention in "eyes-open" conditions, we taped a little toy at the appropriate height to the Equi Test cabin (Figure 9–5; also see the companion website for details). Under these specific conditions, which tests the reliability of the visual cue, the children were instructed to look toward the toy.

Two trials of 20 seconds each were performed for each of the six conditions. We systematically used only two trials, since in a preliminary study conducted in this population, we observed a significant rank effect when comparing ES between the second and third trials, as requested in the standard SOT. This modification in the SOT protocol still allows us to obtain the composite index (CI), as it is evaluated as a weighted average of the scores from the six conditions of the two trials with more emphasis on conditions 3 through 6. Actual data were collected during this assessment.

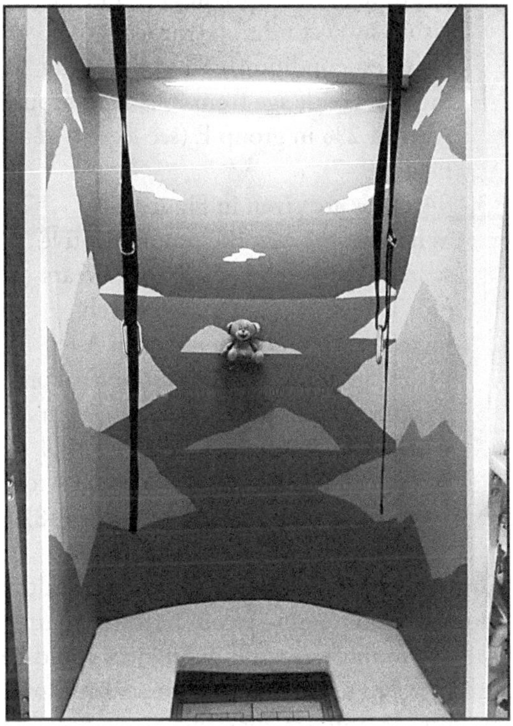

Figure 9–5. EquiTest cabin with the little toy to keep the children's visual attention.

EquiTest Normative Data: Comments

Between 2001 and 2004, we assessed for our department use, equilibrium parameters through SOT (ES and SA ratios) on EquiTest in 186 normal children. The motor control test or the adaptation test classically related to CDP assessment was not included because our main goal was to observe the SOT hierarchy and its maturation through age groups.[18]

The normative data provided rely on a series of 186 healthy children divided into four age groups: 6 to 7 years (n = 35), 8 to 9 years (n = 32), 10 to 11 years (n = 65), and 12 to 13 years (n = 54). A control group of 66 healthy young adults aged 20 to 22 years was also included to compare vestibular characteristics through those five age groups. Characteristics of the studied groups are given in Table 9–2. All subjects met the 7 inclusion criteria used by NeuroCom to produce normative data for EquiTest, plus one additional criterion[23] as provided in Table 9–3. Subjects were excluded if any one of the inclusion criterion were unmet or transiently evoked otoacoustic emissions were abnormal. The studied parameters (ES and SOT) were compared between groups using analysis of variance.

Table 9–2. Physical and Anthropologic Characteristics in the Five Studied Groups According to Age, Height, Weight, and Gender[a]

	Group A	*Group B*	*Group C*	*Group D*	*Group E*
Age (years)	6 to 7	8 to 9	10 to 11	12 to 13	20 to 22
Number	35	32	65	54	66
Mean Age	6.8 ± 0.01	8.6 ± 0.01	10.3 ± 0.06	12.3 ± 0.01	20.7 ± 0.5
Height (cm)	123.5 ± 0.91	134.9 ± 1.52	141.6 ± 2.39	155.9 ± 1.24	170.9 ± 1.14
Weight (kg)	24.2 ± 0.75	30.4 ± 0.93	36.5 ± 0.90	45.1 ± 1.3	61.2 ± 1.23
Males (%)	34	56	51	53.7	45.5
Females (%)	66	44	49	46.3	54.5

[a]With regard to these characteristics, all of the studied groups differed significantly (analysis of variance: $p < 0.05$).

Table 9–3. Criteria for Normative Sensory Organization Test Data in Young Healthy Subjects

Criteria
No current or past medical diagnosis or injury affecting balance
No use of medication affecting the central nervous system or known to affect balance/coordination
No symptoms of dizziness or lightheadedness
No symptoms suggestive of vestibular or neurologic disorders
No psychological disorders including depression
No history of two or more unexplained falls within the past 6 months
Normal vision with or without glasses
Normal hearing status as serous otitis media was reported to decrease postural stability[a]

[a]For additional criteria, see Casselbrant et al.[23]

Differences between each group were considered as significant when $p < 0.05$.

The equilibrium characteristics expressed by SOT for the five studied groups are given in Figure 9–6. The main conclusions of our study are as follows:

1. When the eyes are open, and the platform is stable, ES significantly increases in subjects 10 to 11 years old. In conditions of visual-cue suppression (eg, eyes closed), ES increases progressively with age from 85.9% in group A to 93.5% in group E. In visual-surrounding condition, ES increases progressively with age from 84.1% in group A to 92.4% in group E (see legend of Figure 9–6).
2. ES on the unstable platform (ES %) is given in Figure 9–7. When eyes are open, ES significantly increases with age from 63.3% in group A to 84.9% in group E. When eyes are closed, ES improves with age from 39.2% in group A to 66.6% in group E. In visual-sway condition (the last SOT EquiTest condition), ES significantly increases with age from 27.9% in group A to 64.2% in group E (see legend of Figure 9–7).
3. SA ratios are given in Figure 9–8. Whatever the age, the proprioceptive score is stable in people 6 to 20 years old. The visual score progressively increases from 68.6% in group A to 91.5% in group E. The vestibular score significantly increases from 41.5% in group A to 71.6% in group E. Visual preference is unchanged in people 6 to 20 years old (see legend of Figure 9–8).

Comparing data obtained for young healthy adults to data obtained from healthy children is useful to understand if differences could be attributed to an immaturity of sensorimotor systems. It appears that the proprioceptive system is already operating at full capacity in children as young as 6 years old, whereas that does not seem to be the case for the visual and labyrinthine systems. This observation highlights the major modifications of both the visual and labyrinthine systems in school-aged children. We have observed that first, visual input increases more slowly, reaching the same values as adults at the ages of 12 to 13 years, and second, the vestibular cue increases more slowly than visual input. Therefore, as reported in previous studies, even at the age of 16, normal subjects did not reach the levels of adults. It is known that in cases of intersensory conflict, the vestibular system acts as a referential function by suppressing input that is not congruent with vestibular information.[14] Due to a presumed mature vestibular function, even

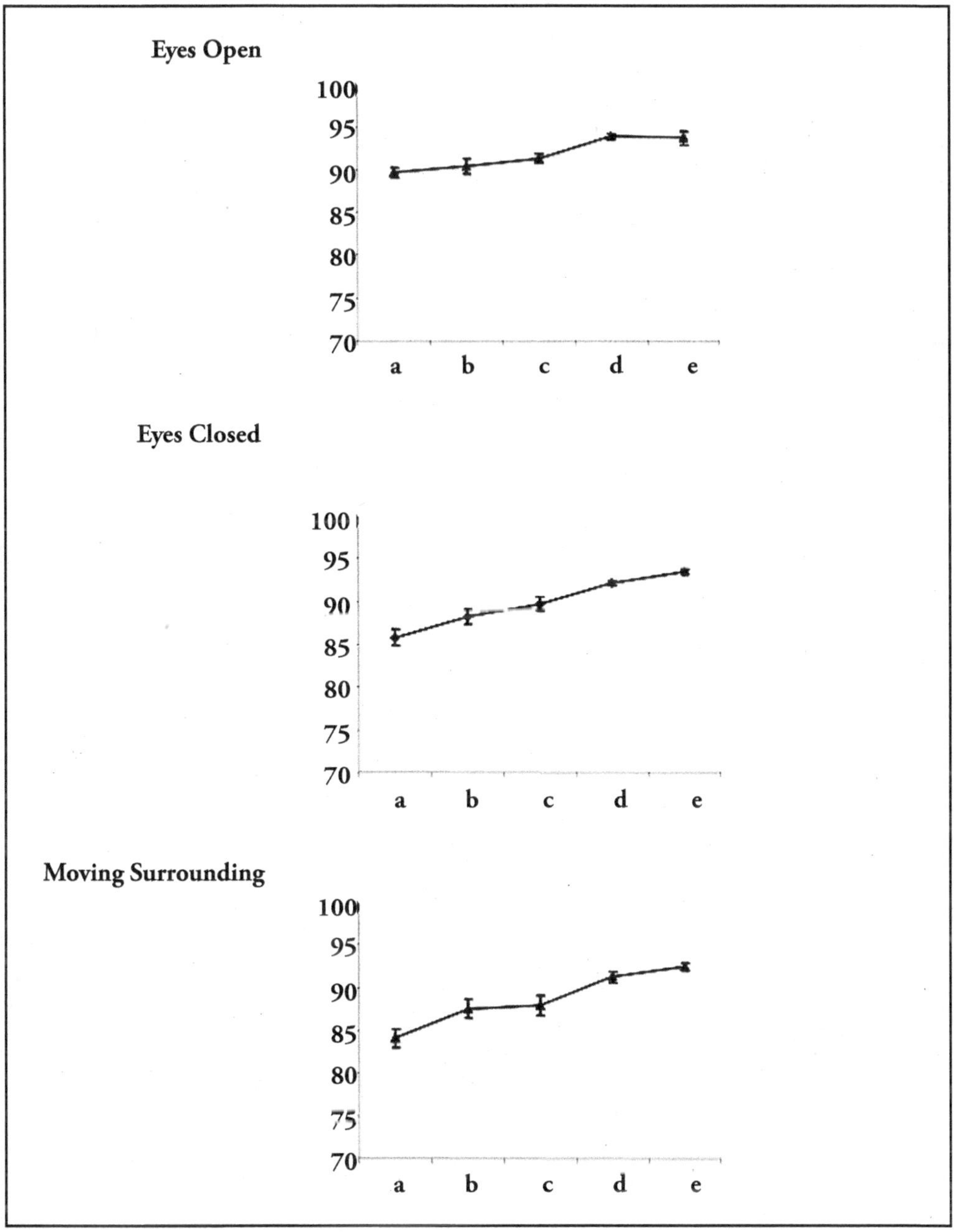

Figure 9–6. Equilibrium scores (%) on the static platform condition in the five groups.

with misleading visual information, adults may improve their postural control; therefore, it can be postulated that by the age of 16 years, children are still not able to select and process misleading visual information, which could be overcome in the adult group. According to other authors,[18] our results suggest that such a maturation process occurs more slowly and

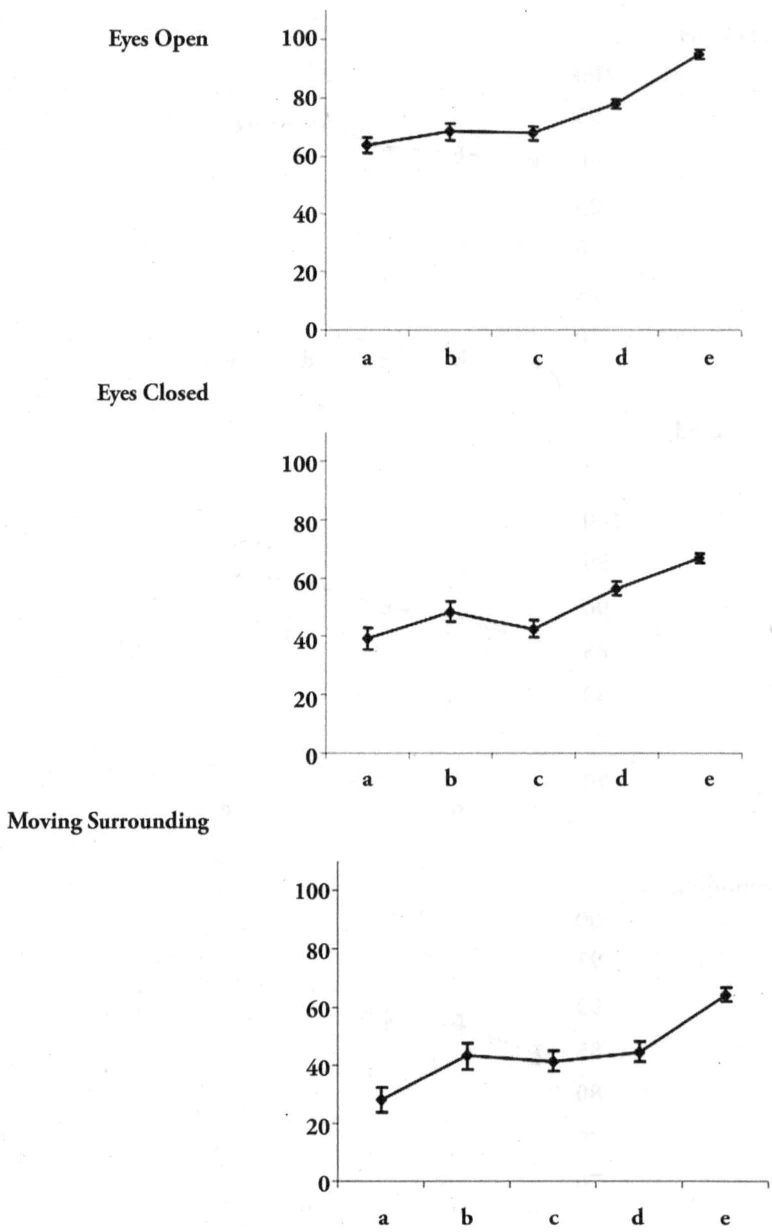

Figure 9–7. Equilibrium scores (%) on the unstable platform condition in the five groups.

continues throughout childhood, at least up to the age of 16 years.

The integration of visual information indeed provides us with a notion of the surrounding-space information. This is particularly relevant to the cognitive function of equilibration. Integration of visual-spatial information changes significantly in school-

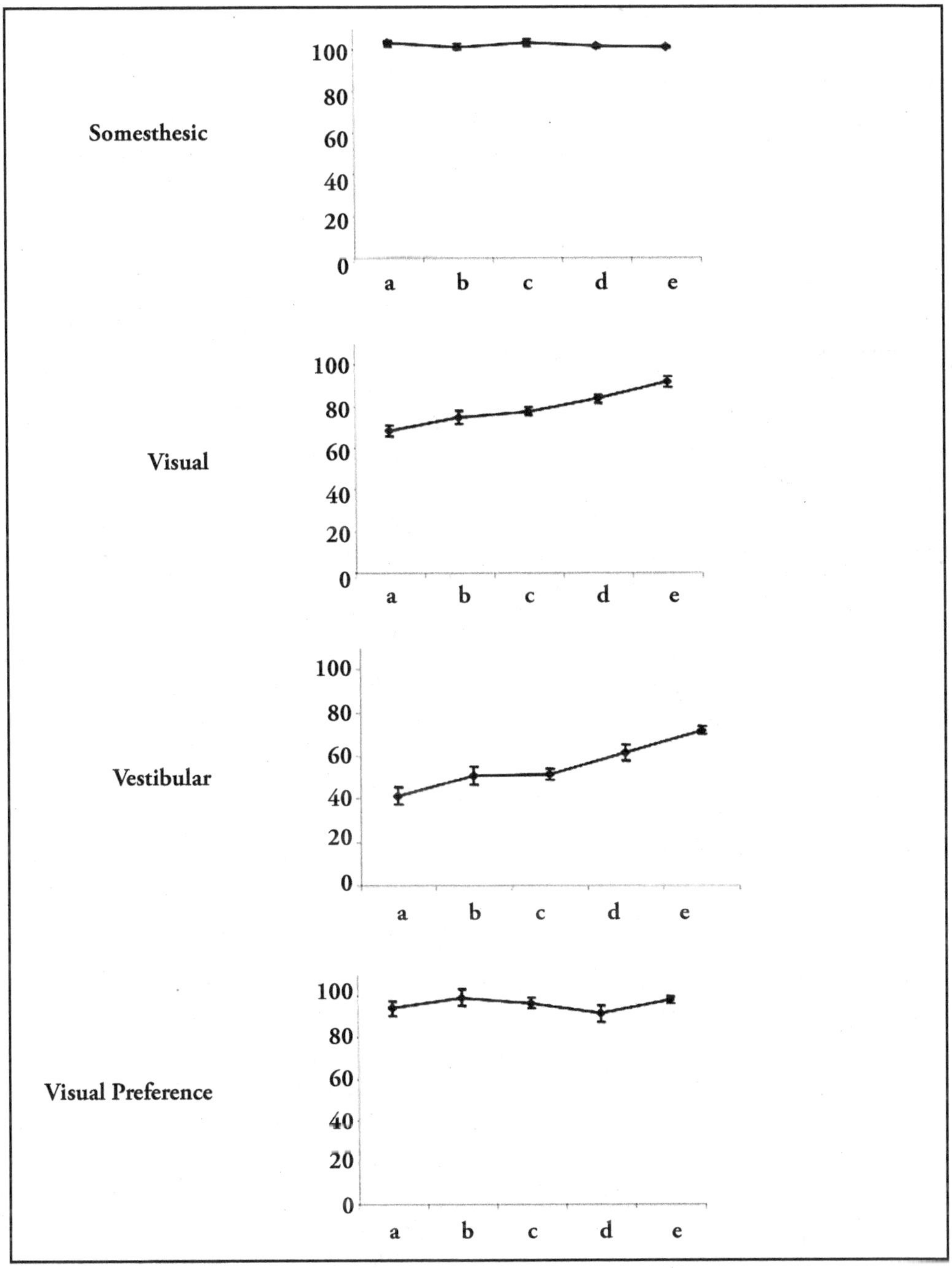

Figure 9–8. Sensory Organization Test (SOT %) in the five tested groups.

aged children. Different sources of visual information are used during visuospatial cognition.[24] They are traditionally classified into two main categories: allocentric and egocentric frames of reference.[25,26] In particular, a right frontal executive network, which develops with age, is strongly involved in inhibiting the aforementioned perceptual bias of length, as demonstrated in a number of comparisons.[27]

These results suggest that there is a progressive maturation of balance control between the ages of 6 and 16 years, especially an improvement in using vestibular inputs. These late maturation processes coincide with the ultimate development of several visual functions, including saccade latency, contrast, or chromatic sensitivity, which do not asymptote to an adult level until about 12 years of age.[28] From these results, it is suggested that between 6 and 16 years of age, children exhibit maturation of both vestibular and ocular pathways, and maturation of sensory-organization strategy of their balance control. These results imply that the vestibular and oculomotor systems are highly functional but still under maturation in this age group. Consequently, due to the development of inhibitory control with age,[29] our results reflect less changes in both visual and labyrinthine perception than in cognitive integration of the sensory inputs. In fact, a previous work[30] has shown that in children, ocular disorders are often responsible for balance abnormalities. The authors reported that 5% of 523 children referred during 5 years for vestibular testing had no other pathologic findings except ocular disorders. For this reason, children with imbalance but with normal neurologic and vestibular findings should undergo complete ocular testing before magnetic resonance imaging.

The Balance Quest Platform

Multitest Equilibre or Balance Quest (BQ), Framiral, Cannes, France, is a dynamic platform designed to mimic the natural range of motion available in the human body while standing. When the platform center support is released from its static position, it essentially floats on a spring suspension allowing dynamic motion with 3° of freedom[31]: Yaw (twist clockwise/counterclockwise), Pitch (tilt forward/backward), and Roll (tilt left/right). The BQ software measures center of pressure (COP) in the x, y, and z planes plus pitch and roll axes for unparalleled information about the direction and amplitude of sway.

In this purpose, a pneumatic and electronic system coupled to the platform allows creating multidirectional suspended and tilted planes, which are displayed graphically in real time. Thus, postural sway can be recorded in six different sensory conditions by attenuating or altering visual and proprioceptive information as in real-life condition—that is, when all sensorial inputs are needed for a good postural control, but some of them are often missing or perturbed (Figure 9–9).

Similar to the EquiTest system, Balance Quest PosturoPro software allows the extraction of usual spatial parameters, the surface area (cm^2) and the mean velocity (mm/s) of the COP, to quantify postural performance and evaluate the displacement of COP. Stability quotients for each sensory condition are produced by the platform's software, which subsequently generates the SOT score. The SOTs show the ability of the central nervous system to compensate for the lack of reliable sensory information by re-weighting across the available ones.[32] Another parameter available with the PosturoPro software is the wavelet analysis, which allows a qualitative evaluation with a three-dimensional (3D) representation of body sway.[33,34] COP displacements, which are dependent not only on time, frequency, and amplitude of oscillation, but also on the energetic expenditure, are displayed as a color code. Cold colors illustrate a small oscillation of postural sway, warm colors greater oscillation, while white holes indicate that there is almost no oscillation for the frequency done and at time considered (Figure 9–10). This 3D cartography allows rapid detection of the energetic

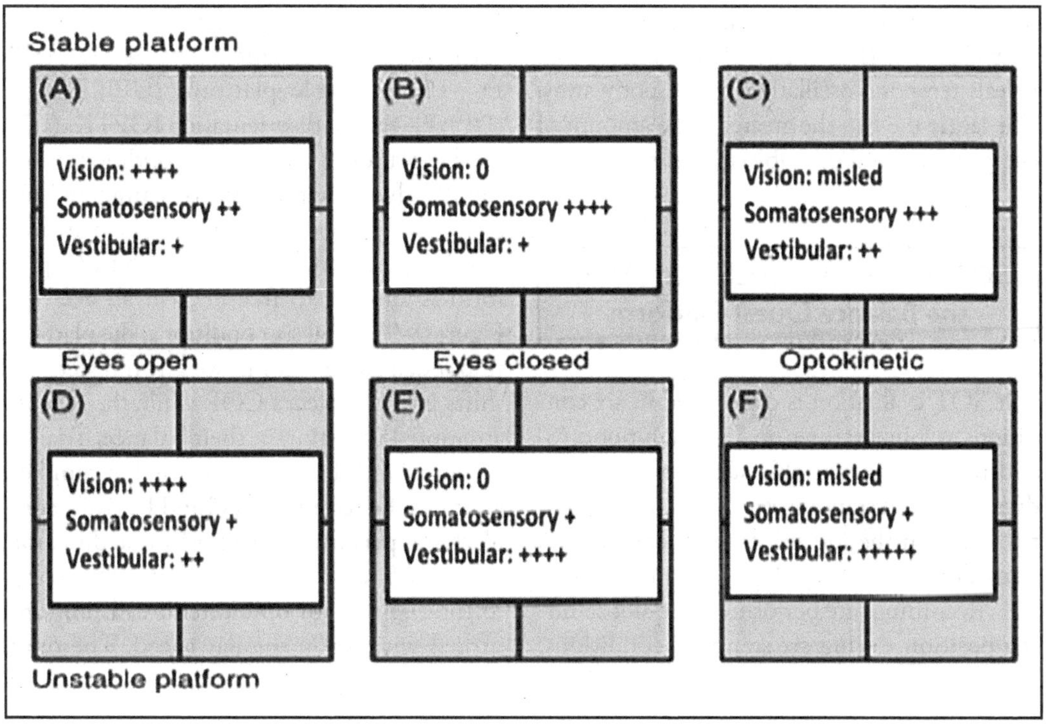

Figure 9–9. Balance Quest: Sensory Organisation Test. The six sensorial conditions with their sensory contribution (vision, somatosensory, vestibular). **A.** Eyes open on stable platform. **B.** Eyes closed on stable platform. **C.** Eyes open with optokinetic field on stable platform. **D.** Eyes open on unstable platform. **E.** Eyes closed on unstable platform. **F.** Eyes open with optokinetic field on unstable platform.

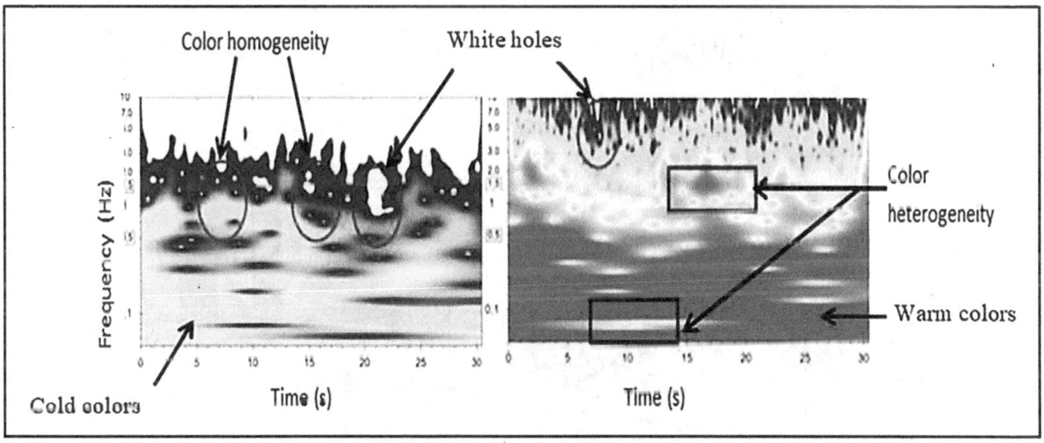

Figure 9–10. Wavelet's analysis also called 3D cartography for Postural Control (PC). *Left:* Good postural control with cold colors. *Right:* poor postural control with high levels of energy dispersion displayed with warm colors.

cost to maintain postural control for each sensory condition. As a result, the postural instability index (PII) is a specific parameter that reveals temporal oscillation in the body sway. The larger the PII, the greater is the amount of energy spent, and the subject is unstable.

SOT Assessment in Children With the Balance Quest Platform

The SOT evaluation is conducted in six conditions as follows: three on a stable support (S) and three on an unstable support (U). Children are tested standing on the platform, with their feet on the footprints, abducted at 30°, arms along their body (Figure 9–11).

Recordings are performed in quiet standing position during six standard conditions: A—eyes open (EO), stable platform (SP); B—eyes closed (EC), (SP); C—visual disorientation (optokinetic field [OPTK]) (SP); D—EO, unstable platform (UP); E—EC (UP); F—visual disorientation (OPTK) (UP). "Stable platform" refers to the conditions where the BQ dynamic platform is maintained in a static, stable position. "Unstable platform" refers to the conditions where the BQ platform is allowed to free-float in all axes (see Figure 9–9). In all six conditions, the platform responded to changes in weight transfers and shifts in the subject's COP while the subjects attempted to maintain their balance. Trials in B and E conditions are conducted in complete darkness. For conditions C and E, visual stimulation is performed in a horizontal direction, moving 15 seconds to the left and 15 seconds to the right by an optokinetic ball projector turned with 15°/s angular speed. The opto-

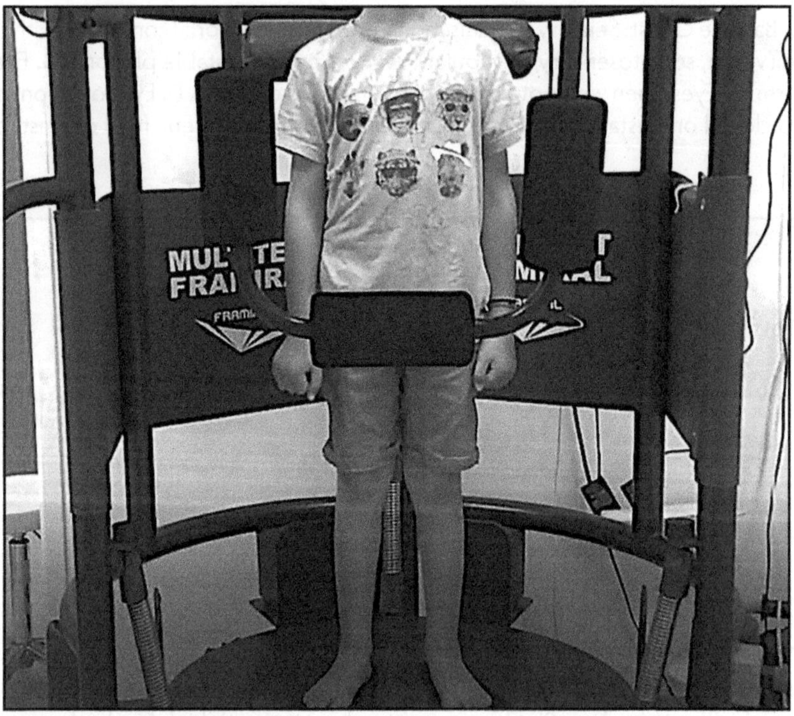

Figure 9–11. Subject's position on the Balance Quest Platform.

kinetic stimulation is projected on a wall at a distance of 250 cm from the subject's eyes. Visual reference including the room's geometry (eg, corners, light spots under the door) is not allowed. Completion of one assessment session included the successful completion of one trial for each of the 6 conditions previously listed. Each assessment lasted 30 seconds with a 15-second rest between each condition. The subject's stability and primary gaze position are monitored by an infrared camera placed overhead in a superior and lateral position. According to previous studies in children, brief instruction to stay as stable as possible are accepted and well understood, including by younger children.[35] If the subject falls or steps on the platform, the trial was considered as failed. The PII is a specific parameter that reveals the temporal oscillation in the body sway during recording. The larger the PII, the greater is the instability. It enables an easy and rapid evaluation of the children's postural performances. PosturoPro software allows us also to obtain the SOT synthesis, showing the degree of efficiency of different sensory inputs, similar to the EquiTest platform.

Normative Data: Comments

Recently, in a multicenter study,[36] postural control was assessed in a large sample of 156 healthy age- and gender-matched children and teenagers from 3.08 to 16.8 years old with a mean age of 9.4 ± 0.27 years. Postural parameters previously mentioned were analyzed (surface, mean velocity of COP, and PII).

All postural parameters (surface, mean velocity of COP, and PII) ameliorated significantly with the age in all conditions on stable support (EO, EC, and OKN), as previously reported.[37,38] Interestingly, contrary to other studies, we observed a significant gender effect (Figure 9–12), since the mean displacement velocity of COP was significantly greater in boys in the OKN-U condition. Growing children were better at using and integrating sensory inputs, and therefore, compensation with

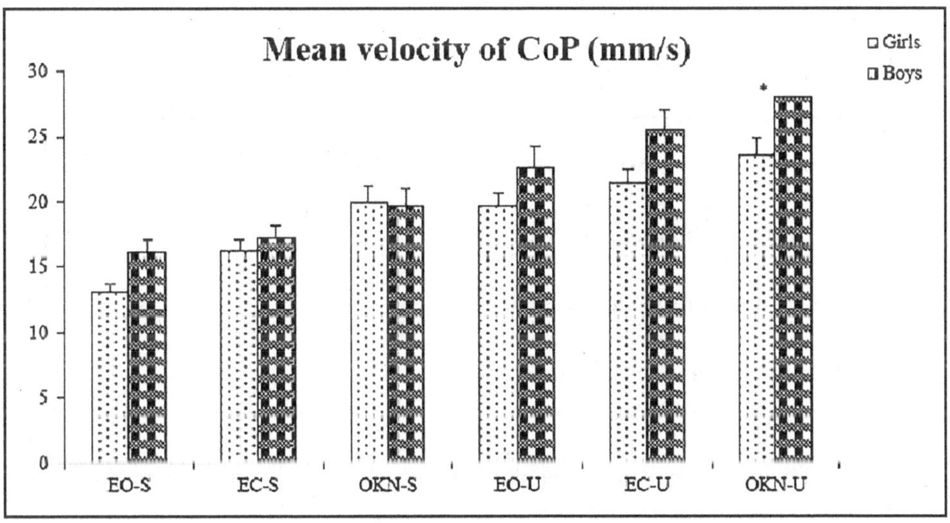

Figure 9–12. Mean velocity of center of pressure (CoP) depending on gender, in all sensory conditions, with a significant difference between boys and girls in condition eyes open with optokinetic field on unstable platform.

an alternative sensory strategy if one was missing or disturbed. In light of these results, this ability does not seem to be completely achieved and is still ongoing beyond age 16.08 years.

Overall, posturographic normative data obtained on large samples and the patterns of the PC maturation process in children observed on each of these two CDP systems are comparable. This would be explained by some technological similarities, although the main difference between the two platforms consists in that on the Neurocom CDP subjects are tested in two conditions, whereas vision is sway referenced to proprioception, while on Balance Quest CDP visual input is only disrupted by optokinetic stimulations in homologues conditions 3 and 6. Furthermore, the visual preference score provided by each platform is then different and, therefore, does not reflect the same adequacy of the PC for a given sensorial condition. However, being less expensive, the Balance Quest platform would be more accessible in the physical therapist's office to assess and/or survey postural compensation in patients complaining of balance disorders.

Conclusion

The CDP is a tool dedicated to globally evaluating the quality of balance control; it does not allow localization of the side of the vestibular impairment, especially in chronic vestibular pathologies. Therefore, CDP evaluation in children with imbalance problems may be an interesting tool, but in daily neurotological practice, this exam is not indispensable because clinical evaluation by RT or the Fukuda test is simple, cheap, and often very relevant in cases of recent vestibular pathology. On the contrary, for research purposes, CDP is indispensable because it is quite sensitive to evaluate PC throughout almost every period of the life span.

Acknowledgments. The authors gratefully acknowledge Michel M. Mazzuca and Chantal Viart-Ferbert for their contribution to the first edition of this chapter. We thank Ruxandra-Cecilia Ionescu for proofreading the last version of the present manuscript.

Self-Assessment Questions

One or more statements may be correct.

1. Postural control depends on:
   a. Proprioceptive, visual, and auditory input
   b. Vestibular, visual, and somesthetic input
   c. Proprioceptive, somesthetic, visual, and vestibular input

2. The presence of a positive Romberg test classically indicates:
   a. Proprioceptive and visual impairment
   b. Vestibular impairment
   c. Proprioceptive impairment

3. Positive vestibular Romberg test associates:
   a. Lateral or axial postural deviation and lateral index deviation toward the labyrinthine impairment
   b. Backward postural deviation and upward index deviation
   c. Lateral deviation, eyes open toward the labyrinthine hypofunction, and contralateral index deviation

4. Computerized dynamic posturography (CDP) objectively assesses:
   a. Static balance control through 6 different, often conflicting, sensorial conditions
   b. Dynamic control of walking mechanisms and imbalance
   c. Equilibrium scores and sensorial ratios (proprioceptive, visual, and vestibular)

5. Equilibrium scores on the CDP EquiTest are calculated:
   a. Using the Romberg quotient in platform-stable and sway-referenced conditions
   b. Comparing the subject's maximum anterior and posterior angle sway to the theoretical limit of the stability
   c. Comparing the subject's maximum sway and comparing it with that of specific age-related normative data

6. The presence of an important degree of instability and ataxia in eyes-open subjects should evoke:
   a. A serious visual impairment
   b. A bilateral vestibular areflexia
   c. A cerebellar pathology

7. The Fukuda maneuver is considered positive when:
   a. The patient falls.
   b. The patient shows an axial deviation/rotation of more than 45°.
   c. The patient spins after 50 steps in place at least 30°.

8. The vestibular system seems to be completely mature:
   a. At age 6 years
   b. At age 18 years or more
   c. Between ages 10 and 14 years

9. In children the visual input:
   a. Is not used for balance control
   b. Is used only in cases of sensorial conflict
   c. Is important for postural control

10. In children with vertigo and/or dizziness:
    a. If otologic and neurologic findings are normal, a magnetic resonance imaging (MRI) exam must be urgently performed.
    b. A complete ophthalmologic exam should be performed before MRI.
    c. In cases of normal neurologic and audiovestibular findings, the origin is probably psychological, and a specific follow-up is necessary.

References

1. Horak FB. Postural orientation and equilibrium: What do we need to know about neural control of balance to prevent falls? *Age Ageing.* 2006;35 (suppl 2):ii7–ii11.
2. Khasnis A, Gokula RM. Romberg's test. *J Postgrad Med.* 2003;49:169.
3. Lanska DJ, Goetz CG. Romberg's sign: Development, adoption, and adaptation in the 19th century. *Neurology.* 2000;55:1201–1206.
4. Garcin R. The ataxias. In: Vinken PJ, Bruyn GW, eds. *Handbook of Clinical Neurology.* New York, NY: Wiley; 1969:311–313.
5. Fukuda T. The stepping test: Two phases of the labyrinthine reflex. *Acta Otolaryngol.* 1959;50:95–108.
6. Unterberger S. Neue objective registrierbare vestibulariskorper-drehreaktion, erhalten durch treten auf der stelle. Der "tretversuch." 1938: 145–478.
7. Winter D. *Biomechanics and Motor Control of Human Movement.* 4th ed. New York, NY: Wiley; 2009:Chapter 5, 127.
8. Nashner LM. Sensory feedback in human posture control. ScD Thesis. Massachusetts Institute of Technology; 1970:76–78.
9. Nashner LM, Black FO. Adaptation to altered support and visual conditions during stance: Patients with vestibular deficits. *Neuroscience.* 1982;536–544.
10. Kaufman GD, Wood SJ, Gianna CC, et al. Spatial orientation and balance control changes induced by altered gravitoinertial force vectors. *Exp Brain Res.* 2001;137:397–410.
11. Black FO. What can posturography tell us about vestibular function? *Ann NY Acad Sci.* 2001;942:446–464.
12. Speers RA, Shepard NT, Kuo AD. EquiTest modification with shank and hip angle measurements: Differences with age among normal subjects. *J Vestib Res.* 1999;9:435–444.
13. Ji Z, Findley T, Chaudhry H, Bukiet B. Computational method to evaluate ankle postural stiffness with ground reaction forces. *J Rehabil Res Dev.* 2004;41:207–214.
14. Forssberg H, Nashner LM. Ontogenetic development of postural control in man: Adaptation to altered support and visual conditions during stance. *J Neurosci.* 1982;2:545–552.
15. Shumway-Cook A, Woollacott MH. The growth of stability: Postural control from a development perspective. *J Mot Behav.* 1985; 17:131–147.
16. Nashner LM, Shupert CL, Horak FB, et al. Organization of posture controls: An analysis of sensory and mechanical constraints. *Prog Brain Res.* 1989;80: 411–418; discussion 395–397.
17. McCollum G, Leen TK. Form and exploration of mechanical stability limits in erect stance. *J Mot Behav.* 1989;21:225–244.
18. Hirabayashi S, IwasakiY. Developmental perspective of sensory organization on postural control. *Brain Dev.* 1995;17:111–113.
19. Baloh RW, Corona S, Jacobson KM, et al. A prospective study of posturography in normal older people. *J Am Geriatr Soc.* 1998;46: 438–443.
20. Cherng RJ, Chen JJ, Su FC. Vestibular system in performance of standing balance of children

and young adults under altered sensory conditions. *Percept Mot Skills.* 2001;92:1167–1179.

21. Ferber-Viart C, Ionescu E, Morlet T, et al. Balance in healthy individuals assessed with Equitest: Maturation and normative data for children and young adults. *Int J Pediatr Otorhinolaryngol.* 2007;71:1041–1046.
22. Foudriat BA, Fabio RPD, Anderson JH. Sensory organization of balance responses in children 3–6 years of age: A normative study with diagnostic implications. *Int J Pediatr Otorhinolaryngol.* 1993;27:255–271.
23. Casselbrant ML, Furman JM, Rubenstein E, et al. Effect of otitis media on the vestibular system in children. *Ann Otol Rhinol Laryngol.* 1995;104;620–624.
24. Nadel L, Hardt O. The spatial brain. *Neuropsychology.* 2004;18:473–476.
25. Ishikawa T, Montello DR. Spatial knowledge acquisition from direct experience in the environment: Individual differences in the development of metric knowledge and the integration of separately learned places. *Cogn Psychol.* 2006; 52:93–129.
26. Rondi-Reig L, Petit GH, Tobin C, et al. Impaired sequential egocentric and allocentric memories in forebrain-specific-NMDA receptor knock-out mice during a new task dissociating strategies of navigation. *J. Neurosci.* 2006;26:4071–4081.
27. Leroux G, Spiess J, Zago L, et al. Adult brains don't fully overcome biases that lead to incorrect performance during cognitive development: An fMRI study in young adults completing a Piaget-like task. *Dev Sci.* 2009;12:326–338.
28. Yang JN, Shevell SK. Stereo disparity improves color constancy. *Vision Res.* 2002;42: 1979–1989.
29. Diamond A, Barnett WS, Thomas J, Munro S. Preschool program improves cognitive control. *Science.* 2007;318:1387–1388.
30. Bucci MP, Kapoula Z, Yang Q, et al. Speed-accuracy of saccades, vergence and combined eye movements in children with vertigo. *Exp Brain Res.* 2004;157:286–295.
31. Ionescu E, Morlet T, Froehlich P, Ferber-Viart C. Vestibular assessment with Balance Quest Normative data for children and young adults. *Int J Pediatr Otorhinolaryngol.* 2006;70:1457–1465.
32. Peterka RJ. Sensorimotor integration in human postural control. *J Neurophysiol.* 2002; 88:1097–1118.
33. Dumistrescu M, Lacour M. Nouveaux critères quantitatifs d'analyse du contrôle postural. In: Perennou D, Lacour M, eds. *Efficience et déficiences du contrôle postural.* Solal Eds. Marseille, France. 2006:65–75.
34. Bernard-Demanze L, Dumitrescu M, Jimeno P, et al. Age-related changes in posture control are differentially affected by postural and cognitive task complexity. *Curr Aging Sci.* 2009; 2:139–149.
35. Zok M, Mazzà C, Cappozzo A. Should the instructions issued to the subject in traditional static posturography be standardised? *Med Eng Phys.* 2008;30:913–916.
36. Goulème N, Debue M, Spruyt K, et al. Changes of spatial and temporal characteristics of dynamic postural control in children with typical neurodevelopment with age: Results of a multicenter pediatric study. *Int J Pediatr Otorhinolaryngol.* 2018;113:272–280.
37. Chiari L, Rocchi L, Cappello A. Stabilometric parameters are affected by anthropometry and foot placement. *Clin Biomech (Bristol, Avon).* 2002;17:666–677.
38. Geurts AC, Nienhuis B, Mulder TW. Intra-subject variability of selected force-platform parameters in the quantification of postural control. *Arch Phys Med Rehabil.* 1993;74: 1144–1150.

CHAPTER 10

Dynamic Balance and Gross Motor Assessment

Anne Scofich and Renée Haldenby

Introduction

When assessing dynamic balance, it is imperative to assess a child's ability to balance as it relates to functional movement and the performance of various motor skills. This can be achieved by performing a gross motor assessment that focuses on functional movement and skills that are fundamental to a child's activity level and participation within their environment. In this context, a comprehensive gross motor assessment will give you invaluable information not only about dynamic balance, but also about the factors that are contributing directly and indirectly to it as well as a starting point when considering how to treat impairments in dynamic balance. Due to continued development throughout childhood, gross motor assessments of infants, children, and adolescents will vary, as these assessments must reflect the stage of development of the child. Although a gross motor assessment would include measures of static balance, this chapter primarily focuses on all other components of a gross motor assessment and how they inform a child's dynamic balance within their overall function. A detailed assessment of static balance can be found in Chapter 9.

Before we start to assess movement, it is important to examine which factors are necessary to the production of movement and to the execution of a functional skill. These include strength, muscle tonus, range of motion, sensation, proprioception, and coordination.

1. Strength

In the clinical setting, strength can be easily measured with manual muscle testing that will provide information about the strength of specific muscles and can be done with an isometric hold (eg, Medical Research Council [MRC] scale) and/or through the functional range of motion (eg, Clarkson Scale). Done isometrically, such testing can provide information about power at mid-range against gravity, and assess symmetry between sides. As most functional movement is performed through various arcs and ranges of motion, it is valuable to look at strength through functional ranges of motion as well. In addition, both proximal and distal strength need to be considered when assessing balance as both the trunk and hips play a large role in dynamic standing and locomotion. Core and trunk strength are necessary to maintain an upright posture against gravity, and the large muscles of the hip and thigh are considered to be principally involved in weight-bearing and are responsible in part for locomotion. However, electromyography (EMG) recordings have shown that proximal muscles are not the primary contributor to balance recovery; in fact, it is the more distal musculature (calf and thigh) that responds first during a threat to balance.[1] In general, the pattern of muscle response to dynamic balance threats occurs in a distal-to-proximal sequence.[2]

2. Muscle Tonus and Spasticity

Muscle tonus refers to the resting state of the muscle. It is generally described qualitatively with such adjectives as hypertonic or high tone, or hypotonic or low tone, or can be graded using such measures as the Modified Ashworth scale[3] or the Tardieu scale.[4] Spasticity refers to a state of hypertonicity, which is a velocity-dependent resistance to stretch. Low tone or hypotonicity through the trunk will impact both static and dynamic balance as it relates to one's ability to maintain core activation and optimal postural alignment for function. Spasticity in the lower extremity, as seen in children with cerebral palsy, for example, can have a significant impact on balance control, particularly in the frontal plane, due to opposing muscle group imbalances (eg, plantarflexors/dorsiflexors) as well as due to deficits in postural control.[5]

3. Range of Motion

Range of motion is measured precisely with goniometry although it is sometimes also documented as approximations (eg, half range, full range). The amount of available range of motion at a joint may impact weight shifting and weight transfer during dynamic activities and may also affect the amplitude of balance reactions elicited.

4. Sensation

An accurate sensory exam is a very important component to a balance assessment. We take sensory information provided to us by our somatosensory, visual, and vestibular systems to adapt our movement to our environment. We use this information to anticipate balance needs, or to react to unexpected disturbances to our equilibrium, such as a slip or a trip.[2] An accurate somatosensory exam includes an assessment of cutaneous sensation (light touch, deep pressure) and proprioception (position sense and vibration sense). This will give information about an individual's ability to react to his or her environment and the surface the individual is moving on. For example, we use sensory information about the compliance and texture of the surface beneath our feet and adapt our muscle stiffness during locomotion. Being unable to feel an uneven surface beneath your feet limits your ability to activate the foot intrinsics and postural muscles necessary to adapt to this change in surface. A lack of proprioception limits your knowledge of where your joints are in space, thus limiting the implementation of a postural reaction in a timely manner. An individual with a sensory impairment may present with an ataxic gait as he or she is unable to coordinate movement using information provided from the environment. The visual and vestibular systems also play a role in proactive strategies for balance, and a full discussion on the physiology and developmental maturation of balance mechanisms can be found in Chapter 2.

5. Coordination

The ability to coordinate muscle activation at all levels (core, lower extremity, proximal and distal) is the crux of maintaining balance both statically and dynamically. Simple tests of coordination such as finger-to-nose or heel-to-shin and rapid alternating movements (RAMs) give us valuable information about coordination. Such measures need to be assessed in an unsupported position (unsupported sit or stand) as the trunk plays a crucial role in the organization of postural reactions.[6] Similarly, this is a position you would want to assume to assess for truncal ataxia in cases of cerebellar dysfunction.

Gross Motor Assessment

Gross motor assessment in infants should center on the acquisition of motor skills that occurs within the first 18 months of life. The assessment will need to include measures of impairment, observation of alignment, weight bearing, and movement in a variety of positions (supine, prone, sitting, standing), and more specific to functional balance, the development of postural control with movement and transitions in and out of these positions. An outcome measure, such as the Alberta Infant Motor Screen (AIMS)[7] or the Movement Assessment of Infants (MAI),[7] that focuses on both posture and movement in a variety of positions is helpful in determining if an infant is at risk for overall gross motor delay and will provide information regarding postural control with movement and developmental skill performance. The assessment of primitive reflexes, equilibrium reactions, and protective reactions will provide additional information regarding postural control. A full description of primitive reflexes, equilibrium reactions, and protective reactions can be found in Chapters 2 and 4.

When assessing a child or adolescent, a gross motor assessment should include impairment measures, basic functional tasks, specific gross motor skills, and high-demand functional tasks that will inform the assessor of the child's level of both functional performance and dynamic balance. For purposes of clarity, a basic functional task would include reaching for an object, a squat, or stair climbing. A specific gross motor skill would encompass items such as throwing, catching, running, and jumping, that a child would use within his or her play environment, and a high-demand functional task would include items such as grapevine walking, a floor-to-stand transfer, or catching on a BOSU Balance Trainer.

Many outcome measures specific to gross motor function are available for use and provide quantitative outcomes that, when paired with impairment measures and qualitative descriptors of gross motor performance, provide a robust gross motor assessment. Standardized assessments such as the Bruininks-Oseretsky Test of Motor Proficiency 2 (BOT2)[9,10] or Peabody Developmental Motor Scales 2 (PDMS2)[11] are discriminative and evaluative and provide information on basic gross motor skill performance and thus function in children. These tests also include a specific balance subset or domain with outcomes related to postural control.[8,10] An example of a healthy 5-year-old child performing the balance subset of the BOT2 can be found on the companion website (Video 10–1). Measures of gross motor function that have been developed for specific populations may be most effective when assessing balance for a child with the particular diagnosis. For example, the Gross Motor Function Measure (GMFM)[12] is a well-known outcome measure that has been validated for use in children with cerebral palsy. Although the measure does not contain a specific balance subset, items included in the measure require postural stability to perform and are reflective of dynamic balance.

The art of performing a good functional motor assessment is to begin with a variety of assessment tools and item options and to adapt and choose the most appropriate tools/items as a child's functional movement is revealed within the assessment. In clinical practice, there are particular assessment components that are extremely useful to inform dynamic balance.

Stance

Generally, functional motor assessments will incorporate the assessment of static standing balance in various positions, including two foot, single leg, tandem stance, and the Romberg position. The variety of stance positions allows for alteration of both the somatosensory input from the standing surface (eg, larger or smaller base of support) and visual input (eg, eyes open and closed). These various standing positions can also be used to assess dynamic balance if a movement component is added within the task. For example, a child with a high level of function can be challenged to stand on one foot and perform knee flexion or throw a ball, placing further demands on the postural control system.

Assessment of stance should include quantitative outcomes such as the duration the position is maintained and qualitative descriptors such as balance strategies used to maintain postural control and symmetry from left to right. It is generally felt that a single leg stance time of at least 5 seconds is required in order to perform the demand of single leg stance within a functional motor task such as a high reach or hopping. Children returning to more demanding leisure activities or sport would require longer single leg stance periods as their task demands would be higher. Lack of single leg stance ability is associated with many problems with community mobility,[13] making it a useful screening tool.

Gait

Observation and analysis of gait on a level surface is a main component of any gross motor assessment and provides many potential factors and measures for analysis. Gait parameters such as heel strike, toe off, stride length symmetry, single leg stance time, and base of support are factors that are specifically of interest when assessing postural control within gait. Gait norms that change over the course of a child's development must be used as comparators during analysis. If video or foot pattern analyses are available, they can be included in a gross motor assessment as analysis of gait can occur at a later time to minimize the overall length of the assessment. Gait parameters such as speed and endurance are often assessed using a treadmill, as these parameters can be more easily measured and manipulated to provide increasing challenges to a child's balance.

Specific to dynamic balance, a variety of gait patterns are included in the gross motor assessment. These include heel, toe, tandem, and backward gait. Each of these gait patterns provides additional information on dynamic balance within function. When performing heel and toe gaits, a child is required to narrow his or her base of support, shift the center of gravity to achieve the position, and maintain his or her postural control while moving in space with these added challenges. The ability to achieve the start position, actual task performance (eg, number of steps), symmetry, and balance strategies used within task performance can all be observed and recorded. Backward gait demands balance control while increasing the demands for a more accurate step pattern from the extensor musculature of the lower extremity and a reversal of the pattern of foot contact all in the presence of altered visual input.

Tandem gait is consistently included in a balance assessment to challenge the balance systems by further narrowing the base of support and requiring targeting to a specific step pattern along a real or imaginary line. Tandem gait can often reveal balance strategy used and asymmetries not uncovered in regular gait, as children tend to perform the gait more slowly, and forward momentum cannot necessarily be used to improve performance. The effects of changes in coordination and motor control, specifically, will be visible and impact performance of this motor task. When a child performs at a high level of gross motor function, an additional challenge can be introduced through the use of a balance beam. Balance beams will introduce a smaller base of support for foot contact and an alternate surface (eg, foam or wood). More accurate foot placement and coordination of the sensory, motor, and biomechanical systems involved in postural control are demanded while performing the tandem gait pattern. An in-depth discussion of gait analysis can be found in Chapter 11.

Basic Functional Tasks

When assessing dynamic balance within a gross motor framework, a variety of functional motor tasks should be included. These include reaching tasks, transitions into and out of positions, tasks with level changes, and stair performance. Alignment, weight shift with movement, base of support, and accomplishment within task performance are all factors to be assessed.

Goal-directed functional reach tasks in sitting and standing are important to include and will provide information on equilibrium and protective reactions. Reaching should be performed in a forward, lateral, and, as possible, posterior direction with the right and left upper extremities. Movements in these three directions will mimic the demands of daily functional reaching and can be compared side to side. Normative data for forward reaching in stand is available from Donahoe et al's work[14] with the Functional Reach Test (FRT) in a pediatric population. The FRT[15] is useful in identifying decreased dynamic balance in children aged 5 to 15 years.

Although the FRT can be used to identify changes in basic functional reach abilities, children have more complex demands placed on them within their everyday lives. Transitions that are composed of sequences of movement must also be included in a gross motor assessment. Transitions in the assessment, such as sit to/from stand and kneel to/from stand, should entail both a change of level in the vertical direction and eccentric muscle work. For example, performance of a squat is a clinically useful assessment task as it demands eccentric lower extremity work in the extensor muscles, graded or controlled movement, and a change in the center of mass and provides richer information on dynamic balance.

Ascending and descending stairs is also an important skill to assess. The number of stairs performed, pattern of stepping, use of aids such as handrails, and evaluation of postural control, when a primarily eccentric muscle demand is required on descent, expands one's information on functional performance, balance, and a child's ability to participate within his or her community.

Specific Gross Motor Skills

Specific motor skills that develop in childhood have been identified on gross motor assessment tools and thoroughly studied, thereby allowing comparisons to normative data with regard to quantitative and qualitative outcomes. These skills include running, jumping, throwing, and catching. Each task demands movement while maintaining equilibrium and is a skill used within daily life in a school environment. Performance of these tasks can be measured from a product and process approach. For example, a throw can be measured in terms of distance or the presence of components that should be incorporated by a certain developmental age. As the performance of each skill is affected by a child's postural control, inclusion of these skills either via a standardized assessment such as the PDMS2[11] or individual task performance is recommended.

Specifically, the inclusion of one-foot hopping and two-foot jumping provides information on postural control when a child is required to produce a period of no foot contact with the floor. Hopping can be viewed as an extension of single leg stance with an additional dynamic demand. Good postural control is necessary for and can be assessed during the initiation and landing of each hop or jump while also assessing the number of repetitions and motor patterns used in performance. Hopping and jumping skills are typical motor activities that children use in school physical education programs, and difficulties in performance can impact participation in the school and community environments.

High-Demand Functional Tasks

Children who present with mild changes in functional movement or balance may require assessment of more complex movement tasks that incorporate components of daily mobility and demand a high level of postural control. These high-demand tasks often reflect skills used to mobilize within the community or school environment and can include complex stepping patterns, turns in space while ambulating, ambulation while maintaining eye contact with an object, and performance of gross motor skills while on a mobile surface.

Grapevine stepping (stepping alternately across and behind the lead foot) is a complex stepping pattern and provides information on a child's ability to move in a lateral direction, coordinate a stepping pattern, use speed and rhythm within gait, and maintain postural control through equilibrium reactions to achieve this task. The crossover steps are similar to lateral avoidance stepping one would use in a crowded environment or lateral evasive steps used in sports.

Problems in performing tasks that incorporate turns while ambulating are associated with decreased balance and risk of falls.[16] Incorporating a turn while walking or turning the head while ambulating increases demands on the somatosensory system and provides a disruption in the regular pattern of ambulation. Including these tasks within a gross motor assessment via the use of the Community Mobility and Balance Scale (CB&M)[17] provides a useful measure of a child's functional performance as would be expected in the community environment. The tool has been shown to be reliable in a pediatric population of children with acquired brain injury.[18] An example of the CB&M scale can be found on the companion website. Generally, the components of a gross motor assessment, previously addressed within this chapter, have occurred on a stable surface (eg, chair, floor). To challenge and optimally assess a child with minor changes in function or balance, it is recommended that the child's ability to maintain postural control while performing functional movement on a mobile surface be assessed. A variety of mobile surfaces exist in clinical environments, including but not limited to wobble boards, rocker boards, balance systems, and BOSU Balance Trainer (Figure 10–1). Maintaining balance on a mobile surface would inform static balance; however, having a child perform a functional task such as throwing and catching a ball on a mobile surface will provide information on high-level balance and dynamic postural control. These tasks are thought to be more representative of functional mobility demands in the community, such as moving on a subway

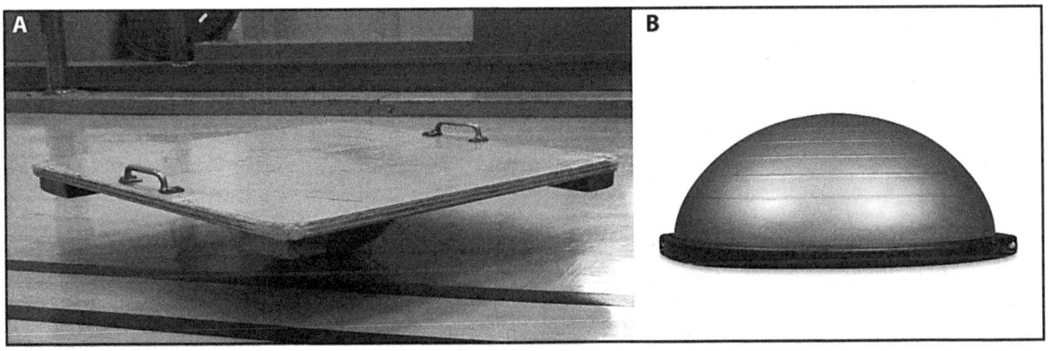

Figure 10–1. Examples of mobile surfaces used for dynamic balance testing and therapy in clinical environments. **A.** Rocker board and **B.** BOSU Balance Trainer.

while it stops or walking on an unstable surface such as a thick mat.

To address the need for an outcome measure for children who present with continued motor impairments and high-level mobility and balance issues, a team of researchers from Holland Bloorview Kids Rehabilitation Hospital in Toronto, Canada, are in the process of developing a challenge assessment for children with acquired brain injury (ABI–CA).[19] The measure is composed of advanced gross motor skills, some of which represent the realm of postural control and balance. The tool is expected to provide standardized data on motor function in individuals who may ceiling on measures of gross motor function and to enable clinicians to more accurately evaluate higher gross motor and balance deficits.

Summary

The assessment of dynamic balance skills in children requires a thorough understanding of a child's ability to balance as it relates to functional movement. This understanding can be achieved through the use of a comprehensive, age-appropriate gross motor assessment that includes assessment of the factors necessary to the production of movement, functional tasks and skills, and standardized outcome measures. A robust gross motor assessment will allow for an improved understanding of dynamic balance and how it impacts the function of a child as well as a starting point when determining the best interprofessional care for a child with altered postural control.

Self-Assessment Questions

Case 1

Jane is a 6-year-old girl who is having difficulty participating in a physical education class at school due to frequent falls. The falls tend to occur when she is playing games such as tag or basketball. The school consults a physiotherapist to assess Jane's level of performance and safety when participating in physical education classes.

The questions are as follows:

1. Is gross motor assessment indicated for this child? Why?
2. What are some specific components that should be included in the assessment?
3. What type of information would a simple measure of dynamic balance, such as an FRT, provide in the assessment?
4. What outcome measure(s) would assist in measuring Jane's gross motor function?
5. Would the assessment of stairs be indicated even though this is not a specific complaint from the school?

Case 2

John is a 12-year-old boy who fell from a tree and sustained a mild traumatic brain injury. He was seen in the emergency room and discharged home. A week later, John continues to complain of headaches and that he is "off balance" when walking. He is being followed by his family physician who has requested a physiotherapy assessment in addition to other investigations.

The questions are as follows:

1. What four areas of focus should be included in the physiotherapy assessment?
2. Due to the nature of the injury, what other system could be a factor to consider when assessing John's gross motor performance and balance?
3. If, upon seeing John walk, you observe an ataxic gait, what specific assessment components should you include in your exam?
4. What outcome measures could you include in your assessment?
5. If John's level of tolerance precludes the use of an outcome measure, what type of functional movements could provide useful information on his dynamic balance?

References

1. Burtner PA, Qualls C, Woollacott MH. Muscle activation characteristics of stance balance control in children with spastic cerebral palsy. *Gait Posture.* 1998;8(3):163–174.
2. Shumway-Cook A, Woollacott MH. The growth of stability: Postural control from a development perspective. *J Mot Behav.* 1985; 17(2):131–147.
3. Bohannon RW, Smith MB. Interrater reliability of a modified Ashworth scale of muscle spasticity. *Phys Ther.* 1987;67(2):206–207.
4. Boyd RN, Graham HK. Objective measurement of clinical findings in the use of botulinum toxin type A for the management of children with cerebral palsy. *Eur J Neurol.* 1999;6:s23–s35.
5. Rose J, Wolff DR, Jones VK, Bloch DA, Oehlert JW, Gamble JG. Postural balance in children with cerebral palsy. *Dev Med Child Neurol.* 2002;44(1):58–63.
6. Verheyden G, Nuyens G, Nieuwboer A, Van Asch P, Ketelaer P, De Weerdt W. Reliability and validity of trunk assessment for people with multiple sclerosis. *Phys Ther.* 2006;86(1): 66–76.
7. Piper M, Darrah J. *Motor Assessment of the Developing Infant.* Philadelphia, PA: WB Saunders; 1994.
8. Chandler J, Andrews M, Swanson M. *Movement Assessment of Infants.* Rolling Bay, WA: Rolling Bay Press; 1980.
9. Bruininks R, Bruininks B. *BOT-2 Bruininks-Oseretsky Test of Motor Proficiency.* 2nd ed. Circle Pines, MN: AGS Publishing; 2005.
10. Cushing SL, Chia R, James AL, Papsin BC, Gordon KA. The vestibular Olympics: A test of dynamic balance function in children with cochlear implants. *Arch Otorhinolaryngol.* 2007;134(1):34–38.
11. Folio R, Fewell R. *Peabody Developmental Motor Scales.* 2nd ed. Austin TX: Pro-Ed; 2000.
12. Russell D, Rosenbaum P, Gowland C, et al. *Gross Motor Function Measure Manual.* 2nd ed. Hamilton, ON: IAHS, McMaster University; 1993.
13. Sutherland DH, Olshen R, Cooper L, Woo SL. The development of mature gait. *J Bone Joint Surg Am.* Apr 1980;62(3):336–353.
14. Donahoe B, Turner D, Worrell T. The use of functional reach as a measurement of balance in boys and girls without disabilities ages 5 to 15 years. *Pediatr Phys Ther.* 1994;6(4): 189–193.
15. Duncan PW, Weiner DK, Chandler J, Studenski S. Functional reach: A new clinical measure of balance. *J Gerontol.* 1990;45(6):M192–197.
16. Berg K, Wood-Dauphinée S, Williams JI, Gayton D. Measuring balance in the elderly: Preliminary development of an instrument. *Physiother Can.* 1989;41(6):304–311.
17. Howe JA, Inness EL, Venturini A, Williams JI, Verrier MC. The Community Balance and Mobility Scale—A balance measure for individuals with traumatic brain injury. *Clin Rehabil.* 2006;20(10):885–895.
18. Wright FV, Ryan J, Brewer K. Reliability of the Community Balance and Mobility Scale (CB&M) in high-functioning school-aged children and adolescents who have an acquired brain injury. *Brain Inj.* 2010;24(13–14):1585–1594.
19. Ibey RJ, Chung R, Benjamin N, et al. Development of a challenge assessment tool for high-functioning children with an acquired brain injury. *Pediatr Phys Ther.* 2010;22(3): 268–276.

CHAPTER 11

Gait Analysis

John Henley, Timothy A. Niiler, and Freeman Miller

Introduction

Computerized motion analysis is a method of analyzing the mechanics of human motion using computers to analyze data from cameras, force plates, and electromyography (EMG) electrodes. These data are augmented by the medical history, physical examination, and functional tasks to generate a complete picture of an individual's movement capabilities and limitations and are also used to develop an accurate and precise plan of treatment. Motion analysis has been applied to virtually every human (and animal) movement. For a more in-depth overview and history of motion analysis, see Baker[1] and Sutherland.[2]

Three-Dimensional Motion Recording

To collect three-dimensional motion analysis, data retro-reflective markers (3M, St Paul, MN) are placed on preestablished anatomical landmarks. The subject then completes a standardized dynamic task (walking) while 12 or more high-speed, high-resolution cameras (eg, Qualisys, Gothenburg, Sweden) simultaneously record data. Processors in each of the cameras examine each individual picture and automatically determine where the markers are in the field of view of that camera. Each camera sends this information to a computer that uses a process called direct linear transformation (DLT)[3–9] to determine the three-dimensional location of each marker. At this point, the computer system can locate each of the markers but cannot identify a marker as an elbow, knee, hip, or any other landmark. This is done by identifying each marker in the first movement or trial and applying this template (relative position of each of the markers) along with expected positions, velocities, and accelerations of each point. Thus, computer software automatically identifies and tracks the location of each of the markers (eg, Qualisys Track Manager). Given the location of each of the markers, we can determine the position of each body segment, the rotation of each joint, and the location of the body's center of mass at each 0.01 of a second (our usual data collection rate for walking) (Figure 11–1).

Standing Task

Walking represents a different balance task than standing. During standing, the task is simply to keep the projection of the body's

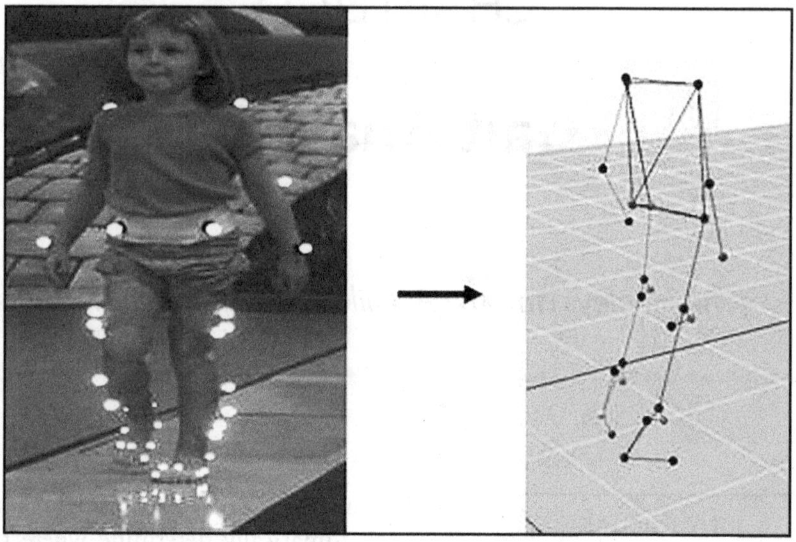

Figure 11–1. A. Child with reflective motion analysis markers over anatomical landmarks. **B.** Computerized transition to three-dimensional stick figure.

center of mass (CM) safely within the base of support (BOS) (Figure 11–2). The CM is the location at which gravitational forces act on the body. The center of pressure (CP) is the location of the net application of the ground reaction forces (GRFs) on the body. With static or near-static stance, horizontal forces are negligible and can be ignored. Therefore, the GRFs and the forces due to gravity (FGs) are parallel. The body can be made to rotate if the GRF and FG are not collinear. In the absence of horizontal forces, this is achieved by moving either the CM or the CP or both. The CP location is altered by changing where one pushes on the ground. For example, if one pushes more with one foot, the CP will move toward that foot. If the CP is moved, the GRF is moved. FG and GRF will no longer be collinear, and a torque will be created acting to tilt the body. Thus, falling can be controlled by altering the relative location of the CP and the CM. If the feet are next to one another, the motion of the CP in the anterior/posterior direction is controlled by ankle dorsiflexors or plantar flexors and in the medial lateral direction by the hip abductors and adductors.[10]

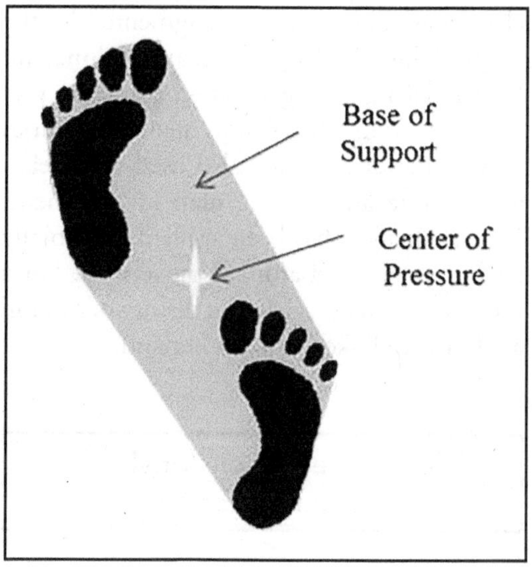

Figure 11–2. Foot-ground contact plus area between equals base of support (BOS) for a person standing with both feet on the ground.

Because no pressure can be applied outside the borders of the BOS, the location of the CP cannot be outside the BOS. Thus, the ability to control falling of the body or equivalently control the motion of the CM is limited by the size and shape of the BOS. The larger the BOS, the more freedom the CM has to move while still maintaining balance. Also with a larger BOS, one can create a greater separation between the CM and CP and thus have a greater influence or control of balance.

Walking Task

When a person walks (gait initiation and termination are beyond the scope of this chapter), the task changes (Figure 11–3). The BOS is constantly changing location, shape, and size. As a person moves forward, the sequence of events follows: they raise their heel, lift their whole foot off the ground, move their foot forward, place that heel on the ground again, and lower the rest of the foot to the ground. They then lift the other foot and repeat the process over again.

During this sequence, the ankle muscles can no longer prevent a fall as effectively as in static stance. These muscles can fine-tune anterior/posterior and medial/lateral acceleration, since the BOS is generally small; however, these effects are limited. The feet are never truly stationary, and the BOS is never as firm during standing. Even when both feet are on the ground during walking, one foot is settling as it accepts the body's weight (usually on the heel) and adjusts to the irregularities of the ground surface and the other foot is actively pushing off (usually on the forefoot) and propelling the body forward. Falls are only averted through safe placement of the swing foot since the area of the BOS and therefore the location of the CP can be dramatically altered by foot placement and transference of the load from one foot to the other.

In light of this background, motion analysis can be used to examine three major areas of walking: a subject's deviation from walking a straight line, the consistency of foot placement, and the consistency of individual joint movements. Stable patients should walk a straight line when requested and should be relatively consistent in their foot placement and general movement, while those with limitations in their stability will likely have difficulty in these three areas.

The path of the body's CM is calculated as the individual walks across the room. This is plotted along with the best-fit straight line from linear regression. From these data, we can calculate the deviation of the CM from the

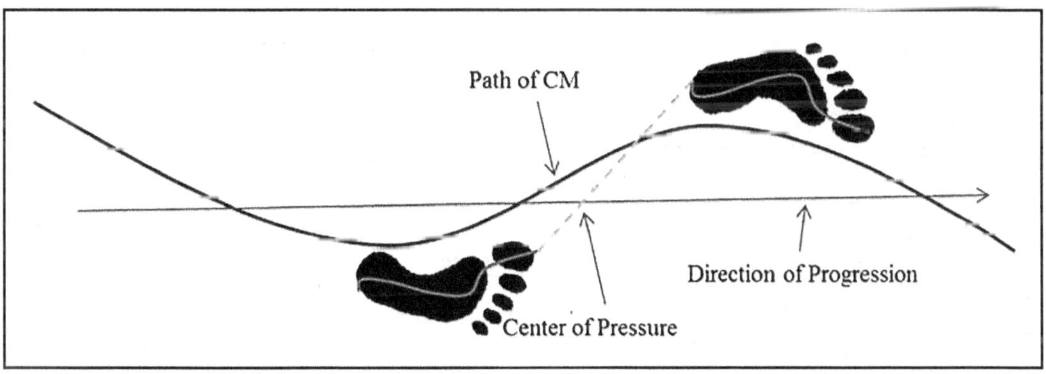

Figure 11–3. Relationship between direction of progression, path of CM and CP during walking.

straight line (Figures 11–4 and 11–5). This is plotted at each frame of data (typically at intervals of 1/60 of a second or 1/120 of a second depending on the data collection rate). Along with this data, two reference lines are produced: a solid black line that represents one average normal route mean-squared deviation from the line (at 2.01cm), and a black dashed line that represents one average normal standard deviation from the straight line (at 2.65 cm). The normal data are calculated from 87 typically developing children ranging in age from 3 to 18 years with no orthopedic or neurologic problems. Additionally, we calculate mean distance from the straight line (1.53 ± 0.49 cm), mean peak deviation from the straight line (1.71 ± 0.93 cm), and the standard deviation of the peak deviations from the straight line (0.93 ± 0.37 cm).

Next the relationship between the placement of the center of the foot and the center of mass in the anterior-posterior and medial-lateral directions during the stance phase can be examined (Figure 11–6). The underlying

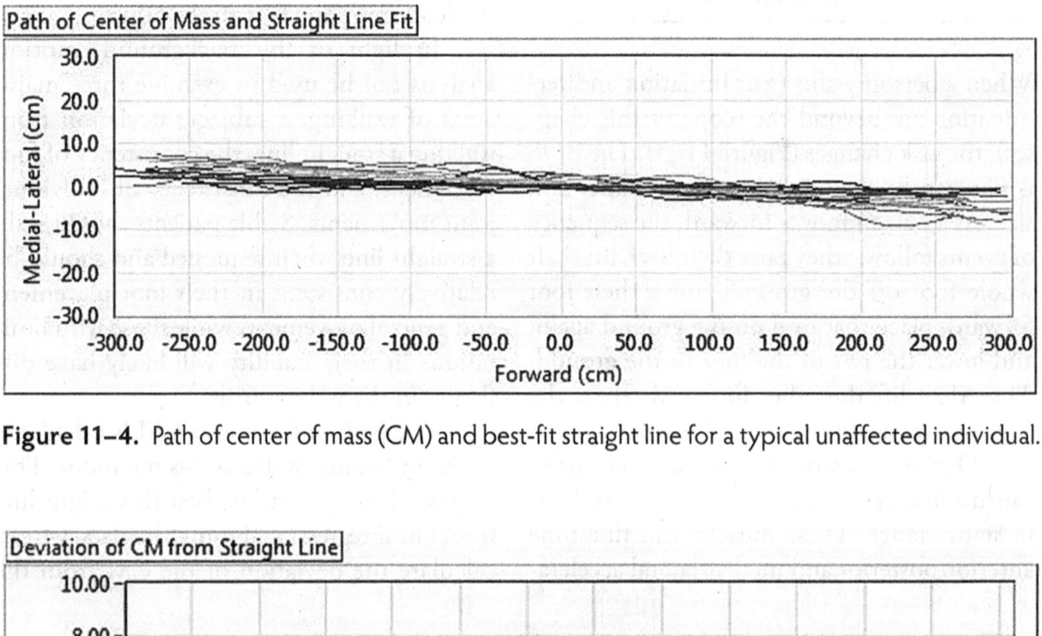

Figure 11–4. Path of center of mass (CM) and best-fit straight line for a typical unaffected individual.

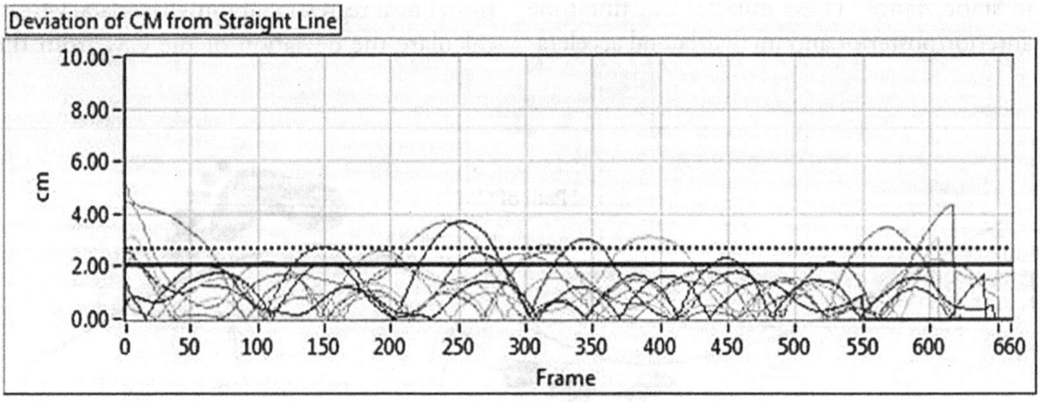

Figure 11–5. The deviation of CM versus frame of data (typically at intervals of 1/60 of a second or 1/120 of a second depending on the data collection rate) for a typical unaffected individual. The solid line indicates level of normal average +SD RMS (2.01 cm). The dashed line indicates level of normal peak + 1 SD (2.65 cm).

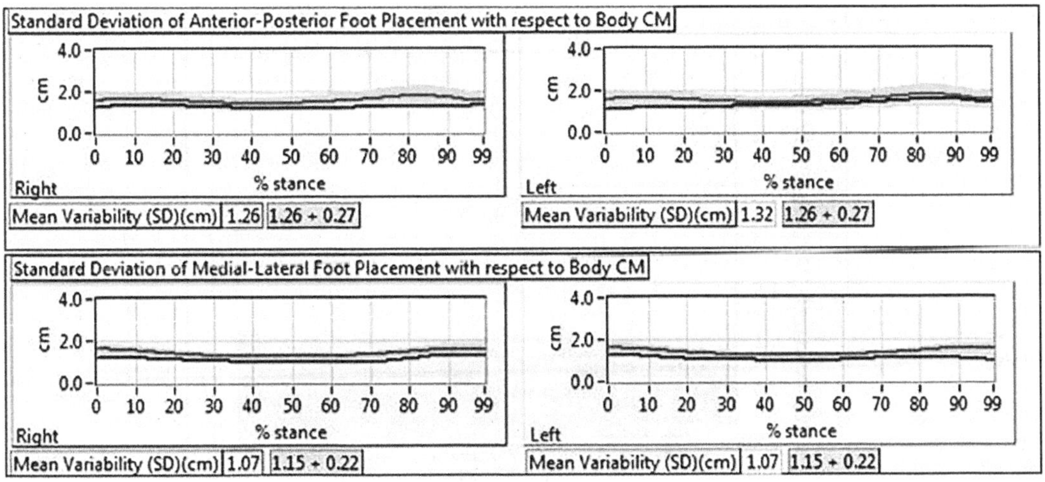

Figure 11–6. The relationship between the location of the foot center and the body center of mass in the anterior-posterior and medial-lateral directions versus the percent of the stance phase of gait in a typically developing child. The lines show the average of many steps (depends on how many were collected) and the typical average deviation at each percent of stance. The gray shaded area is +/–1 SD variability in the typical deviation.

rationale is that the foot is the device that the body is using to interact with the environment, and it is utilized to control the body's progression as represented by the path of the CM. For each step, there should be a typical pattern of foot placement relative to the CM with some minimal variance.

Because this variance in foot placement is not necessarily the same at all times (eg, initial foot contact, mid-stance, toe off), we plot the standard deviation of the foot and body CM relationship as a percentage of stance. One line is the average standard deviation of the distance between the foot and the body CM, while the other line is generated from normative data. Under each graph is the mean variability across the whole stance phase along with the normal mean and one standard deviation. Note that in the figure, the background for the boxes is shaded: clear for less than one standard deviation of the normative data (present for all data in this figure), lightest gray for between one and two standard deviations, light gray for between two and three standard deviations, and dark gray for greater than three standard deviations from the normative data (abnormal shaded results are shown in the case study section). This presentation is utilized for all outputs for easy identification.

The variability of motion at each joint can also be determined by calculating the average standard deviation of each angle over a gait cycle and then normalizing this by the normal average standard deviation. A score of 1 indicates that the average deviation of that subject's joint angle matches the deviation that is seen in typically developing children (Figure 11–7). An overall mean variability for all joints and directions can also be calculated.

Although straight-line walking tasks can expose balance deficits under ideal conditions, in younger subjects, deviations in gait may be due to attention deficits rather than stability changes. Additionally, it may sometimes be desirable to assess balance during turns or other conditions. An alternative way in which to assess balance that considers these

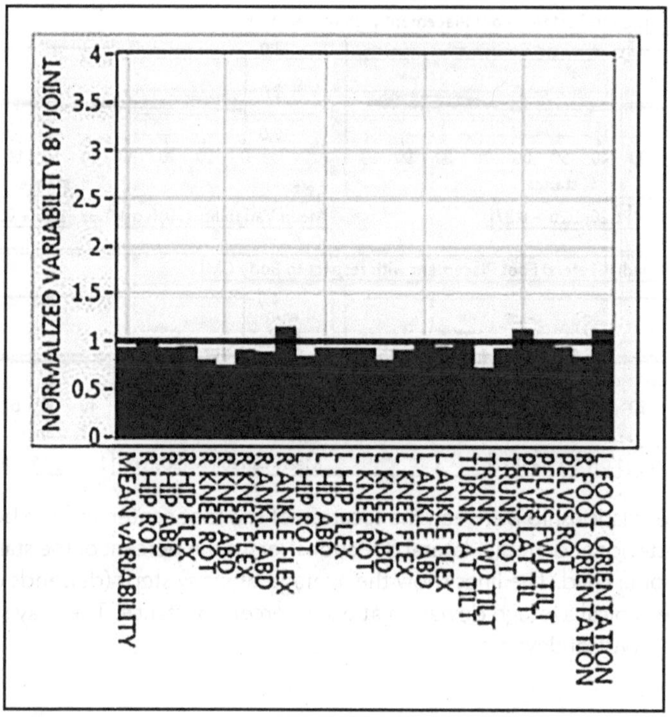

Figure 11–7. Normalized variability by joint in a typically developing child.

complications measures the CM motion with respect to the foot positioning rather than with respect to the lab.[11] In this case, the baseline for measurement is a line joining the centers of the feet termed the *interfoot* line. The shortest distance between this baseline and the CM is then calculated (Figure 11–8). This quantity can then be normalized to half the foot length to indicate when the CM lies outside the region between the feet. When this normalized parameter then exceeds unity, it indicates increased threat to balance. In evaluation of the gait of 66 typically developing children between the ages of 3 and 18 years, a study that considered over 101,000 frames of kinematic data, the normalized parameter exceeded unity in only 33 frames, indicating that during balanced gait, the CM stayed within the region shown in Figure 11–8 even when both feet are not grounded. But during falls due to slips, the normalized parameter quickly increases beyond unity as the walker becomes more unstable. This type of analysis of the CM can be more sensitive than the traditional lab-frame-based anterior-posterior and medial-lateral analysis in that the distance considered is not broken into its vectoral components. Finally, since the majority of real-life falls are either trips or slips, the directionality of the vector from the interfoot line to the CM can indicate when medial-lateral balance or anterior-posterior balance is most at risk.

In addition to the motion analysis, patients are routinely videotaped with a standard video camera while walking. The serial standardized video recordings provide excellent documentation of progress and form a basis for qualitative assessment.[12]

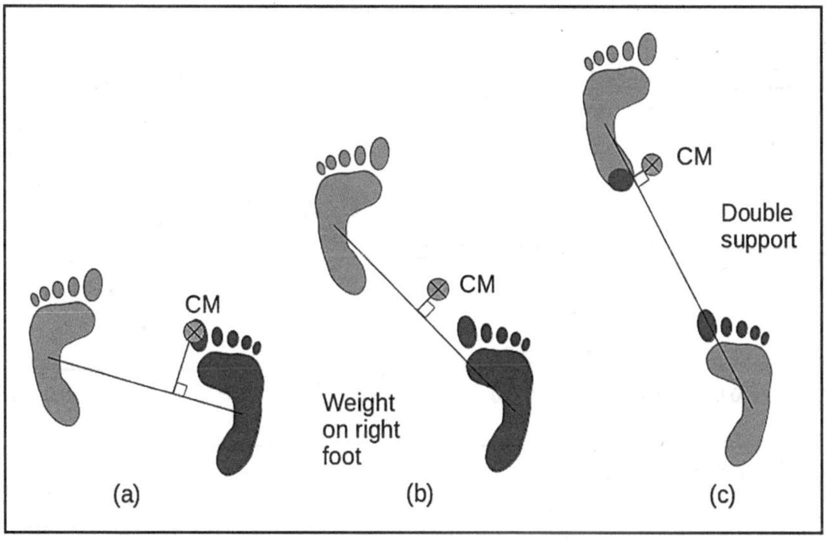

Figure 11–8. Geometry showing foot-centered evaluation of balance. During mid-swing when the weight is on the right foot (**A**), the CM is projected anteriorly, and its distance from the line joining the feet is the largest. This corresponds to when tripping is most likely to occur and when falls are likely to proceed in the forward direction. As the gait cycle progresses, the CM travels along the interfoot line toward the forward foot, and its distance from this line decreases (**B**). Finally at heel strike (**C**), the vector from the interfoot line to the CM is nearly lateral in direction. This positioning corresponds to when slipping is most likely to occur and when falls will be in the lateral or posterior direction as the body begins to rotate. Areas of the foot that are colored red are weight bearing.

Conclusion

Motion analysis is clinically useful for a variety of purposes in patients with balance deficits. Quantitative motion analysis can be utilized as an outcome measure in functional activity. Unlike the questionable relevance of other functional measures, walking is functional for nearly all patients. Serial evaluations can be used to determine not only the natural history but also the effectiveness of intervention such as medication, physical therapy, and surgery.

Motion analysis can also be diagnostic by suggesting reasons for gait instability. Evaluations generally group walking instability into one of three categories for purposes of directing treatment. Category 1 includes instability of central origin (ataxia or vestibular dysfunction resulting in instability) as shown in Figures 11–9, 11–10, and 11–11.

Category 2 includes motor control or movement disorder resulting in instability as shown in Figures 11–12, 11–13, 11–14, and 11–15.

Category 3 includes instability resulting from an unstable base of support (eg. high toe walking, severe foot deformity, pain) as shown in Figures 11–16, 11–17, and 11–18.

Unstable base of support is often addressed with orthotics or surgical procedure, movement disorders can be improved with a variety of medical management, and central instability dysfunction is often managed with therapy.[13,14]

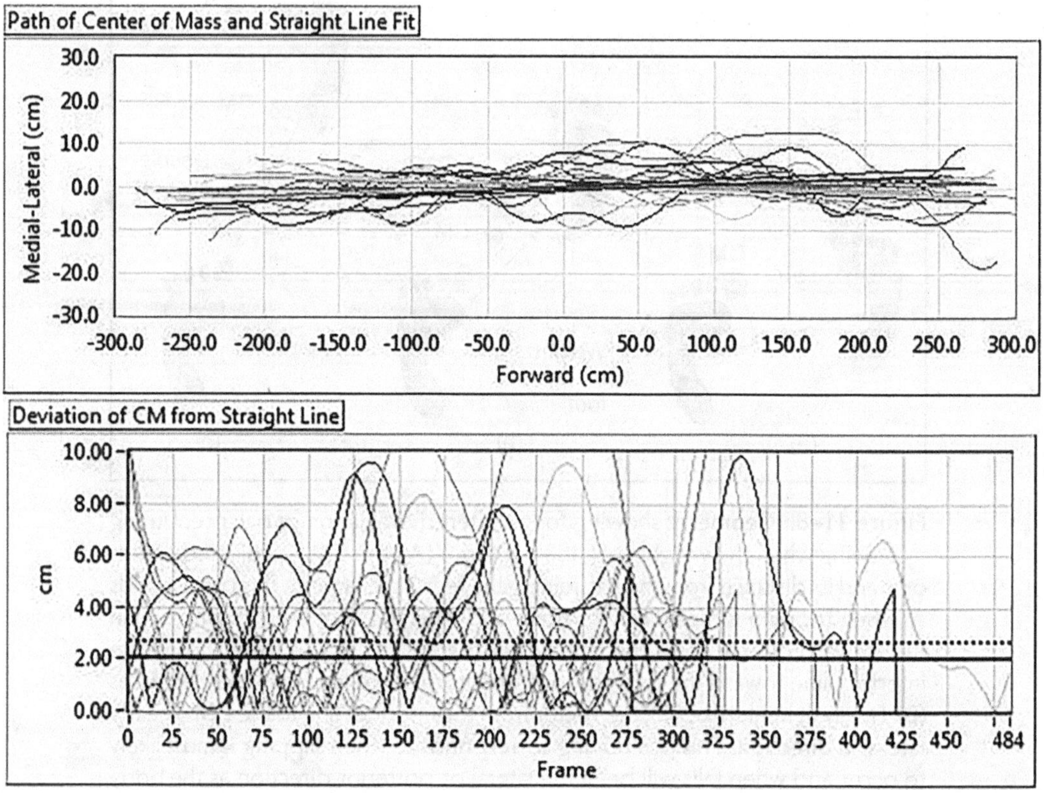

Figure 11–9. Central stability problem (ataxia): path of CM.

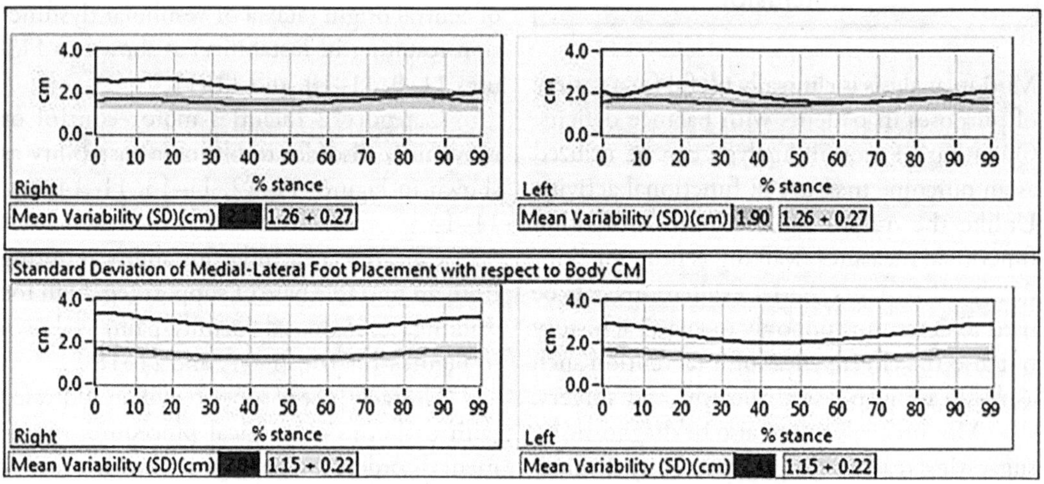

Figure 11–10. Central stability problem (ataxia): variability in foot placement.

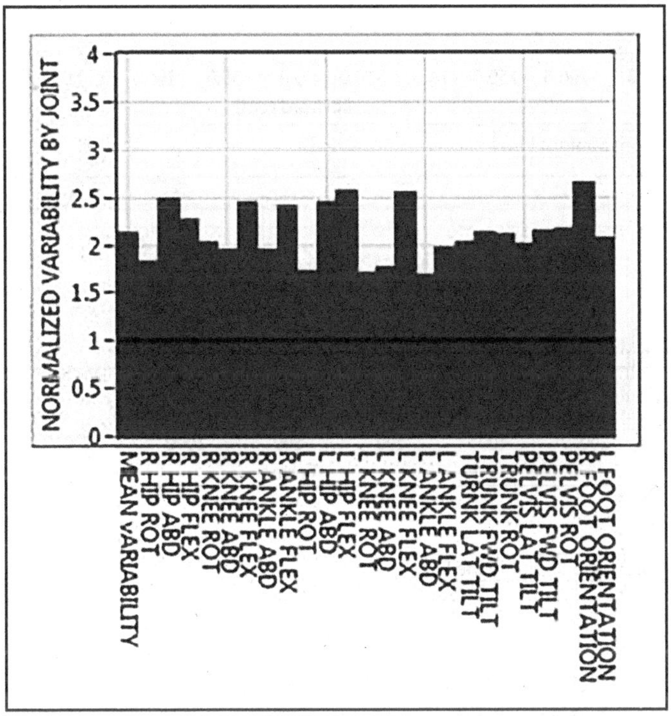

Figure 11–11. Central stability problem (ataxia): joint motion variability.

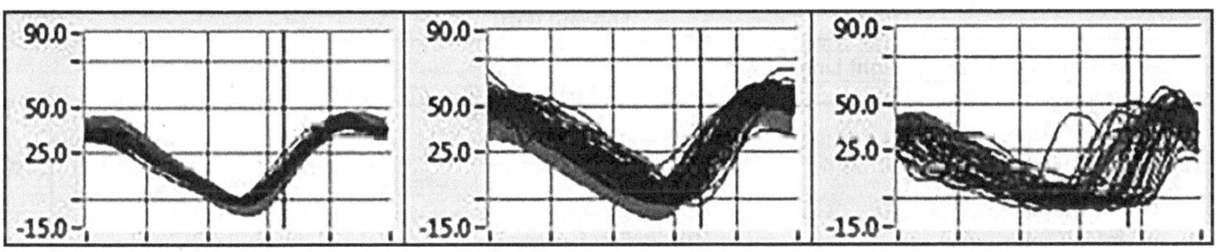

A B C

Figure 11–12. Hip sagittal plane kinematic motion during gait in (**A**) typical development (normal variability); (**B**) ataxia (high variability, normally distributed); (**C**) dystonia (high variability, nonnormally distributed).

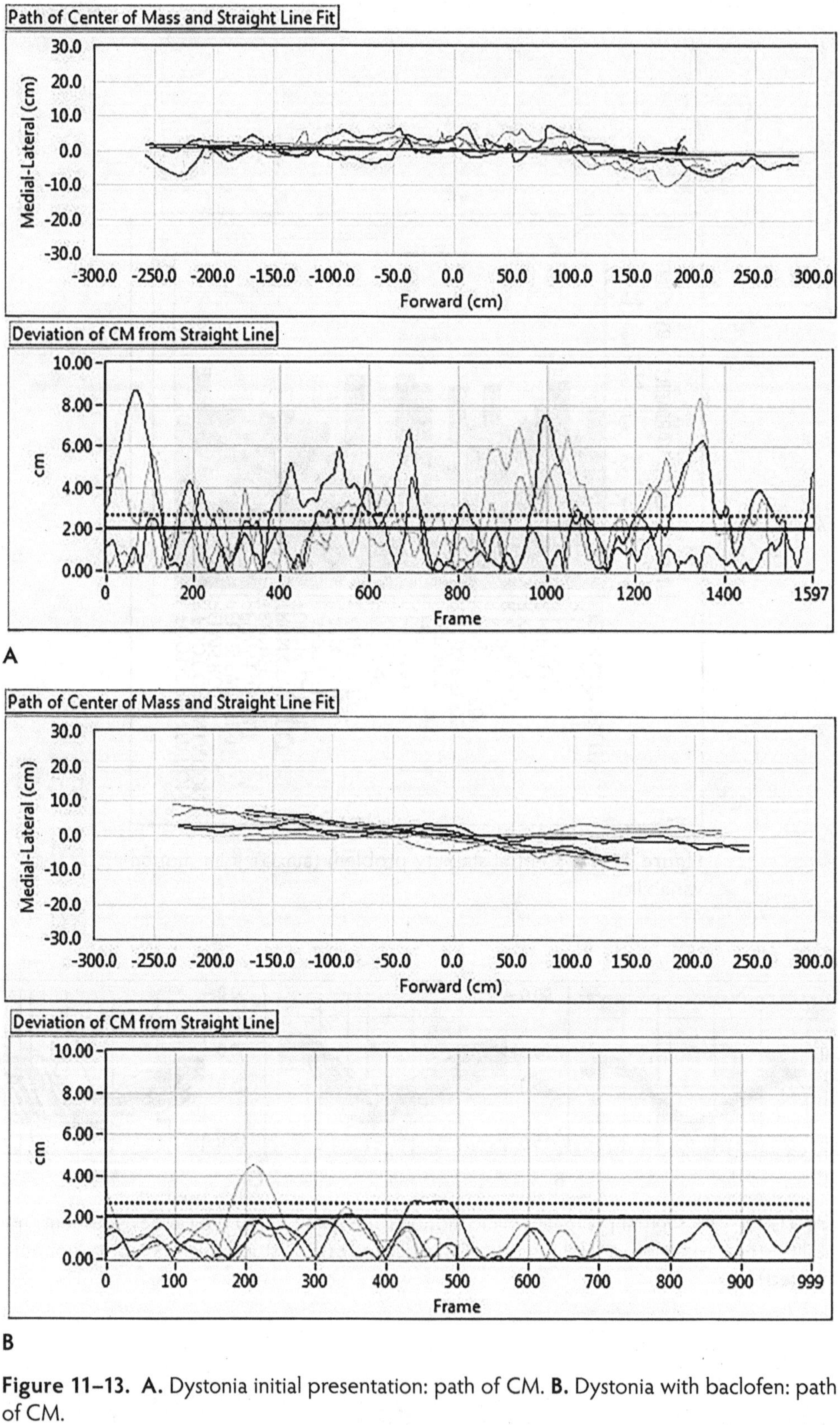

Figure 11–13. **A.** Dystonia initial presentation: path of CM. **B.** Dystonia with baclofen: path of CM.

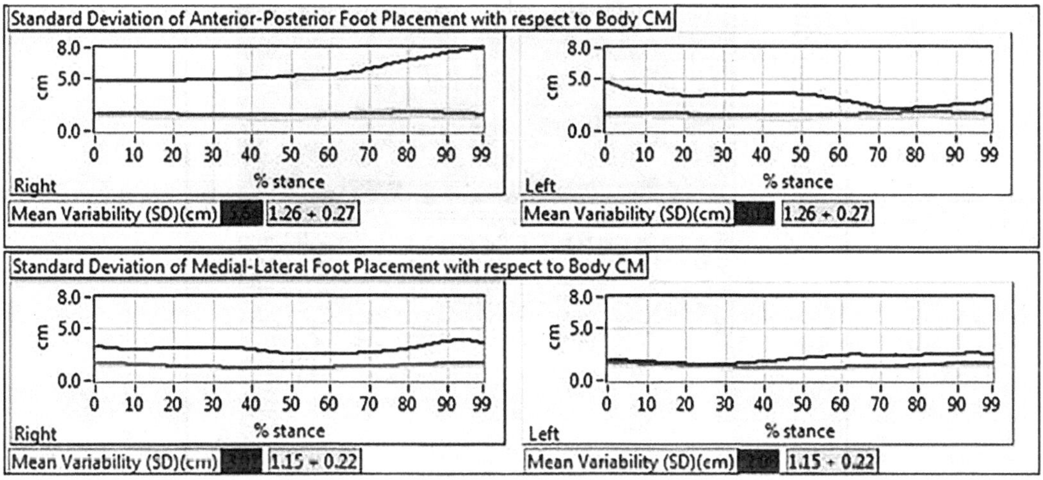

A

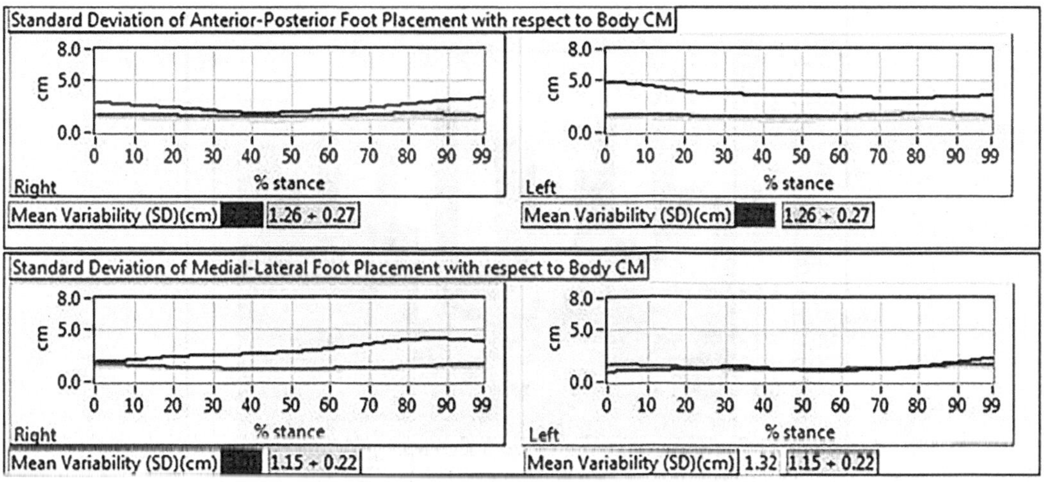

B

Figure 11–14. A. Dystonia initial presentation: Variability of foot placement. **B.** Dystonia with baclofen: variability of foot placement.

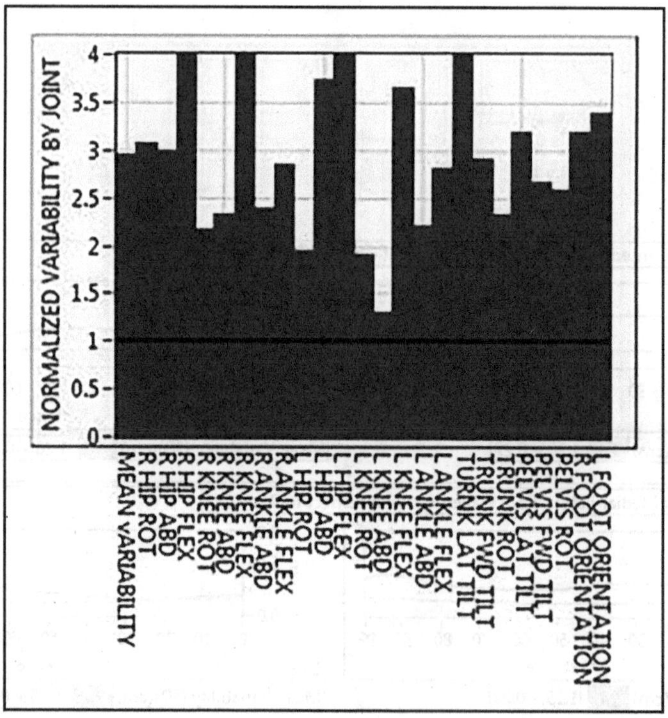

A

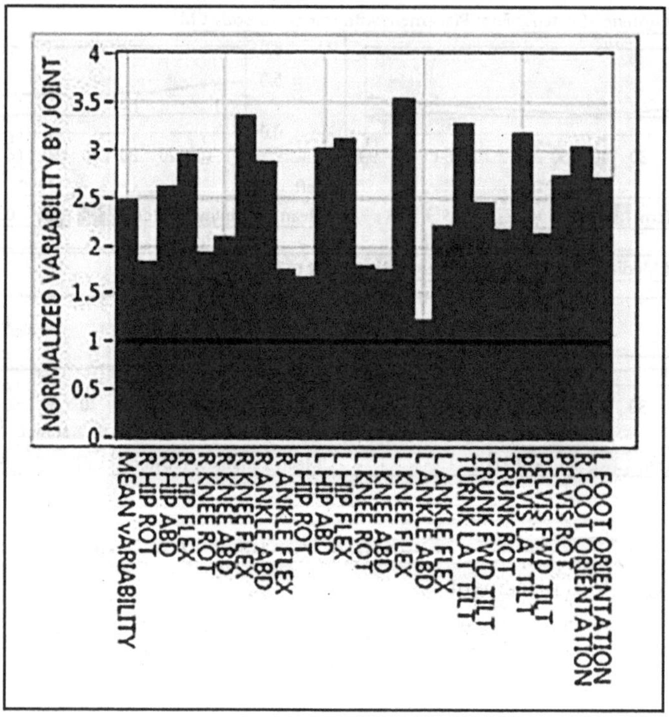

B

Figure 11–15. A. Joint variability dystonia. **B.** Joint variability dystonia with baclofen.

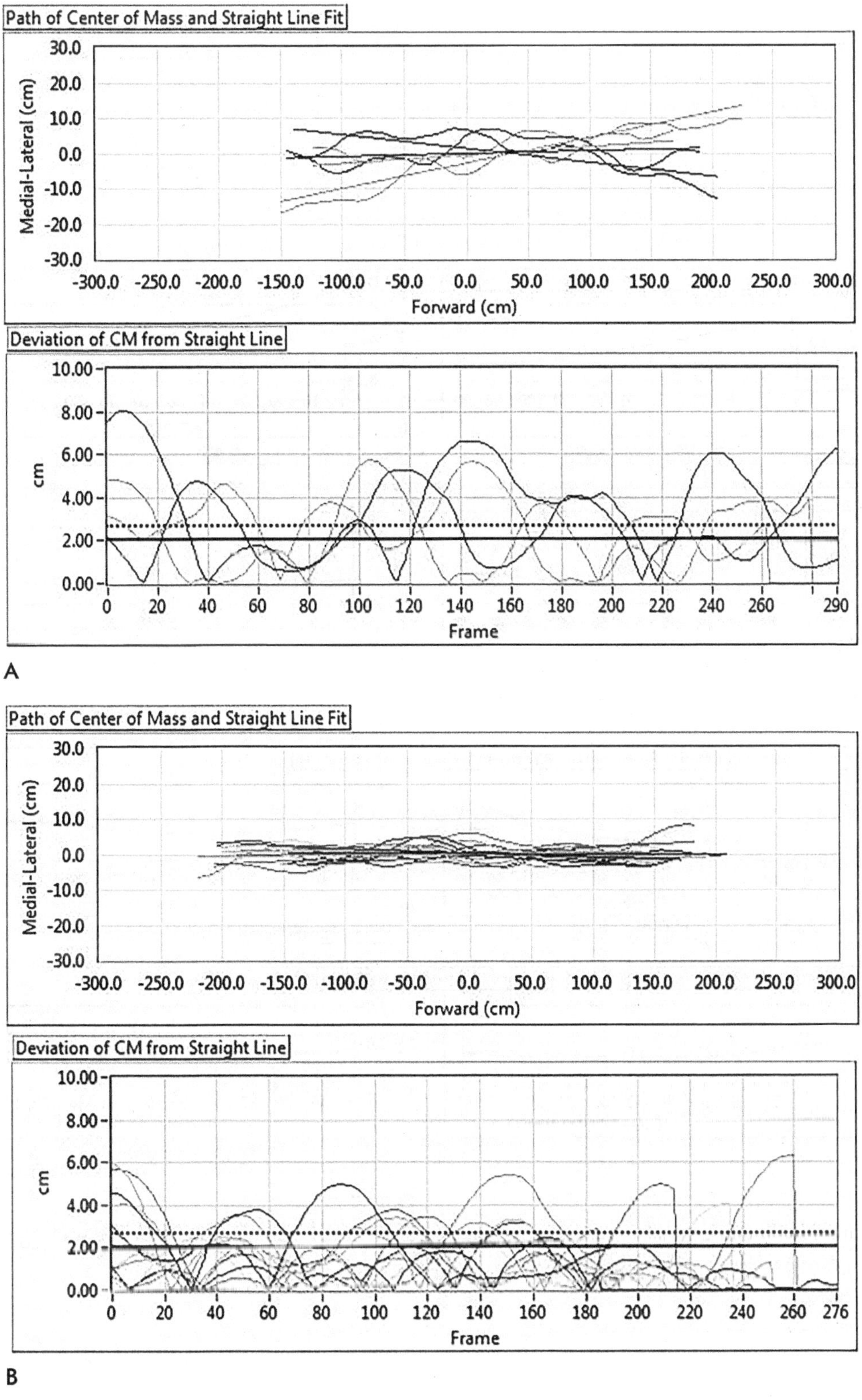

Figure 11–16. **A.** Toe walking initial presentation: path of CM. **B.** Toe walking postoperative: path of CM.

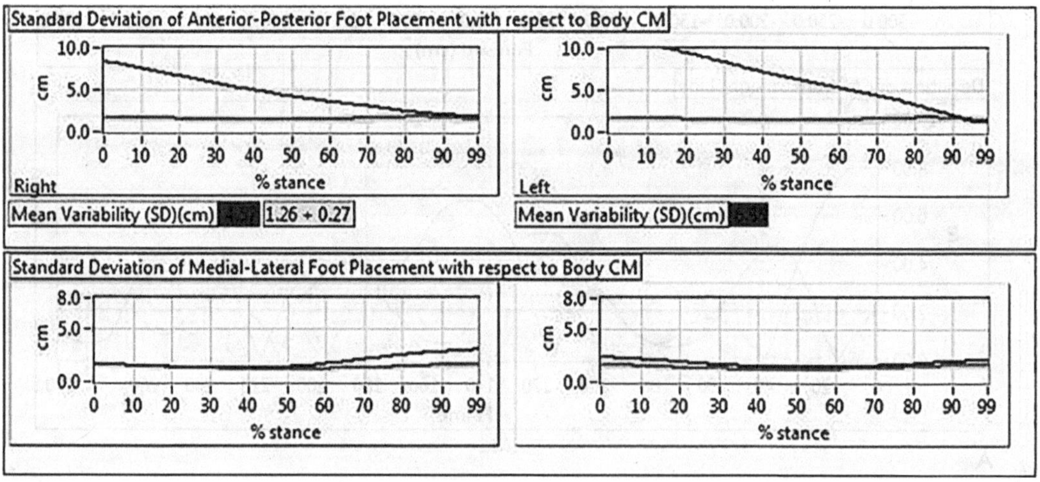

A

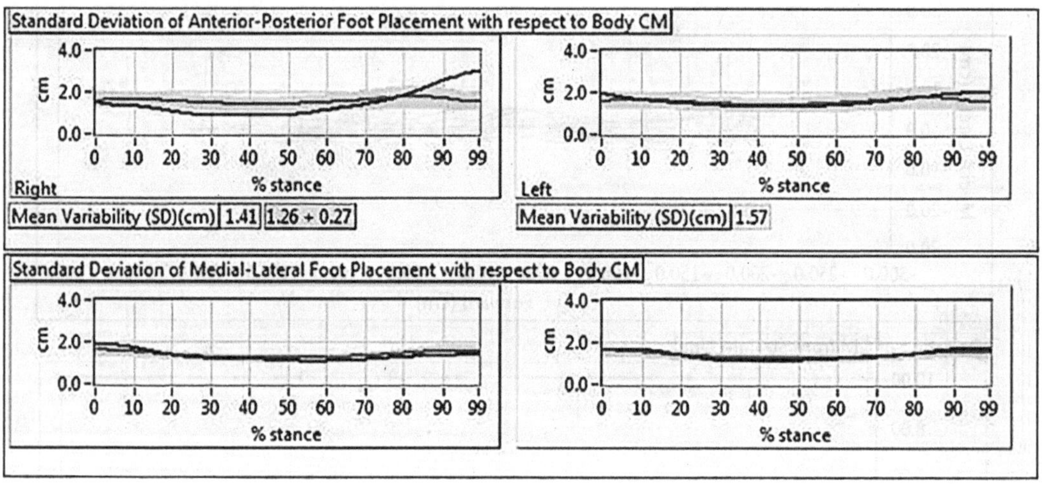

B

Figure 11–17. A. Toe walking initial presentation: variability of foot placement. **B.** Toe walking post-operative: variability of foot placement.

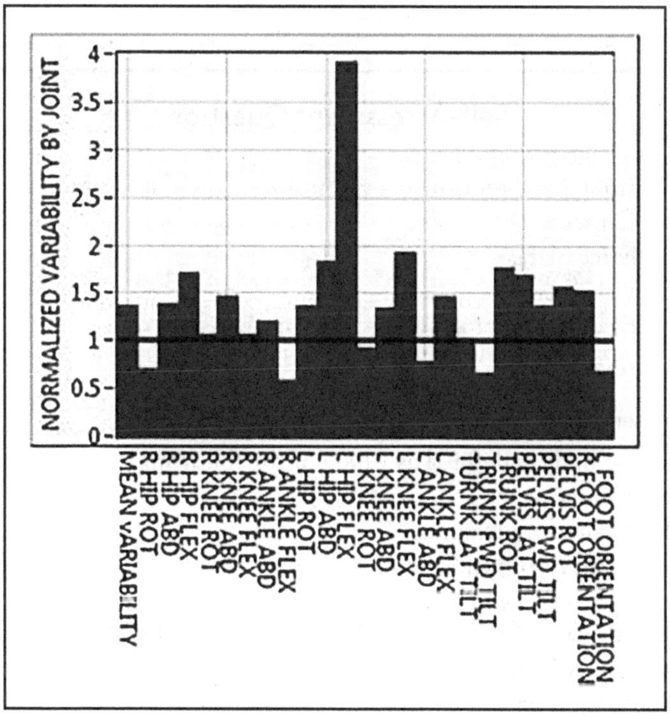

A

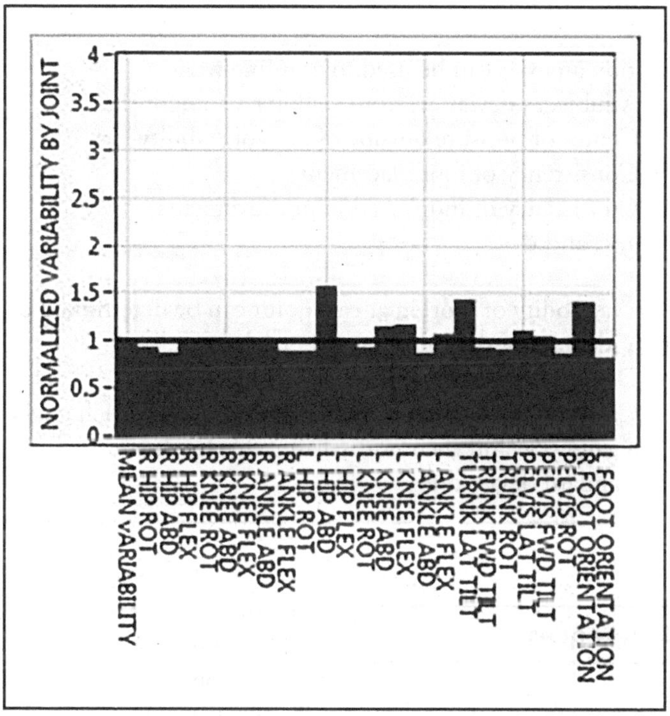

B

Figure 11–18. A. Toe walking pre-op: joint variability. **B.** Toe walking post-op: joint variability.

Self-Assessment Questions

1. Computerized motion analysis utilizes which of the following?
   a. Cameras
   b. Force plates
   c. Video recordings
   d. Electromyography (EMG) electrodes
   e. a, b, and d

2. The location of the net application of the ground-reaction forces on the body is defined as which of the following?
   a. Center of mass
   b. Center of pressure
   c. Point of proprioception

3. A large base of stability includes which of the following?
   a. Ability to move freely and move the CM
   b. A larger separation of CP from CM
   c. A greater influence on maintenance of balance
   d. All of the above

4. Motion analysis can be used to examine what?
   a. A subject's deviation from walking a straight line
   b. Center of pressure outside of base of stability
   c. Consistency of foot placement
   d. Consistency of individual joint movements
   e. a, c, and d

5. The variability of motion at each joint can be determined by what?
   a. Videotaping the subject over 3 trials of walking
   b. Determining the ratio of the CM to the center of gravity
   c. Calculating the average standard deviation of each angle over a gait cycle and then normalizing this by the normal average standard deviation

References

1. Baker R. The History of gait analysis before the advent of modern computers. *Gait Posture.* 2007;26:331–342.
2. Sutherland D. The evolution of clinical gait analysis: Part II Kinematics. *Gait Posture.* 2002;26:159–179.
3. Abdel-Aziz YI, Karara HM. Direct linear transformation from comparator coordinates into object space coordinates in close-range photogrammetry. *Proceedings of the Symposium on Close-Range Photogrammetry.* Falls Church, VA: American Society of Photogrammetry; 1971:1–18.
4. Chen L, Armstrong CW, Raftopoulos DD. An investigation on the accuracy of three-

dimensional space reconstruction using the direct linear transformation technique. *J Biomech. 1994;*27:493–500.

5. Hatze H. High-precision three-dimensional photogrammetric calibration and object space reconstruction using a modified DLT-approach. *J Biomech. 1988;21:*533–538.
6. Marzan GT, Karara HM. A computer program for direct linear transformation solution of the collinearity condition, and some applications of it. *Proceedings of the Symposium on Close-Range Photogrammetric Systems.* Falls Church, VA: American Society of Photogrammetry; 1975:420–476.
7. Miller NR, Shapiro R, McLaughlin TM. A technique for obtaining spatial kinematic parameters of segments of biomechanical systems from cinematographic data. *J Biomech.* 1980;13:535–547.
8. Shapiro R. Direct linear transformation method for three-dimensional cinematography. *Res Q.* 1978;49:197–205.
9. Walton JS. *Close-Range Cine-Photogrammetry: A Generalized Technique for Quantifying Gross Human Motion* [dissertation]. University Park, PA: Pennsylvania State University, University Park; 1981.
10. Winter DA. *Anatomy Biomechanics and Control of Balance During Standing and Walking.* Waterloo, Ontario, Canada: Waterloo Biomechanics; 1995.
11. Niiler T, Henley J, Miller F. (2017) Center of mass perturbation as a normalizable estimate of dynamic balance in gait: An application comparing typically developing children with spastic cerebral palsy. *arXiv.org.* 2017;arXiv: 1701.00507 [physics].
12. Niiler T. Using posture recognition to characterize real life slipping in YouTube videos. *Gait Posture.* 2017;57:121–122. doi:10.1016/j.gaitpost.2017.06.323
13. Barrett MJ, Bressman S. Genetics and pharmacological treatment of dystonia. *Int Rev Neurobiol.* 2011;98:525–549.
14. Hillier SL, Hollohan V. Vestibular rehabilitation for unilateral peripheral vestibular dysfunction. *Cochrane Database Syst Rev.* 2007;(4):CD005397.

CHAPTER 12

New Horizons for the Evaluation of Functional Balance, Self-Motion Perception, Navigation, and Mobility

Jennifer L. Campos, Claire McSweeny, Karen A. Gordon, and Sharon L. Cushing

Overview

The vestibular system plays several important roles in how we navigate through and interact with our environment. These include but are not limited to maintaining a stable visual view of the world through controlled eye movements; estimating and perceiving self-motion including parameters of speed, distance, and heading direction; maintaining standing balance; supporting mobility (walking, cycling, driving); and developing and guiding spatial navigational behaviors, strategies, and memories. Notably, all of these aspects of perception and performance typically require multiple sensory inputs (eg, auditory, visual, proprioceptive) and occur across a variety of complex conditions, including when overall sensory information is impoverished (eg, darkness) or challenged (movement/balance perturbations), and during multitasking (eg, walking while talking, physically navigating while route planning).

While these conditions and constraints are experienced broadly across all ages and sensory abilities, they may have particularly significant effects on the perceptions and behaviors of individuals experiencing sensory loss. As such, considering how vestibular function interacts with other sensory and cognitive functions under realistic and challenging conditions could be advantageous when evaluating how vestibular impairment can affect common, everyday behaviors and overall quality of life. Despite the complex and multifaceted role of the vestibular system, clinical assessments of vestibular and balance function are often narrowly focused on peripheral end-organ testing, reflexive vestibular-ocular responses, or basic balance/mobility testing under ideal clinical conditions (eg, well lit, quiet, void of distractions). As such, there may be additional value in introducing assessment and intervention techniques that are more closely aligned with everyday behaviors and conditions. Further, systematically increasing sensory, motor, and cognitive challenges during assessment/intervention has the potential to provide increased sensitivity to measuring and targeting subtle impairments or subclinical deficits. Common and standardized clinical tests may be diagnostic for more significant or specific impairments but may be less sensitive to slight or multifaceted impairments and/or impairments that become evidenced only when having to accommodate the multisensory, multimodal challenges typical of everyday life. This could also partially explain why some patient complaints about problems during everyday functioning may not be evidenced by test results on typical clinical measures. For children, this could mean missing impairments with potential developmental consequences.

The role of the vestibular system for overall development is beginning to be recognized, and further understanding across the life span is needed. The vestibular system plays an underacknowledged role in developmental neurocognition by providing perceptual and visuospatial input important for memory and executive function. A number of studies have demonstrated that children with a variety of vestibular impairments demonstrate deficits in memory and executive function,[1] and an association between vestibular dysfunction and poor school performance has been documented.[2] A thoughtful review of the cognitive impact of vestibular impairment in children suggests that there is likely a critical period to develop accurate spatial representations.[3] It is essential to further our understanding of the link between vestibular and cognitive dysfunction if we are to expand or develop new pediatric tests of vestibular functioning that are well tolerated, age appropriate, and provide diagnostic value.[4]

Novel methods of assessment should aim to generalize to everyday functioning. These methods may therefore focus on tasks that require the integration of, and interactions between (multi)sensory, motor, and cognitive inputs in behaviors taking place during navigation (eg, across space and over time). While other chapters in this book, as well as other published resources have provided comprehensive summaries describing how vestibular function is assessed at the level of end-organ functioning, reflexive responses (eg, eye movements, see Chapters 5 through 8), and balance function (eg, posturography, BOT-2, see Chapters 9 through 11), here we focus on potential novel methods of measuring perceived self-motion and self-orientation and other behaviors for which vestibular inputs are important. Although many of these tasks have been used extensively in fundamental experimental literature, they have rarely been used to address clinical objectives, and we are not aware of any specific uses in pediatric populations.

Vestibular Perception of Self-Motion Parameters

The otoliths and semicircular canals sense accelerations from linear and rotational movements of the head, respectively. Once detected, the brain must integrate and interpret these signals to generate percepts of self-motion through space and percepts of orientation in space (see Chapters 1 and 2). The ability of the brain to detect, differentiate, and interpret vestibular percepts of self-motion has been studied in the context of self-orientation (eg, subjective upright),[5,6] heading direction,[7–10] traveled distance,[11–13] and velocity.[13–15] Typically, observers are asked to either detect changes/differences in these parameters (eg, movement detection or discrimination tasks), or judge these movement/orientation parameters with respect to some reference frame (eg, gravitational vertical) or reference units (eg, meters or meters per second). For example, tasks used to measure perceptions of subjective upright include the Subjective Visual Vertical (SVV) task,[6] the Subjective Postural Vertical (SPV) task,[16] the Oriented Character Recognition Test (OCHART),[17] and the Rod in Frame test.[18] The most commonly used clinically applied test of subjective upright is currently the SVV task. During the SVV task, participants are typically asked to align a visually presented luminous vertical line with gravitational vertical in the absence of any other external visual reference frames (eg, in otherwise total darkness). Gravity introduces a constant acceleration, which is sensed by the otolith organs. Therefore, with normal otolith function and accurate percepts, participants are able to align the line vertically with generally high precision (typically a <2° bias in nonclinical adult populations).[17,19] Although this degree of precision can be observed in typically developing children,[20,21] there is also evidence that the biases in the SVV of healthy children are greater and more variable than in adults.[21,24] Additionally, SVV biases are larger in females compared to males across all age groups,[25,26] and these biases are often much greater with vestibular dysfunction.[20] The SVV has been used to assess vestibular or visual-vestibular dysfunction across a range of different patient populations, including individuals with stroke, concussion, prematurity, and peripheral vestibular loss.[6,20–23] It has been shown to have very good sensitivity and specificity for identifying peripheral vestibular dysfunction in pediatric populations specifically.[20,27] Furthermore, clinical implementation of the SVV task has been made simpler by the development of mobile device applications that have been shown to achieve high specificity (97%) compared to conventional SVV tasks in detecting peripheral vestibular dysfunction in children.[20]

Children who are deaf and use cochlear implants have a high rate of concurrent vestibular deficits as measured by standard clinical tools. The SVV revealed errors in vertical perception beyond the clinical standard of ±2° in a large proportion (45%) of cochlear implant users ranging in age from 7.9 to 27 years. Biases in this group were reduced by cochlear implant stimulation, suggesting a role for electrical stimulation to help alleviate functional impairments.[6] A more in-depth discussion regarding using CI stimulation as a possible therapeutic tool in this manner can be found in Chapter 28.

Self-motion can be judged using primarily vestibular inputs when other sensory input is not available (eg, during blindfolded, passive movements). It is clear, for example, that when moving along simple linear motion profiles, adults can use vestibular information alone to judge displacement,[12,28–33] velocity,[13,34,35] and acceleration.[13] During visually directed self-motion (eg "blind walking") tasks, observers can view an in-depth target up to 20 m, and walk, or be passively transported along a forward linear trajectory in the dark to estimate the target position with good accuracy.[12,30,34,36–42] Children from ages 4 to 8 can also estimate the extent of walked self-motion in the dark but are not as accurate or consistent as adults,[43] with error and variability decreasing with increasing age.[43] Interestingly, one study demonstrated that children do not make use of visual landmark cues when they are available along with vestibular and proprioceptive cues; whereas the added input was beneficial to the performance of adults.[43]

In another task referred to as the "continuous pointing task," blindfolded participants are asked to point continuously to a previously viewed target while walking or being passively transported forward past the target on a linear trajectory.[13,36,44] Measuring the pointing direction of the arm provides a continuous indicator of perceived location, velocity, and acceleration at every moment in time. Using this highly informative technique, it has been shown that during simple movements, observers are able to perceive direction, displacement, and velocity when walking blindfolded, or during passive transport.[12,36] The capacity for spatial updating during passive movements (when primarily vestibular inputs are available) however, may be reduced for longer or more complex movements.[13,45] Heading detection and discrimination tasks have also shown that observers can detect and differentiate heading direction based on passive movements in the dark.[8,10,46] For instance, when asked to compare two presented passive movements in slightly different directions, observers can discriminate relative heading directions with high levels of precision.[8,10,46]

These skills appear to be impaired in individuals with vestibular dysfunction. For instance, individuals with unilateral vestibular hypofunction underestimate the magnitude of walked distances to a greater extent than those with normal vestibular function,[47] and individuals with chronic vestibular pathologies demonstrate greater veer during blindfolded walking to a previously viewed target.[48–50] In terms of an individual's perception of simple passive rotations around one axis, those with unilateral vestibular deficits have also demonstrated more difficulty (ie, higher detection thresholds) detecting yaw rotations (turning around a vertical axis).[51]

In addition to characterizing vestibular percepts during simple movement trajectories like the ones just described (eg, discrete linear or rotational segments), vestibular percepts can guide more complex behaviors, such as spatial updating and navigational tasks involving multiple translations and turns. There is some indication that individuals with vestibular impairments may demonstrate greater errors on more complex navigational tasks (eg, those requiring the integration/updating of both translations and rotations) compared to simpler linear or rotational movements.[14,50,52]

Vestibular Contributions to Complex Spatial Updating and Navigation

Humans' natural strategies for navigating their environments typically involve moving along complex trajectories, including combined axes and planes of motion. The ability to keep internal track of one's position in space without using visual or auditory landmark cues is referred to as path integration or dead reckoning.[40] Effective path integration allows humans and other animals to return to a starting position (eg, homing) using familiar or novel routes and/or to orient their heading direction to point back to start. The primary sensory inputs used for path integration during walking include dynamic visual and acoustical flow, proprioceptive/efference copy, and vestibular inputs. Many tasks have been implemented to study path integration, including the *triangle completion task*,[53–57] *the novel shortcut task*,[58] and variants of the *Morris water maze test*.[59] In the triangle completion task, participants are asked to move along a straight distance interval, rotate some degree, move along a second interval, and then point, or move back to the start position to complete the triangle.[38,54,57] It has been shown that participants with normal sensory functions are accurate in the triangle completion task during blindfolded walking, but not when watching another person walking the path, or when imagining walking the path through a verbal description.[54] Interestingly, when only visual inputs are available (simulated optic flow presented via a head-mounted display), performance is very poor, but when vestibular inputs are introduced to the visual inputs during the rotations alone, errors are greatly reduced and approximate the actual walking trials.[54] Other studies have also demonstrated an important role for vestibular inputs for path integration by showing no differences in error between blindfolded walking (proprioceptive + vestibular inputs available) and passive transport (primarily vestibular inputs available) during the triangle completion task.[57] Vestibular inputs during navigation are also known to be important for spatial memory encoding,[59–62] and vestibular impairment has been associated with changes to neural substrates important for spatial memory and navigation, including the hippocampus.[59]

In contrast to individuals with normal vestibular functioning, individuals with vestibular dysfunction demonstrate greater and more variable errors in path integration as evidenced through blindfolded triangle completion and triangle reproduction tasks.[14,52] The characteristics of these errors suggest that it is the rotational elements in particular that are misestimated to a greater degree than the translational elements of the path. Further, human and other animal studies have provided evidence that vestibular deficits, particularly bilateral, are associated with impaired spatial memory and navigation.[59,63–65]

Multisensory Self-Motion Perception

It is now well established that integrating redundant inputs from across the sensory systems (multisensory integration) typically leads to perceptual and behavioral benefits.[8,66–68] Specifically, because there is noise inherent in our environments and in our sensory and neural systems, combining redundant inputs is generally advantageous. For example, combining sensory inputs across modalities (eg, visual + tactile cues) typically leads to more *precise* estimates (for instance, when estimating the size of a grasped object) compared to the sensory input alone (eg, visual cues alone or tactile cues alone).[69] Also, when sensory inputs are integrated, the more reliable sensory estimate is typically weighted higher than the less reliable sensory estimate(s). These characteristics of "optimal multisensory integration" have also been observed in the context of self-motion perception.[8,12,44,46,70–72] For instance, combining vestibular estimates with visual estimates leads to more precise judgments of passive heading[8,71] and more robust firing in brain areas associated with motion perception[73] than when either visual or vestibular cues are available in isolation. Whereas it is clear that visual and auditory loss have significant effects on multisensory percepts, mediated by neuroplastic changes in sensory cortices,[74,75] potentially similar effects of vestibular loss are likely but have not yet been defined. These examples of sensory plasticity are clearest during development. It is likely that sensory compensation or recalibration does occur in individuals with vestibular loss, perhaps due to a greater reliance on other sensory inputs such as vision and proprioception, but may be modulated with age.

Defining how the brain weighs individual sensory inputs to support self-motion will be important for developing targeted assessments and rehabilitation interventions. However, it is difficult to tease apart the influence of individual sensory inputs when several are simultaneously available and provide both congruent and redundant information. For instance, during walking, vestibular inputs are necessarily linked directly to dynamic visual flow and proprioceptive inputs.[76] Adding or removing individual sensory inputs and observing the resultant percepts or behaviors may provide some insight into which are sufficient to perceive self-motion, but not necessarily which are actually being used and integrated when more than one is available. A common experimental strategy for dissociating naturally congruent cues has been the "cue conflict approach." This approach involves providing individual modalities with slightly incongruent information about a single perceptual event at the same time. For example, a classic approach to introduce cue conflicts during goal-directed actions is by using displacement prisms.[77,78] Displacement prisms cause the visual field to be shifted (left, right, up, or down), thereby introducing changes to perceptual-motor coupling during visually guided movements. Further, in the context of self-motion perception specifically, the "swinging room" paradigm has been used to dissociate optic flow from vestibular/proprioceptive inputs. Specifically, in this paradigm, observers are asked to stand stationary on a stable floor while the walls of the room (ie, global visual flow) shift/slide in the fore-and-aft directions around them.[79–81] In response to this global visual motion, observers adjust their posture such that their body sways synchronously with the movement of the room. The effects of the swinging room are more pronounced in young children compared to adults,[80,82] with the majority of toddlers falling completely over when the room is quickly moved several centimeters.[80] Within rotational axes (primarily yaw axis), optokinetic drums have also been used to dissociate visual inputs from vestibular/proprioceptive inputs by rotating the visible walls of a cylinder around a physically stationary observer.[33] During optokinetic stimulation, observations associated with eye movements, postural responses, and subjective reports (eg, of vertigo, motion sickness) can provide insight into visual-vestibular interactions. An example of a clinical test that has considered multisensory interactions supporting postural control during conflicting sensory conditions is the Sensory Organization Test[83] and its pediatric variants.[84–87]

Modern technologies such as virtual reality (VR) and motion simulators are also providing new ways of systematically introducing these cue conflicts during tasks involving self-motion perception.[94] For instance, visual inputs presented via head-mounted displays or multiwalled projection displays can be used to systematically vary the content and movement parameters of the visual environment.[72,88–90,94] Motion platforms such as hexapod motion simulators (6° of freedom), sleds (translational), and yaw platforms (rotations) can be combined with VR systems to introduce and control physical movements.[94] The decreasing cost and increasing accessibility and availability of VR hardware, software, and content are making some of these technologies viable and valuable options for novel clinical assessment and intervention strategies. Another advantage of VR beyond manipulating cue congruencies is that it allows for the realistic mimicking of everyday conditions and challenges. This can provide an important middle ground between controlled and safe laboratory/clinical settings and the real world and can potentially enhance generalizability of assessments and interventions. Because the content of the virtual environments is completely customizable, it can be used to present common experiences such as standing in a classroom, walking through a grocery store, traveling in a car, or navigating a busy city intersection.

The reliability of simulated sensory information can also be more easily and strategically manipulated in VR (eg, simulated nighttime); realistic sensory incongruencies can be introduced (eg, moving visual stimuli such as large vehicles or crowds of people), and distracting stimuli can be incorporated, including unexpected objects or events. Cognitive loads can also be introduced by asking individuals to complete two or more tasks at the same time (eg, have a conversation or hold information in memory while standing/walking/driving).[95]

It may be the case that these more complex challenges can most clearly reveal deficits in self-motion perception and associated behaviors.[91] For example, in one study conducted within a fully immersive VR environment (simulated busy city intersection), children with and without unilateral hearing loss performed various balance tasks ranging in difficulty.[92] Specifically, the Bruininks-Oseretsky Test-2 (BOT-2) was administered and scored, and center of pressure (COP) path length was also measured. Results demonstrated poorer BOT-2 scores and greater variability in COP in children with unilateral hearing loss compared to normal hearing peers, particularly during moderately difficult tasks (eg, standing on one foot with eyes closed).[92]

Special Considerations for Children/Pediatric Populations

Our clinical and research toolbox for examining functional balance, self-motion perception, navigation, and mobility is deep and expanding. The necessity of applying these tools to the pediatric patient presenting with vestibular and balance concerns is critical to measuring the "real-world" impact of these deficits and the resultant effects of any interventions that we apply. Much of the work to date in this domain has focused on the fully developed adult with an acquired loss of sensory function. This is very different from applying such techniques to the still developing child with primarily congenital or early acquired sensory deficits. In addition to the fact that the time course of deficit acquisition is often different between children and adults, the onset of the hearing loss (eg. congenital versus acquired), the etiology of these sensory deficits is also frequently different (eg, cytomegalovirus versus stroke). In this context, we need not only to consider the impact of development on the measures we are using but also the impact of the deficit we are aiming to measure on development itself. Much is already known about the developmental trajectory of the vestibular apparatus (Chapter 1), as well as the physiology and maturation of balance mechanisms (Chapter 2), highlighting the changes that occur within the first decades of life in the mechanisms that govern balance and movement in children. We need to consider not only the maturation of the vestibular system (Chapters 1–2) but also maturation of multisensory integration mechanisms, as well as of cognitive abilities. Although this provides challenges in adapting these measures to children, we should not shy away from their application, as much of this variability may be resolved through the collection of age-standardized normative data. Beyond the developmental considerations, the administration and limits of such testing also need to be studied using a pediatric lens, with adaptations considered to ensure compliance and comprehension in children.

Summary and Future Challenges

As humans, our ability to safely and effectively navigate our environment allows us to be interconnected and productive within society. Learning to do so is as important as learning to communicate. Despite its importance, the complexity and redundancy of the sensory systems themselves and the mechanisms of sensory integration can create challenges to meaningfully measure the impact that deficits occurring anywhere within the system create. Add on the additional challenge of obtaining measures in children, whose developmental trajectories create a moving target for evaluation, and one might easily throw up their hands in defeat. Indeed, at this stage, there are more questions than answers; however, acknowledging these questions is key in advancing our clinical and research efforts. Many important open questions remain and are ripe for investigation. For instance, how are impairments in self-motion percepts and behaviors associated with other outcomes, such as gross motor skills, academic performance, and cognitive abilities?[93] How are deficits in self-motion percepts and associated behaviors affected by factors such as the etiology of vestibular impairment, unilateral versus bilateral loss, chronic versus acute stages, congenital versus acquired loss and age of onset, central versus peripheral function, and otolith versus canal function? It is also unknown how common clinically used screening and diagnostic tools are associated with novel functional task performance and what the ideal ways are to adapt approaches traditionally used in research for use in the clinical setting. Finally, identifying vestibular-associated deficits in self-motion perception and spatial orientation/memory and understanding their impact on functional outcomes lays the important groundwork for ultimately understanding how the lives of children who experience them can be improved with the use of appropriate rehabilitative interventions.

Self-Assessment Question

1. How do the assessment and intervention techniques outlined in this chapter differ from typically used clinical measures of vestibular function?
2. Signals from which two vestibular end organs provide the brain with information used during the generation of self-motion through space and orientation in space percepts?
3. Which measure of the perception of subjective upright is available for use through a mobile application?
4. One assessment technique described measures perceived location, velocity, and acceleration during dynamic movement. Name this technique, and describe how it is executed.
5. Describe path integration (dead reckoning) and the primary sensory inputs used for path integration during walking.
6. Which part of memory relies on information provided by vestibular inputs during navigation?
7. During path integration tasks, which element of the task produces the greatest difficulty (evidenced by greatest error) for those with vestibular dysfunction?

8. What is multisensory integration, and how does it provide perceptual and behavioral benefits?
9. Which strategy is used to disassociate naturally congruent sensory inputs in an effort to tease apart which inputs have the greatest influence on the sensory percept?
10. What are some advantages to using virtual reality (VR) to introduce cue conflicts during tasks involving self-motion perception?
11. What are two main differences between children and adults that are important to consider when applying clinical vestibular assessments and interventions?

References

1. Bigelow RT, Agrawal Y. Vestibular involvement in cognition: Visuospatial ability, attention, executive function, and memory. *J Vestib Res*. 2015;(2):73–89.
2. Franco ES, Panhoca I. Vestibular function in children underperforming at school. *Brazilian J Otorhinolaryngol*. 2008;74(6):815–825.
3. Wiener-Vacher SR, Hamilton DA, Wiener SI. Vestibular activity and cognitive development in children: Perspectives. *Front Integr Neurosci*. 2013;7:1–13.
4. Ciolek PJ, Kang E, Honaker JA, Woodson EA, Hopkins BS, Anne S. Pediatric vestibular testing: Tolerability of test components in children. *Int J Pediatr Otorhinolaryngol*. 2018; 113:29–33.
5. Fraser LE, Mansfield A, Harris LR, Merino DM, Knorr S, Campos JL. The weighting of cues to upright following stroke with and without a history of pushing. *Can J Neurol Sci*. 2018;45(4):405–414.
6. Gnanasegaram JJ, Parkes WJ, Cushing SL, McKnight CL, Papsin BC, Gordon KA. Stimulation from cochlear implant electrodes assists with recovery from asymmetric perceptual tilt: Evidence from the Subjective Visual Vertical test. *Front Integr Neurosci*. 2016;10:1–12.
7. Fetsch CR, Wang S, Gu Y, DeAngelis GC, Angelaki DE. Spatial reference frames of visual, vestibular, and multimodal heading signals in area MSTd. *J Neurosci*. 2007;27(3):700–712.
8. Butler JS, Smith ST, Campos JL, Bülthoff HH. Bayesian integration of visual and vestibular signals for heading. *J Vis*. 2010;10(11):1–13.
9. Cullen KE. The vestibular system: Multimodal integration and encoding of self-motion for motor control. *Trends Neurosci*. 2012;35(3): 185–196.
10. Ramkhalawansingh R, Keshavarz B, Haycock B, Shahab S, Campos JL. Examining the effect of age on visual–vestibular self-motion perception using a driving paradigm. *Perception*. 2017;46(5):566–585.
11. Lappe M, Jenkin M, Harris LR. Travel distance estimation from visual motion by leaky path integration. *Exp Brain Res*. 2007;180(1): 35–48.
12. Campos JL, Butler JS, Bülthoff HH. Multisensory integration in the estimation of walked distances. *Exp Brain Res*. 2012;218(4): 551–565.
13. Siegle JH, Campos JL, Mohler BJ, Loomis JM, Bülthoff HH. Measurement of instantaneous

perceived self-motion using continuous pointing. *Exp Brain Res.* 2009;195(3):429–444.

14. Glasauer S, Amorim M-A, Viaud-Delmon I, Berthoz A. Differential effects of labyrinthine dysfunction on distance and direction during blindfolded walking of a triangular path. *Exp Brain Res.* 2002;145(4):489–497.
15. Durgin FH, Pelah A, Fox LF, Lewis J, Kane R, Walley KA. Self-motion perception during locomotor recalibration: More than meets the eye. *J Exp Psychol Gen.* 2005;31(3):398–419.
16. Mansfield A, Fraser L, Rajachandrakumar R, Danells CJ, Knorr S, Campos J. Is perception of vertical impaired in individuals with chronic stroke with a history of "pushing"? *Neurosci Lett.* 2015;590:172–177.
17. Dyde RT, Jenkin MR, Harris LR. The subjective visual vertical and the perceptual upright. *Exp Brain Res.* 2006;173(4):612–622.
18. Sholl MJ. The relation between horizontality and rod-and-frame and vestibular navigational performance. *J Exp Psychol Learn Mem Cogn.* 1989;15(1):110–125.
19. Akin FW, Murnane OD. Clinical assessment of otolith function. *ASHA Leader.* 2009;14(2):14–17.
20. Brodsky JR, Cusick BA, Kawai K, Kenna M, Zhou G. Peripheral vestibular loss detected in pediatric patients using a smartphone-based test of the subjective visual vertical. *Int J Pedatr Otorhinolaryngol.* 2015;79(12):2094–2098.
21. Gaertner C, Bucci MP, Obeid R, Wiener-Vacher S. Subjective visual vertical and postural performance in healthy children. *PLoS One.* 2013;8(11):e79623.
22. Karnath H-O. Pusher syndrome—A frequent but little-known disturbance of body orientation perception. *J Neurol.* 2007;254(4):415–424.
23. Fraser LE, Makooie B, Harris LR. The subjective visual vertical and the subjective haptic vertical access different gravity estimates. *PLoS One.* 2015;10(12):1–20.
24. Tringali M, Wiener-Vacher S, Bucci MP. Developmental study identifies the ages at which the processes involved in the perception of verticality and in postural stability occur. *Acta Paediatrica.* 2017;106(1):55–60.
25. Toupet M, Nechel CV. Subjective visual vertical tilt attraction to the side of rod presentation: Effects of age, sex, and vestibular disorders. 2015;36(6):1074–1080.
26. Toupet M, Van Nechel C, Grayeli AB. Maturation of subjective visual vertical in children. *Otol Neurotol.* 2016;37(6):761–766.
27. Brodsky JR, Cusick BA, Kenna MA, Zhou G. Subjective visual vertical testing in children and adolescents: SVV in children. *Laryngoscope.* 2016;126(3):727–731.
28. Bertin RJV, Berthoz A. Visuo-vestibular interaction in the reconstruction of travelled trajectories. *Exp Brain Res.* 2004;154(1):11–21.
29. Bülthoff H, Little J, Poggio T. A parallel algorithm for real-time computation of optic flow. *Nature.* 337(6207):549–553.
30. Harris LR, Jenkin M, Zikovitz DC. Visual and non-visual cues in the perception of linear self motion. *Exp Brain Res.* 2000;135(1):12–21.
31. Israël I, Chapuis N, Glasauer S, Charade O, Berthoz A. Estimation of passive horizontal linear whole-body displacement in humans. *J Neurophysiol.* 1993;70(3):1270–1273.
32. Israël I, Grasso R, Georges-François P, Tsuzuku T, Berthoz A. Spatial memory and path integration studied by self-driven passive linear displacement. I. Basic properties. *J Neurophysiol.* 1997;77(6):3180–3192.
33. Jürgens R, Becker W. Perception of angular displacement without landmarks: Evidence for Bayesian fusion of vestibular, optokinetic, podokinesthetic, and cognitive information. *Exp Brain Res.* 2006;174(3):528–543.
34. Sun H-J, Campos JL, Young M, Chan GSW, Ellard CG. The contributions of static visual cues, nonvisual cues, and optic flow in distance estimation. *Perception.* 2004;33(1):49–65.
35. Wallis G, Chatziastros A, Bülthoff H. An unexpected role for visual feedback in vehicle steering control. *Curr Biol.* 2002;12(4):295–299.
36. Campos JL, Siegle JH, Mohler BJ, Bülthoff HH, Loomis JM. Imagined self-motion differs from perceived self-motion: Evidence from a novel continuous pointing method. *PLoS One.* 2009;4(11):125–151.
37. Elliott D. Continuous visual information may be important after all: A failure to replicate

Thomson (1983). *J Exp Psychol Hum Percept Perform.* 1986;12(3):388–391.
38. Fukusima SS, Loomis JM. Visual perception of egocentric distance as assessed by triangulation. 1997;23(1):86–100.
39. Loomis JM, da Silva JA, Fujita N, Fukusima SS. Visual space perception and visually directed action. *J Exp Psychol Gen.* 1992; 18(4):906–921.
40. Mittelstaedt M-L, Mittelstaedt H. Idiothetic navigation in humans: Estimation of path length. *Exp Brain Res.* 2001;139(3):318–332.
41. Rieser JJ. Development of perceptual-motor control while walking without vision: The calibration of perception and action. In: Bloch H, Bertenthal BI, eds. *NATO Advanced Science Institutes series, D: Behavioural and Social Sciences, vol 56. Sensory-Motor Organizations and Development in Infancy and Early Childhood.* New York, NY: Kluwer Academic/Plenum Publishers; 1990:379–408.
42. Thomson JA. Is continuous visual monitoring necessary in visually guided locomotion? *J Exp Psychol Hum Percept Perform.* 1983; 9(3):427–443.
43. Nardini M, Jones P, Bedford R, Braddick O. Development of cue integration in human navigation. *Curr Biol.* 2008;18(9):689–693.
44. Frissen I, Campos JL, Souman JL, Ernst MO. Integration of vestibular and proprioceptive signals for spatial updating. *Exp Brain Res.* 2011;212(2):163–176.
45. Waller D, Greenauer N. The role of body-based sensory information in the acquisition of enduring spatial representations. *Psychol Res.* 2007;71(3):322–332.
46. Gu Y, Fetsch CR, Adeyemo B, DeAngelis GC, Angelaki DE. Decoding of MSTd population activity accounts for variations in the precision of heading perception. *Neuron.* 2010;66(4): 596–609.
47. Schubert MC, Arthur JC, Shelhamer M, Kortte KB. Linear path integration deficits in patients with abnormal vestibular afference. *Seeing Perceiving.* 2012;25(2):155–178.
48. Cohen HS. Vestibular disorders and impaired path integration along a linear trajectory. *J Vestib Res.* 2000;10(1):7–15.
49. Cohen HS, Sangi-Haghpeykar H. Walking speed and vestibular disorders in a path integration task. *Gait Posture.* 2011;33(2):211–213.
50. Glasauer S, Amorim M-A, Vitte E, Berthoz A. Goal-directed linear locomotion in normal and labyrinthine-defective subjects. *Exp Brain Res.* 1994;98(2):323–335.
51. Cousins S, Kaski D, Cutfield N, et al. Vestibular perception following acute unilateral vestibular lesions. *PLoS One.* 2013;8(5):e61862.
52. Péruch P, Borel L, Magnan J, Lacour M. Direction and distance deficits in path integration after unilateral vestibular loss depend on task complexity. *Cog Brain Res.* 2005;25(3):862–872.
53. Klatzky RL. Path completion after haptic exploration without vision: Implications for haptic spatial representations. *Percept Psychophys.* 1999;61(2):220–235.
54. Klatzky RL, Loomis JM, Beall AC, Chance SS, Golledge RG. Spatial updating of self-position and orientation during real, Imagined, and virtual locomotion. *Psychol Sci.* 1998;9(4):293–298.
55. Loomis JM, Klatzky RL, Golledge RG, Philbeck JW. Human navigation by path integration. In: *Wayfinding Behavior: Cognitive Mapping and Other Spatial Processes.* Vol 10; Baltimore, MD: Johns Hopkins University Press; 1999.
56. Xie Y, Bigelow RT, Frankenthaler SF, Studenski SA, Moffat SD, Agrawal Y. Vestibular loss in older adults is associated with impaired spatial navigation: Data from the triangle completion task. *Front Neurol.* 2017;8:1–9.
57. Marlinksky VV. Vestibular and vestibulo-proprioceptive perception of motion in the horizontal plane in blindfolded man—III. Route inference. *Neuroscience.* 90(2):403–411.
58. Wang RF, Spelke ES. Human spatial representation: Insights from animals. *Trends Cogn Sci.* 2002;6(9):376–382.
59. Brandt T, Schautzer F, Hamilton DA, et al. Vestibular loss causes hippocampal atrophy and impaired spatial memory in humans. *Brain.* 2005;128(11):2732–2741.
60. Schautzer F, Hamilton D, Kalla R, Strupp M, Brandt T. Spatial memory deficits in patients with chronic bilateral vestibular failure. *Ann NY Acad Sci.* 2003;1004(1):316–324.

61. Stackman RW, Herbert AM. Rats with lesions of the vestibular system require a visual landmark for spatial navigation. *Behav Brain Res.* 2002;128(1):27–40.
62. Russell NA, Horii A, Smith PF, Darlington CL, Bilkey DK. Long-term effects of permanent vestibular lesions on hippocampal spatial firing. *J Neurosci.* 2003;23(16):6490–6498.
63. Brandt T, Zwergal A, Glasauer S. 3-D spatial memory and navigation: Functions and disorders. *Curr Opin Neurol.* 2017;30(1):90–97.
64. Smith PF, Darlington CL, Zheng Y. Move it or lose it—Is stimulation of the vestibular system necessary for normal spatial memory? *Hippocampus.* 2010;20:36–43.
65. Kremmyda O, Hüfner K, Flanagin VL, et al. Beyond dizziness: Virtual navigation, spatial anxiety and hippocampal volume in bilateral vestibulopathy. *Front Hum Neurosci.* 2016;10.
66. Ernst MO, Bülthoff HH. Merging the senses into a robust percept. *Trends Cogn Sci.* 2004; 8(4):162–169.
67. Alais D, Newell F, Mamassian P. Multisensory processing in review: From physiology to behaviour. *Seeing Perceiving.* 2010;23(1):3–38.
68. Krueger Fister J, Stevenson RA, Nidiffer AR, Barnett ZP, Wallace MT. Stimulus intensity modulates multisensory temporal processing. *Neuropsychologia.* 2016;88:92–100.
69. Ernst MO, Banks MS. Humans integrate visual and haptic information in a statistically optimal fashion. *Nature.* 2002;415(6870): 429–433.
70. Butler JS, Campos JL, Bülthoff HH, Smith ST. The role of stereo vision in visual–vestibular integration. *Seeing Perceiving.* 2011;24(5): 453–470.
71. Fetsch CR, Turner AH, DeAngelis GC, Angelaki DE. Dynamic re-weighting of visual and vestibular cues during self-motion perception. *J Neurosci.* 2009;29(49):15601–15612.
72. Ramkhalawansingh R, Butler JS, Campos JL. Visual–vestibular integration during self-motion perception in younger and older adults. *Psychol Aging.* 2018;33(5):798–813.
73. Gu Y, DeAngelis GC, Angelaki DE. A functional link between area MSTd and heading perception based on vestibular signals. *Nat Neurosci.* 2007;10(8):1038–1047.
74. G. Lomber S. Crossmodal Cortical Plasticity in the Developing Brain Following Sensory Loss. *Multisensory Research.* 2013; 26(0): 34.
75. Nava E, Röder B. Adaptation and maladaptation. *Prog Brain Res.* 2011;191:177–194.
76. Lee H-M, Liau J-J, Cheng C-K, Tan C-M, Shih J-T. Evaluation of shoulder proprioception following muscle fatigue. *Clin Biomech.* 2003;18(9):843–847.
77. Pick HL, Warren DH, Hay JC. Sensory conflict in judgments of spatial direction. *Percept Psychophys.* 1969;6(4):203–205.
78. Welch RB, Warren DH. Immediate perceptual response to intersensory discrepancy. *Psychol Bull.* 88(3):638–667.
79. Lee DR, Lishman JR. Visual proprioceptive control of stance. *J Hum Mov Stud.* 1975;18:83–94.
80. Lee DN, Aronson E. Visual proprioceptive control of standing in human infants. *Percept Psychophys.* 1974;15(3):529–532.
81. Dokka K, Kenyon RV, Keshner EA. Influence of visual scene velocity on segmental kinematics during stance. *Gait Posture.* 2009;30(2): 211–216.
82. Gibson EJ, Riccio G, Schmuckler MA, Stoffregen TA, Rosenberg D, Taormina J. Detection of the traversability of surfaces by crawling and walking infants. *J Exp Psychol Hum Percept Perform.* 1987;13(4):533–544.
83. Cohen H, Heaton LG, Congdon SL, Jenkins HA. Changes in sensory organization test scores with age. *Age Ageing.* 1996;25(1):39–44.
84. McFall SA. Children with learning disabilities. *Am J Occup Ther.* 1993;47(9):819–824.
85. Deitz JC, Richardson P, Atwater SW, Crowe TK, Odiorne M. Performance of normal children on the pediatric clinical test of sensory interaction for balance. *Occ Ther J Res.* 1991; 11(6):336–356.
86. Westcott SL, Lowes LP, Richardson P. Evaluation of postural stability in children: Current theories and assessment tools. *Phys Ther.* 1997;77(6):629–645.
87. Richardson PK, Atwater SW, Crowe TK, Deitz JC. Performance of preschoolers on the pediatric clinical test of sensory interaction for balance. *Am J Occ Ther.* 1992;46(9):793–800.
88. Keshner EA, Kenyon RV, Langston J. Postural responses exhibit multisensory dependencies

with discordant visual and support surface motion. *J Vestib Res*. 2004;14:307–319.

89. Keshavarz B, Riecke BE, Hettinger LJ, Campos JL. Vection and visually induced motion sickness: How are they related? *Front Psychol.* 2015;6:472.
90. Quinlivan B, Butler JS, Beiser I, et al. Application of virtual reality head mounted display for investigation of movement: A novel effect of orientation of attention. *J Neural Eng.* 2016;13(5):056006.
91. Borel L, Lopez C, Péruch P, Lacour M. Vestibular syndrome: A change in internal spatial representation. *Clin Neurophysiol.* 2008;38(6): 375–389.
92. Wolter NE, Cushing SL, Madrigal LDV, et al. Unilateral hearing loss is associated with impaired balance in children: A pilot study. *Otol Neurotol.* 2016;37(10):1589–1595.
93. Lucieer F, Duijn S, Van Rompaey V, et al. Full spectrum of reported symptoms of bilateral vestibulopathy needs further investigation—A systematic review. *Front Neurol.* 2018;9:1–7.
94. Campos JL, Bülthoff HH. Multimodal integration during self-motion in virtual reality. In: Murray MM, Wallace MT, eds. *The Neural Bases of Multisensory Processes*. Boca Raton, FL: CRC Press/Taylor and Francis Group; 2012: Chap 30.
95. Lau ST, Pichora-Fuller MK, Li KZ, Singh G, Campos JL. Effects of hearing loss on dual-task performance in an audiovisual virtual reality simulation of listening while walking. *J Am Acad Audiol.* 2016;27(7):567–587.

SECTION III

Pediatric Vestibular Disorder

CHAPTER 13

Genetics and Metabolism in Pediatric Balance Disorders

Lance H. Rodan and Melissa B. Ramocki

Most genetic balance disorders are individually rare, but their recognition is crucial for providers evaluating children with balance or vestibular dysfunction. The determination of a specific genetic diagnosis allows for prognostication, surveillance, and anticipatory guidance regarding disease-related complications, in addition to often directing therapeutic intervention and guiding family planning.

Diagnostic Approach

Genetic Testing Methodologies

Single gene testing is indicated if a specific monogenic condition is suspected, based on clinical features or known family history. Gene-sequencing detects point mutations, small base-pair insertions, and deletions in the coding portions of the gene (called exons). It does not generally detect larger-sized deletions or duplications spanning an entire exon or multiple exons. Gene deletion/duplication testing detects larger gene deletions or duplications (the size of an entire exon or larger). Finally, trinucleotide repeat testing detects repeat disorders, in which the abnormal increased number of repeating elements within a gene disrupts gene function and causes disease.[1]

Multiple gene testing is indicated if a patient's phenotype is nonspecific or when many genes are known to cause an overlapping phenotype. Targeted gene panels generally provide sequencing of a select group of genes associated with a known phenotype. Panels vary considerably between labs, and the ordering provider should become familiar with which genes and testing modalities are included in each panel. The broadest form of multiple gene testing is whole exome sequencing (WES), where the coding regions of all 20,000 nuclear genes are sequenced.[1] Samples for WES are often obtained from both biological parents in addition to the affected proband for segregation analysis.

Chromosome testing is indicated if a specific chromosome disorder is suspected, in patients with multiple congenital anomalies, or for the evaluation of developmental delay or autism.[2] The standard genetic test to evaluate chromosome content is the chromosome microarray, a test that evaluates for chromosome losses (deletions) and gains (duplications), but does not evaluate chromosome structure. In contrast, a karyotype (chromosome microscopy), can evaluate for abnormalities of chromosome structure such as chromosome translocations, inversion, and rings, but can only detect very large losses or gains (5 Mb or greater).[1]

Family History Interpretation

It is crucial to obtain a three-generation pedigree in the evaluation of a genetic disorder. A provider evaluating a child with a potentially genetic balance disorder should particularly determine any family history of ataxia, motor impairment, movement disorder, epilepsy, neuropathy, cognitive decline, dementia, developmental regression, vision loss, or hearing loss. It is also useful to assess for a family history of recurrent miscarriage, fetal demise, infertility, birth defects, developmental delays, or intellectual disability. A family history of "cerebral palsy" should receive particular attention, since many early onset genetic disorders affecting motor function may be misdiagnosed as cerebral palsy. Familial consanguinity or common origin from a geographic isolate should also be considered.

If there are other family members who are similarly affected, then the mode of inheritance can sometimes be established. If no other family members are affected, then the possibilities include a recessive disorder, an X-linked disorder (if the proband is male), or an autosomal dominant disorder with a de novo (new) mutation or with reduced penetrance (only some carriers manifest symptoms).[1]

When to Suspect a Genetic Balance Disorder

In addition to the family history, there are many other important clues to consider in determining whether a balance or vestibular problem may be genetic in origin.

The disease course may suggest a genetic balance disorder. Normal early motor development followed by chronically progressive ataxia over years is suggestive of a genetic balance disorder. Alternatively, an acute-episodic course of ataxia with recovery between episodes can suggest a genetic inborn error of metabolism, a mitochondrial disorder, or a channelopathy. Finally, global developmental delay since birth associated with ataxia can point toward a genetic cerebellar malformation syndrome, an early cerebellar degeneration, or a genetic neurodevelopmental disorder.

Associated symptoms can sometimes also indicate a genetic disorder. Dysmorphic features, congenital anomalies, or global developmental delay can indicate a chromosome disorder or numerous monogenic disorders. A genetic inborn error of metabolism can be suggested by developmental regression, multiple organ dysfunction, basic biochemical abnormalities (acidosis, hypoglycemia, etc), episodic encephalopathy, epilepsy, or unusual odors of urine or sweat.[3]

Particular imaging findings may also suggest a genetic balance disorder, including progressive cerebellar atrophy, gliosis of the cerebellar cortex, or a cerebellar malformation. Symmetric involvement of the basal ganglia and/or brainstem can suggest a genetic inborn error of metabolism or mitochondrial disorder, while prominent involvement of cerebral white matter can suggest a leukodystrophy.[4]

Lesion Localization

Balance is a complex process that requires integration of the visual, proprioceptive, and vestibular systems, so the first step in the evaluation of a child with a balance disorder is basic localization of the lesion(s). A full approach to lesion localization in balance disorders is covered in other sections of this book and will not be further discussed in this chapter. To reflect the significance of lesion localization, the subsequent section on specific genetic balance disorders is divided into *cerebellar (central) ataxias* and *peripheral vestibular disorders*. Most inherited peripheral vestibular disorders are associated with sensorineural hearing loss (SNHL), and are therefore also covered in detail in the SNHL chapter of this book (Chapter 14), so the majority of the current chapter focuses on the central ataxias. Balance disorders resulting exclusively from genetic forms of vision loss or peripheral neuropathy are beyond the scope of this book.

Cerebellar (Central) Ataxia Disorders

The cerebellar ataxia disorders are generally separated into the following four categories, which can mostly be distinguished by age of onset, disease course, and neuroimaging findings: (1) cerebellar malformations, (2) neurodevelopmental disorders associated with ataxia, (3) chronically progressive ataxias in previously normal individuals, and (4) episodic ataxias.

1. Cerebellar Malformations

Many genetic disorders are associated with distinct malformations of the cerebellum. These disorders are generally associated with developmental delay and abnormal tone from birth, with ataxia becoming apparent in the first year of life that may be static or progressive, depending on the specific disorder.

- **Cerebellar dysplasias** include the ciliopathies, which result from the genetic disruption of ciliary function. The most common ciliopathy affecting the cerebellum is **Joubert syndrome**, which is associated with hypoplasia of the cerebellar vermis, thickening and elongation of the superior cerebellar peduncles, and an enlarged interpeduncular space, which collectively give the hindbrain the appearance of a tooth ("molar tooth sign").[5] Clinically, affected patients have nonprogressive congenital ataxia, oculomotor apraxia, variable intellectual disability, and abnormalities of respiratory pattern in early infancy. Variable associated features include renal cysts/nephronophthisis, hepatic fibrosis, retinal disease, limb anomalies, and encephalocele formation.[5] Over 20 known genes have been associated with Joubert syndrome, which are autosomal recessive or X-linked, and gene panel testing is available.[5] Additional cerebellar dysplasias include **LAMA1 gene-related disorder (Poretti-Boltshauser syndrome)** and **GSPM2 gene-related disorder (Chudley-McCullough syndrome)**.[6,7]
- **Dandy-Walker malformation (DWM)** is a specific posterior fossa malformation that consists of hypoplasia and upward rotation of the cerebellar vermis, enlarged fourth ventricle, and enlargement of the posterior fossa.[8] The cerebellar hemispheres and brainstem are relatively spared. DWM can occur as an isolated anomaly (nonsyndromic) or in association with other brain malformations or congenital anomalies (syndromic form). Nonsyndromic forms often do not have an identifiable genetic basis, and the empiric recurrence risk is 1% to 5%.[8] The *ZIC1* and *ZIC4* genes have been implicated in rare cases.[8] Syndromic forms are associated with chromosome disorders, ciliopathy disorders, *FOXC1*

gene-related disorder, and Ritscher-Schinzel syndrome.[8]

- **Cerebellar hypoplasia** refers to a congenitally small cerebellum in a normal-sized posterior fossa.[8] It may preferentially affect the cerebellar vermis or hemispheres, or it may affect both equally. It may occur as an isolated anomaly or in association with additional brain malformations. Most affected individuals exhibit some degree of cognitive and motor impairment, and it may also be associated with cortical malformations.[8] **Lissencephaly with cerebellar hypoplasia** is a well-recognized malformation pattern that is associated with mutations in the RELN (autosomal recessive), LIS1 (autosomal dominant), or DCX (X-linked) genes.[8] **Tubulinopathies** are a group of genetic disorders affecting isotypes of tubulin protein that may be associated with various cortical malformations (lissencephaly, pachygyria, polymicrogyria), cerebellar and pontine hypoplasia, corpus callosum dysgenesis, abnormal cleavage of the basal ganglia, and abnormal formation of the internal capsule.[8] **Dystroglycanopathies** are a group of genetic disorders that alter the O-glycosylation of α-dystroglycan and which are associated with a distinct cortical malformation called *cobblestone lissencephaly* as well as cerebellar hypoplasia, cerebellar cysts, kinked brainstem, enlarged tectum, and abnormal myelination. Associated features include congenital muscular dystrophy with variably elevated CPK, and ophthalmological abnormalities including cataracts and colobomas.[8]
- **Pontocerebellar hypoplasia (PCH)** refers to a group of progressive neurodegenerative disorders of prenatal onset associated with hypoplasia of the cerebellum and pons.[9] Associated neuroimaging features include progressive cerebellar atrophy, cerebral hypomyelination, and sometimes dysgenesis of the corpus callosum. Clinically, patients present with abnormal tone, global developmental delay, and progressive ataxia from birth. Variable features include progressive microcephaly, spasticity, choreoathetosis, and motor neuronopathy (anterior horn disease).[9] Eleven subtypes of pontocerebellar hypoplasia (PCH1-11) have been delineated based on distinct clinical features.[9] Inheritance is autosomal recessive. Both single-gene and gene panel testing are available.
- **Congenital disorders of glycosylation (CDG), type 1a** has the characteristic neuroimaging finding of the "shrunken bright cerebellum," a hypoplastic cerebellum that undergoes progressive atrophy and gliosis (T2 hyperintensity) of the cerebellar cortex.[10] Associated features include hypotonia, intellectual disability, lipodystrophy, effusions (pleural, cardiac), protein-losing enteropathy, coagulopathies, dysmorphic features, and peripheral neuropathy.[11] Congenital disorders of glycosylation can be diagnosed biochemically by evaluation of glycosylated transferrin (transferrin isoelectric focusing or mass spectrometry). Inheritance is autosomal recessive or X-linked, and gene panel testing is available.[11]
- **Cerebellar ataxia, mental retardation, disequilibrium (CAMRQ) syndrome** is associated with hypoplasia of the cerebellar vermis and hemispheres associated with congenital, nonprogressive ataxia and intellectual disability. There are 4 known genes

implicated in this disorder (*VLDLR*, *WDR81*, *CA8*, *ATP8A2*), all of which exhibit autosomal-recessive inheritance.[12–15]

- **CASK gene-related disorder** is associated with hypoplasia of the cerebellum that affects the vermis and hemispheres equally. The cerebellar hemispheres may be asymmetrically affected. The pons and midbrain tegmentum may also appear hypoplastic. The cerebellar hypoplasia phenotype uniquely shows X-linked dominant inheritance, and generally only affects females. Associated features include congenital nonprogressive ataxia, intellectual disability, progressive microcephaly, epilepsy, short stature, sensorineural hearing loss, and variable dysmorphic facial features.[16]
- **OPHN1 gene-related disorder** is associated with hypoplasia of the cerebellum, but it primarily affects the cerebellar vermis. The disorder follows X-linked recessive inheritance and generally affects males, although females may have a hypomorphic presentation. Associated features include nonprogressive congenital ataxia, intellectual disability, macrocephaly, microphallus, and distinct dysmorphic features.[17]
- Other cerebellar hypoplasia genes include DKC1 (**Hoyeraal-Hreidarsson syndrome**), PTF1A, RAB11B, RORA, and *BRF1*.[8,18–20]

2. Neurodevelopmental Disorders Associated With Ataxia

A number of genetic neurodevelopmental disorders may have ataxia as an associated feature in the absence of overt cerebellar malformation. In this category, individuals show neurologic signs from birth, including developmental delays and abnormal tone, with ataxia ultimately manifesting as a feature. The ataxia may be progressive or static, but progression may be slow enough to seem static in the short term. Interestingly, many of the disorders with apparently nonprogressive ataxia in this category may still show progressive cerebellar atrophy on neuroimaging. Many disorders in this category are also associated with dysmorphic facial features or other congenital anomalies.

- **Angelman syndrome** is characterized by severe global developmental delay/intellectual disability, speech impairment, behavioral peculiarities (including fascination with water and "krinkly" textures), happy affect, postnatal microcephaly, epilepsy, distinct facial features, nonprogressive ataxia, and tremulousness.[21] Neuroimaging is typically normal. The disorder results from abnormal methylation or mutations in the maternally imprinted *UBE3A* gene. Diagnosis is made by methylation analysis of chromosome 15q11.2-13, and if negative, sequencing and deletion/duplication testing of the *UBE3A* gene.[21]
- **Christianson syndrome** shares some similarities with Angelman syndrome. It is associated with global developmental delay, intellectual disability, minimal speech, epilepsy, eye movement abnormalities (eg, eye abduction limitations), progressive microcephaly, and truncal ataxia.[22] Neuroimaging may demonstrate progressive cerebellar atrophy and cerebellar cortical gliosis. The disorder follows X-linked recessive inheritance.[22]
- **CACNA1A gene-related disorder** was identified in 8% of patients with congenital nonprogressive ataxia

in one cohort study.[23] Associated features include developmental delay, supranuclear eye movement abnormalities, migraine, and epilepsy. Imaging demonstrates cerebellar hemispheric or vermis atrophy.[23] This is an autosomal-dominant disorder, and it is allelic to episodic ataxia type 2, SCA6, and familial hemiplegic migraine type 1.[23]

- **Marinesco Sjögren syndrome** is an autosomal-recessive disorder associated with infantile hypotonia, global developmental delay, intellectual disability, early onset cataracts, progressive myopathy beginning in the first decade, and eventual development of progressive ataxia.[24] Imaging demonstrates progressive cerebellar atrophy with cerebellar cortical gliosis.[24]
- Additional genes in this category include ***WDR73***, ***OSGEP***, ***TP53RK***, ***TPRKB***, ***LAGE3***, ***SSADH***, ***PMPCA***, ***CAMTA1***, ***ITPR1***, ***EBF3***, ***GPAA1***, ***DNAJC19***, ***ATCAY***, ***CTBP1***, ***SPTBN2***, ***SNX14***, ***GRM1***, ***GRID2***, ***KCNJ10***, ***CWF19L1***, and ***PUM1***.[25–43]

3. Chronically Progressive Ataxia in Previously Normal Individuals

This category represents a distinct group of genetic neurodegenerative disorders affecting the cerebellum or central cerebellar pathways. Unlike the prior two categories previously discussed, in these disorders the individual has normal cognitive and motor development prior to disease onset with a subsequently progressive disease course. These disorders are classified in this chapter by the typical age of onset. These disorders are not generally associated with dysmorphic features or organ malformations, although organ dysfunction is possible in many of these disorders. There are hundreds of disorders in this category, comprising all modes of inheritance. Differential diagnosis is established by considering family history, inheritance pattern, age of onset, disease frequency, associated features, neuroimaging pattern, and biochemical findings, in some cases. A select number of these disorders have disease-modifying treatments. The leukodystrophies are genetic disorders primarily affecting the cerebral white matter that often present with ataxia in combination with spasticity and cognitive impairment. Further detailed discussion of the leukodystrophies is beyond the scope of this text.

Infantile-Onset Ataxia (<2 Years of Age)

Infantile-onset ataxia following a period of normal development is uncommon and should make the clinician consider the disorders **ataxia telangiectasia, X-linked sideroblastic anemia and ataxia,** or an **inborn error of** metabolism.[44]

Childhood Onset Ataxia (2 to 18 Years of Age)

Most genetic forms of childhood-onset progressive ataxia follow autosomal recessive inheritance.[44] There may be affected siblings, but most often there is no family history. Less commonly, children may manifest autosomal-dominant ataxias, including trinucleotide repeat disorders. In these cases, there is usually a family history in parents or grandparents. The one exception is SCA7, which can demonstrate extreme anticipation.[45] X-linked progressive ataxias following a period of normalcy are uncommon in children and have a limited differential diagnosis: X-linked sideroblastic anemia and ataxia (*ABCB7*) and X-linked ataxia (*ATP2B2* gene).[46] Fragile-X tremor ataxia syndrome is exclusively an adult-onset disorder.[46] Ataxias resulting from mutations in mitochondrial DNA (mtDNA) are another cause of chronically progressive ataxia in children and should be considered in cases associated with additional organ dysfunction, vision or hearing loss, diabetes, myopathy, bilateral ptosis, stroke-like episodes, certain neuroimaging patterns (Leigh syndrome), or unexplained lactic acidosis.[47]

For a child with progressive ataxia and a history suggesting autosomal-recessive inheritance, or without a family history, then the most likely considerations include **Friedreich ataxia**, **ataxia telangiectasia**, and **ataxia oculomotor apraxia types 1 and 2**.[48] Other less common but treatable disorders include **ataxia with vitamin E deficiency, disorders of CoQ10 metabolism, and late-infantile neuronal ceroid lipofuscinosis (*CLN2* gene)**.[49,50]

- **Friedreich ataxia** is the most common recessively inherited ataxia disorder, although it is very uncommon in Asia.[48] In its classic form, Friedreich ataxia presents at a mean age of 10 to 15 years (range 2 to 80 years). Symptoms include chronically progressive gait and limb ataxia, dysarthria, abnormal proprioception, spasticity/upper motor neuron signs, polyneuropathy, scoliosis, and variable presence of hypertrophic cardiomyopathy, diabetes mellitus, optic atrophy, and deafness. Reflexes in the lower extremities are reduced early in the disease course and are often associated with upgoing plantar responses.[51] Neuroimaging of the cerebellum is typically normal in the early course of disease, although there may be cervical cord atrophy.[52] In advanced stages, there is cerebellar atrophy involving the superior vermis first. The disorder is an autosomal-recessive trinucleotide repeat disorder resulting from biallelic GAA repeat expansions in the *FXN* gene, or less often from sequence alterations. Friedreich ataxia does not show anticipation.[51]
- **Ataxia telangiectasia** typically presents between 1 and 4 years of age with progressive ataxia, oculomotor apraxia, choreoathetosis, skin/conjunctival telangiectasias, immunodeficiency, and increased cancer risk. Routine lab findings demonstrate elevated α-fetoprotein and reduced immunoglobulins. Neuroimaging demonstrates early cerebellar atrophy. The disorder results from biallelic mutations in the *AT* gene.[53]
- **Ataxia oculomotor apraxia (AOA)** is phenotypically similar to ataxia telangiectasia. AOA type 1 presents between 2 and 10 years of age with progressive ataxia, oculomotor apraxia, choreoathetosis, dystonia, and peripheral neuropathy. Imaging demonstrates early cerebellar atrophy.[49] The disorder results from biallelic mutations in the *APTX* gene. AOA2 presents between 3 and 30 years of age with similar clinical characteristics to AOA1. Patients with AOA2 may also have elevated serum α-fetoprotein. AOA2 results from biallelic mutations in the *SETX* gene.[49]

Adult-Onset Ataxia (>18 Years of Age)

In an adult, autosomal-dominant forms of ataxia are most common.[54] Of these, the most common are **SCA1**, **SCA2**, **SCA3**, **SCA6**, and **SCA7**.[48] These are all trinucleotide repeat disorders with average age of onset in the fourth or fifth decades.[55] Of the recessive ataxias that present in adulthood, Friedreich ataxia is one of the most common.[48] The adult-onset form of Friedreich ataxia may follow a more attenuated and slower clinical course than the childhood-onset form.[51] An adult-onset ataxia with X-linked inheritance is **Fragile X tremor ataxia syndrome** until proven otherwise.[56] Rare but treatable ataxias that can present in adulthood include **Refsum disease, cerebrotendinous xanthomatosis**, and **CoQ10 deficiency** syndromes.[49]

Associated Features

Beyond ataxia, associated neurologic and nonneurologic features can facilitate narrowing of the differential diagnosis. Associated neurologic signs and symptoms may include spasticity/upper motor neuron signs, peripheral neuropathy, extrapyramidal signs (choreoathetosis, dystonia, or parkinsonism), dementia, epilepsy, myoclonus, and eye movement abnormalities.[44] The triad of progressive ataxia, epilepsy, and cortical myoclonus suggests a form of **progressive myoclonus ataxia,** which has a limited differential diagnosis (Table 13–1).[57] Nonneurologic features include retinal degeneration, cataracts, hearing loss, cardiomyopathy, gastrointestinal dysmotility, liver disease, kidney disease, skin lesions, and endocrinopathy.[44] Table 13–1 summarizes additional neurologic and nonneurologic features that can be used to refine the differential diagnosis.

Neuroimaging Pattern

In most progressive ataxias, neuroimaging demonstrates nonspecific cerebellar atrophy. Cerebellar atrophy associated with gliosis (T2 hyperintensity) of the cerebellar cortex is seen in infantile neuroaxonal dystrophy, disorders of coenzyme Q10 biosynthesis, and late-infantile neuronal ceroid lipofuscinosis.[58] Pontine and/or brainstem atrophy can be seen in some of the autosomal-dominant trinucleotide repeat ataxias.[55] Abnormalities of the basal ganglia, thalami, or brainstem can be seen in mitochondrial and metabolic disorders.[47] Cerebellar atrophy–associated abnormal T2 hypointensity of the thalami, cortical atrophy, and dysmyelination may suggest neuronal ceroid lipofuscinosis.[59] Autosomal-recessive spastic ataxia of Charlevoix-Saguenay is associated with atrophy of the superior cerebellar vermis and hemispheres and pathognomonic linear T2 hypointensities in the pons.[60] Cereberotendinous xanthomatosis is associated with symmetric T2 hyperintensities in the cerebellar dentate nuclei, and in the cerebral and cerebellar white matter.[61] Fragile-X tremor ataxia syndrome is associated with symmetric T2 hyperintensities in bilateral middle cerebellar peduncles.[56] Uniquely, a normal appearing cerebellum is characteristic in Friedreich ataxia until an advanced stage of the disorder and in FLVCR1 gene-related disorder.[52, 62] FLVCR1 gene-related disorder may be associated with T2 hyperintensity of the dorsal column of the spinal cord.[62]

Biochemical Screening

A number of progressive ataxias can be screened for or diagnosed with biochemical testing. As previously mentioned, ataxia telangiectasia and ataxia oculomotor apraxia type 2 are frequently associated with elevated α-fetoprotein levels.[49] Refsum disease is associated with elevated levels of plasma phytanic acid.[49] Genetic forms of coenzyme Q10 deficiency are associated with decreased CoQ10 levels in leukocytes.[63] Ataxia vitamin E deficiency is associated with reduced levels of vitamin E.[49] Abeta-/hypobetalipoproteinemia is associated with abnormal lipoprotein electrophoresis and reduced levels of vitamin E.[64] Cerebrotendinous xanthomatosis is associated with elevated levels of serum cholestenol.[49] The infantile and late-infantile forms of neuronal ceroid lipofuscinosis can be diagnosed via enzyme testing of PPT1 and TPP1 enzymes, respectively.[65] Niemann-Pick type C can be screened for with plasma oxysterols.[66] Mitochondrial disorders may be associated with elevated lactate in blood and

Table 13–1. Additional Neurological and Nonneurological Signs[44]

Clinical Features	*Disorder*
Spasticity/pyramidal signs	SCA1, SCA3, SCA42, PNPLA6 gene-related disorder, ARSACS, SYNE1, VAMP1, KIF1C, MARS2, MTPAP, AFG3L2, SPG7
Peripheral neuropathy	Friedreich ataxia, SCA1, SCA2, SCA4, SCA18, SCA25 (sensory), IOSCA, Refsum disease, ARSACS, ataxia oculomotor apraxia type 2, SYNE1, PHARC syndrome, STUB1 gene-related disorder, ataxia oculomotor apraxia type 4, mitochondrial disorders, TDP1 gene-related disorder, TFSM gene-related disorder, TXN gene-related disorder, abetalipoproteinemia, ataxia vitamin E deficiency
Choreoathetosis and/or dystonia	Ataxia telangiectasia, ataxia oculomotor apraxia type 1, ataxia oculomotor apraxia type 3, DRPLA, SCA17, SCA20 (spasmodic dysphonia), cerebrotendinous xanthomatosis, Gordon Holmes syndrome, TXN2
Parkinsonism	SCA3, POLG
Dementia	SCA12, SCA17, SCA21, Gordon Holmes syndrome, cerebrotendinous xanthomatosis, Neimann-Pick type C, Gaucher disease, mitochondrial disease
Epilepsy +/− myoclonus	**Progressive myoclonus ataxias:** Neuronal ceroid lipofuscinosis, MERRF syndrome, sialidosis, Lafora disease, Unverricht-Lundborg disease, PRICKLE1 gene disorder, DRPLA, GOSR2, SCARB2, KCTD7, KCNC1. SCA10 (rarely), SCA17, SCA19/22 (myoclonus only), IOSCA, CoQ10 deficiency, TXN2, mitochondrial disorders
Abnormality of eye movement	Oculomotor apraxia: ataxia telangiectasia, ataxia oculomotor apraxia types 1–4 Supranuclear gaze palsy: Niemann-Pick type C, Gaucher disease (types II and III), SCA1, SCA2, SCA3, SCA28, SCA37, SQSTM1 Progressive external ophthalmoparesis: POLG-related disorders, IOSCA, other mitochondrial disorders
Retinal degeneration	Refsum disease, neuronal ceroid lipofuscinosis, mitochondrial disease, infantile cerebellar-retinal degeneration, PHARC syndrome, SCA7, PNPLA6 gene-related disorder, ataxia vitamin E deficiency, abetalipoproteinemia, FLVCR1 gene-related disorder
Cataract	PHARC, Refsum, cerebrotendinous xanthomatosis
Hearing loss	Mitochondrial disorder, Friedreich ataxia, Refsum disease, PHARC syndrome, PNPLA6 gene-related disorder, SNX14 gene-related disorder, SCA4, IOSCA, SLC9A1, DNMT1
Cardiac disease	Cardiomyopathy: Friedreich ataxia, mitochondrial disease, TSFM Arrhythmia: Friedreich ataxia, Refsum, mitochondrial
Liver disease	Niemann-Pick type C, Gaucher disease, mitochondrial disease

continues

Table 13–1. *continued*

Clinical Features	*Disorder*
Kidney disease	CoQ10 metabolism disorders, SCARB2 gene-related disorder
Gastrointestinal dysmotility	Mitochondrial disease, cerebrotendinous xanthomatosis, abeta-/hypobetalipoproteinemia, FLVCR1 gene-related disorder
Skin lesions	Refsum disease (ichthyosis), cerebrotendinous xanthomatosis (tendon xanthomas), SCA34
Hematologic	X-linked sideroblastic anemia, abetalipoproteinemia (acanthocytes), ataxia-pancytopenia syndrome, ABCB7 (sideroblastic anemia), mitochondrial disease
Immunologic	Ataxia telangiectasia
Endocrine	Hypogonadism: POLR3-related disorder, Perrault syndrome, Gordon Holmes syndrome, IOSCA, POLG. Diabetes: mitochondrial disorders, Friedreich ataxia, ataxia telangiectasia
Other	Narcolepsy: DNMT1

cerebrospinal fluid, elevated alanine and proline on plasma amino acids (and sometimes reduced arginine), elevated or reduced Kreb cycle metabolites on urine organic acids, and elevations in serum GDF-15 levels. Muscle biopsy is occasionally required to measure enzyme activity of the respiratory chain, to quantify mitochondria, and to evaluate mitochondrial ultrastructure.[67,68]

4. Episodic Ataxias

A number of genetic disorders are associated with ataxia that presents episodically. The individual is often asymptomatic between episodes or may have a persistent slowly progressive ataxia. At first presentation, these disorders can mimic acquired etiologies of acute cerebellar ataxia such as infectious/parainfectious cerebellitis, cerebrovascular events, and acute intoxications. Episodic ataxias are typically caused by either genetic disorders impairing cerebral ion channels, termed **channelopathies**, or by inborn errors of metabolism.

Channelopathies

There are various forms of "Episodic Ataxia," numbered episodic ataxia (EA) types 1 to 8; only four of these are associated with known genes:

- **Episodic ataxia type 1** is associated with mutations in the *KCNA1* gene. It presents in childhood (mean 8 years) with episodes of ataxia and muscle twitching/stiffening lasting seconds to minutes (maximum hours). Episodes may be provoked by startle, stressors, vestibular stimulation, exercise, certain foods (eg, caffeine, alcohol, chocolate, etc). Frequency of events is variable. There is no ataxia between episodes; however, there is typically myokymia (fine muscle twitching) and cramps between events. Variable associated features include cognitive abnormalities, epilepsy, and muscle hypertonia leading to contractures and orthopedic abnormalities. Episodes may decrease in frequency with treatment with acetazolamide or various anticonvulsants. Neuroimaging is normal. Inheritance is autosomal dominant with incomplete penetrance.[69]

- **Episodic ataxia type 2** is associated with mutations in the *CACNA1A* gene. It presents in childhood or adolescence with episodes of ataxia, vertigo, and nausea. Variable features include headache, hemiplegia, dystonia, or torticollis. Episodes last hours to days. Episodes may be provoked by stress, exertion, fever, and certain foods (eg, caffeine, alcohol). Frequency of episodes is variable. In between episodes, individuals may be asymptomatic, but most eventually develop fixed cerebellar ataxia (80%), nystagmus (90%), and eye movement abnormalities. Episodes may decrease in frequency with acetazolamide or 4-aminopyridine. Neuroimaging may be normal or may demonstrate atrophy of the cerebellar vermis. Interictal videonystagmography typically shows oculomotor dysfunction and spontaneous downbeat nystagmus. Inheritance is autosomal dominant with incomplete penetrance.[70]
- Less common forms of episodic ataxia with known loci include episodic ataxia 5 (CACNB4) and episodic ataxia 6 (SLC1A3). Episodic ataxia 3, 4, 7, and 8 have no known gene locus.[71]

Inborn Errors of Metabolism Associated With Episodic Ataxia

A number of inborn errors of metabolism can present with episodic neurologic manifestations, including ataxia. The pathophysiology of these disorders relates to intermittent intoxication from endogenous metabolites, nutritional deficiency, or intermittent cerebral energy failure.

- **Urea cycle disorders** are a group of genetic disorders related to defects in the individual enzymes of the urea cycle, the metabolic pathway in the liver that converts neurotoxic ammonia into urea that can be excreted in the urine. These disorders generally present with intermittent episodes of hyperammonemia provoked by illness, prolonged fasting, or high protein intake. Hyperammonemic episodes may be associated with headache, psychiatric signs, encephalopathy, ataxia, and seizures. Untreated hyperammonemia can result in progressive cerebral edema, altered level of consciousness, and death. The most common urea cycle disorder is ornithine transcarbamylase (OTC) deficiency, which is associated with X-linked inheritance (females may be affected). The other urea cycle disorders follow autosomal recessive inheritance. In addition to the finding of hyperammonemia, specific diagnosis is made by measuring plasma amino acids that demonstrate characteristic abnormalities of citrulline and arginine and urine organic acids that may demonstrate elevations of orotic acid or arginosuccinic acid depending on the specific disorder. Acute treatment includes cessation of dietary protein, provision of high-dextrose-containing intravenous fluids, and treatment with ammonia scavenging medications under the guidance of a biochemical geneticist.

- The **intermittent form of maple syrup urine disease (MSUD)** can also present with episodic ataxia. MSUD is a genetic disorder affecting the enzyme complex that oxidizes branched-chain α-keto acids, the metabolites of the branched-chain amino acids leucine, isoleucine, and valine. Biochemically, the disorder presents with episodes of extremely elevated plasma leucine, isoleucine, and valine. Leucine is neurotoxic and results in encephalopathy, headache, nausea, ataxia, dystonia, and epilepsy. Untreated, it can result in cerebral edema, decreased level of consciousness, and death. Episodes of decompensation are provoked by illness, fasting, or high protein intake. In between episodes, individuals are typically asymptomatic. The disorder follows autosomal-recessive inheritance. Specific diagnosis is made by finding highly elevated levels of plasma leucine, isoleucine, valine, and alloisoleucine. Urine organic acids may demonstrate elevations in branched-chain keto acids. Acute treatment requires provision of a special branched-chain amino acid–free medical formula combined with measured amounts of isoleucine and valine under the guidance of a biochemical geneticist. Some individuals may also be responsive to thiamine.[73]
- **Hartnup disease** is a transportopathy affecting intestinal and renal transport of large neutral amino acids due to biallelic mutations in the *SLC6A19* gene. Clinical symptoms result from deficiency of tryptophan, the precursor for niacin. Symptoms include episodic ataxia, chorea, encephalopathy, and pellagra skin rash. Episodes may last weeks and are often provoked by emotional stress, sunlight, or sulfonamide medications. Inheritance is autosomal recessive. Diagnosis is made by finding elevated excretion of large neutral amino acids on urine amino acid measurement. Treatment is with niacin supplementation.[70,74]
- **X-linked pyruvate dehydrogenase complex (PDH) deficiency** is the best example of a variety of mitochondrial disorders that can present with episodic ataxia. In males, PDH deficiency can present with episodic ataxia, neuropathy/weakness, and extrapyramidal movement disorders with interictal well periods. Typically, affected individuals eventually develop fixed neurologic deficits. Biochemical evaluation typically demonstrates elevated serum lactate with a normal lactate:pyruvate ratio (<15). Lactate elevation may be carbohydrate sensitive. PDH enzyme activity can be measured in cultured skin fibroblasts. Potential treatments include the ketogenic diet, dichloroacetate (a PDH kinase inhibitor), and thiamine supplementation.[75]

Peripheral Vestibular Disorders

A number of distinct genetic balance disorders present with prominent peripheral vestibular dysfunction. Some of these disorders are also associated with cerebellar dysfunction, but this is overshadowed by the peripheral involvement. Hearing loss may be an associated feature.

- **Usher syndrome** is a group of genetic disorders associated with sensorineural hearing loss and retinal degeneration. Usher syndrome gene panels are clinically available.
    - **Usher syndrome type 1** is associated with congenital profound bilateral sensorineural hearing loss, congenital vestibular areflexia, and later development of retinitis pigmentosa. Due to the vestibular dysfunction, gross motor milestones are delayed, and older children have balance difficulties. This ataxia is nonprogressive. Inheritance is autosomal recessive, and six genes have been discovered to date (ordered from most to least frequent): MYO7A, USH1C, CDH23, PCDH15, USH1G, CIB2.[76]
    - **Usher syndrome type 2** is by definition not associated with vestibular dysfunction.[76]
    - **Usher syndrome type 3** is associated with postlingual, progressive bilateral sensorineural hearing loss; late onset of retinitis pigmentosa; and variable vestibular dysfunction. Inheritance is autosomal recessive, and two genes have been implicated: *CLNR1* and *HARS*.[76]
- **CHARGE syndrome** is a multiple congenital anomaly syndrome associated with colobomas, heart defects, choanal atresia, growth retardation, developmental delay, genitourinary anomalies, and dysmorphic features. Vestibular dysfunction is a common finding in CHARGE syndrome. The semicircular canals are typically seen to be absent or severely malformed on temporal bone imaging. Some individuals may also have hypoplasia of the cerebellar vermis and abnormal cerebellar foliation. The disorder results from de novo mutations in the *CHD7* gene, and rarely the *SEMA3E* gene.[77,78]
- **Cerebellar ataxia, neuropathy, and vestibular areflexia (CANVAS) syndrome** is a late-adult–onset neurodegenerative disorder associated with slowly progressive ataxia, loss of vestibular reflexes including impaired vestibuloocular (VOR) reflex, and peripheral sensory neuropathy. Imaging may demonstrate cerebellar atrophy. Inheritance is presumed to be autosomal recessive, but no gene has been identified to date.[79]

Summary

There are a vast number of genetic disorders affecting balance and coordination. Most disorders are associated with central ataxia from cerebellar or cerebellar-pathway dysfunction. When approaching these patients, the clinician should strive to place the patient into one of the following four categories: cerebellar malformation, neurodevelopmental disorder associated with ataxia, chronically progressive ataxia in a previously normal individual, and episodic ataxia. Family history, age of disease onset, disease course, associated findings, neuroimaging, and corollary lab tests can further refine the diagnosis. Clinicians should focus on those genetic central ataxia disorders that are amenable to disease-modifying treatments. In the evaluation of patients with genetic ataxia disorders, the clinician should carefully consider the roles of single gene testing, panel testing, specialized molecular testing, chromosome testing, and biochemical analysis/metabolic testing. These methodologies all have specific strengths and weaknesses, and test selection should be tailored to the specific case.

Self-Assessment Questions

1. Which of the following disorders is generally *not* associated with a cerebellar malformation?
   a. Pontocerebellar hypoplasia type 1
   b. Joubert syndrome
   c. Angelman syndrome
   d. Congenital disorder of glycosylation type 1a
   e. CASK gene-related disorder

2. What is the most common autosomal recessive form of progressive ataxia worldwide?
   a. Ataxia telangiectasia
   b. Ataxia oculomotor apraxia 1
   c. Ataxia oculomotor apraxia 2
   d. Friedreich ataxia
   e. Fragile-X tremor ataxia syndrome

3. Which of the following disorders can generally be diagnosed with whole exome sequencing?
   a. Fragile-X tremor ataxia syndrome
   b. Friedreich ataxia
   c. SCA1
   d. SCA3
   e. Ataxia telangiectasia

4. Which of the following progressive ataxias has disease-modifying therapy?
   a. Refsum disease
   b. Ataxia with vitamin E deficiency
   c. Cerebrotendinous xanthomatosis
   d. Disorders of coenzyme Q10 biosynthesis
   e. All of the above

5. Which of the following disorders is *not* associated with episodic ataxia?
   a. Intermittent maple syrup urine disease
   b. X-linked pyruvate dehydrogenase deficiency
   c. Marinesco Sjögren syndrome
   d. CACNA1A gene-related disorder
   e. KCNA1 gene-related disorder

6. Which of the following disorders is *not* associated with peripheral vestibular dysfunction?
   a. Usher syndrome type 1
   b. Usher syndrome type 2
   c. Usher syndrome type 3
   d. CHARGE syndrome
   e. CANVAS syndrome

References

1. Valente EM, Nuovo S, Doherty D. Cerebellar disorders. *Handbook Clin Neurol.* 2018;154: 267–286.
2. Miller DT, Adam MP, Aradhya S, et al. Consensus statement: Chromosomal microarray is a first-tier clinical diagnostic test for individuals with developmental disabilities or congenital anomalies. *Am J Hum Genet.* 2010;86(5): 749–764.
3. De Meirleir L, Rodan LH. Approach to the patient with a metabolic disorder. In: *Swaiman's Pediatric Neurology.* 6th ed. New York, NY: Elsevier; 2017:277–285.
4. Poretti A, Wolf NI, Boltshauser E. Differential diagnosis of cerebellar atrophy in childhood: An update. *Neuropediatrics.* 2015;46(6):359–370.
5. Romani M, Micalizzi A, Valente EM. Joubert syndrome: Congenital cerebellar ataxia with the "molar tooth." *Lancet Neurol.* 2013;12(9): 894–905.
6. Aldinger KA, Mosca SJ, Tétreault M, et al. Mutations in *LAMA1* cause cerebellar dysplasia and cysts with and without retinal dystrophy. *Am J Hum Genet.* 2014;95:227–234.
7. Doherty D, Chudley AE, Coghlan G, et al. GPSM2 mutations cause the brain malformations and hearing loss in Chudley-McCullough syndrome. *Am J Hum Genet.* 2012;90:1088–1093.
8. Aldinger KA, Doherty D. The genetics of cerebellar malformations. *Semin Fetal Neonatal Med.* 2016;21(5):321–332.
9. van Dijk T, Baas F, Barth PG, et al. What's new in pontocerebellar hypoplasia? An update on genes and subtypes. *Orphanet J Rare Dis.* 2018;13(1):92.
10. Feraco P, Mirabelli-Badenier M, Severino M, et al. The shrunken, bright cerebellum: A characteristic MRI finding in congenital disorder of glycosylation type 1a. *Am J Neuroradiol.* 2012;33(11):2062–2067.
11. Freeze HH, Eklund EA, Ng BG, et al. Neurology of inherited glycosylation defects. *Lancet Neurol.* 2012 May;11(5):453–466.
12. Ali BR, Silhavy JL, Gleeson MJ, et al. A missense founder mutation in VLDLR is associated with dysequilibrium syndrome without quadrupedal locomotion. *BMC Med Genet.* 2012;13:80.
13. Kaya N, Aldhalaan H, Al-Younes B, et al. Phenotypical spectrum of cerebellar ataxia associated with a novel mutation in the CA8 gene, encoding carbonic anhydrase (CA) VIII. *Am J Med Genet B Neuropsychiatr Genet.* 2011; 156B:826–834.
14. Cacciagli P, Haddad MR, Mignon-Ravix C, et al. Disruption of the ATP8A2 gene in a patient with a t(10;13) de novo balanced translocation and a severe neurological phenotype. *Eur J Hum Genet.* 2010;18:1360–1363.
15. Onat OE, Gulsuner S, Bilguvar K, et al. Missense mutation in the aTPase, aminophospholipid transporter protein ATP8A2 is associated with cerebellar atrophy and quadrupedal locomotion. *Eur J Hum Genet.* 2013;21:281–285.
16. Moog U, Uyanik G, Kutsche K. CASK-related disorders. 2013 Nov 26. In: Adam MP, Ardinger HH, Pago RA, et al., eds. *Gene-*

Reviews. Seattle, WA: University of Washington, Seattle; 1993–2019. Available from: https://www.ncbi.nlm.nih.gov/books/NBK169825/

17. Zanni G, Saillour Y, Nagara M, et al. Oligophrenin 1 mutations frequently cause X-linked mental retardation with cerebellar hypoplasia. *Neurology*. 2005;65:1364–1369.
18. Pearson T, Curtis F, Al-Eyadhy A, et al. An intronic mutation in DKC1 in an infant with Hoyerall-Hreidarsson syndrome. *Am J Med Genet*. 2008;146A:2159–2161.
19. Lamers IJC, Reijnders MRF, Venselaar H, et al. Recurrent de novo mutations disturbing the GTP/GDP binding pocket of RAB11B cause intellectual disability and a distinctive brain phenotype. *Am J Hum Genet*. 2017; 101:824–832.
20. Guissart C, Latypova X, Rollier P, et al. Dual molecular effects of dominant RORA mutations cause two variants of syndromic intellectual disability with either autism or cerebellar ataxia. *Am J Hum Genet*. 2018; 102:744–759.
21. Bird LM. Angelman syndrome: Review of clinical and molecular aspects. *Appl Clin Genet*. 2014;7: 93–104.
22. Schroer RJ, Holden KR, Tarpey PS, et al. Natural history of Christianson syndrome. *Am J Med Genet A*. 2010;152A(11):2775–2783.
23. Travaglini L, Nardella M, Bellacchio E, et al. Missense mutations of CACNA1A are a frequent cause of autosomal dominant nonprogressive congenital ataxia. *Eur J Paediatr Neurol*. 2017;21(3):450–456.
24. Senderek J, Krieger M, Stendel C, et al. Mutations in *SIL1* cause Marinesco-Sjögren syndrome, a cerebellar ataxia with cataract and myopathy. *Nature Genet*. 2005;37:1312–1314.
25. Jinks, RN, Puffenberger EG, Baple E, et al. Recessive nephrocerebellar syndrome on the Galloway-Mowat syndrome spectrum is caused by homozygous protein-truncating mutations of WDR73. *Brain*. 2015;138:2173–2190.
26. Braun DA, Rao J, Mollet G, et al. Mutations in KEOPS-complex genes cause nephrotic syndrome with primary microcephaly. *Nature Genet*. 2017;49:1529–1538.
27. Gibson KM, Christensen E, Jakobs C, et al. The clinical phenotype of succinic semialdehyde dehydrogenase deficiency (4-hydroxybutyric aciduria): Case reports of 23 new patients. *Pediatrics*. 1997;99:567–574.
28. Jobling RK, Assoum M, Gakh O, et al. PMPCA mutations cause abnormal mitochondrial protein processing in patients with non-progressive cerebellar ataxia. *Brain*. 2015; 138:1505–1517.
29. Thevenon J, Lopez E, Keren B, et al. Intragenic CAMTA1 rearrangements cause nonprogressive congenital ataxia with or without intellectual disability. *J Med Genet*. 2012;49: 400–408.
30. Huang L, Chardon JW, Carter MT, et al. Missense mutations in ITPR1 cause autosomal dominant congenital nonprogressive spinocerebellar ataxia. *Orphanet J Rare Dis*. 2012;7:67.
31. Chao HT, Davids M, Burke E, et al. A syndromic neurodevelopmental disorder caused by de novo variants in EBF3. *Am J Hum Genet*. 2017;100:128–137.
32. Nguyen TTM, Murakami Y, Sheridan E, et al. Mutations in GPAA1, encoding a GPI transamidase complex protein, cause developmental delay, epilepsy, cerebellar atrophy, and osteopenia. *Am J Hum Genet*. 2017;101:856–865.
33. Ojala T, Polinati, P, Manninen T, et al. New mutation of mitochondrial DNAJC19 causing dilated and noncompaction cardiomyopathy, anemia, ataxia, and male genital anomalies. *Pediat Res*. 2012;72:432–437.
34. Nystuen A, Benke PJ, Merren, J, et al. A cerebellar ataxia locus identified by DNA pooling to search for linkage disequilibrium in an isolated population from the Cayman Islands. *Hum Mol Genet*. 1996;5:525–531.
35. Beck DB, Cho MT, Millan F, et al. A recurrent de novo CTBP1 mutation is associated with developmental delay, hypotonia, ataxia, and tooth enamel defects. *Neurogenetics*. 2016;17: 173–178.
36. Lise S, Clarkson Y, Perkins E, et al. Recessive mutations in SPTBN2 implicate beta-III spectrin in both cognitive and motor development. *PLOS Genet*. 2012;8:e1003074.
37. Thomas AC, Williams H, Seto-Salvia N, et al. Mutations in SNX14 cause a distinctive autosomal-recessive cerebellar ataxia and intel-

lectual disability syndrome. *Am J Hum Genet.* 2014;95:611–621.
38. Guergueltcheva V, Azmanov DN, Angelicheva D, et al. Autosomal-recessive congenital cerebellar ataxia is caused by mutations in metabotropic glutamate receptor 1. *Am J Hum Genet.* 2012;91:553–564.
39. Hills LB, Masri A, Konno K, et al. Deletions in GRID2 lead to a recessive syndrome of cerebellar ataxia and tonic upgaze in humans. *Neurology.* 2013;81:1378–1386.
40. Guissart C, Latypova X, Rollier P, et al. Dual molecular effects of dominant RORA mutations cause two variants of syndromic intellectual disability with either autism or cerebellar ataxia. Am J Hum Genet. 2018;102:744–759.
41. Scholl UI, Choi M, Liu T, et al. Seizures, sensorineural deafness, ataxia, mental retardation, and electrolyte imbalance (SeSAME syndrome) caused by mutations in KCNJ10. *Proc Nat Acad Sci.* 2009;106:5842–5847.
42. Evers C, Kaufmann L, Seitz A, et al. Exome sequencing reveals a novel CWF19L1 mutation associated with intellectual disability and cerebellar atrophy. *Am J Med Genet.* 2016; 170A:1502–1509.
43. Gennarino VA, Palmer EE, McDonel LM, et al. A mild PUM1 mutation is associated with adult-onset ataxia, whereas haploinsufficiency causes developmental delay and seizures. *Cell.* 2018;172:924–936.
44. Bird TD. Hereditary ataxia overview. 1998 Oct 28 [updated 2019 Apr 18]. In: Adam MP, Ardinger HH, Pagon RA, et al., eds. *GeneReviews.* Seattle, WA: University of Washington; 1993–2019. Available from: https://www.ncbi.nlm.nih.gov/books/NBK1138/
45. Martins JJ. Spinocerebellar ataxia type 7. *Handb Clin Neurol.* 2012;103:475–491.
46. Zanni G, Bertini E. X-linked ataxias. *Handb Clin Neurol.* 2018;155:175–189.
47. Vernon HJ, Bindoff LA. Mitochondrial ataxias. *Handb Clin Neurol.* 2018;155:129–141.
48. Rauno L, Melo C, Silva MC, Coutinho P. The global epidemiology of hereditary ataxia and spastic paraplegia: A systematic review of prevalence studies. *Neuroepidemiology.* 2014; 42(3):174–183.
49. Synofzik M, Nemeth AH. Recessive ataxias. *Handb Clin Neurol.* 2018;155:73–89.
50. Schulz A, Ajayi T, Specchio N, et al. Study of intraventricular cerliponase alfa for CLN2 disease. *N Engl J Med.* 2018;378(20):1898–1907.
51. Parkinson MH, Boesch S, Nachbauer W, Mariotti C, Giunti P. Clinical features of Friedreich's ataxia: Classical and atypical phenotypes. *J Neurochem.* 2013;126(Suppl 1):103–117.
52. Mascalchi M. The cerebellum looks normal in Friedreich ataxia. *Am J Neuroradiol.* 2013; 34:E22.
53. Rothblum-Oviatt C, Wright J, Lefton-Greif MA, McGrath-Morrow SA, Crawford TO, Lederman HM. Ataxia telangiectasia: A review. *Orphanet J Rare Dis.* 2016;11(1):159.
54. Jayadev S, Bird TD. Hereditary ataxias overview. *Genet Med.* 2013;15:673–683.
55. Soong BW, Morrison PJ. Spinocerebellar ataxias. *Handb Clin Neurol.* 2018;155:143–174.
56. Hall DA, Berry-Kravis E. Fragile X syndrome and fragile X-associated tremor ataxia syndrome. *Handb Clin Neurol.* 2018;147: 377–391.
57. Kälviäinen R. Progressive myoclonus epilepsies. *Semin Neurol.* 2015;35(3):293–299.
58. Poretti A, Wolf NI, Boltshauser E. Differential diagnosis of cerebellar atrophy of childhood. *Neuropediatrics.* 2015;46(6):359–370.
59. Haltia M. The neuronal ceroid lipofuscinoses. *J Neuropathol Exp Neurol.* 2003;62(1):1–13.
60. Synofzik M, Soehn AS, Gburek-Augustat J, et al. Autosomal recessive spastic ataxia of Charlevoix Saguenay (ARSACS): Expanding the genetic, clinical and imaging spectrum. *Orphanet J Rare Dis.* 2013;8:41.
61. Nie S, Chen G, Cao X, Zhang Y. Cerebrotendinous xanthomatosis: A comprehensive review of pathogenesis, clinical manifestations, diagnosis, and management. *Orphanet J Rare Dis.* 2014;9:179.
62. Rajadhyaksha AM, Elemento O, Puffenberger E, et al. Mutations in *FLVCR1* cause posterior column ataxia and retinitis pigmentosa. *Am J Hum Genet.* 2010;87(5):643–654.
63. Malicdan MCV, Vilboux T, Ben-Zeev B, et al. A novel inborn error of the coenzyme Q10 biosynthesis pathway: Cerebellar ataxia

and static encephalomyopathy due to COQ5 C-methyltransferase deficiency. *Hum Mutat.* 2018;39(1):69–79.
64. Burnett JR, Hooper AJ, Hegele RA. Abetalipoproteinemia. 2018 Oct 25. In: Adam MP, Ardinger HH, Pagon RA, et al., eds. *GeneReviews.* Seattle, WA: University of Washington; 1993–2019. Available from: https://www.ncbi.nlm.nih.gov/books/NBK532447/
65. Sheth J, Mistri M, Bhavsar R, et al. Batten disease: Biochemical and molecular characterization revealing novel PPT1 and TPP1 gene mutations in Indian patients. *BMC Neurol.* 2018;18(1):203.
66. Deodato F, Boenzi S, Taurisano R, et al. The impact of biomarkers analysis in the diagnosis of Niemann-Pick C disease and acid sphingomyelinase deficiency. *Clin Chim Acta.* 2018; 486:387–394.
67. Mitochondrial Medicine Society's Committee on Diagnosis, Haas RH, Parikh S, et al. The in-depth evaluation of suspected mitochondrial disease. *Mol Genet Metab.* 2008;94(1):16–37.
68. Davis RL, Liang C, Sue CM. Mitochondrial diseases. *Handb Clin Neurol.* 2018;147: 125–141.
69. Hasan SM, D'Adamo MC. Episodic ataxia type 1. 2010 Feb 9 [updated 2018 Nov 1]. In: Adam MP, Ardinger HH, Pagon RA, et al., eds. *GeneReviews.* Seattle, WA: University of Washington; 1993–2019. Available from: https://www.ncbi.nlm.nih.gov/books/NBK25442/
70. Spacey S. Episodic ataxia type 2. 2003 Feb 24 [updated 2015 Oct 15]. In: Adam MP, Ardinger HH, Pagon RA, et al., eds. *GeneReviews.* Seattle, WA: University of Washington; 1993–2019. Available from: https://www.ncbi.nlm.nih.gov/books/NBK1501/
71. Jen JC, Wan J. Episodic ataxias. *Handb Clin Neurol.* 2018;155:205–221.
72. Ah Mew N, Simpson KL, Gropman AL, et al. Urea cycle disorders overview. 2003 Apr 29 [updated 2017 Jun 22]. In: Adam MP, Ardinger HH, Pagon RA, et al., eds. *GeneReviews.* Seattle, WA: University of Washington; 1993–2019. Available from: https://www.ncbi.nlm.nih.gov/books/NBK1217/
73. Strauss KA, Puffenberger EG, Morton DH. Maple syrup urine disease. 2006 Jan 30 [updated 2013 May 9]. In: Adam MP, Ardinger HH, Pagon RA, et al., eds. *GeneReviews.* Seattle, WA: University of Washington; 1993–2019. Available from: https://www.ncbi.nlm.nih.gov/books/NBK1319/
74. Seow HF, Bröer S, Bröer A, et al. Hartnup disorder is caused by mutations in the gene encoding the neutral amino acid transporter SLC6A19. *Nature Genet.* 2004;36:1003–1007.
75. Barnerias C, Saudubray JM, Touati G, et al. Pyruvate dehydrogenase complex deficiency: Four neurological phenotypes with differing pathogenesis. *Dev Med Child Neurol.* 2010; 52(2):e1–e9.
76. Gettelfinger JD, Dahl JP. Syndromic hearing loss: A brief review of common presentations and genetics. *J Pediatr Genet.* 2018;7(1):1–8.
77. Lalani SR, Hefner MA, Belmont JW, Davenport SLH. CHARGE syndrome. 2006 Oct 2 [updated 2012 Feb 2]. In: Adam MP, Ardinger HH, Pagon RA, et al., eds. *GeneReviews.* Seattle, WA: University of Washington; 1993–2019. Available from: https://www.ncbi.nlm.nih.gov/books/NBK1117/
78. Lalani SR, Safiullah AM, Molinari LM, et al. *SEMA3E* mutation in a patient with CHARGE syndrome. *J Med Genet.* 2004;41:e94.
79. Szmulewicz DJ, McLean CA, MacDougall HG, et al. CANVAS an update: Clinical presentation, investigation and management. *J Vestib Res.* 2014;24(5–6):465–474.

CHAPTER 14

Peripheral Vestibular Dysfunction

Sharon L. Cushing and Jane Lea

Introduction

When children present with true vertigo or disequilibrium, much effort is often spent determining whether these symptoms originate from a central versus peripheral cause or a combination thereof. This important distinction is made through the combination of history, physical examination (see Chapter 4), imaging studies, and ancillary testing findings (Chapters 5–12). The current chapter focuses on those causes of vertigo and disequilibrium that can be attributed to the peripheral vestibular end organs. A number of institutions have examined the underlying diagnoses given to children presenting with complaints of vertigo or dizziness.[1–6] The most common diagnoses are listed in Table 14–1; those of peripheral etiology are reviewed in this chapter, with the exception of benign paroxysmal positional vertigo, which is covered separately in Chapter 15.

Ménière's Disease

Definition, Prevalence, and Etiology

The underlying histopathologic correlate in Ménière's disease (MD) is felt to be endolymphatic hydrops (EH); however, this association remains theoretical. The cause of hydrops remains unknown and may be variable across patients, representing cytochemical abnormalities (eg, autoimmune, viral) or anatomic anomalies (ie, vascular), or a combination thereof. MD is exceedingly uncommon in children in general (<4%) (see Table 14–1).[7] It is possible that this incidence is underestimated and that at presentation the child lacks a full complement of signs and symptoms. Many of the children who are labeled as having "recurrent vestibulopathy" may over time develop into recognizable or confirmed MD. Likewise, given that MD in children is rare, care must be taken to rule out other inner ear anomalies (enlarged vestibular aqueduct syndrome) and autoimmune inner ear disease that may present with an overlapping "hydropic" picture clinically.

Diagnosis

The Committee on Hearing and Equilibrium of the American Academy of Otolaryngology-Head and Neck Surgery (AAO-HNS) initially published guidelines of MD in 1995 (Table 14–2A).[8] In 2015, revised diagnostic criteria of MD were published, tightening the criteria for definite MD, and eliminating "certain" and

Table 14–1. Summary of Series Within the Literature Reporting on the Most Common Causes of Vertigo/Dizziness in Pediatric Patients

O'Reilly et al. 2011[154]				*Wiener-Vacher, S. et al. 2008 (Wiener-Vacher, 2008)*		*Bower et al. 2007 (Bower & Cotton, 1995)*[155]		*Balatsouras et al. 2007*		*Niemensivu, R. et al. 2006 (Niemensivu, Pyykko, Wiener-Vacher, & Kentala, 2006)*	
132		***39***		***> 2000***		***34***		***54***		***119***	
Diagnosis	***%***	***Diagnosis***	***%***	***Diagnosis***	***%***	***Diagnosis***	***%***	***Diagnosis***	***%***	***Diagnosis***	***%***
Peripheral Vestibulopathy	30 →	Cochleovestibular anomaly	23	Migraine	25	OME	15	Viral infection	28	BPVC	19
Migraine/BPVC	24	SNHL	10	BPVC	20	BPVC	15	Migraine	20	Migraine	14
Motor delay	11	BPPV	8	Trauma	10	Migraine	12	BPVC	17	VN	12
Trauma	10	MD	8	VN	5	Vestibulopathy (unclassified)	12	OME	9	OME	10
CNS lesion	9	OME	8			Trauma	9	Vestibulopathy (unclassified)	9	Psychogenic	5
Psychogenic	6	Progressive cochleovestibulopathy	5			VN	9	Trauma	6	Vestibulopathy (unclassified)	5
Idiopathic	3	CMV	5			MD	6	BPPV	9	Trauma	5
Movement Disorders	3	Temporal bone fracture	5					MD	2	SSNHL	3
Encephalopathy	1.5	Congenital vestibular hypofunction	5					Tumor	2	DEH	3
Vascular	1.5	Post CI	5							Neck Tension	3
Peripheral	1	Vestibulopathy (unclassified)	5							Orthostatis	3
Neuropathy	1	VN	5							Epilepsy	3
		Autoimmune	5							MD	2
		Viral labyrinthitis	3							Cholesteatoma	2

Erbek et al. 2006		Weisleder et al. 2005 (Weisleder & Fife, 2001)[156]		Ravid, S. et al. (Ravid, Bienkowski, & Eviatar, 2003)		Choung, Y.H. et al. 2003 (Choung, Park, Moon, Kim, & Ryu, 2003)		D'Agostino et al. 1997 (D'Agostino, Tarantino, Melagrana, & Taborelli, 1997)[157]	
50		**31**		**62**		**55**		**282**	
Diagnosis	***%***	***Diagnosis***	***%***	***Diagnosis***	***%***	***Diagnosis***	***%***	***Diagnosis***	***%***
Migraine	34	Migraine	36	Migraine	39	Migraine	31	Trauma	30
BPVC	12	BPVC	19	BPVC	16	BPVC	26	BPVC	21
BPPV	12	Vestibulopathy (unclassified)	13	VN	14	Vestibulopathy (unclassified)	18	Labyrinthitis	18
Psychogenic	10	Anxiety	10	Psychogenic	13	Trauma	7	Tumor	9
Vestibulopathy (unclassified)	10	MD	6	Orthostasis	9	MD	4	Ototoxicity	8
Seizure	6			Concussion	3	DEH	4	Migraine	5
Metabolic	5			Seizure	3	BPPV	4	Seizure	4
VN	4			Syncope	3	CPA tumor	2	Demyelination	3
MD	2					Seizure	2	VN	1.1
PLF	2					VN	2	PLF	0.8
Amblyopia	2					Autoimmune	2		

Abbreviations: BPPV, benign paroxysmal positional vertigo; BPVC, benign paroxysmal vertigo of childhood; CI, cochlear implant; CMV, cytomegalovirus; CNS, central nervous system; MD, Ménière's disease; OME, otitis media with effusion; PLF, perilymphatic fistula; SNHL, sensorineural hearing loss; VN, vestibular neuronitis.

Sources: Balatsouras DG, Kaberos A, Assimakopoulos D, Katotomichelakis M, Economou NC, Korres SG Etiology of vertigo in children. *Int J Pediatr Otorhinolaryngol.* 2007;71(3):487–494. doi:10.1016/j.ijporl.2006.11.024 / Bower CM, Cotton RT. The spectrum of vertigo in children. *Arch Otolaryngol Head Neck Surg.* 1995;121(8): 911–915 / Choung YH, Park K, Moon SK, Kim CH, Ryu SJ. Various causes and clinical characteristics in vertigo in children with normal eardrums. *Int J Pediatr Otorhinolaryngol.* 2003;67(8):889–894 / D'Agostino, R., Tarantino, V., Melagrana, A., & Taborelli, G. Otoneurologic evaluation of child vertigo. *Int J Pediatr Otorhinolaryngol,* 1997;40(2–3):133–139 / Erbek SH, Erbek SS, Yilmaz I, Topal O, Ozgirgin N, Ozluoglu LN, Alehan F. Vertigo in childhood: a clinical experience. *Int J Pediatr Otorhinolaryngol.* 2006;70(9):1547–1554. doi:10.1016/j.ijporl.2006.04.001 / Niemensivu R, Pyykko I, Wiener-Vacher SR, Kentala E. Vertigo and balance problems in children—an epidemiologic study in Finland. *Int J Pediatr Otorhinolaryngol.* 2006;70(2):259–265 / O'Reilly RC, Greywoode J, Morlet T, et al. Comprehensive vestibular and balance testing in the dizzy pediatric population. *Otolaryngol Head Neck Surg.* 2011;144(2):142–148. doi:10.1177/0194599810393679 / Ravid S, Bienkowski R, Eviatar L. A simplified diagnostic approach to dizziness in children. *Pediatr Neurol.* 2003;29(4):317–320 / Weisleder P, Fife TD. Dizziness and headache: a common association in children and adolescents. *J Child Neurol.* 2001;16(10): 727–730 / Wiener-Vacher SR. Vestibular disorders in children. *Int J Audiol.* 2008;47(9):578–583.

Table 14–2A. Classification of Ménière's Disease According to the 1995 Guidelines of the Committee on Hearing and Equilibrium of the American Academy of Otolaryngology and Head and Neck Surgery[8]

Definition	*Symptoms*
Certain Ménière's disease	Definite Ménière's disease plus histopathologic confirmation
Definite Ménière's disease	Two or more definitive spontaneous episodes of vertigo 20 min or longer
	Audiometrically documented hearing loss on at least one occasion
	Tinnitus or aural fullness in the treated ear
	Other causes excluded
Probable Ménière's disease	One definitive episode of vertigo
	Audiometrically documented hearing loss on at least one occasion
	Tinnitus or aural fullness in the treated ear
	Other causes excluded
Possible Ménière's disease	Episodic vertigo without documented hearing loss, or sensorineural hearing loss fluctuating or fixed, with disequilibrium but nonepisodic
	Others causes excluded

Table 14–2B. Classification of Ménière's Disease According to the International Classification of Vestibular Disorders Committee 2015 Guidelines[10]

Definition	*Symptoms*
Definite Ménière's disease	A. Two of more spontaneous episodes of vertigo, each lasting 20 minutes to 12 hours
	B. Audiometrically documented low- to medium-frequency sensorineural hearing loss, in the affected ear on at least one occasion before, during, or after one of the episodes of vertigo
	C. Fluctuating aural symptoms (hearing, tinnitus, or fullness) in the affected ear
	D. Not better accounted for by another vestibular diagnosis
Probable Ménière's disease	A. Two of more episodes of vertigo or dizziness, each lasting 30 minutes to 24 hours
	B. Fluctuating aural symptoms (hearing, tinnitus, or fullness) in the reported ear
	C. Not better accounted for by another vestibular diagnosis

"possible" MD categories (Table 14–2B).[9,10] Classically, audiometric testing reveals a fluctuating, typically low-frequency sensorineural hearing loss (SNHL). In recent years, several diagnostic tests have been proposed to study the presence of EH and complement the diagnosis of MD. Electrocochleography (EcoG) allows for the intra- or extratympanic recording of the summation potential (SP) and action potential (AP) of the eighth nerve. An increased SP/AP ratio (>0.4) and/or a widened AP width (>3 ms) are considered to be diagnostic of EH. The cervical VEMP (cVEMP) (see Chapter 8 for details) measures the integrity of the saccule and, thus, a portion of the inferior vestibular nerve. Reduced amplitude or absent air-conducted cVEMP and oVEMP responses have been demonstrated in patients with MD as well as a shift in the optimal AC VEMP frequency from 500 to 1000 Hz; "tuning shifts" thought to reflect mechanical alterations secondary to endolymphatic hydrops.[11–14] Significant lateral canal weakness detected by either caloric testing or head thrust testing is present in 42% to 73% of patients with MD with areflexia occurring in 6% to 11%.[15]

Management

Medical Management

The medical management of MD includes both lifestyle modifications and medications. Lifestyle modifications include a low-salt diet, and avoidance of caffeine derivatives and alcohol. Medical therapies include the use of diuretics, vasodilators, and steroids. The challenge in assessing the effect of a management paradigm in the setting of MD remains the natural history of the disease and a strong placebo effect. In individual studies, diuretics and low-sodium diet appeared to be effective in controlling the symptoms of MD in 71% to 79% of patients.[16,17] However, a Cochrane database review of all prospective randomized controlled trials (RCTs), between 1966 and 2005 comparing diuretics with placebo failed to show a single trial of sufficient quality to meet standard criteria set for review.[18] Another Cochrane database review of all RCT comparing betahistine (a vasodilator) with placebo between 1966 and 1999 (six trials with 162 patients) failed to show any benefit.[19] A more recent study examined the dose response of betahistine and demonstrated that while all groups saw a reduction in their attacks over a 12-month period, the high-dose group (48 mg three times a day) saw a significantly larger reduction in attacks. No children, however, were included in this study.[20]

Nondestructive Management

Treatment of MD with the Meniett device and endolymphatic sac surgery falls into this category. Much debate exists as to the efficacy of either procedure; however, despite this debate, in a recent survey 9% of otologists report using the Meniett device and 50% report performing endolymphatic sac decompression.[21] A new surgical technique involving blocking off the endolymphatic duct has recently been published suggesting improved outcomes when compared to endolymphatic sac decompression among adult patients.[22]

Ablative Management

Ablative management of MD includes modalities such as intratympanic (IT) injections of gentamycin and surgical ablation such as labyrinthectomy and vestibular nerve section. Gentamicin is a selective vestibulotoxic aminoglycoside antibiotic that causes apoptotic cell death of the vestibular dark cells, resulting in partial or complete ablation of peripheral vestibular function.[23,24] Its cochleotoxic effects vary considerably, and hearing deterioration occurs in 13% to 35% of patients.[25] In general, vertigo control relates to the completeness of the ablation of the vestibular end organ, which in turn increases the risk of the associated hearing loss.[25] It would be exceedingly rare to perform any type of ablative therapy in the pediatric population.

Recurrent Vestibulopathy

Definition, Prevalence, and Etiology

Recurrent vestibulopathy (RV) is a clinical syndrome initially described in 1981[26] and is defined by multiple episodes of vertigo lasting for minutes to hours, without auditory or neurologic signs or symptoms and the attacks are not provoked by changes in head position. The underlying cause of recurrent vestibulopathy is unknown, while some suggest that it relates to periodic reductions in the afferent rate of discharge and is potentially virally mediated.[27] A number of studies have claimed that episodic vertigo is causally related to migraine[28] (see Chapter 16); other considerations include recurrent vestibular neuritis and a precursor of MD.[27] Indeed, long-term follow-up studies suggest that up to 30% of patients given a diagnosis of recurrent vestibulopathy subsequently develop MD or benign positional vertigo, while the remainder retain their original diagnosis.[27] Over a follow-up period of 5 years, one recent review noted symptom resolution in 80 patients (82%) (inactive RV), continued symptoms in 12 (12%) (active RV), MD in 4 (4%), and migraine in 2 (2%).[29] Few pediatric patients appear among the reported series in the literature; however, it may be that a portion of those children figuring in the "unknown" category in pediatric series (see Table 14–1) indeed fit the criteria for RV.

Diagnosis

This diagnosis of recurrent vestibulopathy requires the following criteria:

- Multiple (>2) vertigo attacks lasting from 5 minutes to a maximum of 24 hours
- No associated hearing loss, no tinnitus or aural pressure sensation
- No provocation by changed head position

The exclusion criteria include the following:

- Presence of migraine, meeting the International Headache Society criteria[30]
- Presence of unilateral sensorineural hearing loss
- Abnormalities at neurologic examination

There may be an associated unilateral loss of lateral canal function in patients with RV, although this occurs in the minority of patients.[26]

Management

Given the benign course and the likelihood for resolution in RV, management typically consists of routine clinical and audiologic follow-up to ensure that those individuals who develop into another clinical entity such as MD are recognized and treated.

Toxicity-Induced Vestibular Dysfunction

Drug-induced ototoxicity can occur secondary to the administration of several groups of antibiotic, chemotherapeutic, and diuretic agents. Monitoring for ototoxicity in children who are of necessity on such therapeutic regimens typically consists of audiometric assessment. Vestibular evaluation is rarely, if ever, considered within the monitoring paradigms. This contradicts the fact that many of these agents are more likely to cause vestibular than cochlear toxicity. For children with ototoxic injuries, disequilibrium is the most common impairment, with vertiginous symptoms being relatively uncommon. Aminoglycosides are the most common category of antibiotic agents that lead to ototoxicity; however, severe vestibular end-organ damage can also occur with vancomycin and viomycin. While uncommon, some individuals present with increased genetic susceptibility to aminoglycoside toxicity as a results of a mitochondrial DNA defect.[31] Likewise, most children with cystic fibrosis routinely receive aminoglycosides via a variety of routes. Some series report that vestibulotoxicity in this group is roughly 12%; however, this is likely an underestimate as this prevalence was determined by survey data, and only 15% of cystic fibrosis units participating in the study routinely performed audiometric and/or vestibular ototoxicity monitoring.[32]

Children receiving chemotherapy are also at risk of ototoxicity. Cisplatin in particular is well documented to have ototoxic effects, with a prevalence ranging from 26% to 90%, where the variability can be accounted for by differences in treatment and monitoring protocols.[33] Most centers monitor ototoxicity through audiometric outcomes including ultra-high-frequency testing (>8 kHz), with few if any concurrently monitoring vestibular toxicity.

Ongoing study is required to better define the incidence of vestibular toxicity in children undergoing necessary therapy with known ototoxins. High-risk groups such as those previously outlined may benefit from screening for vestibulotoxicity, which may be feasible through the use of dynamic visual acuity testing, high-frequency head impulse testing (see Chapter 7), or the use of computerized testing, such as the vestibular autorotation test or rotational testing including high-frequency rotation.[34]

Balance Dysfunction Associated With Middle Ear Effusion/ Otitis Media With Effusion

Otitis media is exceedingly common in the pediatric population. The impact of persistent otitis media with effusion (OME) on the acquisition of language is well studied and well accepted as a risk factor for poor development. However, the impact that persistent OME has on motor skills acquisition, particularly if present during critical periods of development, has been studied but is less pervasive among clinicians looking after these children. Eustachian tube dysfunction and associated middle ear effusion (MEE) are arguably the most common causes and risk factors for the development of balance disturbances in the pediatric population.[35–39] Multiple sources have documented that vestibular end-organ, balance, and general motor function are acutely worse in the presence of a MEE[40–45] and that this deterioration reverses upon either spontaneous resolution or treatment of the MEE.[40,41,43–45] Different theories have been proposed as to how middle ear pathologies can affect the vestibular labyrinth. Golz and colleagues[43] postulated that toxins present in middle ear fluid enter the inner ear fluid and cause serous labyrinthitis. Other researchers have proposed that pressure changes in the middle ear cause displacement of the round and oval window, leading to secondary movement of labyrinthine fluids.[46,47]

While the acute effects of MEE on balance have been well established, the consequences of recurrent MEE on balance function following resolution are less clear. There is some evidence to suggest that vestibular and balance function remains impaired following resolution of the MEE, although 2 of these studies did not assess middle ear function at the time of testing.[38,48,49] However, other studies have not demonstrated a significant difference following resolution of MEE.[37] It is certainly possible that recurrent and/or persistent MEEs that occur early and/or during the time of critical transitions (learning to sit, walk, etc) could translate into overall delays that persist beyond the resolution of the MEE. Children with underlying motor or vestibular dysfunction at baseline may be at particular risk of such effects. While more research is required, balance and motor skills should be weighed along with other factors when considering tympanostomy tube placement for children presenting with MEE.[50]

Peripheral Vestibular Dysfunction Associated With Hearing Loss

The cochlea shares an anatomic proximity as well as histologic and physiologic similarities to the neighboring vestibular end organs. It has been well established that the relationship between auditory and vestibular function is complex. The importance of studying the relationship between peripheral vestibular function in the setting of deafness is underlined by the fact that SNHL is the most common congenital sensory impairment occurring in 3 out of every 1000 live births.[51] Should even a small proportion of these individuals with SNHL exhibit concurrent vestibular involvement, this would still account for large numbers of individuals with vestibular dysfunction requiring identification, education, and therapy. A number of studies have examined both vestibular and balance function in large cohorts of children with hearing impairment. The challenge of summarizing these results relates to the heterogeneity inherent both to the population as well as to the measures utilized to assess vestibular and balance function. Likely the most important population factors that contribute to this heterogeneity include etiology of the underlying hearing loss as well as severity and time course of the hearing loss. In the literature, the categorization of etiology has obviously evolved from a generic label such as congenital onset or genetic, to a more specific diagnosis such as Connexin 26–related deafness, where even the specific mutation can be identified. Despite these advancements, a specific etiology is still not identified in a significant proportion of children with SNHL with this proportion accounting for somewhere between 40% and 70% depending on the unknown role of monoallelic mutations. As a result, all studies tend to still include a large and heterogeneous subgroup of children in whom the etiology of deafness is unknown. In addition, some children with uncommon causes of SNHL (ie, mitochondrial or metabolic disorders) have not studied in sufficient numbers to draw population conclusions.

As with etiology, when the severity of the SNHL is considered, many of the early studies included a very heterogeneous group. More recently and with the advent of cochlear implantation (CI) and in particular bilateral CI, numerous studies have included a more homogeneous cohort of children with severe to profound SNHL. The time course of the hearing loss (progressive versus nonprogressive) may also play a role in the functional outcomes and needs to be considered.

With respect to measures of vestibular and balance function, large variation also exists throughout the literature. Most studies include either a clinical or ancillary measure of horizontal canal function (ie, head thrust testing, pre-/post-rotary nystagmus, caloric testing, rotational chair testing), and more recent studies may examine the vestibulocollic pathway using cVEMP. In some studies, end-organ testing may be coupled with an assessment of static and dynamic balance, and again the tests used are quite variable. With these caveats in mind, we attempt to provide an overview of the general relationship of SNHL and vestibular and balance dysfunction in children.

Documentation of vestibular function and dysfunction in children with hearing impairment has a long and rich history that has indicated that somewhere in the range of 20% to 85% of children with hearing loss demonstrate some form of vestibular end-organ dysfunction.[52–66] Some cohorts demonstrated a mix of partial versus complete vestibular dysfunction,[65] while others suggested that a partial vestibular lesion in the presence of total deafness is rare.[55] Numerous studies have also shown that vestibular dysfunction can be unilateral versus bilateral and does not always correlate with the sidedness of the auditory loss.[54,55,61,65] There has been increasing interest in the functional deficits of children with unilateral SNHL to include vestibular evaluation. Children with unilateral profound SNHL demonstrate vestibular function that is worse in comparison to normal-hearing peers but better than that of children with bilateral deafness.[67] More than 50% of children with unilateral profound SNHL displayed an abnormality of the vestibular end organs, usually occurring only on the deaf side.[68–76] Just as the degree of hearing loss can span the spectrum of mild to profound, unilateral to bilateral, vestibular function similarly has a wide spectrum of findings.

Relationship Between Hearing Threshold and Vestibular Function

Although the relationship between vestibular and auditory function is not simple, there does appear to be an association. A number of studies have shown that, at least on a group level, the likelihood of a vestibular impairment relates to the degree of the hearing loss.[54,57,61,65,66] As a group, children with normal vestibular function, as measured by caloric stimulation, have lower pure-tone averages (PTAs) than those with unilateral vestibular hypofunction, who in turn have higher PTAs than those with bilateral vestibular hypofunction.[54] Likewise, in some studies, the proportion of individuals with vestibular impairment is significantly lower (20% to 36%) in children with a hearing threshold of less than 90 dB and higher (80%) in those with more severe hearing loss.[61,66] Although the literature supports the significant relationship known to exist between concurrent depression of hearing sensitivity and vestibular responsiveness, hearing thresholds are not predictive for the individual case. This is underlined by the findings in one study that 16.1% of children with relatively good auditory sensitivity demonstrated complete absence of vestibular function, while 43.3% of the children with the poorest auditory sensitivity had normal responses.[65] The advent of bilateral CI prompted an increase in the interest of examining vestibular function in children with SNHL. By definition, most children who are candidates for CI have severe to profound SNHL. Across several studies, the prevalence of vestibular end-organ function in this category ranges from roughly 50% to 70%.[77–80]

Relationship Between Etiology and Combined Audiovestibular Loss

Variability Across Etiology

The variability in vestibular responsiveness across different etiologies of SNHL is readily apparent in the available literature. The vestibular phenotypes of a number of congenital, hereditary, and acquired causes of SNHL have been defined. Several genetic causes of SNHL have a high prevalence of vestibular dysfunction, the most important of which is type 1 Usher syndrome (USH1). USH1 is a recessive disorder characterized by congenital SNHL, vestibular impairment, and progressive visual impairment due to retinitis pigmentosa (RP). As multigene panels for evaluation of childhood hearing loss often include Usher syndrome genes, Usher syndrome may be diagnosed pre-symptomatically prior to onset of the RP. Alternatively, Usher syndrome may be diagnosed by its clinical manifestations, prompting genetic evaluation and testing. Any child with profound SNHL and vestibular/balance impairments of unknown etiology should be referred to a specialized ophthalmologist and geneticist with the specific question of USH1 in mind.[81] Further discussion regarding Usher syndrome can be found in Chapter 13.

Likewise, bacterial meningitis is another etiology where the SNHL is often accompanied by profound vestibular dysfunction.[62,82–85] Well-defined syndromes and acquired infectious losses, however, account for only a small percentage of all SNHL, with the etiology of deafness being either unknown or due to a nonsyndromic genetic cause in the majority of children.[86] Despite very little literature on the topic, there is a general feeling that nonsyndromic recessive causes of deafness, of which the most common are defects in the *GJB2* gene, are not typically associated with concurrent deficits in vestibular end-organ function.[87] A large cohort ($N = 153$) of children with CI examined vestibular end-organ function according to etiology and demonstrated that all children with meningitis and 46% with cochleovestibular anomalies had horizontal canal dysfunction, while 45% and 46%, respectively, displayed saccular dysfunction.[88] Table 14–3 presents an overview of vestibular end-organ function by etiology for this cohort.

Variability Within Etiology

Meningitis. While tremendous variability exists across etiology, an incredible degree of variability is also present within a single etiologic category such as deafness secondary to meningitis, even though the relationship between auditory and vestibular function in this setting is thought to be better understood. Meningitis is known to cause progressive but variable ossification of the inner ear structures (Figure 14–1). Children with SNHL due to meningitis demonstrate a disproportionately large degree of vestibular non-responsiveness; however the degree of non-responsiveness does range from unilateral weakness to bilateral areflexia of the horizontal canals.[61] Similarly, cases have been documented where nearly half of the children with profound SNHL due to meningitis demonstrated normal horizontal canal function as measured by a caloric stimulation.[64]

Abnormal Cochleovestibular Anatomy. One might expect the relationship between vestibular and auditory dysfunction to be relatively straightforward in the setting of inner ear dysplasia. In many cases, vestibular dysfunction correlates well with the presence of inner ear dysplasia on computed tomography (CT) imaging; however, overall, equal numbers of children with normal vestibular function were found in both the radiologically normal group as in the radiologically abnormal group.[89] Not all children with hearing loss due to inner ear dysplasia demonstrate complete vestibular areflexia.[64,89] Pendred syndrome is another autosomal-recessive cause of vestibular dysfunction. This syndrome is a constellation of incomplete partition type 2 (IP-2) of the cochlea and enlarged vestibular aqueduct

Table 14–3. Vestibular End-Organ Function by Etiology of Sensorineural Hearing Loss

Etiology (n)	*Horizontal Canal*[a]		*Saccule*[b]
	Caloric	*Rotation*	
	□ *Normal* ▒ *Abnormal* ■ *Areflexia*	□ *Normal* ■ *Abnormal*	□ *Normal* ▒ *Unilateral* ■ *Bilateral*
Cochleovestibular anomaly (28)	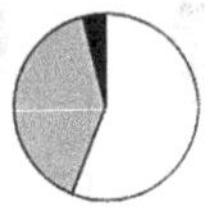	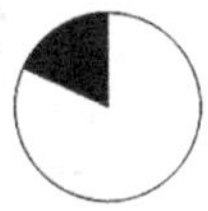	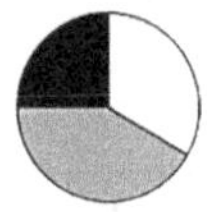
Homozygous connexin-26 (25)	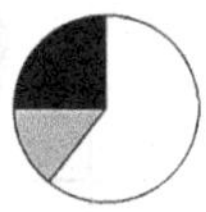	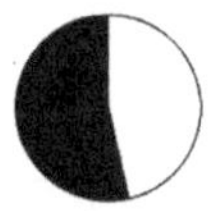	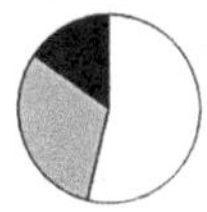
Meningitis (11)	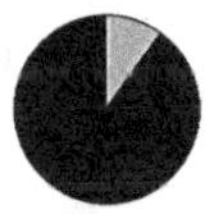	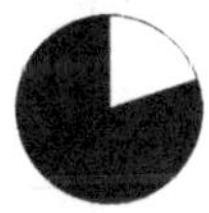	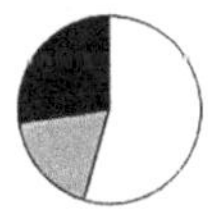
Cytomegalovirus (5)	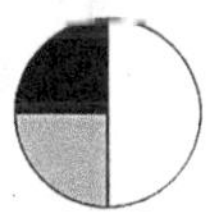	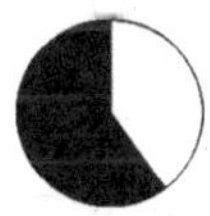	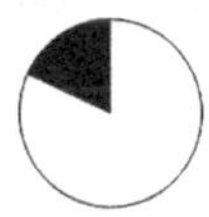
Usher's (4)	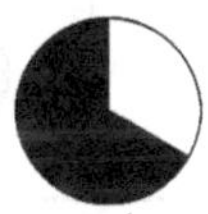		
Pendred (3)	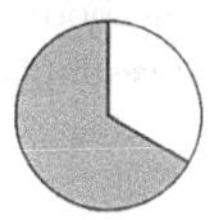	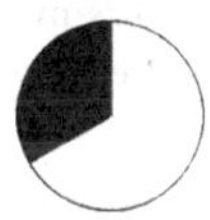	
Phelps (2)			
Auditory neuropathy (2)	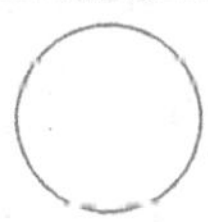	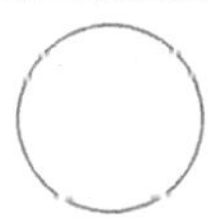	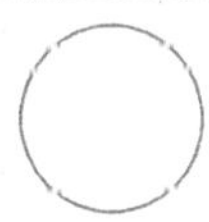
Autoimmune (1)			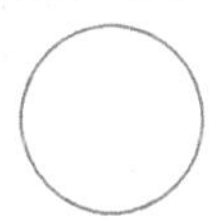
Ototoxicity (1)			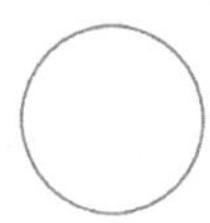

continues

Table 14–3. *continued*

Etiology (n)	*Horizontal Canal*[a]		*Saccule*[b]
	Caloric	*Rotation*	
	□ *Normal* ▩ *Abnormal* ■ *Areflexia*	□ *Normal* ■ *Abnormal*	□ *Normal* ▩ *Unilateral* ■ *Bilateral*
Klippel-Feil (1)			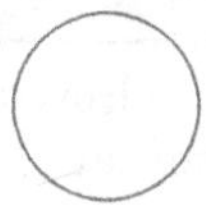
Mitochondrial (1)	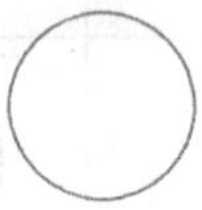		
Stickler (1)	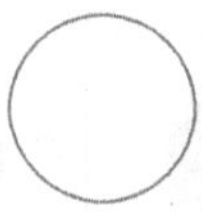		
Waardenburg (1)			
Unknown (64)	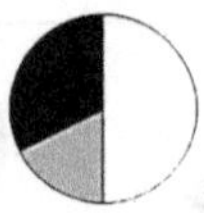	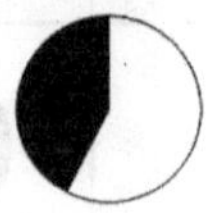	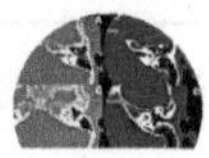

[a]Horizontal canal function is measured using both a caloric and rotational stimulus.
[b]Saccule function is measured using cervical vestibular-evoked myogenic potentials.

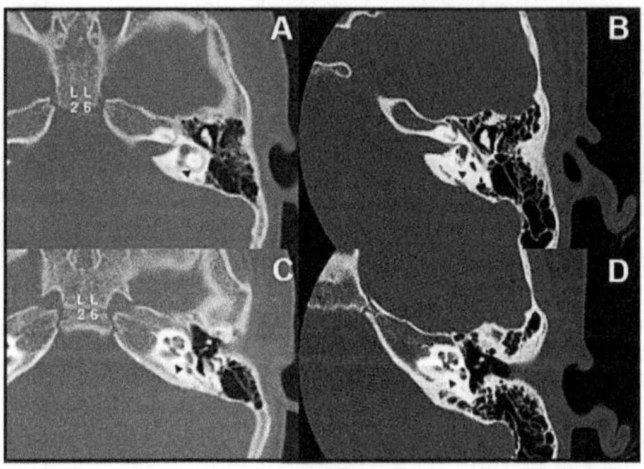

Figure 14–1. Axial, nonenhanced high-resolution computed tomography of the left petrous temporal bone demonstrating a normal horizontal semicircular canal (**A**, *black arrowhead*) which underwent progressive ossification (**B**, *black arrowhead*) following meningitis as an infant. Similar ossification of the posterior semicircular canal is noted (**D**, *black arrowhead*) compared to the baseline scan (**C**, *black arrowhead*). Interscan interval was greater than 10 years.

(EVA). Vestibular dysfunction maybe present in up to one-third of cases.[90]

Congenital Cytomegalovirus Infection. A number of acquired infectious causes of SNHL such as meningitis and congenital CMV (cCMV) infection also present with associated vestibular and balance impairment.[91] Congenital CMV is increasingly recognized as an important cause of SNHL and motor delay. Congenital CMV infection is estimated to affect 0.4% to 2.3% of live births in the United States. Similarly, the seroprevalence in Ontario, Canada, was found to be 0.6%.[92] Up to 90% of those are asymptomatic at birth. Eight to 15% of asymptomatic patients will present later in life with SNHL, while symptomatic cCMV infection will lead to SNHL in 30% to 65% of patients.[93] Vestibular insult in the setting of cCMV can be expected in patients who are severely affected but can also occur in those children who are classified as "asymptomatic." The impact of the virus on the labyrinth has recently been confirmed histopathologically, where cytomegalic cells containing inclusion bodies, inflammation, and active infection produced extensive injury throughout the inner ear in addition to the central nervous system.[94,95] This dual peripheral and central insult may worsen the functional deficit as well as impair or limit central compensation. The sensory deficits resulting from cCMV are acquired, most commonly in the third trimester, and progressive, which may reflect that the underlying injury is degenerative and vascular in nature.[96] Progressive, partial, or complete vestibular dysfunction is more common than SNHL in infants with symptomatic cCMV.[97–99] This peripheral dysfunction along with the associated central nervous system dysfunction leads to the significant balance disturbances seen in this population with the majority of the children with cCMV infection experiencing a later age at walking.[100] Congenital CMV infection should be considered in the differential diagnosis for children with SNHL and/or balance disturbance as well as neurodevelopmental disabilities.[101]

Other Etiologies Associated With Vestibular Loss. Similarly, some children whose SNHL is not due to meningitis have bilateral vestibular dysfunction.[61] In the literature, reports of complete bilateral loss of vestibular function have been associated with SNHL due to thalidomide fetopathy, kernicterus, as well as nonsyndromic autosomal recessive–type hearing loss and hearing loss of unknown etiology.[61] The prevalence of vestibular disorders among these other etiologies is highlighted in studies that excluded children whose deafness was secondary to meningitis or other severe infantile infection.[65] Despite this exclusion, Rosenblut and colleagues reported that a large proportion (43%) of the remaining cohort demonstrated vestibular dysfunction.[65] Cogan syndrome is an autoimmune disorder that presents with non-syphylitic interstitial keratitis, acute SNHL, and vestibulopathy. The hearing loss may be progressive. The timing and association of symptoms of Cogan syndrome can be highly variable, making diagnosis difficult. Despite this, accurate and prompt diagnosis is essential, as high-dose steroids may help to limit the degree of SNHL and vestibulopathy.[102]

Relationship Between Vestibular End-Organ and Balance Function

Many of the studies mentioned previously included a measure of not only vestibular end-organ function but also of balance function, and the immense heterogeneity and variability within and across etiologic subgroups was preserved for this measure. In general, as a group, children with SNHL have poorer balance skills than their normal hearing peers

(Figure 14–2).[60,78,103–110] In a recent cohort of over 200 children with severe to profound SNHL, balance function was examined, and while there were significant differences between different etiologies of hearing loss, the within-group variability remained high (Figure 14–3).

Impact of Cochlear Implantation on Vestibular and Balance Function

With the advent of bilateral cochlear implantation (CI), the concern for bilateral vestibular impairment led to increased awareness and interest in measuring vestibular function in children with SNHL. There are a number of potential mechanisms by which surgically induced injuries to the labyrinth may occur, including (1) induction of a serous labyrinthitis due to opening of the membranous labyrinth, (2) introduction of blood into the inner ear, (3) mechanical injury due to the insertion of the electrode array,[68–72,74–76,111] and (4) high-speed drilling within the temporal bone.[112,113] Diminished end-organ function following CI occurs in anywhere from 0 to 77% of the cohort examined, depending on the population tested and the type and timing of testing.[73,77,109,114–134] Based on careful pre- and postoperative study of vestibular function in children undergoing delayed sequential CI, the theoretical risk of total bilateral vestibular loss following bilateral simultaneous CI is estimated at 2%.[135–138] While this 2% risk may appear modest, parents and patients considering bilateral CI should be counseled appropriately. Put in perspective, total bilateral vestibular loss is far more likely to result from the underlying etiology of the deafness itself than from bilateral CI surgery.

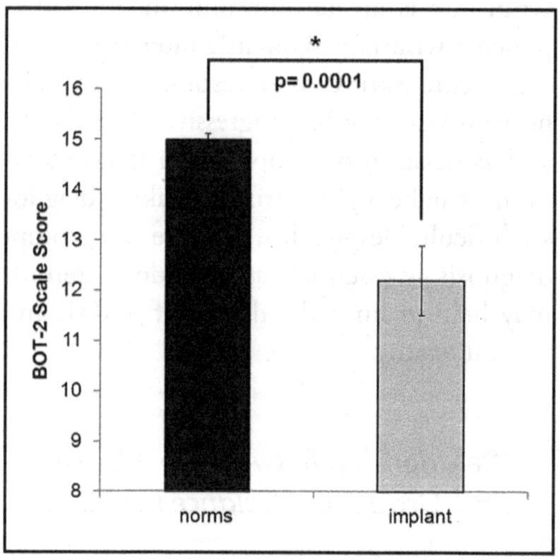

Figure 14–2. Comparison of balance skills between children with normal hearing (norms) versus children with severe to profound sensorineural hearing loss. Differences in balance scores between the 2 groups are statistically significant. Balance skills were measured using the balance subset of the Bruininks-Oseretsky Test of Motor Proficiency 2.

Conversely, children with poor balance function are at increased risk for CI device failure. Specifically, an absence of bilateral horizontal canal function (areflexia) increases the odds of CI device failure 7.6 times,[139] where failure is defined as mechanical or electrical malfunction of the surgically implanted internal component. Likewise, poor balance measured on objective tests of function and saccular dysfunction measured by absence of vestibular evoked myogenic potentials, were also significantly more common in children with CI failure. The likely mechanism is an increase in falls leading to repetitive device damage. Vestibular dysfunction is therefore the largest patient-related factor contributing to CI failure identified to date.[139]

Summary and Conclusions

Variability in the relationship between auditory and vestibular function can certainly be linked to differences in the etiology and the

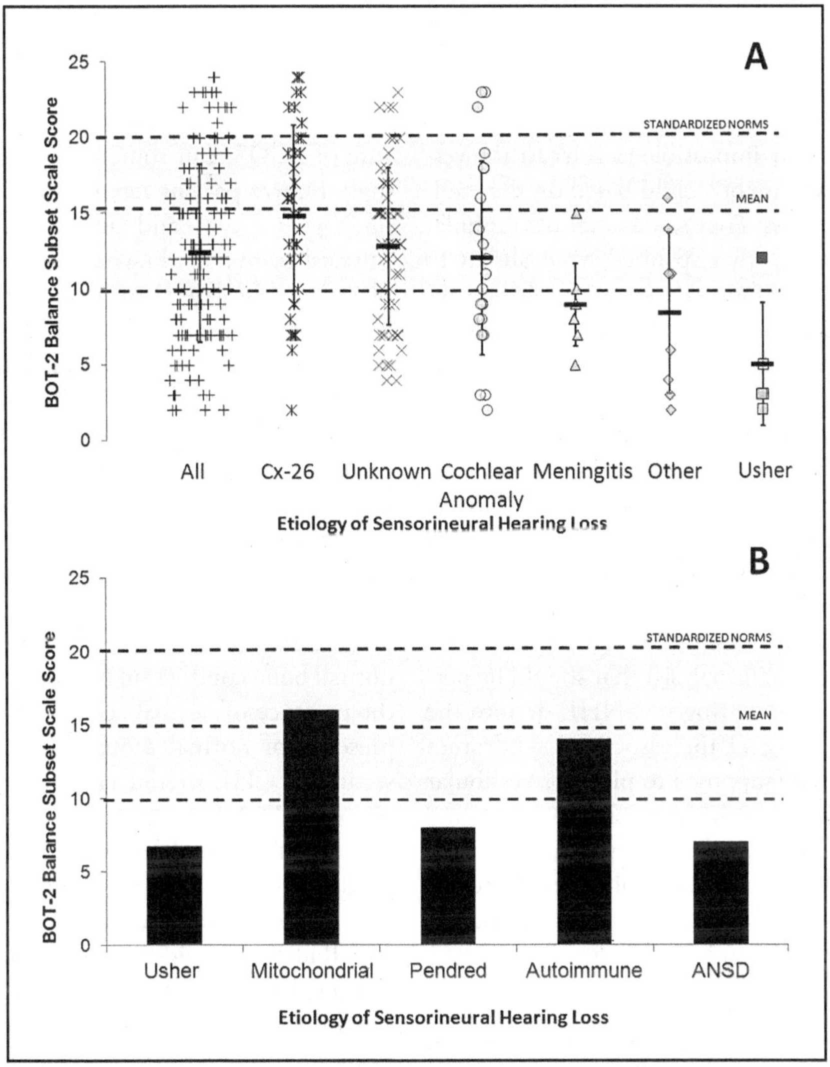

Figure 14–3. Balance skills in children with severe to profound sensorineural hearing loss according to the etiology. The most common etiologies are shown in **A**. The etiologies comprising the "Other" category are expanded in **B**. Comparison is made with the mean age and gender adjusted score (mean = 15 ± 5 (SD); dotted lines, gray box). Balance skills were measured using the balance subset of the Bruininks-Oseretsky Test of Motor Proficiency 2.

severity of the inner ear disorder. Children with severe to profound SNHL, particularly if the underlying etiology is (1) an acquired infectious cause (ie, meningitis), (2) syndromic (CHARGE association), or related to (3) abnormal cochleovestibular anomalies are at very high risk of vestibular and balance dysfunction. While on a group level etiology and severity are predictive, this does not hold true on the individual level. Remarkably, the overall conclusion that can be drawn from much of the current literature was insightfully summarized by Guilder and Hopkins in their 1935 study examining vestibular responses in children attending a school for the deaf. They noted that with the exception of meningitis, it was absolutely impossible to forecast the vestibular response of a child based on the etiology of deafness. They saw a range of vestibular responsiveness that spanned from absent to normal across their designated etiologic subgroups, as well as across different categories of residual hearing.[58]

Despite the variability, the prevalence of vestibular and balance dysfunction in children with SNHL is high. The take-home message is that an assessment of vestibular end-organ function and balance should be performed in all children presenting with SNHL. Clinicians will often debate the content of the laundry list of tests and evaluations (ie, electrocardiogram, urinalysis) that should be performed in the setting of SNHL despite the low prevalence of the associated syndromes these tests are supposed to pick up. Vestibular and balance assessment rarely figures among that list despite the high prevalence of associated dysfunction, and this likely speaks to the challenges and lack of expertise in evaluating vestibular function in children.

Superior Semicircular Canal Dehiscence Syndrome

Superior semicircular canal dehiscence syndrome (SCDS) was first described by Minor in 1998[140] and encompasses an unusual subset of audiovestibular symptoms, including aural fullness, conductive hyperacusis, and pressure-/sound-induced vertigo.

The disease causes a "third window phenomenon," whereby sound energy is redistributed and the vestibular system is inadvertently stimulated. Patients may present with isolated hearing or vestibular symptomatology, or a combination of both. SCDS is the great mimicker and can easily be mistaken as a variety of other pathologies to the untrained clinician.

Conductive hyperacusis, a common feature of SCDS, can sometimes lead to seemingly bizarre patient reports such as hearing one's eyes move, and unusual abilities on physical exam including hearing a tuning fork placed on the lateral malleolus of the ankle in the affected ear. Vertigo and nystagmus are induced by loud sounds (Tullio phenomenon), pressure changes in the middle ear (Hennebert's sign), or Valsalva against closed glottis or pinched nostrils. Physical examination in the absence of fixation reveals eye movements evoked by sound or pressure that align with the plane of the affected superior semicircular canal.

Audiometric data classically reveal supranormal bone conduction (<0 db) and CHL in the presence of normal acoustic reflexes. The presence of normal acoustic reflexes in the setting of CHL should raise diagnostic suspicion of SCDS, even without supranormal bone conduction thresholds. VEMP testing produces a low-threshold, high-amplitude response in the affected ear.

Radiologic evidence of dehiscence is an integral diagnostic feature. SCDS is best identified on high-resolution CT temporal bone studies reformatted in the plane of the superior semicircular canal (Figure 14–4).

Although SCDS has been well delineated in the adult literature, the pediatric literature is still relatively sparse, the first case series of 7 patients only recently emerging in 2011.[141] The radiologic prevalence of SCDS in those undergoing CT temporal scans in a tertiary care setting ranges from 2% to 10%, but the largest study to date in pediatric patients (n = 334) suggests a radiologic prevalence rate of 3.3%.[142–144] The etiology of SCDS is unknown, with congenital, developmental, and traumatic theories postulated throughout the literature.

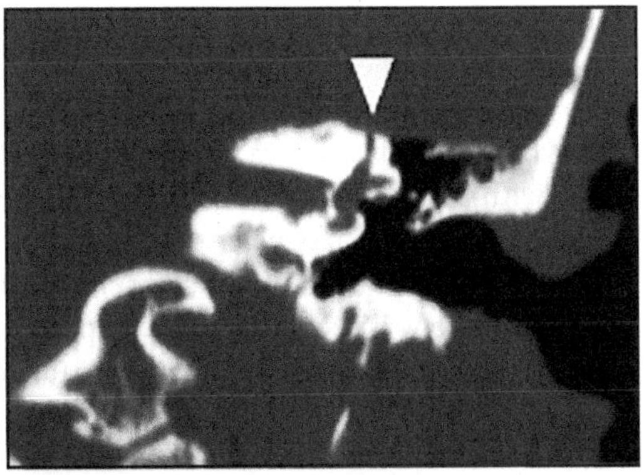

Figure 14–4. Coronal nonenhanced high-resolution computed tomography of the left petrous temporal bone demonstrating dehiscence of the left superior semicircular canal (*white arrowhead*).

Management is individualized according to symptomatology, with surgical repair of the dehiscence through a middle cranial fossa or transmastoid approach reserved for those with intractable vestibular symptoms or troublesome autophony.

Ramsay Hunt Syndrome

Ramsay Hunt syndrome (RHS) is characterized by acute facial palsy and herpetic eruptions on the auricle +/– cochleovestibular dysfunction. The presence of herpetic eruptions distinguishes it from Bell's palsy. The etiology is secondary to reactivation of the latent varicella-zoster virus in the geniculate ganglion. Although an exceedingly rare cause of peripheral vestibulopathy in children, we feel this condition deserves brief mention.

RHS accounts for 17% of cases of facial nerve palsy in pediatrics, with pediatric cases classically having a milder presentation and improved prognosis, with less facial weakness, and 50% less cochleovestibular manifestations than their adult counterparts.[145] Only a small subset (17%) of pediatric RHS develop vertigo, and unlike in adults, vesicle eruption can also be delayed, occurring several days after facial nerve symptoms in 50% of cases (Figure 14–5).[145]

Milder disease symptomatology and improved prognosis have been attributed to stronger immunity in children, likely secondary to shorter periods between the onset of chicken pox and reactivation in the form of RHS.

Debate exists regarding the proper management of this condition with insufficient and underpowered literature causing uncertainty. Despite two recent Cochrane reviews on the subject citing a lack of benefit with antivirals alone and combined with corticosteroids, the general consensus based on the literature available and expert opinion is that combination therapy with antivirals and steroids provides benefit in terms of facial nerve outcomes in

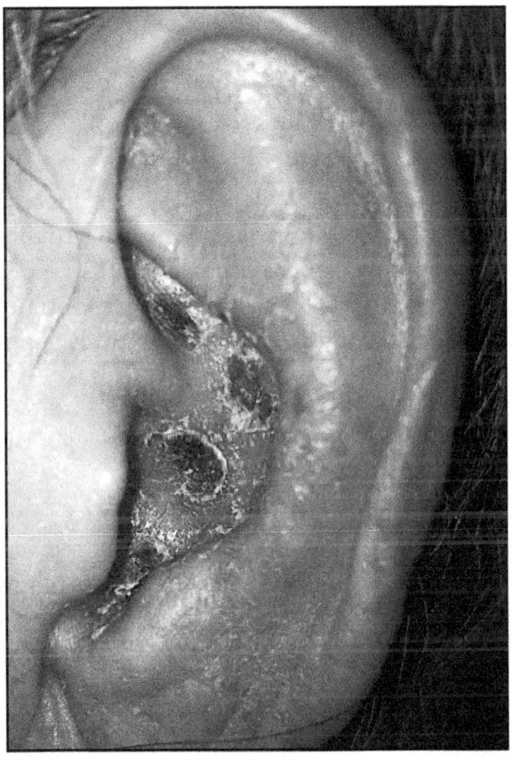

Figure 14–5. Healing lesions in the conchal bowl in the setting of Ramsay-Hunt syndrome.

the adult population.[146] Given the improved prognosis among pediatrics and the absence of literature evaluating treatment regimens, we are unable to ascertain whether the same recommendation holds true in pediatrics.

Vestibular Neuronitis

Definition, Prevalence, and Etiology

Vestibular neuronitis (VN), also termed vestibular neuritis, is a sudden idiopathic unilateral vestibular loss. Classically, VN presents with an acute onset of intense rotatory vertigo lasting several days, with associated nausea, vomiting, and imbalance in the absence of hearing loss. As with other similar diagnoses, such as Bell's palsy, VN is a diagnosis of exclusion, requiring an absence of central neurologic deficits, and an absence of ear pathology. It most often affects the superior vestibular nerve.

In children, VN is relatively uncommon, accounting for less than 5% of all children presenting with vertigo (see Table 14–1). A viral prodrome occurs in 50% of children affected by VN, and it is overwhelmingly believed that the neurotropic herpes simplex virus type 1 (HSV-1) is the etiologic agent responsible, although conclusive evidence is still lacking.

Clinical Course

Vertigo is initially constant and present at rest, exacerbated with movement, and improved with immobility or visual fixation, fitting a classic peripheral etiology. The most important question on history, like most vestibular disorders, is the duration of the vertigo, with VN characteristically lasting "days." Patients tend to veer and fall toward the affected side. Given the difficulty of obtaining a history of vertigo in very young children, VN can easily be confused with gastroenteritis; however, an appropriate physical exam should deliver findings that are diagnostic.

The clinical course is typical in that vertigo symptoms subside over a period of several days, with residual sensations of imbalance or nonspecific dizziness persisting, especially with rapid movements. Persistent residual symptomatology is exceedingly rare in pediatrics as children recover and compensate much more efficiently than adults.[147,148] Recurrent VN is exceedingly rare.

Diagnosis

The diagnosis is primarily clinical, relying on a thorough history and physical examination. Classic signs of an acute unilateral peripheral vestibular loss (affecting the superior vestibular nerve) can be elicited on bedside examination, with common examination findings outlined in Table 14–4. When assessing for spontaneous and post head shake nystagmus, it is essential to remove fixation (Frenzel goggles or video goggles) to increase diagnostic accuracy, as nystagmus can be masked in the presence of fixation.

The clinical diagnosis is often corroborated with audiovestibular testing, with a normal audiogram being characteristic. While vestibular function tests are not essential for diagnosis, they are often performed and classically reveal a unilateral canal paresis. Given the predilection of VN for the superior vestibular nerve, classic findings on VFTs and video head impulse testing can be elicited and are outlined in Table 14–5. As a cautionary note, normal VFTs do not preclude the diagnosis of VN; calorics solely test for low-frequency vestibular losses, and children can compensate quite quickly yielding normal results in less than 2 weeks.[147] It is for this reason that the authors strongly advocate for video head impulse testing (high-frequency test), as both overt and covert saccades can be detected; covert saccades are especially beneficial in highlighting

Table 14–4. Classic Bedside Findings in Left Vestibular Neuronitis (affecting the left superior vestibular nerve)

Test	*Finding*
Spontaneous nystagmus	Right-beating[a]; obeys Alexander's Law
Head thrust	Abnormal catch-up saccade on leftward head turn (similar finding on testing left superior canal)
Head shake	Right-beating post head shake nystagmus
Rhomberg	Fall toward left side
Subjective visual vertical/horizontal	Leftward deviation
Fukuda/Unterberger step test	Leftward deviation ≥45°

[a]Direction of nystagmus, by convention, refers to fast phase.

Table 14–5. Classic Findings on VFT and Video Head Impulse Testing in Left Vestibular Neuronitis (affecting the left superior vestibular nerve)

Test	*Finding*
Caloric	Left canal paresis
cVEMP	Normal
oVEMP	Reduced or absent[157]
Head impulse testing	Reduced gain of left horizontal and superior canal, and abnormal catch-up saccades of these respective canals

subtle or compensated vestibular losses not detectable by the bedside head thrust.

Although imaging studies are not required in classic cases of vestibular neuritis, magnetic resonance imaging is often used given the rarity of this condition in pediatrics and concerns about missing a diagnosis of central etiology. Niemensivu et al. explored the value of imaging studies among children with vertigo and recommended imaging in those with neurologic deficits, head trauma, or persistent headaches, concluding that "when vertigo is the only symptom, imaging studies are unlikely to aid diagnostic work up."[149] It is the opinion of the authors that MRI be restricted to those with atypical, protracted, or noncompensated symptomatology, significant vascular risk factors, or in the presence of central neurologic signs and symptoms, with high-resolution CT temporal bone imaging reserved for those with recent trauma (± MRI), or acute/chronic ear disease to rule out an otologic source.

Serologic testing is not recommended as it does not prove a causal relationship and does not affect management or treatment decisions.

Management

Management in the acute phase of VN is supportive, including antiemetics, hydration, and vestibular suppressants. Intravenous hydration and hospitalization are key elements in the pediatric population given susceptibility to dehydration. Vestibular rehabilitation exercises should be instigated early, as this is key to central compensation. Vestibular suppressants should be utilized only in the acute phase as prolonged use prevents central compensation.

Debate exists regarding treatment with steroids and antivirals. In adults, conflicting evidence exists regarding the benefit of steroids.[150–152] Some benefit in terms of rate of recovery (reduced hospital stay) and degree of vestibular recovery based on caloric paresis has been demonstrated; however, great debate exists as to whether this translates to any perceivable patient benefit. There is an absence of definitive evidence for the use of antivirals alone or as an adjunct to steroids. Because of the paucity of pediatric data to direct treatment decisions and the realization that most patients spontaneously recover with little to no residual symptomatology, the authors feel the decision to treat with steroids should be individualized. The physician's role should comprise dissemination of current evidence, rationale, and risks, ultimately leaving treatment decisions to the discretion of the patient or caregiver.

Summary

A variety of peripheral vestibular causes can lead to vertigo and disequilibrium in the pediatric population. The underlying etiologic distribution is considerably different than the adult population and in general children compensate much more rapidly to acute changes in vestibular function. The biggest risk factors for the development of peripheral vestibular dysfunction in children include an associated SNHL and head trauma. A thorough and age-appropriate evaluation of both balance and vestibular end-organ function should be performed in children presenting with such complaints.

Perilymphatic fistulas are rare and difficult to diagnose because they often present in a nonuniform fashion. Although perilymphatic fistulas (PLFs) are often found in the setting of head trauma and barotrauma, it is important to recognize that multiple other mechanisms for this condition exist (ie, erosive masses, congenital conditions, surgical trauma/iatrogenic, spontaneous/idiopathic). Audiologic symptoms include fluctuating or progressive hearing loss, aural fullness, and tinnitus. Vestibular symptoms include brief recurring episodes of vertigo, lasting anywhere from several seconds to hours. Worsening of symptoms with straining, exercise, Valsalva, or nose blowing can be elicited with history and result due to increased intracranial or middle ear pressure. As this is essentially a "third window phenomenon" similar to superior canal dehiscence, Tullio phenomenon and Hennebert's sign may be present on physical examination (see Chapter 4). The varied presentation overlaps with superior SCDS, MD, and syphilis. A strong suspicion for this condition should be raised in the setting of recent trauma. Treatment is similar to a traumatic cerebrospinal fluid leak, with conservative measures being first line (bed rest, head elevation, and avoidance of straining/exertion). PLFs that do not resolve with this conservative treatment may require middle ear exploration and plugging of the defect.

Conclusion

A variety of peripheral vestibular causes can lead to vertigo and disequilibrium in the pediatric population. The underlying etiologic distribution is considerably different than in the adult population, and in general children compensate much more rapidly to acute changes in vestibular function. The biggest risk factors for the development of peripheral vestibular dysfunction in children include an associated SNHL and head trauma. A thorough and age-appropriate evaluation of both balance and vestibular end-organ function should be performed in children presenting with such complaints.

Self-Assessment Questions

1. Outline the treatment options for Ménière's disease.
2. What percentage of individuals given a diagnosis of recurrent vestibulopathy go on to develop Ménière's disease?
3. In general, which part of the inner ear (cochlea versus vestibular end organs) is more susceptible to injury from ototoxic agents?
4. What clinical tests can be performed to detect bilateral vestibular loss?
5. Which etiologies of hearing loss are most likely to be associated with vestibular end-organ dysfunction?
6. What are the clinical features of superior semicircular canal dehiscence syndrome?
7. What are the characteristics of the vertigo and nystagmus induced in benign paroxysmal positional vertigo?
8. What is the underlying etiology of Ramsay Hunt syndrome? How is it distinguished from Bell's palsy?
9. What types of peripheral vestibular injury are associated with traumatic brain injury with and without temporal bone fracture?
10. How is definite Ménière's disease defined?

References

1. Choung YH, Park K, Moon SK, Kim CH, Ryu SJ. Various causes and clinical characteristics in vertigo in children with normal eardrums. *Int J Pediatr Otorhinolaryngol.* 2003; 67(8):889–894.
2. Niemensivu R, Pyykko I, Wiener-Vacher SR, Kentala E. Vertigo and balance problems in children—An epidemiologic study in Finland. *Int J Pediatr Otorhinolaryngol.* 2006; 70(2):259–265.
3. O'Reilly R, Grindle C, Zwicky EF, Morlet T. Development of the vestibular system and balance function: Differential diagnosis in the pediatric population. *Otolaryngol Clin North Am.* 2011;44(2):251–271, vii.
4. O'Reilly RC, Morlet T, Nicholas BD, et al. Prevalence of vestibular and balance disorders in children. *Otol Neurotol.* 2010;31(9):1441–1444.
5. Ravid S, Bienkowski R, Eviatar L. A simplified diagnostic approach to dizziness in children. *Pediatr Neurol.* 2003;29(4):317–320.
6. Wiener–Vacher SR. Vestibular disorders in children. *Int J Audiol.* 2008;47(9):578–583.
7. Akagi H, Yuen K, Maeda Y, et al. Ménière's disease in childhood. *Int J Pediatr Otorhinolaryngol.* 2001;61(3):259–264.
8. Committee on Hearing and Equilibrium guidelines for the diagnosis and evaluation of therapy in Ménière's disease. American Academy of Otolaryngology-Head and Neck Foundation. *Otolaryngol Head Neck Surg.* 1995;113:181.
9. Goebel JA. 2015 Equilibrium Committee Amendment to the 1995 AAO-HNS Guidelines for the Definition of Ménière's Disease. *Otolaryngol Head Neck Surg.* 2016;154(3): 403–404.
10. Lopez-Escamez JA, Carey J, Chung WH, et al. Diagnostic criteria for Ménière's disease. *J Vestib Res.* 2015;25(1):1–7.
11. Rauch SD, Zhou G, Kujawa SG, Guinan JJ, Herrmann BS. Vestibular evoked myogenic potentials show altered tuning in patients with Ménière's disease. *Otol Neurotol.* 2004; 25(3):333–338.
12. Taylor RL, Wijewardene AA, Gibson WP, Black DA, Halmagyi GM, Welgampola MS. The vestibular evoked-potential profile of Ménière's disease. *Clin Neurophysiol.* 2011; 122(6):1256–1263.
13. Taylor RL, Zagami AS, Gibson WP, et al. Vestibular evoked myogenic potentials to sound and vibration: Characteristics in vestibular migraine that enable separation from Ménière's disease. *Cephalalgia.* 2012;32(3): 213–225.
14. Winters SM, Berg IT, Grolman W, Klis SF. Ocular vestibular evoked myogenic potentials: Frequency tuning to air-conducted acoustic stimuli in healthy subjects and Ménière's disease. *Audiol Neurootol.* 2012; 17(1):12–19.
15. Park HJ, Migliaccio AA, Della Santina CC, Minor LB, Carey JP. Search-coil head-thrust and caloric tests in Ménière's disease. *Acta oto-laryngologica.* 2005;125(8):852–857.
16. Santos PM, Hall RA, Snyder JM, Hughes LF, Dobie RA. Diuretic and diet effect on Ménière's disease evaluated by the 1985 Committee on Hearing and Equilibrium guidelines. *Otolaryngol Head Neck Surg.* 1993;109(4):680–689.
17. Silverstein H, Smouha E, Jones R. Natural history vs. surgery for Ménière's disease. *Otolaryngol Head Neck Surg.* 1989;100(1): 6–16.
18. Thirlwall AS, Kundu S. Diuretics for Ménière's disease or syndrome. *Cochrane Database Syst Rev.* 2006;(3):CD003599.
19. James AL, Burton MJ. Betahistine for Ménière's disease or syndrome. *Cochrane Database Syst Rev.* 2001;(1):CD001873.
20. Strupp M, Hupert D, Frenzel C, et al. Long-term prophylactic treatment of attacks of vertigo in Ménière's disease—Comparison of a high with a low dosage of betahistine in an open trial. *Acta Otolaryngol.* 2008;128(5): 520–524.
21. Kim HH, Wiet RJ, Battista RA. Trends in the diagnosis and the management of Ménière's disease: Results of a survey. *Otolaryngol Head Neck Surg.* 2005;132(5):722–726.
22. Saliba I, Gabra N, Alzahrani M, Berbiche D. Endolymphatic duct blockage: A

randomized controlled trial of a novel surgical technique for Ménière's disease treatment. *Otolaryngol Head Neck Surg.* 2015;152(1):122–129.

23. Forge A, Li L. Apoptotic death of hair cells in mammalian vestibular sensory epithelia. *Hear Res.* 2000;139(1–2):97–115.
24. Nedzelski JM, Chiong CM, Fradet G, Schessel DA, Bryce GE, Pfleiderer AG. Intratympanic gentamicin instillation as treatment of unilateral Ménière's disease: Update of an ongoing study. *Am J Otol.* 1993;14(3):278–282.
25. Chia SH, Gamst AC, Anderson JP, Harris JP. Intratympanic gentamicin therapy for Ménière's disease: A meta-analysis. *Otol Neurotol.* 2004;25(4):544–552.
26. Leliever W, Barber H. Recurrent vestibulopathy. *Laryngoscope.* 1981;91(1):1–6.
27. Rutka JA, Barber H. Recurrent vestibulopathy: Third review. *J Otolaryngol.* 1986;15(2):105–107.
28. Dieterich M, Brandt T. Episodic vertigo related to migraine (90 cases): Vestibular migraine? *J Neurol.* 1999;246:883–892.
29. Lee HK, Ahn SK, Jeon SY, et al. Clinical characteristics and natural course of recurrent vestibulopathy. *Laryngoscope.* 2012;122(4):883–886.
30. Headache Classification Committee of the International Headache Society. The International Classification of Headache Disorders. *Cephalgia.* 2004;24:1–160.
31. Talaska AE, Schacht J, Fischel-Ghodsian N. Molecular and genetic aspects of aminoglycoside-induced hearing loss. *Drug Discov Today Dis Mech.* 2006,3(1):119–124.
32. Phillips JA, Bell SC. Aminoglycosides in cystic fibrosis: A descriptive study of current practice in Australia. *Intern Medic J.* 2001;31(1):23–26.
33. Knight KR, Kraemer D, Winter C, Neuwelt EA. Early changes in auditory function as a result of platinum chemotherapy: Use of extended high-frequency audiometry and evoked distortion product otoacoustic emissions. *J Clin Oncol.* 2007;25:1190–1195.
34. Kitsigianis GA, O'Leary DP, Davis LL. Active head-movement analysis of cisplatin-induced vestibulotoxicity. *Otolaryngol Head Neck Surg.* 1988;98(1):82–87.
35. Mercia F. Vertigo due to obstruction of the eustachian tube. *JAMA.* 1942;118:1282–1284.
36. Busis SN. Vertigo in children. *Pediatr Ann.* 1976;5(8):478–481.
37. Von T, Deitz JC, McLaughlin J, DeButts S, Richardson M. The effects of chronic otitis media on motor performance in 5- and 6-year-old children. *Am J Occup Ther.* 1988;42(7):421–426.
38. Casselbrant ML, Furman JM, Mandel EM, Fall PA, Kurs-Lasky M, Rockette HE. Past history of otitis media and balance in four-year-old children. *Laryngoscope.* 2000;110(5 pt 1):773–778.
39. Casselbrant ML, Villardo RJ, Mandel EM. Balance and otitis media with effusion. *Int J Audiol.* 2008;47(9):584–589.
40. Casselbrant ML, Black FO, Nashner LM, Panion R. Vestibular function assessment in children with otitis media. *Ann Otol Rhinol Laryngol.* 1983;107:46–47.
41. Casselbrant ML, Furman JM, Rubenstein E, Mandel EM. Effects of otitis media on the vestibular system in children. *Ann Otol Rhinol Laryngol.* 1995;104:620–624.
42. Casselbrant ML, Redfern MS, Furman J, Fall PA, Mandel EM. Visual-induced postural sway in children with and without otitis media. *Ann Otol Rhinol Laryngol.* 1998;107:401–405.
43. Golz A, Netzer A, Angel-Yeger B, Westerman ST, Gilbert LM, Joachims HZ. Effects of middle ear effusion on the vestibular system in children. *Otolaryngol Head Neck Surg* 1998;119(6):695–699.
44. Hart MC, Nichols DS, Butler EM, Barin K. Childhood imbalance and chronic otitis media with effusion: Effect of tympanostomy tube insertion on standardized tests of balance and locomotion. *Laryngoscope.* 1998;108(5):665–670.
45. Jones NS, Radomskij P, Prichard AJ, Snashall SE. Imbalance and chronic secretory otitis media in children: Effect of myringotomy and insertion of ventilation tubes on body sway. *Ann Otol Rhinol Laryngol.* 1990;99(6 pt 1):477–481.

46. Carlborg BI, Konradsson KS, Carlborg AH, Farmer JC, Jr, Densert O. Pressure transfer between the perilymph and the cerebrospinal fluid compartments in cats. *Am J Otol.* 1992; 13(1):41–48.
47. Suzuki M, Kitano H, Yazawa Y, Kitajima K. Involvement of round and oval windows in the vestibular response to pressure changes in the middle ear of guinea pigs. *Acta Otolaryngol.* 1998;118(5):712–716.
48. Denning J, Mayberry W. Vestibular dysfunction in preschool children with a history of otitis media. *Occup Ther J Res.* 1987;7: 335–348.
49. Schaarf RC. The frequency of vestibular disorders in developmentally delayed preschoolers with otitis media. *Am J Occup Ther.* 1985;4:247–252.
50. Rosenfeld RM, Schwartz SR, Pynnonen MA, et al. Clinical practice guideline: tympanostomy tubes in children—Executive summary. *Otolaryngol Head Neck Surg.* 2013; 149(1):8–16.
51. NCHAM. National Center for Hearing Assessment and Management. http://www.infanthearing.org/summary/prevalence.html. Last updated 2010.
52. Arnvig J. Vestibular function in deafness and severe hardness of hearing. *Acta Otolaryngol Head Neck Surg.* 1955;45(4):283–288.
53. Black FO, Shupert CL, Peterka RJ, Nashner LM. Effects of unilateral loss of vestibular function on the vestibulo-ocular reflex and postural control. *Ann Otol Rhinol Laryngol.* 1989;98(11):884–889.
54. Brookhouser PE, Cyr DG, Beauchaine KA. Vestibular findings in the deaf and hard of hearing. *Otolaryngol Head Neck Surg.* 1982; 90(6):773–777.
55. Everberg G. Unilateral total deafness in children clinical problems with a special view to vestibular function. *Acta Otolaryngol.* 1960; 52:253–269.
56. Gasparini P, Estivill X, Fortina P. Vestibular and hearing loss in genetic and metabolic disorders. *Curr Opin Neurol.* 1999;12(1): 35–39.
57. Goldstein R, Landau E, Kleffner F. Neurological assessment of some deaf and aphasic children. *Ann Otol Rhinol Laryngol.* 1958; 67:468–479.
58. Guilder R, Hopkins L. Auditory function studies in an unselected group of pupils at the Clarke School for the Deaf. *Laryngoscope.* 1936;46:190–197.
59. Holderbaum FM, Ritz S, Hassanein KM, Goetzinger CP. A study of otoneurologic and balance tests with deaf children. *Am Ann Deaf.* 1979;124(6):753–759.
60. Horak FB, Shumway-Cook A, Crowe TK, Black FO. Vestibular function and motor proficiency of children with impaired hearing, or with learning disability and motor impairments. *Dev Med Child Neurol.* 1988; 30(1):64–79.
61. Huygen PL, van Rijn PM, Cremers CW, Theunissen EJ. The vestibulo-ocular reflex in pupils at a Dutch school for the hearing impaired; findings relating to acquired causes. *Int J Pediatr Otorhinolaryngol.* 1993; 25(1–3):39–47.
62. Kaplan SL, Goddard J, Van Kleeck M, Catlin FI, Feigin RD. Ataxia and deafness in children due to bacterial meningitis. *Pediatrics.* 1981;68(1):8–13.
63. Potter CN, Silverman LN. Characteristics of vestibular function and static balance skills in deaf children. *Phys Ther.* 1984;64(7): 1071–1075.
64. Rapin I. Hypoactive labyrinths and motor development. *Clin Pediatr (Phila).* 1974; 13(11):922–923, 926–929, 934–927.
65. Rosenblut B, Goldstein R, Landau WM. Vestibular responses of some deaf and aphasic children. *Ann Otol Rhinol Laryngol.* 1960; 69:747–755.
66. Sandberg L, Terkildsen K. Caloric tests in deaf children. *Arch Otorhinolaryngol.* 1965; 81:350–354.
67. Sokolov M, Gordon K, Polonenko MJ, Blaser S, Papsin B, Cushing S. Vestibular and balance function is often impaired in children with unilateral sensorineural hearing loss. *Hear Res.* 2019;372:52–61.
68. Eshraghi AA, Yang NW, Balkany TJ. Comparative study of cochlear damage with three perimodiolar electrode designs. *Laryngoscope.* 2003;113(3):415–419.

69. Gstoettner W, Plenk H, Jr, Franz P, et al. Cochlear implant deep electrode insertion: Extent of insertional trauma. *Acta Otolaryngol.* 1997;117(2):274–277.
70. Kennedy DW. Multichannel intracochlear electrodes: Mechanism of insertion trauma. *Laryngoscope.* 1987;97(1):42–49.
71. Richter B, Jaekel K, Aschendorff A, Marangos N, Laszig R. Cochlear structures after implantation of a perimodiolar electrode array. *Laryngoscope.* 2001;111(5):837–843.
72. Richter B, Aschendorff A, Lohnstein P, Husstedt H, Nagursky H, Laszig R. The nucleus contour electrode array: A radiological and histological study. *Laryngoscope.* 2001;111(3):508–514.
73. Rossi G, Solero P, Rolando M, Spadola Bisetti M. Vestibular function and cochlear implant. *ORL J Otorhinolaryngol Relat Spec.* 1998;60(2):85–87.
74. Welling DB, Hinojosa R, Gantz BJ, Lee JT. Insertional trauma of multichannel cochlear implants. *Laryngoscope.* 1993;103(9):995–1001.
75. Kamakura T, Nadol JB, Jr. Correlation between word recognition score and intracochlear new bone and fibrous tissue after cochlear implantation in the human. *Hear Res.* 2016;339:132–141.
76. Tien HC, Linthicum FH, Jr. Histopathologic changes in the vestibule after cochlear implantation. *Otolaryngol Head Neck Surg.* 2002;127(4):260–264.
77. Buchman CA, Joy J, Hodges A, Telischi FF, Balkany TJ. Vestibular effects of cochlear implantation. *Laryngoscope.* 2004;114(10 Pt 2 suppl 103):1–22.
78. Cushing SL, Papsin BC, Rutka JA, James AL, Gordon KA. Evidence of vestibular and balance dysfunction in children with profound sensorineural hearing loss using cochlear implants. *Laryngoscope.* 2008; 118(10):1814–1823.
79. Licameli G, Zhou G, Kenna MA. Disturbance of vestibular function attributable to cochlear implantation in children. *Laryngoscope.* 2009;119(4):740–745.
80. Selz PA, Girardi M, Konrad HR, Hughes LF. Vestibular deficits in deaf children. *Otolaryngol Head Neck Surg.* 1996;115(1):70–77.
81. Kletke S, Batmanabane V, Dai T, et al. The combination of vestibular impairment and congenital sensorineural hearing loss predisposes patients to ocular anomalies, including Usher syndrome. *Clin Genet.* 2017;92: 26–33.
82. Karjalainen S, Terasvirta M, Karja J, Kaariainen H. Usher's syndrome type III: ENG findings in four affected and six unaffected siblings. *J Laryngol Otol.* 1985;99(1): 43–48.
83. Kumar A, Fishman G, Torok N. Vestibular and auditory function in Usher's syndrome. *Ann Otol Rhinol Laryngol.* 1984;93(6 pt 1): 600–608.
84. Otterstedde CR, Spandau U, Blankenagel A, Kimberling WJ, Reisser C. A new clinical classification for Usher's syndrome based on a new subtype of Usher's syndrome type I. *Laryngoscope.* 2001;111(1):84–86.
85. Samuelson S, Zahn J. Usher's syndrome. *Ophthalmic Paediatr Genet.* 1990;11(1):71–76.
86. Propst EJ, Papsin BC, Stockley TL, Harrison RV, Gordon KA. Auditory responses in cochlear implant users with and without GJB2 deafness. *Laryngoscope.* 2006;116(2): 317–327.
87. Todt I, Hennies HC, Basta D, Ernst A. Vestibular dysfunction of patients with mutations of Connexin 26. *Neuroreport.* 2005; 16(11):1179–1181.
88. Cushing SL, Gordon KA, Rutka JA, James AL, Papsin BC. Vestibular end-organ dysfunction in children with sensorineural hearing loss and cochlear implants: An expanded cohort and etiologic assessment. *Otol Neurotol.* 2013;34:422–428.
89. Diepeveen JE, Jensen J. Differential caloric reactions in deaf children. *Acta Otolaryngol.* 1968;65(6):570–574.
90. Luxon L, Pagarkar W. The dizzy child. In: Graham J, Scadding G, Bull P, eds. *Pediatric ENT.* Berlin (Heidelberg, Germany): Springer; 2008:459–478.
91. Dollard SC, Grosse SD, Ross DS. New estimates of the prevalence of neurological and sensory sequelae and mortality associated with congenital cytomegalovirus infection. *Rev Med Virol.* 2007;17(5):355–363.

92. Bulman DE, Yeh E, Durie D, et al. MG-129 The development of a genetic newborn screening assay for permanent hearing loss using blood spots—A collaboration between Newborn Screening Ontario (NSO) and the Infant Hearing Program (IHP). *J Med Genet.* 2015;52(Suppl 1):A8–A8.
93. Teissier N, Delezoide AL, Mas AE, et al. Inner ear lesions in congenital cytomegalovirus infection of human fetuses. *Acta Neuropathol.* 2011;122:763–744.
94. Carraro M, Park AH, Harrison RV. Partial corrosion casting to assess cochlear vasculature in mouse models of presbycusis and CMV infection. *Hear Res.* 2016;332:95–103.
95. Carraro M, Almishaal A, Hillas E, Firpo M, Park A, Harrison RV. Cytomegalovirus (CMV) infection causes degeneration of cochlear vasculature and hearing loss in a mouse model. *J Assoc Res Otolaryngol.* 2017;18(2):263–273.
96. Zagolski O. Vestibular-evoked myogenic potentials and caloric stimulation in infants with congenital cytomegalovirus infection. *J Laryngol Otol.* 2008;122:574–579.
97. Teissier N, Bernard S, Quesnel S, Van Den Abbeele T. Audiovestibular consequences of congenital cytomegalovirus infection. *Eur Ann Otorhinolaryngol Head Neck Dis.* 2016;133(6):413–418.
98. Nassar MN, Elmaleh M, Cohen A, Van Den Abbeele T, Wiener-Vacher SR, Teissier N. Vestibular calcification in a case of congenital cytomegalovirus infection. *Otol Neurotol.* 2015;36(6):e107–109.
99. Bernard S, Wiener-Vacher S, Van Den Abbeele T, Teissier N. Vestibular disorders in children with congenital cytomegalovirus infection. *Pediatrics.* 2015;136(4):e887–895.
100. Karltorp E, Lofkvist U, Lewensohn-Fuchs I, et al. Impaired balance and neurodevelopmental disabilities among children with congenital cytomegalovirus infection. *Acta Paediatr.* 2014;103:1165–1173.
101. Wolter NE, Cushing SL, Vilchez-Madrigal LD, et al. Unilateral hearing loss is associated with impaired balance in children: A pilot study. *Otol Neurotol.* 2016;37(10):1589–1595.
102. Migliori G, Battisti E, Pari M, Vitelli N, Cingolani C. A shifty diagnosis: Cogan's syndrome. A case report and review of the literature. *Acta Otorhinolaryngol Ital.* 2009;29(2):108–113.
103. Crowe TK, Horak FB. Motor proficiency associated with vestibular deficits in children with hearing impairments. *Phys Ther.* 1988;68(10):1493–1499.
104. Cushing SL, Chia R, James AL, Papsin BC, Gordon KA. A test of static and dynamic balance function in children with cochlear implants: The Vestibular Olympics. *Arch Otolaryngol Head Neck Surg.* 2008;134(1):34–38.
105. Cushing SL, Papsin BC, Rutka JA, James AL, Blaser SL, Gordon KA. Vestibular end-organ and balance deficits after meningitis and cochlear implantation in children correlate poorly with functional outcome. *Otol Neurotol.* 2009;30(4):488–495.
106. Cushing SL CR, James AL, Papsin BC, Gordon KA. The Vestibular Olympics: A test of dynamic balance function in children with cochlear implants. *Arch Otorhinolaryngol.* 2007;134.(1):34–38.
107. Davey PR. Observations on equilibrium in deaf children. *J Laryngol Otol.* 1954;68(5):329–331.
108. Enbom H, Magnusson M, Pyykko I. Postural compensation in children with congenital or early acquired bilateral vestibular loss. *Ann Otol Rhinol Laryngol.* 1991;100(6):472–478.
109. Enticott JC, Tari S, Koh SM, Dowell RC, O'Leary SJ. Cochlear implant and vestibular function. *Otol Neurotol.* 2006;27(6):824–830.
110. Magnusson M, Enbom H, Pyykko I. Postural compensation of congenital or early acquired vestibular loss in hearing disabled children. *Acta Otolaryngol Suppl.* 1991;481:433–435.
111. Rossi G, Bisetti MS. Cochlear implant and traumatic lesions secondary to electrode insertion. *Rev Laryngol Otol Rhinol (Bord).* 1998;119(5):317–322.

112. Molony NC, Marais J. Balance after stapedectomy: The measurement of spontaneous sway by posturography. *Clin Otolaryngol Allied Sci.* 1996;21(4):353–356.
113. Spector M. Electronstagmography after stapedectomy. *Ann Otol Rhinol Laryngol.* 1973; 82(3):374–377.
114. Black FO. Present vestibular status of subjects implanted with auditory prostheses. *Ann Otol Rhinol Laryngol Suppl.* 1977;86(3 pt 3 suppl 38):49–56.
115. Black FO. Effects of the auditory prosthesis on postural stability. *Ann Otol Rhinol Laryngol Suppl.* 1977;86(3 pt 2 suppl 38): 141–164.
116. Black FO, Lilly DJ, Peterka RJ, Fowler LP, Simmons FB. Vestibulo-ocular and vestibulospinal function before and after cochlear implant surgery. *Ann Otol Rhinol Laryngol Suppl.* 1987;96(1 pt 2 suppl 128):106–108.
117. Cohen NL, Hoffman RA, Stroschein M. Medical or surgical complications related to the Nucleus multichannel cochlear implant. *Ann Otol Rhinol Laryngol Suppl.* 1988;135: 8–13.
118. Huygen PL, van den Broek P, Spies TH, Mens LH, Admiraal RJ. Does intracochlear implantation jeopardize vestibular function? *Ann Otol Rhinol Laryngol.* 1994;103(8 pt 1): 609–614.
119. Ito J. Influence of the multichannel cochlear implant on vestibular function. *Otolaryngol Head Neck Surg.* 1998;118(6):900–902.
120. Kempf HG, Johann K, Lenarz T. Complications in pediatric cochlear implant surgery. *Eur Arch Otorhinolaryngol.* 1999;256(3): 128–132.
121. Kubo T, Yamamoto K, Iwaki T, Doi K, Tamura M. Different forms of dizziness occurring after cochlear implant. *Eur Arch Otorhinolaryngol.* 2001;258(1):9–12.
122. Ribari O, Kustel M, Szirmai A, Repassy G. Cochlear implantation influences contralateral hearing and vestibular responsiveness. *Acta Otolaryngol.* 1999;119(2):225–228.
123. Webb RL, Lehnhardt E, Clark GM, Laszig R, Pyman BC, Franz BK. Surgical complications with the cochlear multiple-channel intracochlear implant: Experience at Hannover and Melbourne. *Ann Otol Rhinol Laryngol.* 1991;100(2):131–136.
124. Black FO, Peterka RJ, Elardo SM. Vestibular reflex changes following aminoglycoside induced ototoxicity. *Laryngoscope.* 1987; 97(5):582–586.
125. Brey RH, Facer GW, Trine MB, Lynn SG, Peterson AM, Suman VJ. Vestibular effects associated with implantation of a multiple channel cochlear prosthesis. *Am J Otol.* 1995;16(4):424–430.
126. Chiong CM, Nedzelski JM, McIlmoyl LD, Shipp DB. Electro-oculographic findings pre- and post-cochlear implantation. *J Otolaryngol.* 1994;23(6):447–449.
127. Chouard CH, Fugain C, Meyer B, Gegu D. Prognostic evaluation of the multichannel cochlear implant. *Acta Otolaryngol Suppl.* 1984;411:161–164.
128. Eisenberg LS, Nelson JR, House WF. Effects of the single-electrode cochlear implant on the vestibular system of the profoundly deaf adult. *Ann Otol Rhinol Laryngol Suppl.* 1982; 91(2 pt 3):47–54.
129. Higgins KM, Chen JM, Nedzelski JM, Shipp DB, McIlmoyl LD. A matched-pair comparison of two cochlear implant systems. *J Otolaryngol.* 2002;31(2):97–105.
130. Huygen PL, Hinderink JB, van den Broek P, et al. The risk of vestibular function loss after intracochlear implantation. *Acta Otolaryngol Suppl.* 1995;520(pt 2):270–272.
131. Kiyomizu K, Tono T, Komune S, Ushisako Y, Morimitsu T. Dizziness and vertigo after cochlear implantation. *Adv Otorhinolaryngol.* 2000;57:173–175.
132. van den Broek P, Huygen PL, Mens LH, Admiraal RJ, Spies T. Vestibular function in cochlear implant patients. *Acta Otolaryngol.* 1993;113(3):263–265.
133. Vibert D, Hausler R, Kompis M, Vischer M. Vestibular function in patients with cochlear implantation. *Acta Otolaryngol Suppl.* 2001; 545:29–34.
134. Migliaccio AA, Della Santina CC, Carey JP, Niparko JK, Minor LB. The vestibulo-ocular reflex response to head impulses rarely

decreases after cochlear implantation. *Otol Neurotol.* 2005;26(4):655–660.

135. Wiener-Vacher SR, Obeid R, Abou-Elew M. Vestibular impairment after bacterial meningitis delays infant posturomotor development. *J Pediatr.* 2012;161(2):246–251, e241.
136. Wiener Vacher S, Petrof N, Francois M, Viala P, Tessier N, Van den Abbeele T. *Impact of cochear implant of vestibular function in children and decision between two steps or one step bilateral implant.* Paper presented at 12th European Symposium on Pediatric Cochlear Implants; 18–21 June 2015; Toulouse, France.
137. Thierry B, Blanchard M, Leboulanger N, et al. Cochlear implantation and vestibular function in children. *Int J Pediatr Otorhinolaryngol.* 2015;79(2):101–104.
138. Jacot E, Van Den Abbeele T, Debre HR, Wiener-Vacher SR. Vestibular impairments pre- and post-cochlear implant in children. *Int J Pediatr Otorhinolaryngol.* 2009;73(2): 209–217.
139. Wolter NE, Gordon KA, Papsin BC, Cushing SL. Vestibular and balance impairment contributes to cochlear implant failure in children. *Otol Neurotol.* 2015;36(6):1029–1034.
140. Minor LB, Solomon D, Zinreich JS, Zee DS. Sound- and/or pressure-induced vertigo due to bone dehiscence of the superior semicircular canal. *Arch Otolaryngol Head Neck Surg.* 1998;124(3):249–258.
141. Lee GS, Zhou G, Poe D, et al. Clinical experience in diagnosis and management of superior semicircular canal dehiscence in children. *Laryngoscope*, 2011;121(10):2256–2261.
142. Chen EY, Paladin A, Phillips G, et al. Semicircular canal dehiscence in the pediatric population. *Int J Pediatr Otorhinolaryngol.* 2009;73(2):321–327.
143. Nadgir RN, Ozonoff A, Devaiah AK, Halderman AA, Sakai O. Superior semicircular canal dehiscence: Congenital or acquired condition? *Ajnr.*, 2011;32(5):947–949.
144. Saxby AJ, Gowdy C, Fandino M, et al. Radiological prevalence of superior and posterior semicircular canal dehiscence in children. *Int J Pediatr Otorhinolaryngol.* 2015; 79(3):411–418.
145. Hato N, Kisaki H, Honda N, Gyo K, Murakami S, Yanagihara N. Ramsay Hunt syndrome in children. *Ann Neurol.* 2000; 48(2):254–256.
146. de Ru JA, van Benthem PP. Combination therapy is preferable for patients with Ramsay Hunt syndrome. *Otol Neurotol.* 2011; 32(5):852–855.
147. Erbek SH, Erbek SS, Yilmaz I, et al. Vertigo in childhood: A clinical experience. *Int J Pediatr Otorhinolaryngol.* 2006;70(9):1547–1554.
148. Taborelli G, Melagrana A, D'Agostino R, Tarantino V, Calveo MG, Calevo. Vestibular neuronitis in children: Study of medium and long term follow-up. *Int J Pediatr Otorhinolaryngol.* 2000;54(2-3):117–121.
149. Niemensivu R, Pyykko I, Valanne L, Kentala E. Value of imaging studies in vertiginous children. *Int J Pediatr Otorhinolaryngol.* 2006;70(9):1639–1644.
150. Fishman JM, Burgess C, Waddell A. Corticosteroids for the treatment of idiopathic acute vestibular dysfunction (vestibular neuritis). *Cochrane Database Syst Rev.* 2011;(5): CD008607.
151. Karlberg ML, Magnusson M. Treatment of acute vestibular neuronitis with glucocorticoids. *Otol Neurotol.*, 2011;32(7):1140–1143.
152. Strupp M, Zingler VC, Arbusow V, et al. Methylprednisolone, valacyclovir, or the combination for vestibular neuritis. *N Engl J Med.* 2004;351(4):354–361.
153. O'Reilly RC, Greywoode J, Morlet T, et al. Comprehensive vestibular and balance testing in the dizzy pediatric population. *Otolaryngol Head Neck Surg.* 2011;144(2):142–148.
154. Bower CM, Cotton RT. The spectrum of vertigo in children. *Arch Otolaryngol Head Neck Surg.* 1995;121(8):911–915.
155. Weisleder P, Fife TD. Dizziness and headache: A common association in children and adolescents. *J Child Neurol.* 2001;16(10): 727–730.
156. D'Agostino R, Tarantino V, Melagrana A, Taborelli G. Otoneurologic evaluation of

child vertigo. *Int J Pediatr Otorhinolaryngol.* 1997;40(2–3):133–139.

157. Manzari L, Tedesco A, Burgess AM, Curthoys IS. Ocular vestibular-evoked myogenic potentials to bone-conducted vibration in superior vestibular neuritis show utricular function. *Otolaryngol Head Neck Surg.* 2010; 143(2):274–280.

CHAPTER 15

Benign Paroxysmal Positional Vertigo (BPPV)

Sophie E. Lipson and Jacob R. Brodsky

Benign paroxysmal positional vertigo (BPPV) is a peripheral vestibular disorder that causes episodes, lasting seconds to minutes, of transient vertigo provoked by position changes. BPPV is the most common peripheral cause of vertigo in adults, and it has a lifetime prevalence of 2.4%.[1] Historically, most chapters and articles on pediatric vertigo have indicated that BPPV is rare in the pediatric population, but recently it has been found to be much more common than previously described and may actually even be one of the most common causes of pediatric vertigo.[2]

Physiology

BPPV occurs when otoconial debris from the macula of the utricle becomes displaced and enters a semicircular canal, which leads to one of two outcomes: canalithiasis or cupulolithiasis. In canalithiasis, otoliths remain suspended in the endolymph in the semicircular canal.[3] In cupulolithiasis, otoliths attach directly to the cupula of the semicircular canal.[4] Both of these underlying pathologies result in abnormal displacement of endolymph when the head orients into a gravity-dependent position in the plane of the affected canal. This stimulation results in vertigo and nystagmus in the plane of the affected canal.

Etiology

The exact etiology of BPPV remains unknown; however, BPPV can present either on its own (idiopathic or primary BPPV) or in conjunction with another disorder or injury (secondary BPPV). Idiopathic BPPV is the most common etiology in adults, which has been theorized to result from age-related degeneration of the utricle, resulting in displacement of otolithic debris.[5] Idiopathic BPPV is rare in children and adolescents, where secondary causes of BPPV are more common.[2] BPPV can occur following a head trauma in which the impact leads to otolith displacement.[6] A study on adult military patients found that nearly a third of patients with dizziness following a concussion had BPPV.[7] Similarly, a study on pediatric patients found BPPV in 21% of patients referred for prolonged dizziness symptoms following a concussion.[8] Moreover, 8.5% to 27% of adult patients with BPPV had sustained a head trauma, so it is evident that such an event can precipitate BPPV.[9] Additionally, BPPV has been found to frequently occur in the setting of other inner ear disorders, including vestibular neuritis, labyrinthitis, and enlarged vestibular aqueduct syndrome.[9–12] BPPV can also present secondary to sensorineural hearing loss or vestibular migraine.[2] The reason for secondary BPPV occurring in the setting of other vestibular disorders such as those listed is not yet known. Possible mechanisms include ischemic or inflammatory changes at the level of the utricle resulting in otoconial displacement or inflammation and associated narrowing of the affected semicircular canals. More study is needed to better establish the mechanisms of secondary BPPV in pediatric patients to allow for more optimal management strategies for treatment-resistant and recurrent cases.

Risk Factors

Vitamin D deficiency and impaired calcium metabolism have been linked to BPPV, which is increasingly relevant as the rate of vitamin D deficiency is rising in the pediatric population.[13] People with vitamin D deficiency are at a greater risk for BPPV and may be more likely to develop treatment-resistant and/or recurrent BPPV.[14,15] One proposed mechanism is that low levels of vitamin D and high bone turnover may affect calcium levels systemically and impact the composition and stability of the otoliths, which are composed of calcium carbonate.[16] This may explain seasonal variations that have been observed in the incidence of BPPV in adults[17], and it may also cause geographic variations that may partially explain the wide variations in reported incidence of BPPV in pediatric patients.

Another risk factor for BPPV is migraine, as adults with migraine are two times more likely to develop BPPV.[1,18,19] Additionally, vestibular migraine and benign paroxysmal vertigo of childhood (see Chapter 16) have been associated with recurrent BPPV.[2] The pathophysiology underlying this connection remains unknown. Migraine has been shown to cause direct effects on the inner ear, possibly through inflammatory mediators triggered by connections of the trigeminovascular system with the vestibular labyrinth, which may have impacts on the utricle and/or semicircular canals as previously described.[20]

Localization

BPPV can affect any semicircular canal and can even affect multiple canals on both sides simultaneously. The reported incidence of multiple canal BPPV in the adult population ranges from 6.8% to 20% of cases; however, multiple canal BPPV is more common in children, accounting for 36% of cases.[2,21] Likewise, approximately 20% of pediatric cases demonstrate bilateral involvement, whereas the percentage of cases that are bilateral in adults is much lower.[22] Approximately 73% of pediatric cases involve the posterior canal, 34% involve the lateral canal, and 19% involve the anterior canal.[2] While this is similar to adults in that the posterior canal is most commonly affected, a larger proportion of pediatric cases involve the lateral and anterior canals than in adults.[22–24] The right and left ears are affected relatively equally in children.[2]

Diagnostic Maneuvers

The presence of BPPV in a given canal is determined by a diagnostic maneuver that rotates the head through the plane of that canal. A positive diagnostic maneuver is characterized by the presence of subjective vertigo and visible nystagmus around the axis of the affected canal(s). The nystagmus is characterized by a latency of up to 20 seconds and fatigability after 30 to 60 seconds as the otoliths eventually stop moving and stimulating the canal. The absence of latency and fatigability should raise concern for alternative diagnoses, such as physiologic positional nystagmus or compressive lesions of the posterior fossa, such as a Chiari malformation or arachnoid cyst.[25] However, it should be noted that fatigability and latency may often be absent with BPPV of the lateral and the anterior canals, possibly due to a higher incidence of cupulolithiasis in these particular canals relative to the posterior canal.[26–30] Additionally, the directionality and plane of the nystagmus should be specific to the canal being tested, and alternative patterns of nystagmus should raise concern for alternative causes. Performing the maneuvers with the patient wearing Frenzel or videonystagmography (VNG) goggles aids in the identification of the nystagmus. Nystagmus may be geotropic (toward the down-facing ear) or apogeotropic (toward the up-facing ear), depending on the canal affected and the position of the otolithic debris within the affected canal. The presence of torsional nystagmus is essential to the diagnosis of posterior canal BPPV but may not be present when the lateral or anterior canals are involved. Nonetheless, ENG (electronystagmography) is much lower yield than VNG in evaluating for BPPV, since ENG detects only horizontal and vertical components of nystagmus and not torsion.

Dix-Hallpike Maneuver—Posterior and Anterior Canals

Steps (Figure 15–1)

1. Patient sits upright with the head tilted slightly back and turned 45° toward the examiner.
2. Patient is quickly lowered to a supine position with the head 30° below the horizontal plane.

Nystagmus Pattern

- Posterior canal—Torsional, upbeating, geotropic nystagmus
- Anterior canal—Torsional, downbeating nystagmus (may be geotropic or apogeotropic)

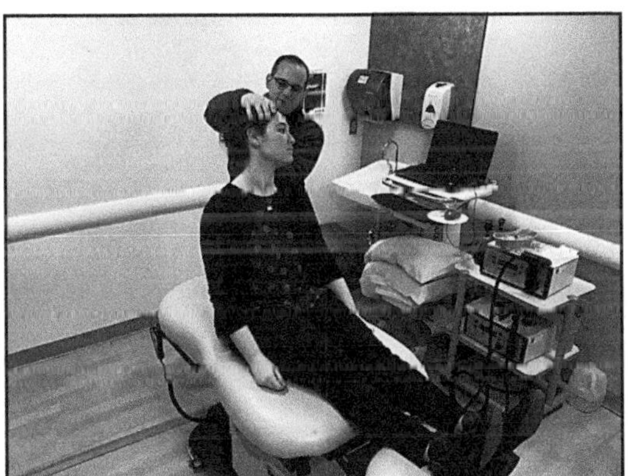

Step 1

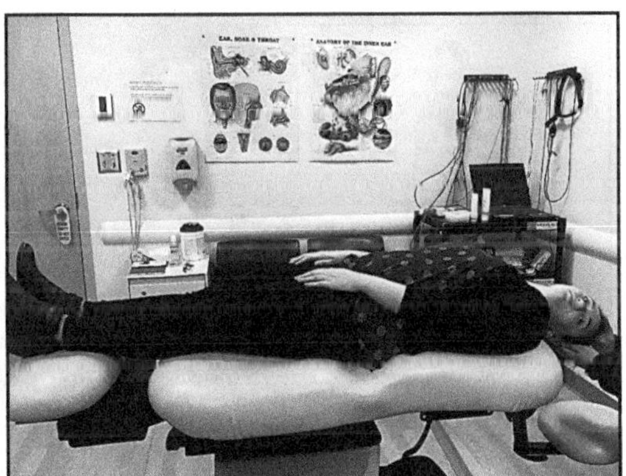

Step 2

Figure 15–1. Left Dix-Hallpike maneuver.

Supine Head Roll Maneuver[31]—Lateral Canals

Steps (Figure 15–2)

1. Patient lies supine and the neck is flexed 30° above the horizontal plane.
2. The head is rotated 90° to the right.
3. The head is returned to the center and then rotated 90° to the left.

Nystagmus Pattern[26,28]

- Horizontal geotropic nystagmus—indicative of canalithiasis in the down-facing ear
- Horizontal apogeotropic nystagmus—indicative of cupulolithiasis in the up-facing ear

Midline Head Hang Maneuver[32]—Anterior Canals

Steps (Figure 15–3)

1. Patient starts in sitting position.
2. The body is moved backward into a supine position, while the head is extended backward as close to 90° below the horizontal plane as possible.

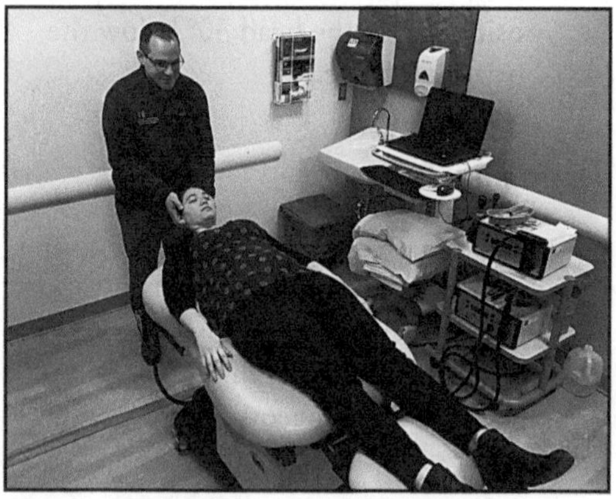

Step 1

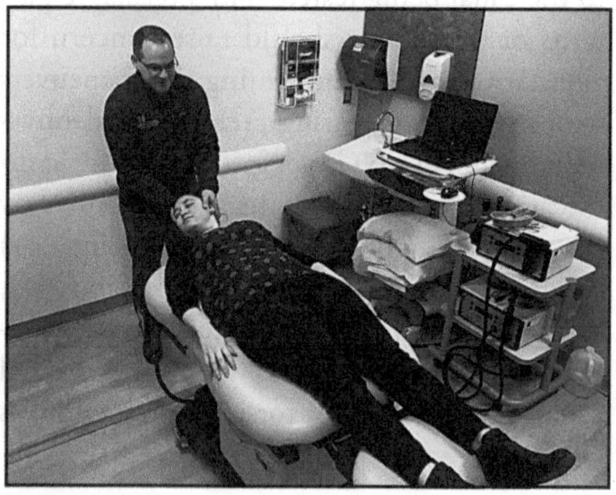

Step 2

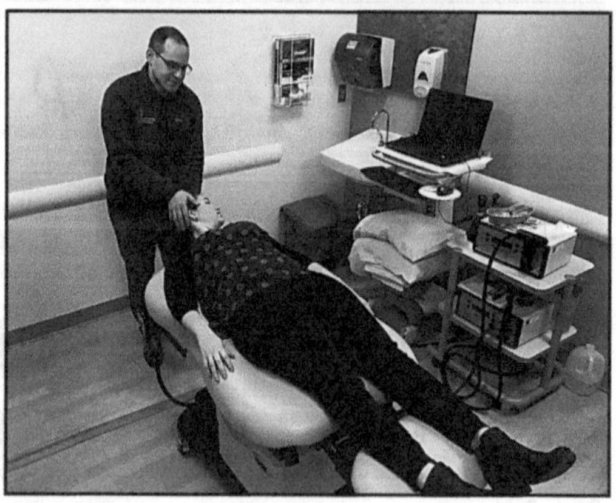

Step 3

Figure 15–2. Supine head roll maneuver (left then right).

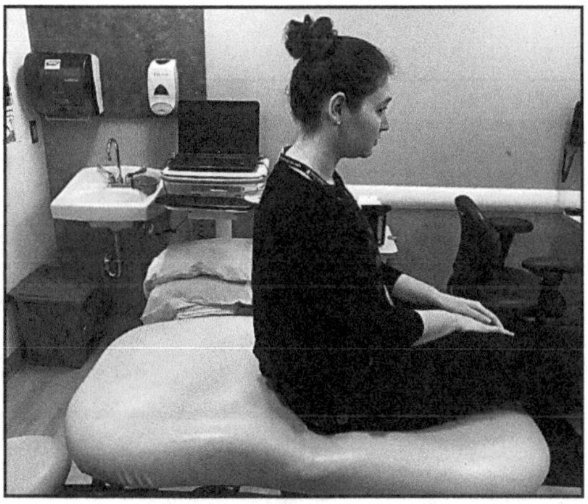

Step 1

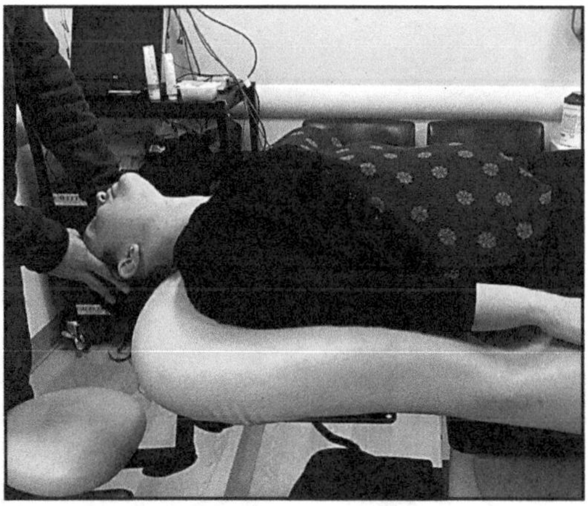

Step 2

Figure 15–3. Midline head hang maneuver.

Nystagmus Pattern

- Downbeating nystagmus, sometimes with a torsional component (this maneuver will not determine the affected side, unless a torsional component is present)

Treatment

BPPV is primarily treated by performing canalith repositioning maneuvers, which utilize gravity to move the otoliths out of the affected canal. There have been numerous maneuvers described for treatment of each canal. Description of all treatment maneuvers is beyond the scope of this chapter, but the most commonly performed maneuvers for each canal are described here.

Additionally, maneuvers are modifiable so patients can perform them at home. Some patients' BPPV may fully resolve following one treatment maneuver, while others require additional maneuvers.

Epley Maneuver[33]—Posterior Canal

Steps (Figure 15–4)

1. A Dix-Hallpike maneuver is performed on the affected side (see previous discussion).
2. The head is turned 90° to face the contralateral side, while still hanging below the horizontal plane.
3. The body is further rotated toward the contralateral side until the patient is lying on the side and the head is further rotated until the patient is facing the floor.
4. The patient is briskly returned to the sitting position.

Each of the previous numbered positions should be maintained until the subjective vertigo resolves and the nystagmus subsides in that position. If vertigo and nystagmus pass quickly or do not occur in a given position, then that position should be maintained for 30 seconds. Another effective maneuver for the posterior canal is the Semont maneuver.[34]

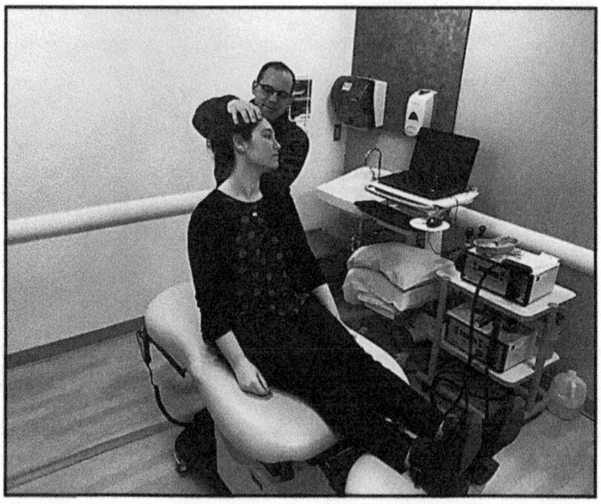

Step 1a

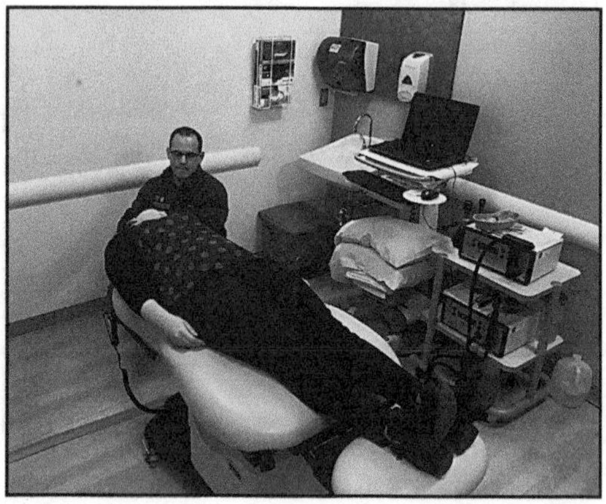

Step 1b

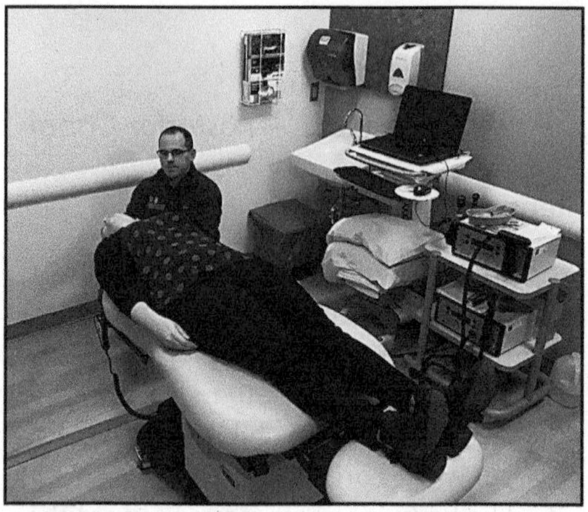

Step 2

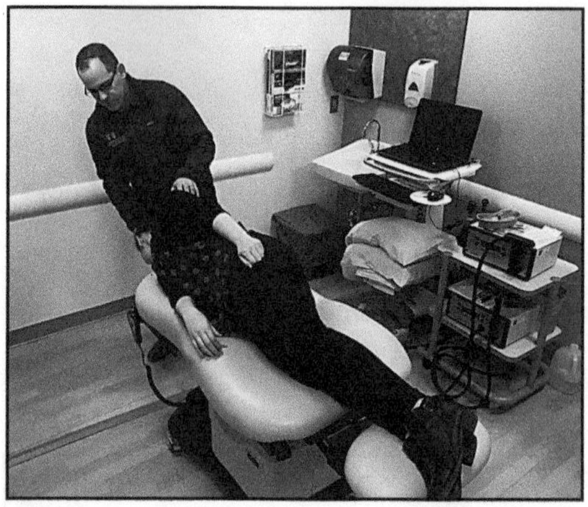

Step 3

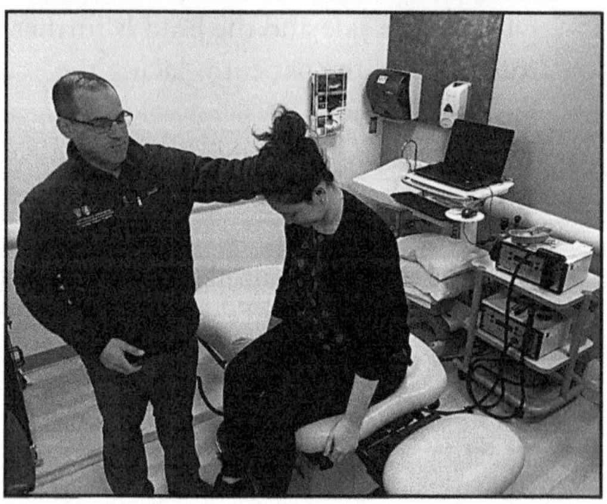

Step 4

Figure 15–4. Left Epley maneuver.

Log Roll (Barbecue/Barrel Roll/ Lempert) Maneuver[35]—Lateral Canal

Steps (Figure 15–5)

1. The patient lies down in the supine position and the head is turned toward the affected ear.
2. The head is turned 90° toward the contralateral side so that the patient is looking up toward the ceiling.
3. The head is turned another 90° toward the contralateral side so that the affected ear is facing the ceiling.
4. The patient's body is turned 180° toward the contralateral side into a prone or kneeling position, and the head is rotated another 90° toward the contralateral side so that the patient is facing the floor.
5. The patient sits upright, and the chin is tilted to the chest.

Each of these numbered positions should be maintained for 30 seconds. This maneuver is primarily intended to treat geotropic lateral canal BPPV. Another maneuver that is effective for lateral canal BPPV is the Gufoni

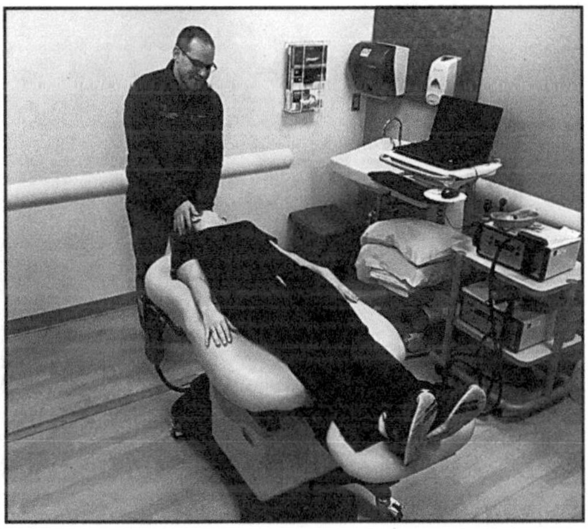

Step 1

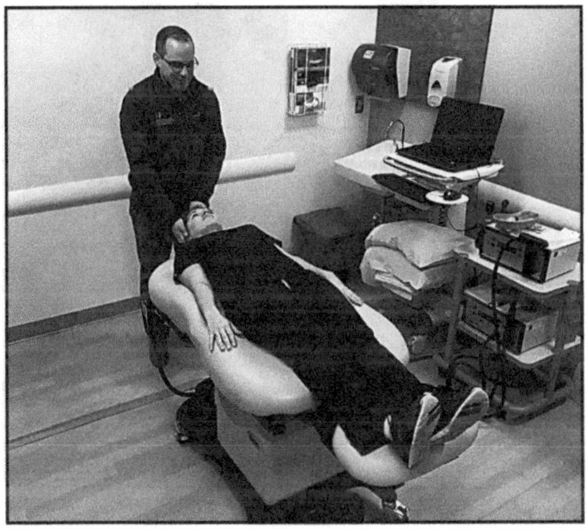

Step 2

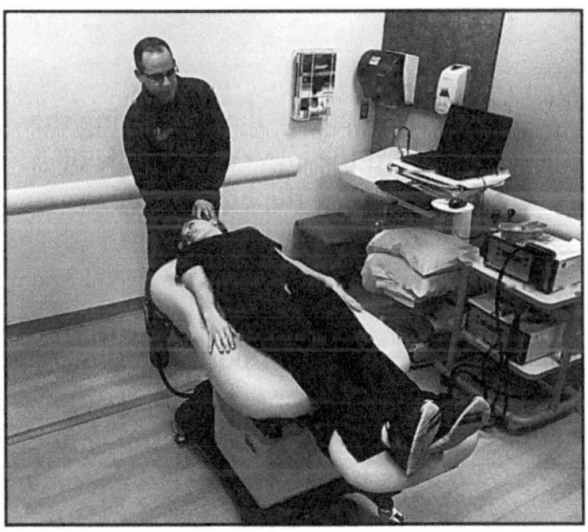

Step 3

Figure 15–5. Left log roll maneuver. *continues*

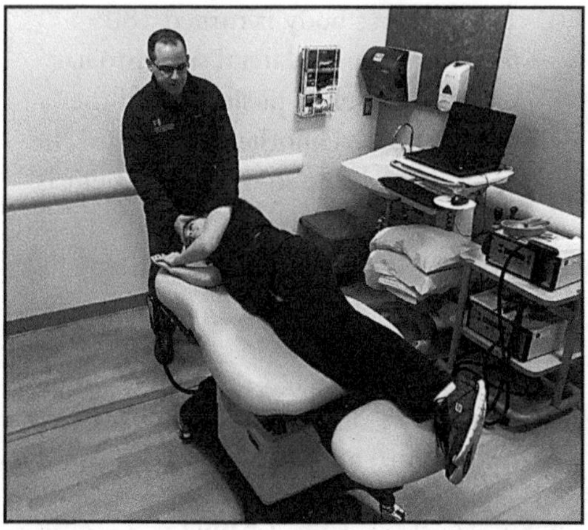

Step 4a

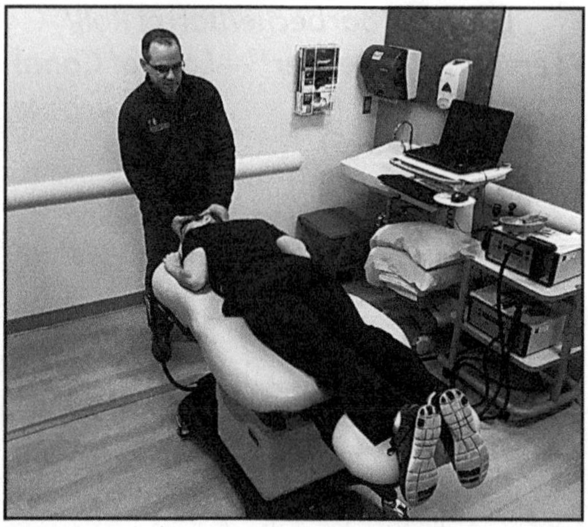

Step 4b

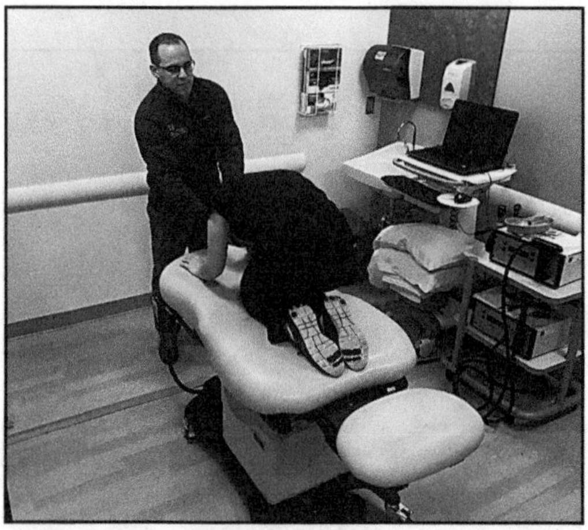

Step 5a

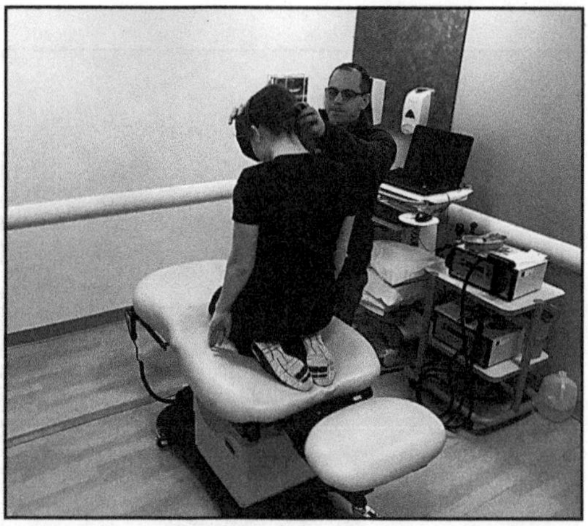

Step 5b

Figure 15–5. *continued*

maneuver, which can be used to treat geotropic or apogeotropic lateral canal BPPV.[36]

Yacavino Maneuver[37]*— Anterior Canal*

Steps (Figure 15–6)

1. A midline head hang maneuver is first performed (see previous discussion).
2. The neck is rapidly flexed to bring the chin toward the chest to an angle of about 30° above the horizontal.
3. The patient rapidly sits upright with the chin to the chest.

Each of these numbered positions should be maintained for 30 seconds. There are numerous other maneuvers intended to treat anterior canal BPPV, including the Rahko, Kim, and reverse Epley maneuvers.[37–39]

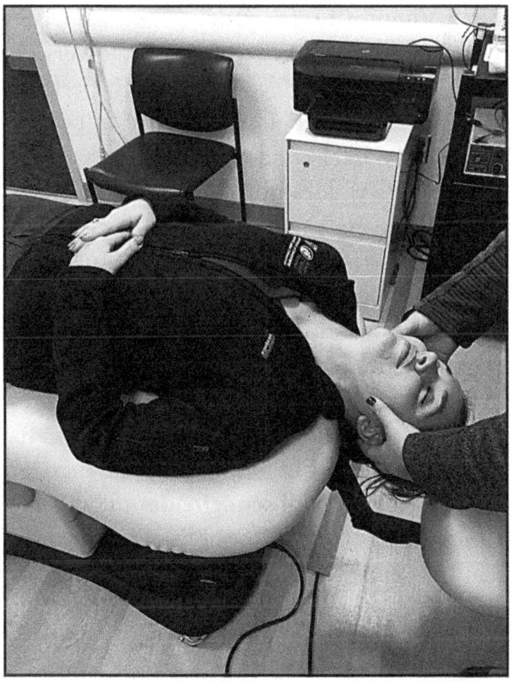

Step 1

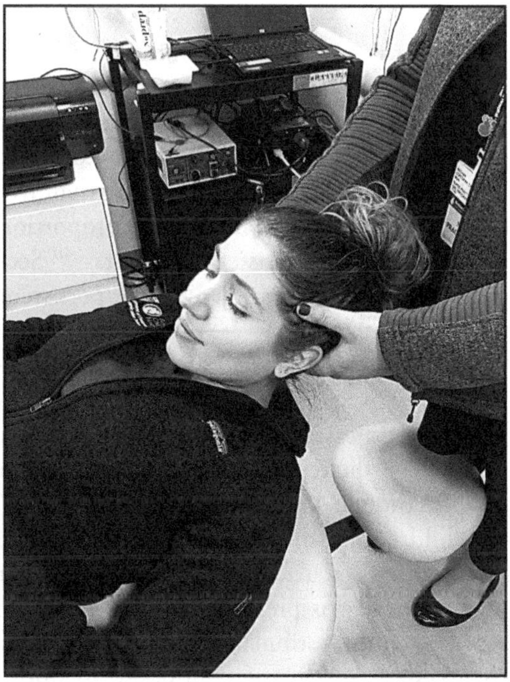

Step 2

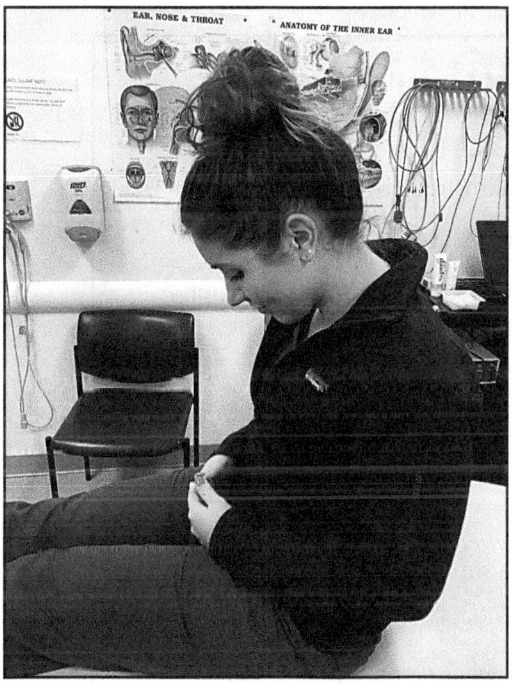

Step 3

Figure 15–6. Yacavino maneuver.

Persistence and Recurrence

While most cases are successfully treated with one or two canalith repositioning maneuvers, some cases of BPPV are treatment resistant and require several maneuvers. Approximately 12% of pediatric cases require more than five maneuvers, which is similar to the proportion of cases that are persistent in adults.[2,40] Secondary BPPV is more likely to be persistent than idiopathic BPPV.[6,40]

BPPV may also recur after successful resolution with maneuvers. Approximately 18% of pediatric cases recur, which is somewhat lower than the reported rate of recurrence in adults, though longitudinal data for BPPV in children are much more limited, so the incidence of recurrence may be higher than described.[41,42] As previously stated, pediatric patients with vestibular migraine or benign paroxysmal vertigo of childhood are more likely to have a recurrence than those without.[2] Vitamin D deficiency is also associated with recurrence, and treating it lowers the risk of recurrence.[43,44] Additionally, performing treatment maneuvers as early as possible reduces the likelihood of recurrence.[45]

If BPPV does not resolve following several maneuvers, then use of the Epley Omniax System (Vesticon, Inc.) may be helpful, where available.[46] In cases that persist despite multiple repositioning maneuvers or frequently recur in the same canal, then surgical intervention may be warranted. Semicircular canal occlusion, developed by Lorne Parnes, has proven successful in adults.[47] While there are no reported cases of semicircular canal occlusion for pediatric BPPV published in the medical literature at the time of this writing, the senior author has had success with this procedure for resolving the symptoms of treatment-resistant BPPV in the pediatric population.

Self-Assessment Questions

1. True/False:
   Cupulolithiasis occurs when otoliths remain suspended within the endolymph of a semicircular canal.

2. The Dix-Hallpike maneuver can identify (circle all that apply):
   a. Posterior canal BPPV
   b. Lateral canal BPPV
   c. Anterior canal BPPV

3. What two features characterize a positive diagnostic maneuver?

4. True/False:
   Geotropic nystagmus during the supine head roll maneuver is indicative of canalithiasis.

5. If the posterior canal is affected, what pattern of nystagmus is expected when a Dix-Hallpike maneuver is performed?
   a. Horizontal, apogeotropic
   b. Torsional, upbeating, geotropic

c. Pure downbeating
d. Torsional, downbeating, geotropic

6. What pattern of nystagmus is expected when a midline head hang maneuver is performed if an anterior canal is affected by BPPV?
   a. Torsional, upbeating, geotropic
   b. Horizontal, geotropic
   c. Horizontal, apogeotropic
   d. Pure downbeating

7. List at least two risk factors for BPPV in the pediatric population.

8. Which of the following correctly matches the affected canal with the appropriate treatment maneuver? (circle all that apply)
   a. Posterior canal—Epley maneuver
   b. Anterior canal—log roll maneuver
   c. Posterior canal—Yacavino maneuver
   d. Lateral canal—log roll maneuver

References

1. von Brevern M, Radtke A, Lezius F, et al. Epidemiology of benign paroxysmal positional vertigo: A population based study. *J Neurol Neurosurg Psychiatry*. 2007;78(7):710–715.
2. Brodsky JR, Lipson S, Wilber J, Zhou G. Benign paroxysmal positional vertigo (BPPV) in children and adolescents: Clinical features and response to therapy in 110 pediatric patients. *Otol Neurotol.* 2018;39(3):344–350.
3. Parnes LS, McClure JA. Free floating endolymph particles: A new operative finding during posterior semicircular canal occlusion. *Laryngoscope.* 1992;102(9):988–992.
4. Schuknecht HF. Cupulolithiasis. *Arch Otolaryngol.* 1969;90(6):765–778.
5. Baloh RW, Honrubia V, Jacobson K. Benign positional vertigo: Clinical and oculographic features in 240 cases. *Neurology.* 1987;37(3): 371–378.
6. Balatsouras DG, Koukoutsis G, Aspris A, et al. Benign paroxysmal positional vertigo secondary to mild head trauma. *Ann Otol Rhinol Laryngol.* 2017;126(1):54–60.
7. Hoffer ME, Gottshall KR, Moore R, Balough BJ, Wester D. Characterizing and treating dizziness after mild head trauma. *Otol Neurotol.* 2004;25(2):135–138.
8. Brodsky JR, Shoshany TN, Lipson S, Zhou G. Peripheral vestibular disorders in children and adolescents with concussion. *Otolaryngol Head Neck Surg.* 2018. https://doi.org/10.1177/0194599818770618
9. Riga M, Bibas A, Xenellis J, Korres S. Inner ear disease and benign paroxysmal positional vertigo: A critical review of incidence, clinical characteristics, and management. *Int J Otolaryngol.* 2011;2011:709469.
10. Balatsouras DG, Koukoutsis G, Ganelis P, et al. Benign paroxysmal positional vertigo secondary to vestibular neuritis. *Eur Arch Otorhinolaryngol.* 2014;271(5):919–924.
11. Karlberg M, Hall K, Quickert N, Hinson J, Halmagyi GM. What inner ear diseases cause benign paroxysmal positional vertigo? *Acta Otolaryngol.* 2000;120(3):380–385.
12. Song JJ, Hong SK, Kim JS, Koo JW. Enlarged vestibular aqueduct may precipitate benign paroxysmal positional vertigo in children. *Acta Otolaryngol.* 2012;132(suppl 1):S109–S117.

13. Holick MF. The vitamin D deficiency pandemic: Approaches for diagnosis, treatment and prevention. *Rev Endocr Metab Disord.* 2017;18(2):153–165.
14. Buki B, Ecker M, Junger H, Lundberg YW. Vitamin D deficiency and benign paroxysmal positioning vertigo. *Med Hypotheses.* 2013; 80(2):201–204.
15. Rhim GI. Serum vitamin D and recurrent benign paroxysmal positional vertigo. *Laryngoscope Investig Otolaryngol.* 2016;1(6):150–153.
16. Lee SB, Lee CH, Kim YJ, Kim HM. Biochemical markers of bone turnover in benign paroxysmal positional vertigo. *PLoS One.* 2017; 12(5):e0176011.
17. Meghji S, Murphy D, Nunney I, Phillips JS. The seasonal variation of benign paroxysmal positional vertigo. *Otol Neurotol.* 2017;38(9): 1315-1318.
18. Chu CH, Liu CJ, Lin LY, Chen TJ, Wang SJ. Migraine is associated with an increased risk for benign paroxysmal positional vertigo: A nationwide population-based study. *J Headache Pain.* 2015;16:62.
19. Faralli M, Cipriani L, Del Zompo MR, Panichi R, Calzolaro L, Ricci G. Benign paroxysmal positional vertigo and migraine: analysis of 186 cases. *B-ENT.* 2014;10(2):133–139.
20. Koo JW, Balaban CD. Serotonin-induced plasma extravasation in the murine inner ear: Possible mechanism of migraine-associated inner ear dysfunction. *Cephalalgia.* 2006;26 (11):1310–1319.
21. Shim DB, Song CE, Jung EJ, Ko KM, Park JW, Song MH. Benign paroxysmal positional vertigo with simultaneous involvement of multiple semicircular canals. *Korean J Audiol.* 2014;18(3):126–130.
22. Caruso G, Nuti D. Epidemiological data from 2270 PPV patients. *Audiol Med.* 2005;3(1): 7–11.
23. Anagnostou E, Kouzi I, Spengos K. Diagnosis and treatment of anterior-canal benign paroxysmal positional vertigo: A systematic review. *J Clin Neurol.* 2015;11(3):262–267.
24. Silva C, Amorim AM, Paiva A. Benign paroxysmal positional vertigo—A review of 101 cases. *Acta Otorrinolaringol Esp.* 2015;66(4): 205–209.
25. Macdonald NK, Kaski D, Saman Y, Al-Shaikh Sulaiman A, Anwer A, Bamiou D-E. Central positional nystagmus: A systematic literature review. *Front Neurol.* 2017;8:141.
26. Balatsouras DG, Koukoutsis G, Ganelis P, Korres GS, Kaberos A. Diagnosis of single- or multiple-canal benign paroxysmal positional vertigo according to the type of nystagmus. *Int J Otolaryngol.* 2011;2011:483965–483965.
27. Crevits L. Treatment of anterior canal benign paroxysmal positional vertigo by a prolonged forced position procedure. *J Neurol Neurosurg Psychiatry.* 2004;75(5):779.
28. Vannucchi P, Pecci R. Pathophysiology of lateral semicircular canal paroxysmal positional vertigo. *J Vestib Res.* 2010;20(6):433–438.
29. Pérez-Vázquez P, Franco-Gutiérrez V. Treatment of benign paroxysmal positional vertigo. A clinical review. *J Otol.* 2017;12(4):165–173.
30. Parnes LS, Agrawal SK, Atlas J. Diagnosis and management of benign paroxysmal positional vertigo (BPPV). *Can Med Assoc J.* 2003; 169(7):681–693.
31. McClure JA. Horizontal canal BPV. *J Otolaryngol.* 1985;14(1):30–35.
32. Casani AP, Cerchiai N, Dallan I, Sellari-Franceschini S. Anterior canal lithiasis: Diagnosis and treatment. *Otolaryngol Head Neck Surg.* 2011;144(3):412–418.
33. Epley JM. The canalith repositioning procedure: For treatment of benign paroxysmal positional vertigo. *Otolaryngol Head Neck Surg.* 1992;107(3):399–404.
34. Semont A, Freyss G, Vitte E. Curing the BPPV with a liberatory maneuver. *Adv Otorhinolaryngol.* 1988;42:290–293.
35. Lempert T, Tiel-Wilck K. A positional maneuver for treatment of horizontal-canal benign positional vertigo. *Laryngoscope.* 1996;106(4): 476–478.
36. Gufoni M, Mastrosimone L, Di Nasso F. [Repositioning maneuver in benign paroxysmal vertigo of horizontal semicircular canal]. *Acta Otorhinolaryngol Ital.* 1998;18(6):363–367.
37. Yacovino DA, Hain TC, Gualtieri F. New therapeutic maneuver for anterior canal benign paroxysmal positional vertigo. *J Neurol.* 2009;256(11):1851–1855.

38. Rahko T. The test and treatment methods of benign paroxysmal positional vertigo and an addition to the management of vertigo due to the superior vestibular canal (BPPV-SC). *Clin Otolaryngol Allied Sci.* 2002;27(5):392–395.
39. Kim YK, Shin JE, Chung JW. The effect of canalith repositioning for anterior semicircular canal canalithiasis. *J Otorhinolaryngol Relat Spec.* 2005;67(1):56–60.
40. Choi SJ, Lee JB, Lim HJ, et al. Clinical features of recurrent or persistent benign paroxysmal positional vertigo. *Otolaryngol Head Neck Surg.* 2012;147(5):919–924.
41. Luryi AL, Lawrence J, Bojrab DI, et al. Recurrence in benign paroxysmal positional vertigo: A large, single-institution study. *Otol Neurotol.* 2018;39:622–627.
42. Perez P, Franco V, Cuesta P, Aldama P, Alvarez MJ, Mendez JC. Recurrence of benign paroxysmal positional vertigo. *Otol Neurotol.* 2012; 33(3):437–443.
43. Sheikhzadeh M, Lotfi Y, Mousavi A, Heidari B, Monadi M, Bakhshi E. Influence of supplemental vitamin D on intensity of benign paroxysmal positional vertigo: A longitudinal clinical study. *Caspian J Intern Med.* 2016; 7(2):93–98.
44. Talaat HS, Kabel AM, Khaliel LH, Abuhadied G, El-Naga HA, Talaat AS. Reduction of recurrence rate of benign paroxysmal positional vertigo by treatment of severe vitamin D deficiency. *Auris Nasus Larynx.* 2016;43(3):237–241.
45. Do YK, Kim J, Park CY, Chung MH, Moon IS, Yang HS. The effect of early canalith repositioning on benign paroxysmal positional vertigo on recurrence. *Clin Exp Otorhinolaryngol.* 2011;4(3):113–117.
46. West N, Hansen S, Moller MN, Bloch SL, Klokker M. Repositioning chairs in benign paroxysmal positional vertigo: Implications and clinical outcome. *Eur Arch Otorhinolaryngol.* 2016;273(3):573–580.
47. Parnes LS, McClure JA. Posterior semicircular canal occlusion for intractable benign paroxysmal positional vertigo. *Ann Otol Rhinol Laryngol.* 1990;99(5 pt 1):330–334.

CHAPTER 16

Vestibular Migraine and the Pediatric Migraine Variants

Henri Traboulsi, Margaretha L. Casselbrant, and Jacob Brodsky

Introduction

Migraine is common in the pediatric population, yet it suffers from a lack of dedicated studies in children, and most recommendations are extrapolated from the adult literature. However, migraine can present quite differently in children compared to adults. For example, migraine headaches tend to be more bilateral in children, as opposed to unilateral in adulthood and late adolescence.[1] The recently released third edition of the *International Classification of Headache Disorders* (*ICHD-3*) defines the "episodic syndromes that may be associated with migraine" as follows: infantile colic, cyclical vomiting syndrome, alternating hemiplegia of childhood, abdominal migraine, benign paroxysmal torticollis of infancy (BPTI), benign paroxysmal vertigo of childhood (BPVC), and vestibular migraine (VM). Of these, the last three are the "migraine variants" that cause vestibular symptoms, so we focus this chapter on these disorders, which are presented in chronological order by typical affected age group. These disorders have been grouped together since they display striking similarities with migraine, such as associated migraine symptoms and a strong family history of migraine.[2,3] For example, some patients with BPTI have demonstrated mutations in the *CACNA1A* gene, a neuronal calcium channel gene associated with familial hemiplegic migraine and episodic ataxia, though most of them had a family history of these disorders.[4–7]

It is unfortunate that these three entities are often unknown or go undiagnosed, since they collectively constitute the most common causes of vertigo in the pediatric population.[8–13] For example, a recent study showed that only 2.4% of a randomly surveyed group of pediatricians were aware that BPTI existed.

Pediatric Migraine Variants

1. Benign Paroxysmal Torticollis of Infancy

BPTI was first described by Snyder and colleagues in 1969 as a self-limiting, benign disorder characterized by episodes of head tilting from cervical dystonia.[14] Affected patients usually wake up with a head tilt. Some studies have reported precipitating factors to include colds, teething, or a change in posture,[15–16] whereas others have not identified such factors.[2] The direction of head tilt may vary with each attack. About half of affected children also demonstrate an asymmetric posture of the trunk (tortipelvis), which bends toward the same side as the head. Attempts to straighten the head are resisted by some children, and they immediately tilt the head back again.[17] During the attack, the child may demonstrate agitation, pallor, nausea, or vomiting. Children who are ambulatory may display gait instability or falls. The onset of symptoms occurs within the first few months of life, and the condition spontaneously resolves in most children by 3 to 4 years of age. Attack duration varies from hours to days, and attack frequency varies from days to months in between episodes. A family history of a similar childhood syndrome has been reported, and a family history of migraine is common.[17–18] The diagnostic criteria for BPTI, as outlined in the *ICHD-3*, are shown in Table 16–1.[1]

Table 16–1. Diagnostic Criteria of BPTI According to ICHD, Third Edition[1]

A. Recurrent attacks in a young child, fulfilling criteria B and C

B. Tilt of the head to either side, with or without slight rotation, remitting spontaneously after minutes to days

C. At least one of the following five associated symptoms or signs:
   - Pallor
   - Irritability
   - Malaise
   - Vomiting
   - Ataxia

D. Normal neurologic examination between attacks

E. Not attributed to another disorder

Physical examination, electroencephalography, and imaging studies are typically normal between episodes. Results of audiometric and vestibular testing vary. Snyder and colleagues reported a reduced ice water caloric response in more than half of patients.[14] In most subsequent studies, caloric and audiometric testing has been normal or inconclusive.[2,17] Brodsky and colleagues have reported abnormal rotary chair testing in 5 out of 12 patients with BPTI, and abnormal cervical vestibular-evoked myogenic potential (cVEMPs) in 2 out of 6 patients.[19] Many authors have recommended routinely obtaining brain imaging in children with BPTI, although these studies are rarely abnormal, so the yield of this approach is debatable. Drigo and colleagues reported normal neurologic findings during and after episodes with no significant change in muscle tone or motor development,[15] but a more recent study with detailed neurodevelopmental assessments has indicated a high incidence of delayed gross and fine motor development in children with BPTI.[2] The resolution of BPTI coincides with a period of catch-up in motor development. In a study that followed 14 patients with BPTI, 6 children developed BPVC later in childhood, and 3 of them eventually developed migraine.[19] Interestingly, the patients with BPTI who had abnormal vestibular testing were much more likely to develop BPVC.

Although migraine is considered the most common etiology of paroxysmal torticollis in infants, an additional important diagnosis to consider is enlargement of the vestibular aqueducts (EVA). Brodsky and colleagues recently performed a retrospective survey of the families of patients who had previously been diagnosed with BPVC, VM, EVA, GJB2 (hearing loss control group), or epistaxis (normal hearing control group).[20] They found that a history of paroxysmal torticollis in infancy was reported in 19% of EVA patients and 21%

of BPVC patients, but only in 6% of patients with VM and in no patients with GJB2 or epistaxis. They also found that symptoms of paroxysmal torticollis were reported to have occurred an average of 35.2 months (nearly 3 years) prior to the identification of hearing loss in the EVA patients. Therefore, the authors recommended ongoing routine audiometric monitoring in children with BPTI, at least until the BPTI has definitively resolved.

2. Benign Paroxysmal Vertigo of Childhood

BPVC was first described by Basser and colleagues in 1964 and presents with recurrent, brief attacks of vertigo usually lasting seconds to minutes.[21] The age of onset is usually 2 to 4 years of age (older age of onset than BPTI) and the disorder resolves spontaneously, generally between 6 and 8 years of age. Symptoms usually consist of pure vertigo and imbalance, with or without associated nausea or vomiting. Hearing loss, tinnitus, and headache are usually absent, and consciousness is not impaired during an attack. The vertigo is not positional, which helps to differentiate it from benign paroxysmal positional vertigo (BPPV). However, it is not unusual for the child to remain still and avoid position change, and a child may become limp and require some support to stand or sit during an attack. Immediately after the attack, the child resumes normal activities and will remain asymptomatic until the next attack, without the interictal period of fatigue and confusion that typically follows a seizure. The intervals between the attacks may vary from a week to 6 months. The frequency of the attacks decreases with age, and there are no known precipitating factors.

Reports have varied on the typical outcomes of vestibular testing in patients with BPVC. Basser and colleagues reported that positional vertigo or nystagmus was not recorded in his series of patients; however, vestibular dysfunction was present in the form of moderate, severe, or complete canal paresis on caloric testing.[21] Balatsouras et al also reported reduced caloric responses in most of their patients,[22] but this has not been reported by others.[13,23,24] O'Reilly et al did not identify any peripheral vestibular abnormalities[13]; however, they noted deficiencies in gross motor development, similar to findings reported by Brodsky et al.[19] Reale et al reported that behavioral and emotional difficulties, anxiety, as well as depressive and hyperactive symptoms were elevated in children with BPVC compared with normal peers.[25] In a 10-year prospective study involving 15 patients, testing was abnormal in 3 patients during the interictal period, and abnormal in 4 of the 6 participants tested during the ictal period.[26] Positional nystagmus and down-beating nystagmus after horizontal head shaking were the most frequent neuro-otological signs, although it is possible that some or all patients with these findings actually had BPPV instead of (or in addition to) BPVC. Rotary chair testing and cVEMP were abnormal in about 25% of the patients in the study by Brodsky et al.[19]

Fenichel was the first to suggest that BPVC "may at times be an early manifestation of migraine."[27] This was based on the high incidence of a family history of migraine in BPVC patients and the observation that the episodes often evolve over time into typical migraine attacks. BPVC is now universally considered to be a migraine precursor. In the 10-year follow-up study by Marcelli et al, 10 out of 15 patients had migraine with or without aura either at the initial encounter or at some point during the course of the study.[26] In the Brodsky et al study, 15.4% of BPVC patients progressed to vestibular migraine at some point.[19] The diagnostic criteria for BPVC according to the *ICHD-3* are outlined in Table 16–2.

Table 16–2. Diagnostic Criteria of BPVC According to ICHD, Third Edition[1]

A. At least five attacks fulfilling criteria B and C

B. Vertigo occurring without warning, maximal at onset and resolving spontaneously after minutes to hours without loss of consciousness

C. At least one of the following five associated symptoms or signs:
- Nystagmus
- Ataxia
- Vomiting
- Pallor
- Fearfulness

D. Normal neurologic examination and audiometric and vestibular functions between attacks

E. Not attributed to another disorder

3. Vestibular Migraine

While BPTI and BPVC are classified under "Episodic syndromes that may be associated with migraine" in the most recent version of *ICHD*, vestibular migraine is only described in the Appendix.[1] The Appendix is for "novel entities that have not been sufficiently validated by research conducted so far." This is surprising, given that vestibular migraine has been well-established in the medical literature as being one of the most common causes of vertigo in both children and adults.[28]

VM episodes are usually associated with a headache, which can last from minutes to days. The *ICHD-3* criteria for VM specify that the "vestibular symptoms" must be either true vertigo or motion sensitivity with nausea. Nausea and vomiting as well as photophobia are also common. The attacks may occur when the patient is tired, and ocular problems may intensify the symptoms. Menstruation, stress, sensory stimuli, such as bright lights, intense smell, and noise may precipitate an attack. A history of motion sickness, a family history of migraine, and an increased sensitivity to movement are all very common.[29] About 30% of patients will not experience a headache, making the migraine-associated symptoms essential for the diagnosis.[30]

Physical examination is typically normal between episodes.[31] There are reports of a reduced unilateral caloric response in approximately 20% to 30% of patients as well as unilateral preponderance in approximately 10% of subjects.[32] Intolerance to caloric testing is very common in patients with VM, and vestibular testing often triggers a migraine. The diagnostic criteria for VM are outlined in Table 16–3.

Numerous comorbidities can occur in conjunction with VM that may also contribute to dizziness symptoms. Posttraumatic migraine is a common sequela of concussion and can have features of VM. BPPV has also been shown to commonly occur in pediatric patients with VM.[33] Functional dizziness, including persistent postural perceptual dizziness ("3PD"), can often occur in conjunction with VM (see Chapter 24). Anxiety is also a common comorbid condition with migraine. It is important to differentiate dizziness from these comorbid conditions from dizziness directly related to VM in order to determine the most effective management plan for a given patient.

4. Migraine With Brainstem Aura

As our understanding of migraine pathophysiology has shifted away from the traditional "vasodilatation" or "vasospastic" theory, "basilar-type migraine" was recently renamed "migraine with brainstem aura" in the third edition of the *ICHD*.[1,34] This disorder is now thought to result from the spread of the corti-

Table 16–3. Vestibular Migraine Diagnostic Criteria as Outlined by the ICHD, Third Edition[1]

A. At least five episodes fulfilling criteria C and D

B. A current or past history of migraine without aura or migraine with aura

C. Vestibular symptoms of moderate or severe intensity, lasting between 5 minutes and 72 hours

D. At least half of episodes are associated with at least one of the following three migrainous features:
   1. Headache with at least two of the following four characteristics:
      a. Unilateral location
      b. Pulsating quality
      c. Moderate or severe intensity
      d. Aggravation by routine physical activity
   2. Photophobia and phonophobia
   3. Visual aura

E. Not better accounted for by another *ICHD-3* diagnosis or by another vestibular disorder

Table 16–4. Diagnostic Criteria of Migraine With Brainstem Aura According to ICHD, Third Edition[1]

A. Attacks fulfilling criteria for 1.2 Migraine with aura and criterion B as follows

B. Aura with both of the following:
   1. At least two of the following fully reversible brainstem symptoms:
      a. Dysarthria
      b. Vertigo
      c. Tinnitus
      d. Hyperacusis
      e. Diplopia
      f. Ataxia not attributable to sensory deficit
      g. Decreased level of consciousness
   2. No motor or retinal symptoms

cal depression that causes migraine aura.[35,36] A recent review of clinical observations and functional mapping studies has found that all symptoms listed in the *ICHD* definition may originate from the cortex and not necessarily from the brainstem (Table 16–4).[37] The authors have argued that migraine with brainstem aura should be reclassified as typical migraine with aura. Migraine with brainstem aura is not considered a migraine variant per se but has been included in this chapter because it is often accompanied by vestibular symptoms.

Migraine with brainstem aura has not been well-described as a distinct entity in the pediatric population. A recent retrospective study did not mention a single case of migraine with brainstem aura in a systematic review of 2276 cases of pediatric vertigo,[28] although such cases may have been lumped together with cases of vestibular migraine and/or BPVC.

5. Familial Hemiplegic Migraine and Episodic Ataxia

Familial hemiplegic migraine (FHM) and episodic ataxia type 2 (EA2) are 2 key entities that must be differentiated from VM and from migraine with brainstem aura. They are treated differently and are discussed in detail in a separate chapter (see Chapters 13 and 19). Briefly, FHM is characterized by episodes of recurrent hemiplegia during the aura phase of a migraine headache. Both are also associated with cerebellar atrophy on magnetic resonance imaging (MRI) and the presence of interictal downbeat nystagmus.[38] Patients with EA2 present with early onset of ataxia and vertigo.

Both entities are most commonly associated with *CACNA1* gene mutations, though other causative genetic mutations have also been described.[4] Acetazolamide and 4-amino-pyridine are effective at preventing the symptoms of EA2 in most affected patients.[39,40] The most effective medications for FHM are more variable across patients and studies, although the calcium channel blocker verapamil has been shown to be particularly effective in many FHM patients.[41]

Pathophysiology

Migraine is now believed to be triggered by an initial "cortical depression," which is a wave of depressed activity that spreads across cortical neurons and glial cells triggering changes in cortical perfusion and enzymatic activity, as well as changes in the molecular environment with the release of caspase, calcitonin gene-related peptide (CGRP), and other mediators.[39] The trigeminovascular system is sensitized by this cortical depression and becomes disproportionally responsive to minimal stimuli from the meningeal nociceptors. Efferent outflow from the trigeminal nuclei to different areas of the brain might explain the different symptoms associated with migraine.[42]

A number of studies have shown evidence of inner ear changes associated with migraine, both acutely during migraine attacks and chronically in migraine patients. The trigeminovascular system has been shown to be intimately connected with the inner ear.[43] A landmark study conducted by Vass et al demonstrated that electrical stimulation of paravascular trigeminal afferents may result in permeability changes in the vessels that supply the inner ear, mainly the basilar, anterior-inferior cerebellar, and spiral modiolar arteries with release of substance P.[44] It was also found that the spiral and vestibular ganglia of animal models contain the same serotonin receptors that are the targets of triptans ($5\text{-}HT_{1B}$ and $5\text{-}HT_{1D}$),[45] and that serotonergic pathways are also believed to be heavily involved in the pathophysiology of migraine.[46] It has been recently shown that up to 15% of patients with VM can have abnormalities on caloric testing and VHIT, indicating that VM is not purely a central neurologic disease but can also be associated with peripheral vestibular dysfunction.[47] The incidence of BPPV has also been shown to be significantly higher in patients with BPVC and VM, and the recurrence rate of BPPV was found to be five times higher in pediatric patients with VM compared to nonmigraine controls.[33]

Management

There are now many well-documented options for the treatment of adult migraine, including abortive and prophylactic medications, in addition to in-clinic procedures. Unfortunately, high-quality studies for the treatment of VM are lacking, and treatment trends for VM in children are primarily based on findings from the adult literature. The treatment of patients should be individualized and should include watchful waiting and education of patients and parents, in addition to reduction of stress, encouraging sufficient and consistent sleep, psychological counseling, and avoidance of dietary triggers. Some common migraine trigger foods that are often consumed by children include yogurt, chocolate, dairy products, nuts, bananas, as well as nitrates in luncheon meats. It is important to iterate that a migraine diet is different from a "healthy" diet.

Although vestibular rehabilitation is the treatment workhorse for many pediatric vestibular disorders, its role in migraine variants is generally limited. Physical therapy may be beneficial for children with BPTI and/or BPVC who also exhibit baseline imbalance or motor delay. Vestibular rehabilitation may be beneficial for patients with VM or migraine with brainstem aura who exhibit significant peripheral vestibular impairments on vestibular testing, who have developed BPPV, or who find motion stimuli to be a major migraine trigger. Other important non-medication–based therapies that have been shown to be effective for migraine in adults are cognitive behavioral therapy and acupuncture, but their roles in the treatment of vestibular migraine and in pediatric migraine variants are yet to be established.[48,49]

For infrequent attacks of migraine, medical treatment is mainly with abortive therapies, which presently include primarily the triptan class. Zolmitriptan and rizatriptan are the only two drugs that have been studied in randomized controlled trials for the treatment of migraine-induced vertigo at the time of this writing.[50,51] All other therapeutic approaches are based on case reports, retrospective cohort studies, and open-label trials.[52] The triptans are the most extensively studied group of migraine-abortive medications, and their effectiveness has been demonstrated in children as young as 6 years of age for classic migraine.[53] Currently most triptans are approved by the U.S. Food and Drug Administration (FDA) for use in children 12 years of age and older, while only rizatriptan is FDA approved for use in children down to 6 years of age. Common side effects of the triptans include drowsiness, tingling and chest tightness, and possible serotonergic symptoms. The efficacy of triptans in VM has been limited and variable in adult studies, and there is presently only one pediatric study describing triptan use in VM.[54] Nonsteroidal anti-inflammatory agents such as ibuprofen or naproxen are acceptable options in children. Meclizine is also sometimes effective at suppressing the vestibular symptoms of VM during an attack.

Prophylactic medications are typically recommended if the child experiences frequent, recurrent, and disabling attacks interfering with schoolwork and social interaction. Options include propranolol, verapamil, topiramate, tricyclic antidepressants (amitriptyline and nortriptyline), valproate, cyproheptadine, and others. Treatment for BPTI has rarely been described in the medical literature, with most authors reporting that treatment is rarely necessary, since attacks are usually infrequent and self-limited. Retrospective reports describe some benefit from the use of cyproheptadine or topiramate in preventing BPTI attacks.[55–58] In a recent report of 28 patients with VM, the drugs that were found to be the most effective were the tricyclics, topiramate, and cyproheptadine.[54] While amitriptyline and topiramate have been reported to be the most commonly used drugs in children and adolescents, the Childhood and Adolescent Migraine Prevention (CHAMP) study recently showed these drugs to offer no advantage over placebo in the prevention of migraine in children aged 8 to 17 years, although it should be noted that this study did not include patients with VM.[59,60] Recent studies have shown the medication venlafaxine, a selective serotonin norepinephrine reuptake inhibitor (SSNRI), to be particularly effective in the treatment of VM in adults.[61] Although SSNRI medications have not yet been studied in pediatric VM, the senior author of this chapter has anecdotally found these medications to be particularly useful in the prophylactic treatment of adolescents with VM.

A newer development in the prophylactic treatment of migraine is the CGRP receptor inhibitor class of medications, which is the first class of medications designed specifically for the prophylactic treatment of migraine. The first of these medications (erenumab-aaoe) was released in 2018 and others are slated for release in the near future at the time of this writing. The true efficacy of these medications in migraine and VM prevention is still not yet known. Currently, none of these medications is FDA approved for use in patients younger than 18 years of age.

The choice of medication should be individualized based on age and clinical background. Therefore, a thorough knowledge of these medications and their side-effect profile is essential. Table 16–5 summarizes the most commonly prescribed prophylactic migraine medications in children, along with their dosages and most common side effects.

Conclusion

Migraine variants collectively constitute the most common causes of vertigo in both adults and children. Children affected with a migraine variant are at risk of developing another later in life, a phenomenon that has been recently referred to as the "vestibular march."[19] A thorough history taking and familiarity with these entities are of utmost importance since the physical examination and vestibular testing are often normal, or may reveal only minor abnormalities. Treatment should be individualized and may include reassurance, sleep optimization, diet modifications, abortive medications, and prophylactic medications.

Table 16–5. Most Commonly Prescribed Prophylactic Migraine Medications in Children[62]

Drug	*Total Daily Dose*	*Frequency of Administration*	*Most Common Side Effects*	*Notes*
Amitriptyline	0.25–1 mg/kg	Daily, at night	Sedation, anticholinergic symptoms, QT prolongation, suicidality	Available only in tablet form
Topiramate	25–200 mg	Twice daily	Fatigue, memory impairment, confusion	Available in tablet, capsule, and extended release forms
Cyproheptadine	2–18 mg	Twice to three times daily	Weight gain, drowsiness	Available in liquid form
Propranolol	80–240 mg	Three to four times daily	Bradycardia, hypotension, asthma exacerbation	Available in liquid form, and extended release tablets
Verapamil	80–240 mg	Three times daily	Constipation, drowsiness, nausea	Available in extended release form

Self-Assessment Questions

1. In what typical order do these migraine variants present in a child?
   a. BPTI, VM, BPVC
   b. VM, BPVC, BPTI
   c. BPVC, VM, BPTI
   d. BPTI, BPVC, VM
   e. BPVC, BPTI, VM

2. Which of the following statements are *false* regarding benign paroxysmal torticollis of childhood?
   a. Affected children are typically a few months to 3 to 4 years old.
   b. Patients are often symptomatic between episodes.
   c. Despite having a normal physical exam, patients can have abnormalities on vestibular testing.
   d. Children with BPTI can have a delay in gross and fine motor development.
   e. Medical treatment is often unnecessary since BPTI is mostly self-limited.

3. Why are BPTI, BPVC, and VM considered migraine variants?
   a. Because they cause episodic symptoms
   b. Because they are associated with others symptoms also found with migraine, such as nausea/vomiting, and motion sickness
   c. Because they can respond to migraine prophylactic medications
   d. Because they can share some genetic mutations with some forms of migraine
   e. Because patients affected with any of these entities are at a higher risk of developing migraine or other migraine variants in the future
   f. All of the above

4. Which of the following correctly associate the migraine variants with their typically affected age group?
   a. BPTI: 6 to 10 years of age
   b. BPVC: 4 to 8 years of age
   c. VM: Variable, but typically older children and adolescents
   d. b. and c.
   e. All of the above

5. Which of the following statements is *true* about vestibular migraine?
   a. Vestibular migraine always presents with a headache.
   b. Patients with vestibular migraine typically tolerate vestibular testing very well.
   c. Since vestibular migraine is purely a central process, vestibular testing is always normal in patients with vestibular migraine.
   d. The duration of the attacks can be very variable from patient to patient and can last from minutes to several days.
   e. Most migraine abortive and prophylactic medications are FDA approved for their use in children.

6. Which of the following is *not* a typical drug used for migraine prophylaxis?
   a. Amitryptiline
   b. Nortryptiline
   c. Desloratadine
   d. Cyproheptadine
   e. Topiramate

References

1. Headache Classification Committee of the International Headache Society. The International Classification of Headache Disorders, 3rd edition. *Cephalalgia*. 2018;38(1):1–211. doi:10.1177/0333102417738202
2. Rosman NP, Douglass LM, Sharif UM, Paolini J. The neurology of benign paroxysmal torticollis of infancy: Report of 10 new cases and review of the literature. *J Child Neurol.* 2009;24(2):155–160. doi:10.1177/0883073808322338
3. Hadjipanayis A, Efstathiou E, Neubauer D. Benign paroxysmal torticollis of infancy: An underdiagnosed condition. *J Paediatr Child Health*. 2015;51(7):674–678. doi:10.1111/jpc.12841
4. Roubertie A, Echenne B, Leydet J, et al. Benign paroxysmal tonic upgaze, benign paroxysmal torticollis, episodic ataxia and CACNA1A mutation in a family. *J Neurol.* 2008;255(10):1600–1602. doi:10.1007/s00415-008-0982-8
5. Giffin NJ, Benton S, Goadsby PJ. Benign paroxysmal torticollis of infancy: Four new cases and linkage to CACNA1A mutation. *Dev Med Child Neurol.* 2002;44(7):490–493. doi:10.1017/S0012162201002407
6. Vila-Pueyo M, Gené GG, Flotats-Bastardes M, et al. A loss-of-function CACNA1A mutation causing benign paroxysmal torticollis of infancy. *Eur J Paediatr Neurol.* 2014;18(3):430–433. doi:10.1016/j.ejpn.2013.12.011
7. Shin M, Douglass LM, Milunsky JM, Paul Rosman N. The genetics of benign paroxysmal torticollis of infancy. *J Child Neurol.* 2016;31(8):1057–1061. doi:10.1177/0883073816636226
8. Bower CM, Cotton RT. The spectrum of vertigo in children. *Arch Otolaryngol Head Neck Surg.* 1995;121:9110–9915.
9. Choung YH, Park K, Moon SK, Kim CH, Ryu SJ. Various causes and clinical characteristics in vertigo in children with normal eardrums. *Int J Pediatr Otorhinolaryngol.* 2003;67(8):889–894. doi:10.1016/S0165-5876(03)00136-8
10. D'Agostino R, Tarantino V, Melagrana A, Taborelli G. Otoneurologic evaluation of child

vertigo. *Int J Pediatr Otorhinolaryngol.* 1997; 40(2-3):133–139. doi:10.1016/S0165-5876(97)00032-3

11. Erbek SH, Erbek SS, Yilmaz I, et al. Vertigo in childhood: A clinical experience. *Int J Pediatr Otorhinolaryngol.* 2006;70(9):1547–1554. doi:10.1016/j.ijporl.2006.04.001
12. Wiener-Vacher SR. Vestibular disorders in children. *Int J Audiol.* 2008;47(9):578–583. doi:10.1080/14992020802334358
13. O'Reilly RC, Greywoode J, Morlet T, et al. Comprehensive vestibular and balance testing in the dizzy pediatric population. *Otolaryngol Head Neck Surg.* 2011;144(2):142–148. doi:10.1177/0194599810393679
14. Snyder CH. Paroxysmal torticollis in infancy: A possible form of labyrinthitis. *Am J Dis Child.* 1969;117(4):458–460. doi:10.1001/archpedi.1969.02100030460013
15. Drigo P, Giavonna C, Laverda AM. Benign paroxysmal torticollis of infancy: A case report. *Brain Dev.* 2000;22:169–172. doi:10.1016/S0387-7604(00)00099-1
16. Cataltepe SU, Barron TF. Benign paroxysmal torticollis presenting as "seizures" in infancy. *Clin Pediatr (Phila).* 1993;32(9):564–565. doi:10.1177/000992289303200913
17. Deonna T, Martin D. Benign paroxysmal torticollis in childhood. *Pediatr Med Chir.* 1997; 19(1):69–70.
18. Sanner G, Bergstrom B, Bergstrom G. Benign paroxysmal torticollis in infancy. *Acta Pediatr Scand.* 1979;68(1):219–223. doi:10.2298/VSP0601069D
19. Brodsky J, Kaur K, Shoshany T, Lipson S, Zhou G. Benign paroxysmal migraine variants of infancy and childhood: Transitions and clinical features. *Eur J Paediatr Neurol.* 2018; 22(4):667–673. doi:10.1016/j.ejpn.2018.03.008
20. Brodsky JR, Kaur K, Shoshany T, et al. *Paroxysmal torticollis in infants with congenital hearing loss in the setting of enlarged vestibular aqueduct syndrome.* Presented at: European Society of Pediatric Otolaryngology Meeting, June 2018; Stockholm, Sweden.
21. Basser LS. Benign paroxysmal vertigo of childhood. *Brain.* 1964;87(1):141–152.
22. Balatsouras DG, Kaberos A, Assimakopoulos D, Katotomichelakis M, Economou NC, Korres SG. Etiology of vertigo in children. *Int J Pediatr Otorhinolaryngol.* 2007;71(3):487–494. doi:10.1016/j.ijporl.2006.11.024
23. Mira E. Benign paroxysmal vertigo in childhood. Diagnostic significance of vestibular examination and headache provocation tests. *Acta Otolaryngol.* 1984;406:271–274.
24. Weisleder P, Fife TD. Dizziness and headache: A common association in children and adolescents. *J Child Neurol.* 2001;16(10):727–730. doi:10.1177/088307380101601004
25. Reale L, Guarnera M, Grillo C, Maiolino L, Ruta L, Mazzone L. Psychological assessment in children and adolescents with benign paroxysmal vertigo. *Brain Dev.* 2011;33(2):125–130. doi:10.1016/j.braindev.2010.03.006
26. Marcelli V, Russo A, Cristiano E, Tessitore A. Benign paroxysmal vertigo of childhood: A 10-year observational follow-up. *Cephalalgia.* 2015;35(6):538–544. doi:10.1177/0333102414547781
27. Fenichel GM. Migraine as a cause of benign paroxysmal vertigo of childhood. *J Pediatr.* 1967;71(1):114–115. doi:10.1016/S0022-3476(67)80239-7
28. Davitt M, Delvecchio MT, Aronoff SC. The differential diagnosis of vertigo in children: A systematic review of 2726 cases. *Pediatr Emerg Care.* 2017 In Press. doi:10.1097/PEC.0000000000001281
29. Jeong SH, Oh SY, Kim HJ, Koo JW, Kim JS. Vestibular dysfunction in migraine: Effects of associated vertigo and motion sickness. *J Neurol.* 2010;257(6):905–912. doi:10.1007/s00415-009-5435-5
30. Stolte B, Holle D, Naegel S, Diener H-C, Obermann M. Vestibular migraine. *Cephalalgia.* 2015;35:262–270. doi:10.1177/0333102414535113
31. Cutrer FM, Baloh RW. Migraine-associated dizziness. *Headache J Head Face Pain.* 1992; 32(6):300–304. doi:10.1111/j.1526-4610.1992.hed3206300.x
32. Çelebisoy N, Gökçay F, Şirin H, Biçak N. Migrainous vertigo: Clinical, oculographic and posturographic findings. *Cephalalgia.* 2008;

28(1):72–77. doi:10.1111/j.1468-2982.2007.01474.x

33. Brodsky JR, Lipson S, Wilber J, Zhou G. Benign paroxysmal positional vertigo (BPPV) in children and adolescents. *Otol Neurotol.* 2017;(15):1. doi:10.1097/MAO.0000000000001673
34. Bickerstaff ER. Basilar artery migraine. *Lancet.* 1961;277:15–17.
35. Tfelt-Hansen PC. Review: History of migraine with aura and cortical spreading depression from 1941 and onwards. *Cephalalgia.* 2010;30(7):780–792. doi:10.1111/j.1468-2982.2009.02015.x
36. Charles A, Hansen JM. Migraine aura: New ideas about cause, classification, and clinical significance. *Curr Opin Neurol.* 2015;28(3):255–260. doi:10.1097/WCO.0000000000000193
37. Demarquay G, Ducros A, Montavont A, Mauguiere F. Migraine with brainstem aura: Why not a cortical origin? *Cephalalgia.* 2017;38(10):1–9. doi:10.1177/0333102417738251
38. Yabe I, Kitagawa M, Suzuki Y, et al. Downbeat positioning nystagmus is a common clinical feature despite variable phenotypes in an FHM1 family. *J Neurol.* 2008;255(10):1541–1544. doi:10.1007/s00415-008-0970-z
39. Ling X, Zhao D, Zhao J, Shen B, Yang X. Episodic ataxia type 2 characterized by recurrent dizziness/vertigo: A report of four cases. *Int J Neurosci.* 2019;129(2):103–109. doi:10.1080/00207454.2018.1486829
40. Feil K, Bremova T, Muth C, Schniepp R, Teufel J, Strupp M. Update on the pharmacotherapy of cerebellar ataxia and nystagmus. *Cerebellum.* 2016;15(1):38–42. doi:10.1007/s12311-015-0733-1
41. Pelzer N, Stam AH, Haan J, Ferrari MD, Terwindt GM. Familial and sporadic hemiplegic migraine: Diagnosis and treatment. *Curr Treat Options Neurol.* 2013;15(1):13–27. doi:10.1007/s11940-012-0208-3
42. Burstein R, Noseda R, Borsook D. Migraine: Multiple processes, complex pathophysiology. *J Neurosci.* 2015;35(17):6619–6629. doi:10.1523/JNEUROSCI.0373-15.2015
43. Furman JM, Marcus DA, Balaban CD. Migrainous vertigo: Development of a pathogenetic model and structured diagnostic interview. *Curr Opin Neurol.* 2003;16(1):5–13. doi:10.1097/00019052-200302000-00002
44. Vass Z, Dai CF, Steyger PS, Jancsó G, Trune DR, Nuttall AL. Co-localization of the vanilloid capsaicin receptor and substance P in sensory nerve fibers innervating cochlear and vertebro-basilar arteries. *Neuroscience.* 2004;124(4):919–927. doi:10.1016/j.neuroscience.2003.12.030
45. Khalmuratova R, Hah YS, Ahn SK, Jeon SY, Kim JP, Balaban CD. Immunohistochemical and biomolecular identification of 5-HT7 receptor in rat vestibular nuclei. *J Vestib Res.* 2010;20(6):401–406. doi:10.3233/VES-2010-0390
46. Sari Y. Serotonin 1B receptors: From protein to physiological function and behavior. *Neurosci Biobehav Rev.* 2004;28(6):565–582. doi:10.1016/j.neubiorev.2004.08.008
47. Kang WS, Lee SH, Yang CJ, Ahn JH, Chung JW, Park HJ. Vestibular function tests for vestibular migraine: Clinical implication of video head impulse and caloric tests. *Front Neurol.* 2016;30(7):166. doi:10.3389/fneur.2016.00166
48. Ernst MM, O'Brien HL, Powers SW. Cognitive-behavioral therapy: How medical providers can increase patient and family openness and access to evidence-based multimodal therapy for pediatric migraine. *Headache.* 2015;55(10):1382–1396. doi:10.1111/head.12605
49. Da Silva AN. Acupuncture for migraine prevention. *Headache.* 2015;55(3):470–473. doi:10.1111/head.12525
50. Neuhauser H, Radtke A, Von Brevern M, Lempert T. Zolmitriptan for treatment of migrainous vertigo: A pilot randomized placebo-controlled trial. *Neurology.* 2003;60(5):882–883. doi:10.1212/01.WNL.0000049476.40047.A3
51. Furman JM, Marcus DA, Balaban CD. Rizatriptan reduces vestibular-induced motion sickness in migraineurs. *J Headache Pain.* 2011;12(1):81–88. doi:10.1007/s10194-010-0250-z
52. Obermann M, Strupp M. Current treatment options in vestibular migraine. *Front Neurol.* 2014;5:257. doi:10.3389/fneur.2014.00257

53. Ho TW, Pearlman E, Lewis D, et al. Efficacy and tolerability of rizatriptan in pediatric migraineurs: Results from a randomized, double-blind, placebo-controlled trial using a novel adaptive enrichment design. *Cephalalgia.* 2012;32(10):750–765. doi:10.1177/0333102412451358
54. Brodsky JR, Cusick BA, Zhou G. Evaluation and management of vestibular migraine in children: Experience from a pediatric vestibular clinic. *Eur J Paediatr Neurol.* 2016;20(1):85–92. doi:10.1016/j.ejpn.2015.09.011
55. Cuvellier JC, Lépine A. Childhood periodic syndromes. *Pediatr Neurol.* 2010;42(1):1–11. doi:10.1016/j.pediatrneurol.2009.07.001
56. Gelfand AA. Migraine and childhood periodic syndromes in children and adolescents. *Curr Opin Neurol.* 2013;26(3):262–268. doi:10.1097/WCO.0b013e32836085c7
57. Tomczak KK, Rosman NP. Torticollis. *J Child Neurol.* 2013;28(3):365–378. doi:10.1177/0883073812469294
58. Yaghini O, Badihian N, Badihian S. The efficacy of topiramate in benign paroxysmal torticollis of infancy: Report of four cases. *Pediatrics.* 2016;137(4):1–9. doi:10.1542/peds.2015-0868
59. Lewis D, Ashwal S, Hershey A, Hirtz D, Yonker M, Silberstein S. *Practice parameter: Pharmacological treatment of migraine headache in children and adolescents.* Report of the American Academy of Neurology Quality Standards Subcommittee and the Practice Committee of the Child Neurology Society. *Am Acad Neurol.* 2004;63(12):2015–2024.
60. Powers SW, Hershey AD, Coffey CS. The Childhood and Adolescent Migraine Prevention (CHAMP) study: "What do we do now?" *Headache.* 2017;57(2):180–183. doi:10.1111/head.13025
61. Salviz M, Yuce T, Acar H, Karatas A, Acikalin RM. Propranolol and venlafaxine for vestibular migraine prophylaxis: A randomized controlled trial. *Laryngoscope.* 2016;126(1):169–174. doi:10.1002/lary.25445
62. Merison K, Jacobs H. Diagnosis and treatment of childhood migraine. *Curr Treat Options Neurol.* 2016;18(11):48. doi:10.1007/s11940-016-0431-4

CHAPTER 17

Vestibular Dysfunction in Pediatric Concussion

Jacob R. Brodsky

Epidemiology and Definitions

Concussion or mild traumatic brain injury (mTBI) is an increasingly well-recognized problem that has received increasing media attention in recent years, primarily due to a combination of its significant impact on military service members and on athletes, including participants in professional, collegiate, and youth sports. Over 1.5 million people experience a concussion in the United States annually.[1] Concussion is the reason for about 1 of every 220 emergency room (ER) visits per year by children in the United States, and the number of ER visits for pediatric traumatic brain injury (TBI) more than doubled in the United States between 2001 and 2012.[2,3] The symptoms after a concussion typically resolve within about a month or less, but approximately 12% to 30% of patients will have a prolonged recovery beyond 4 weeks, which is designated as postconcussion syndrome (PCS).[4–7] Concussion's high prevalence and broad reach have numerous downstream implications beyond health care, including major negative impacts on education, the workforce, the economy, public safety, and national security.[1]

Despite all of the attention around concussion, it is surprising to note that it currently has no universally accepted definition, which is a major issue for concussion epidemiology and research. Currently, the "working definition" agreed upon by the Centers for Disease Control and Prevention, World Health Organization, and U.S. Department of Defense is most widely accepted and is summarized as follows[8]:

> Mild traumatic brain injury is the occurrence of injury to the head arising from blunt trauma or acceleration or deceleration forces with one or more of the following:
>
> - Any period of observed or self-reported:
>   - Impaired consciousness, disorientation, or transient confusion
>   - Memory dysfunction surrounding injury time
>   - Loss of consciousness for less than 30 minutes
> - Other observed signs of neuropsychological or neurologic dysfunction
>   - Seizures acutely after head injury
>   - Presence of lethargy, irritability, or vomiting after head injury
>   - Presence of headache, dizziness, irritability, poor concentration, fatigue

Vestibular specialists have a particularly important role to play in the care of children with concussion. Dizziness is the second most common symptom of concussion and of PCS, after headache.[9,10] A study of on-field symptoms of sports-related concussion showed that only dizziness was predictive of a prolonged recovery, resulting in six times the risk of developing PCS relative to those without on-field dizziness.[10] Balance impairment is also one of the most commonly reported initial symptoms of concussion, and it has important implications for the monitoring of recovery and in clearance for return to sport or work. Postconcussive dizziness and imbalance can result from any combination of a variety of different processes affecting the brain and/or the inner ear, which are described in further detail in a later section of this chapter. Most primary pediatric concussion providers are in fields such as emergency medicine, general pediatrics, neurology, and sports medicine. The training programs for these fields typically do not include extensive education in vestibular medicine. Therefore, children with prolonged dizziness or imbalance following a concussion may often benefit from consultation with a vestibular specialist. The objective of this chapter is to help guide primary concussion providers and vestibular specialists in the effective evaluation and management of children with postconcussive vestibular symptoms.

Pathophysiology

Much of our current understanding of the pathophysiological mechanisms of concussion is based on studies of animal models. The signs and symptoms of a concussion have been attributed to multiple processes that occur at the cellular level in the brain following a head injury. A head trauma of adequate rotational acceleration results in the sudden release of excitatory neurotransmitters in conjunction with a diffuse neuronal egress of potassium and influx of calcium in multiple areas of the brain.[11] The metabolic demands on the brain subsequently increase as cellular membrane ion pumps work to counteract this effect. This hypermetabolic state is associated with increased lactate production, impaired neuronal function, reduced blood flow, and impaired glucose metabolism.

These processes typically resolve within a few days, but the hypermetabolic state and impaired cerebral blood flow can last much longer in some patients. The brain is at a higher risk of long-standing or even permanent damage if it is reinjured while still in this recovery state.[11–13] This is the proposed basis for the "second impact syndrome," which is the primary impetus for delaying clearance for return-to-play in concussed athletes until the point of complete recovery is reached. Unfortunately, it is often difficult to determine when the brain has fully recovered from the concussion itself, especially since numerous other comorbid factors can cloud the picture. Prolonged mitochondrial calcium retention following concussion can result in diffuse axonal injury (DAI) causing more long-standing impairments even after the brain has otherwise recovered. The impaired state of the brain during concussion recovery also frequently reduces its ability to effectively manage baseline comorbid neurologic and psychological conditions, which in turn can further impact concussion recovery. Additionally, secondary conditions may occur as a result of the concussion recovery process, such as deconditioning, depression, anxiety, and posttraumatic migraine. There is much overlap between the mechanisms that cause cortical spreading depression following head trauma and migraine, making posttraumatic migraine a particularly prevalent issue in concussed patients.[11,14] Last, damage to nearby extracranial structures, such as the neck, eyes, and ears, may also occur concurrently with concussion, leading to symptoms that can persist even after the brain has recovered from the concussion itself.

The effects of concussion on the vestibular system include damage to both the peripheral vestibular organs and the central vestibular pathways in the brain. Posttraumatic disorders of the inner ear are discussed in further detail in a later section of this chapter. The exact processes leading to postconcussive central vestibulopathy remain poorly defined, and studies on this topic are surprisingly limited. A histopathological study of adult major TBI victims showed a high incidence of damage to Purkinje cells in the cerebellum and vestibular nuclei in the brainstem along with lacerations of the vestibulocochlear nerve.[15] A more recent study used magnetic resonance imaging scans of the brain with a modality known as diffusion tensor imaging to evaluate adult patients with vestibular symptoms after concussion, which demonstrated relatively consistent evidence of DAI in the cerebellum and fusiform gyri.[16] Further study in this area is greatly needed.

Primary Concussion Management

A detailed discussion of primary concussion management is beyond the scope of this book. However, some key points deserve brief mention.

Diagnosis/Monitoring

The initial diagnosis of concussion is a clinical one and sometimes can be difficult. A number of tools are available to aid in the initial diagnosis of concussion, quantification of impact, and monitoring of recovery. Some of the most commonly used tools are summarized as follows:

- **The Sport Concussion Assessment Tool (SCAT-5)** has both adult and pediatric versions that include a battery of well-validated tests that aid in the initial diagnosis and assessment of the possibly concussed athlete, but the SCAT-5 is also applicable to nonathletic injuries as well.[17,18]
- **The Post-Concussion Symptom Scale (PCSS)** is a symptom profile that rates common postconcussive symptoms on a 6-point scale.[19] The PCSS is frequently used to monitor symptom impact and to track concussion recovery.
- **The Immediate Post-Concussion Assessment and Cognitive Testing (ImPACT) test** is a computer-based neurocognitive assessment that is often used to aid in both concussion diagnosis and recovery tracking.[20] However, the utility of ImPACT testing is limited in patients who have not had preinjury baseline testing, which is fortunately becoming a more frequent requirement for young athletes.
- **The Balance Error Scoring System (BESS)** is a bedside evaluation of balance that is not only helpful in assessing postconcussive balance impairment but is also a well-validated marker of concussion recovery and is part of the SCAT-5 test battery.[17,18,21]
- **The Vestibular Oculo-Motor Screening (VOMS) Test** was designed primarily to track concussion recovery.[22,23] Unfortunately, it has also generated a lot of interest as a tool to diagnose binocular vision deficits and vestibular dysfunction in concussed

patients, which it is not designed to do reliably.

- **Imaging studies** play a limited role in the evaluation of concussion patients, unless focal neurologic signs, sustained loss of consciousness, seizures, or signs of major TBI are present.

Physical and Cognitive Rest

Strict physical and cognitive rest until symptom resolution has recently fallen out of favor due to increasing evidence that such an approach may be detrimental.[5,8] The likelihood of a prolonged recovery is actually reduced by early initiation (about 1 to 2 days postinjury) of progressively increasing levels of cognitive and physical activity that are kept just below the threshold of symptom provocation.[24]

Multispecialty Concussion Clinic Model

Typical concussion recovery can generally be effectively managed by a single primary concussion provider. However, patients with PCS may have symptoms and secondary disorders affecting their recovery that cross multiple specialties. The multispecialty concussion clinic model is gaining increasing popularity at many centers, since this model may improve collaboration between providers and increase convenience for patients and their families. However, further study is needed to determine the optimal components of such clinics, as well as their impact on concussion recovery and cost of care.

Return to Learn/Sport/Work

A number of important factors are taken into consideration when clearing a concussed patient to return to full-time school participation, sports, or work. Such clearance is generally beyond the scope of practice of most vestibular specialists and should typically be left to the patient's primary concussion provider. However, the vestibular specialist often plays an important role in the clearance process by determining whether any ongoing vestibular symptoms are a result of the concussion recovery itself, or instead a result of other secondary processes, as further discussed later in this chapter. Such ongoing vestibular disorders may require specific accommodations in the classroom and may prevent clearance to return to sport for safety reasons, even if the child is otherwise considered cleared from a concussion recovery standpoint.

Postconcussive Vestibular Disorders

Persistent dizziness and imbalance after a concussion may occur from central processes resulting from the concussive effects on the brain itself or from peripheral vestibular dysfunction resulting from impacts to the nearby inner ear structures. Although central causes make up the majority of cases, peripheral causes may be present in approximately one of every three patients with persistent postconcussive dizziness in the pediatric population.[25] Paying attention to specific key symptoms and physical examination findings will facilitate an accurate diagnosis and effective treatment plan in most cases; however, confirmatory tests may also sometimes be necessary. A summary of the common peripheral and central causes of postconcussive dizziness follows. The clinical algorithm in Figure 17–1 is designed to aid the concussion provider in establishing which of these causes are at play in a given patient. It is important to recognize that these diagnoses are not mutually exclusive, and more than one of them are often present in a single concussed patient. A breakdown of the relative

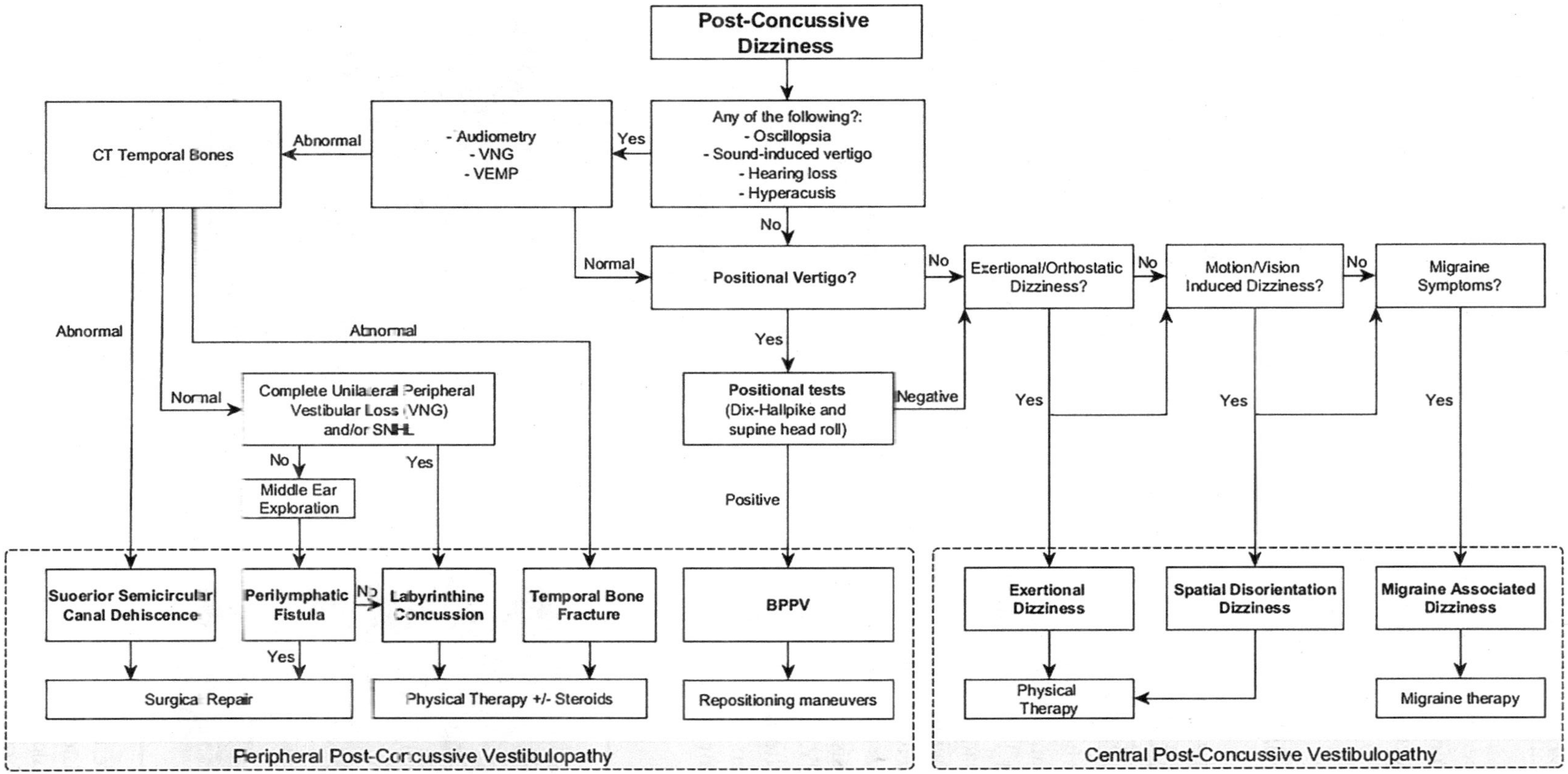

Figure 17–1. Clinical algorithm for the diagnosis and management of postconcussive dizziness.[25] (BPPV, benign paroxysmal positional vertigo; CT, computed tomography; SNHL, sensorineural hearing loss; VEMP, vestibular-evoked myogenic potential; VNG, videonystagmography.)

incidences of peripheral vestibular disorders in children with persistent postconcussive dizziness from a recent study by Brodsky and colleagues is shown in Figure 17–2.[25]

Peripheral Vestibular Disorders

- **Benign paroxysmal positional vertigo (BPPV)** is caused by the displacement of otolith debris into the semicircular canals (SCs) resulting in transient vertigo whenever the head is rotated in the plane of the affected canal(s) (Chapter 15). Hoffer and Gottshall found that one of every three military patients with postconcussive dizziness had evidence of BPPV.[14] Brodsky and colleagues found that 17% of children with persistent postconcussive dizziness had BPPV.[25] BPPV is typically treated effectively with repositioning maneuvers of the head to facilitate movement of the debris back out of the affected SC(s). Such maneuvers can be easily performed in an office setting, often resulting in rapid resolution of dizziness symptoms, making early recognition important in facilitating appropriate treatment.
- **Superior semicircular canal dehiscence (SSCD)** occurs when a patient has an abnormally thin bony covering between the superior SC and the middle cranial fossa dura directly above it.[26,27] Symptoms occur when the already thinned bone becomes frankly dehiscent, which can occur either from progressive thinning over time or from an acute fracture of the thinned bone from a head trauma, including concussion. The prevailing theory of the mechanism of SSCD symptoms is the "third window effect," where the dehiscence causes a third opening to the inner ear (in addition to the oval and round windows). This causes an additional route for sounds to enter

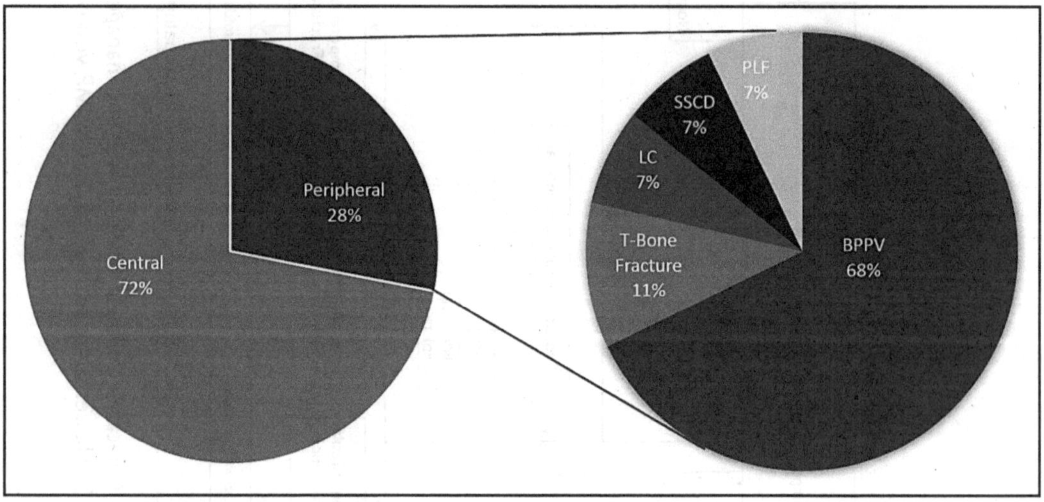

Figure 17–2. Peripheral vestibular disorders diagnosed in 28 patients out of 109 children and adolescents with persistent postconcussive dizziness. (BPPV, benign paroxysmal positional vertigo; LC, labyrinthine concussion; PLF, perilymphatic fistula; SSCD, superior semicircular canal dehiscence; T-Bone Fracture, temporal bone fracture.)

the inner ear causing conductive hyperacusis and autophony, where many patients report that their own voice and sounds from their own body (eg, eye blinks, hair brushing, footsteps, etc) sound amplified. This also causes sound to be rerouted through the superior SC resulting in sound-induced vertigo ("Tullio's phenomenon") and often also in hearing loss. Patients will also often have some degree of oscillopsia. SSCD is diagnosed by high-resolution computed tomography (CT) of the temporal bone with oblique cuts through the plane of the superior SC (Figure 17–3). Diagnosis is also aided by vestibular-evoked myogenic potential (VEMP) testing demonstrating a "third window" pattern, where the response threshold is reduced and the signal amplitude is increased (Chapter 8). SSCD can be effectively treated by surgical occlusion or resurfacing of the superior SC through either a middle cranial fossa approach or a transmastoid approach.

- **Traumatic perilymphatic fistula (PLF)** occurs when one or both of the two existing windows of the inner ear (round and oval windows) is violated, either from spontaneous rupture from excess pressure induced into the inner ear from a sudden impact or from a traumatic injury to the ossicular chain resulting in displacement or fracture of the stapes footplate. Symptoms are often similar to those experienced with SSCD. Conductive hearing loss is often present, but sensorineural hearing loss (SNHL) may also develop and become severe if a traumatic PLF goes untreated for even a brief period of time. Therefore, early recognition and management of a PLF are essential. Unfortunately, a traumatic PLF can be very tricky to identify, since vestibular testing and temporal bone imaging are often normal in the setting of a traumatic PLF. Therefore, a high degree of clinical suspicion is key, and a PLF should always be considered when an unexplained conductive or mixed hearing loss occurs after a concussion

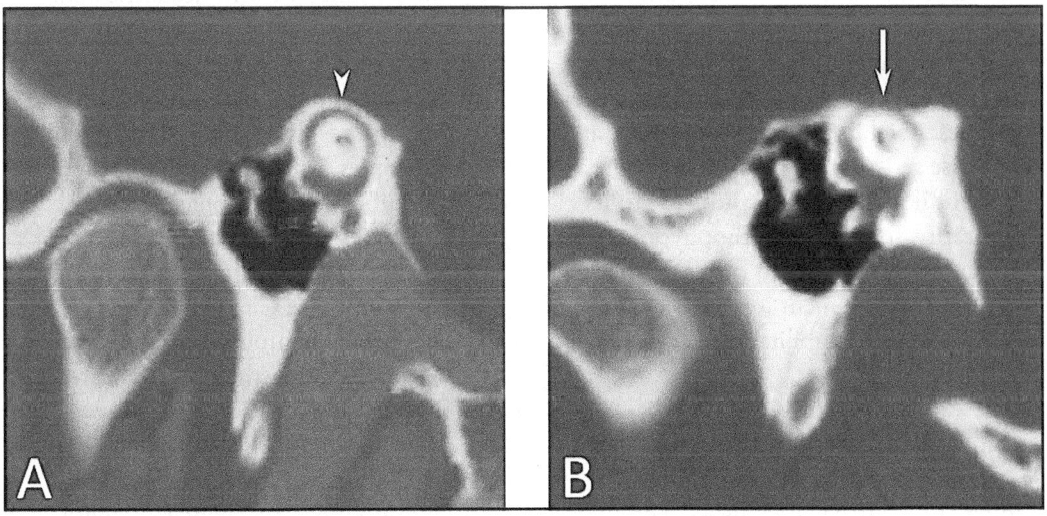

Figure 17–3. High-resolution computed tomography images of the temporal bone in long-axis reformats demonstrating (**A**) normal (*arrowhead*) and (**B**) dehiscent (*arrow*) superior semicircular canals.

in a pediatric patient. Traumatic PLF will occasionally resolve spontaneously, but early surgical exploration of the middle ear and repair of the fistula are recommended whenever the suspicion for a PLF is high to prevent progressive SNHL.

- **Temporal bone fracture** technically defines a head injury as a major TBI instead of a concussion, but occasionally occult fractures may be present in patients diagnosed with a concussion, since high-resolution temporal bone imaging is not a routine component of the initial workup of concussion patients. A temporal bone fracture involving the otic capsule may cause SNHL, vestibular loss, vertigo, imbalance, and/or oscillopsia. Surgical treatment of temporal bone fractures is not typically indicated or possible, so the management of the resulting vestibular deficits typically consists primarily of vestibular rehabilitation with a physical therapist.
- **Labyrinthine concussion** causes severe unilateral peripheral vestibular loss and usually also severe SNHL following a head injury, but without evidence of temporal bone fracture on imaging. This phenomenon has primarily been described in assorted case reports and case series in the medical literature, but it is difficult to study due to its rarity, so an exact pathophysiological mechanism is yet to be established. The management is primarily with vestibular rehabilitation.

Central Dizziness

Hoffer and Gottshall established a useful classification system for postconcussive dizziness, which includes three categories of central causes as well as positional dizziness (BPPV).[14] This classification system excludes the other peripheral vestibular causes of postconcussive dizziness outlined previously, but our algorithm (see Figure 17–2) incorporates their three central categories, as we have found these to be particularly useful in clinical practice.

- **Exertional dizziness** causes a lightheaded, presyncopal type of dizziness symptom that is induced by upright positioning, ambulation, and/or exertional activities. Although it primarily results from the impaired state of the brain during concussion recovery, it is also typically exacerbated by deconditioning, poor sleep, dehydration, and malnourishment in many concussed patients. Therefore, it is primarily treated by aggressive hydration and a gradual reconditioning regimen.
- **Migraine-associated dizziness** or vestibular migraine (see Chapter 16) causes dizziness that may consist of either motion sensitivity or true vertigo. It occurs in flares that last for minutes to hours at a time, typically in conjunction with headache and/or other migrainous symptoms, such as photophobia, phonophobia, nausea, or visual aura. Migraine-associated dizziness is managed with migraine therapies, which may include lifestyle modifications, nonpharmaceutical therapies, and/or medications.
- **Spatial disorientation–related dizziness** (see Chapter 24) is a functional neurologic disorder that now falls under the umbrella category of persistent postural perceptual dizziness ("3PD"). Dizziness is chronic with flares that can be triggered by motion, position changes, activity, standing, noise, and/or visual flow. Physical examination and testing are

often normal, although other peripheral or central vestibular disorders can occur concurrently. Treatment primarily includes habituation-based vestibular rehabilitation but also often requires cognitive behavioral therapy (CBT) and/or selective serotonin reuptake inhibitor medications.

Summary

Dizziness and balance impairment are two of the most common symptoms of concussion and PCS, but their causes are often multiple. Most causes relate to the direct impacts of concussion on the brain itself, but nearly a third of patients with persistent postconcussive dizziness may also have a peripheral vestibular disorder. A careful history and physical examination, as well as the selective use of supplemental tests when needed, will allow providers to determine the unique combination of causative factors in each child with postconcussive vestibular symptoms. This will facilitate a more comprehensive and effective treatment plan to hasten recovery and minimize long-term morbidity in children and adolescents with concussion.

Self-Assessment Questions

1. Which of the following is not a sign of a concussion following a head injury?
   a. Impaired consciousness, disorientation, or transient confusion
   b. Presence of lethargy, irritability, or vomiting after head injury
   c. Bruising or laceration of the scalp or face
   d. Presence of headache, dizziness, irritability, poor concentration, or fatigue

2. Which of the following is not a physiological process that has been associated with concussion?
   a. Neuronal egress of potassium and influx of calcium
   b. Tearing of nerve fibers causing neurotransmitter leakage
   c. Mitochondrial calcium retention resulting in diffuse axonal injury in the brain.
   d. Hypermetabolic state of the brain
   e. Decreased cerebral blood flow

3. Which of the following is a tool that is commonly used in diagnosing and monitoring concussion?
   a. The Sport Concussion Assessment Tool (SCAT-5)
   b. The Concussion Diagnostic Inventory (CDI-3)
   c. The Brain Injury Grading Scale (BIGS-4)
   d. The Head Trauma Impact Assessment Test (HTIAT-6)

4. Strict cognitive and physical rest until complete resolution of postconcussive symptoms is associated with a shortened recovery.
   a. True
   b. False

5. Which of the following is a peripheral vestibular disorder that has been associated with head trauma?
   a. Ménière's disease
   b. Vestibular paroxysmia
   c. Superior semicircular canal dehiscence
   d. Vestibular neuronitis

References

1. Gerberding JL, Binder S. Report to Congress on mild traumatic brain injury in the United States. In: *Steps to Preventing a Serious Public Health Problem*. Atlanta, GA: Centers for Disease Control and Prevention; 2003.
2. Meehan WP, 3rd, Mannix R. Pediatric concussions in United States emergency departments in the years 2002 to 2006. *J Pediatr.* 2010;157:889–893.
3. Coronado VG, Haileyesus T, Cheng TA, et al. Trends in sports- and recreation-related traumatic brain injuries treated in US emergency departments: The National Electronic Injury Surveillance System–All Injury Program (NEISS-AIP) 2001–2012. *J Head Trauma Rehab.* 2015;30:185–197.
4. Barlow KM, Crawford S, Brooks BL, Turley B, Mikrogianakis A. The incidence of postconcussion syndrome remains stable following mild traumatic brain injury in children. *Pediatr Neurol.* 2015;53:491–497.
5. McCrory P, Meeuwisse W, Dvorak J, et al. Consensus statement on concussion in sport—the 5(th) international conference on concussion in sport held in Berlin, October 2016. *Br J Sports Med.* 2017;51:838–847.
6. Babcock L, Byczkowski T, Wade SL, Ho M, Mookerjee S, Bazarian JJ. Predicting postconcussion syndrome after mild traumatic brain injury in children and adolescents who present to the emergency department. *JAMA Pediatr.* 2013;167:156–161.
7. Grubenhoff JA, Deakyne SJ, Comstock RD, Kirkwood MW, Bajaj L. Outpatient follow-up and return to school after emergency department evaluation among children with persistent post-concussion symptoms. *Brain Inj.* 2015;29:1186–1191.
8. McCrea MA, Nelson LD, Guskiewicz K. Diagnosis and management of acute concussion. *Phys Med Rehabil Clin N Am.* 2017;28:271–286.
9. Eisenberg MA, Meehan WP, 3rd, Mannix R. Duration and course of post-concussive symptoms. *Pediatrics.* 2014;133:999–1006.
10. Guerriero RM, Proctor MR, Mannix R, Meehan WP, 3rd. Epidemiology, trends, assessment and management of sport-related concussion in United States high schools. *Curr Opin Pediatr.* 2012;24:696–701.
11. Mullally WJ. Concussion. *Am J Med.* 2017; 130:885–892.
12. Giza CC, Hovda DA. The neurometabolic cascade of concussion. *J Athl Train.* 2001;36: 228–235.
13. Giza CC, Hovda DA. The new neurometabolic cascade of concussion. *Neurosurgery.* 2014;75(suppl 4):S24–S33.
14. Gottshall KR, Gray NL, Drake AI, Tejidor R, Hoffer ME, McDonald EC. To investigate the influence of acute vestibular impairment following mild traumatic brain injury on sub-

sequent ability to remain on activity duty 12 months later. *Mil Med.* 2007;172:852–857.
15. Makishima K, Sobel SF, Snow JB, Jr. Histopathologic correlates of otoneurologic manifestations following head trauma. *Laryngoscope.* 1976;86:1303–1314.
16. Alhilali LM, Yaeger K, Collins M, Fakhran S. Detection of central white matter injury underlying vestibulopathy after mild traumatic brain injury. *Radiology.* 2014;272:224–232.
17. Davis GA, Purcell L, Schneider KJ, et al. The Child Sport Concussion Assessment Tool 5th Edition (Child SCAT5): Background and rationale. *Br J Sports Med.* 2017;51:859–861.
18. Echemendia RJ, Meeuwisse W, McCrory P, et al. The Sport Concussion Assessment Tool 5th Edition (SCAT5): Background and rationale. *Br J Sports Med.* 2017;51:848–850.
19. Merritt VC, Meyer JE, Arnett PA. A novel approach to classifying postconcussion symptoms: The application of a new framework to the Post-Concussion Symptom Scale. *J Clin Exp Neuropsychol.* 2015;37:764–775.
20. Alsalaheen B, Stockdale K, Pechumer D, Broglio SP. Validity of the Immediate Post Concussion Assessment and Cognitive Testing (ImPACT). *Sports Med.* 2016;46:1487–1501.
21. Bell DR, Guskiewicz KM, Clark MA, Padua DA. Systematic review of the Balance Error Scoring System. *Sports Health.* 2011;3: 287–295.
22. Anzalone AJ, Blueitt D, Case T, et al. A positive Vestibular/Ocular Motor Screening (VOMS) is associated with increased recovery time after sports-related concussion in youth and adolescent athletes. *Am J Sports Med.* 2017;45:474–479.
23. Mucha A, Collins MW, Elbin RJ, et al. A brief Vestibular/Ocular Motor Screening (VOMS) assessment to evaluate concussions: Preliminary findings. *Am J Sports Med.* 2014; 42:2479–2486.
24. Schneider KJ. Early return to physical activity post-concussion associated with reduced persistent symptoms. *J Pediatr.* 2017;184: 235–238.
25. Brodsky JR, Shoshany TN, Lipson S, Zhou G. Peripheral vestibular disorders in children and adolescents with concussion. *Otolaryngol Head Neck Surg.* 2018;159(2):365–370.
26. Minor LB, Solomon D, Zinreich JS, Zee DS. Sound- and/or pressure-induced vertigo due to bone dehiscence of the superior semicircular canal. *Arch Otolaryngol Head Neck Surg.* 1998;124:249–258.
27. Ward BK, Carey JP, Minor LB. Superior canal dehiscence syndrome: Lessons from the first 20 years. *Front Neurol.* 2017;8:177.

CHAPTER 18

Structural Lesions of the Central Nervous System

Shelly Wang and George M. Ibrahim

Introduction

Although the majority of children with vestibular and balance disorders do not have offending structural lesions in the central nervous system (CNS), awareness of this possibility is critical to inform patient care. Attending practitioners must be familiar with the potential diagnoses as well as useful diagnostic imaging modalities.

In general, CNS lesions leading to balance disorders can be dissociated into those causing disequilibrium or vertigo. Disequilibrium, or imbalance, can be related to dysfunction in a number of pathways involving the vestibular, visual, cerebellar, basal ganglia, or dorsal column systems. Vertigo (the illusory sensation of movement) typically involves the posterior fossa, particularly the cerebellopontine angle (CPA) or craniocervical junction. In this chapter, we present an overview of common CNS structural lesions leading to balance disorders. These diagnoses are organized first anatomically and subsequently by etiology. Awareness of the possibility of these CNS structural lesions in children presenting with vestibular and balance disorders will facilitate patient evaluation, referral, and subsequent management.

Cerebellum

Various pathologies may manifest in the cerebellum, leading to vestibular and balance disorders. In pediatric populations, cerebellar pathologies include neoplasms, developmental anomalies, vascular abnormalities leading to either infarct or hemorrhage, and less commonly, structural lesions of infectious or inflammatory etiologies. The presenting symptoms in these children may be subtle or extreme, often depending on the speed at which these lesions evolve and the extent to which they obstruct circulation of cerebrospinal fluid (CSF), leading to hydrocephalus. Children with elevated intracranial pressure (ICP) from hydrocephalus can present with headaches, vomiting, and drowsiness, while infants may display macrocephaly, bulging fontanelles, irritability, poor feeding, and restricted growth and development. Focal neurologic findings with respect to lesions within and near the cerebellum include cranial nerve deficits, diplopia, vertigo, and nystagmus.

Neoplasms

Tumors of the CNS account for approximately 20% of childhood neoplasms. While the majority of adult CNS tumors are supratentorial, roughly 70% of pediatric tumors are infratentorial.[1] In the pediatric population, the three most common cerebellar tumors are astrocytomas, ependymomas, and medulloblastomas.

Juvenile pilocytic astrocytoma (JPA) comprises approximately 15% of pediatric brain tumors and is commonly found in the cerebellum. They are usually slow growing, and can involve the midline or cerebellar hemispheres, but rarely invade the CPA or brainstem. With appropriate management and gross total resection, the long-term prognosis is excellent.[3]

In contrast, ependymomas arise from glial cells of the fourth ventricular ependymal lining, and often extend through the foramen of Lushka and Magendie. Although the majority of ependymomas are World Health Organization (WHO) grade II tumors and pathologically benign, they often involve important structures around the brainstem, cranial nerves, and fourth ventricular floor, leading to increased morbidity of an aggressive surgical resection. As gross total resection is strongly correlated with improved long-term prognosis, it is often necessary to aggressively separate the tumor from individual cranial nerves to achieve maximal safe resection.[4] Children may, however, sustain postoperative deficits, including those associated with the vestibulocochlear nerve.

Last, medulloblastomas are aggressive, small blue round cell tumors that present with a shorter clinical course and increased probability of metastasis. Although they are most likely found in the midline, some medulloblastomas invade the brainstem through the floor of the fourth ventricle.[2] As a WHO grade IV tumor, medulloblastomas require more aggressive management and are associated with worse prognoses.

Given the appropriate clinical suspicion, children should undergo magnetic resonance (MR) imaging of the entire craniospinal axis with gadolinium to establish a diagnosis and define the extent of disease. The primary management often involves surgical resection and potential adjuvant chemoradiation therapy, depending on the age and risk profile of the tumor, including the molecular classification. Postoperatively, children may experience posterior fossa syndrome, which is characterized by emotional lability, worsening ataxia, disequilibrium, and mutism or speech disturbances. It is thought to result from injury to the dentate nuclei, cerebellar peduncles, or fourth ventricular floor, and the management is supportive.[5]

Arachnoid Cyst

The arachnoid membrane is a leptomeningeal layer surrounding the brain and spinal cord that contains CSF. During development, the arachnoid may split to form a separate CSF space, which enlarges through a hypothesized ball-valve mechanism. Although many arachnoid cysts are thought to be congenital in nature, there are reports of acquired, symptomatic arachnoid cysts following trauma.[10] These lesions are most commonly found in the middle cranial fossa, but they can also involve other compartments of the CNS. In the posterior fossa, arachnoid cysts are often incidental findings with no clinical consequence.

Rarely, these lesions may compress the cerebellum and brainstem, leading to symptoms of ventricular obstruction, cranial nerve deficits, or cerebellar dysfunction. These lesions also rarely lead to hemorrhage, either spontaneously or following trauma, resulting in rapidly progressive symptoms. There are reports of patients with posterior fossa arachnoid cysts who present with typical symptoms of Ménière's disease, consisting of episodic vertigo, tinnitus with aural fullness and hearing loss,[11] or hearing loss with facial weakness,[12] who subsequently improved with treatment of the cyst.

Although some arachnoid cysts are incidental findings, symptomatic lesions may benefit from treatment. The two options of the management of these cysts are fenestration or fluid diversion via shunt placement. Cyst fenestration may be performed either endoscopically or via open microsurgery. Cysts that either fail or are not anatomically favorable for fenestration are treated most commonly with a cystoperitoneal shunt to divert the CSF into the peritoneal cavity.

Vascular

Although vascular pathologies are rare in the pediatric populations, the sudden onset of headaches, balance disorders, and other neurologic deficits should prompt suspicion for vascular conditions associated with either hemorrhagic or ischemic stroke. An arteriovenous malformation (AVM) is a tangled mass of abnormal connections between arteries and veins. The annual risk of rupture is approximately 4% and may lead to sudden-onset headaches, ataxia, nausea and vomiting, decreased levels of consciousness, and focal neurologic deficits. Other vascular malformations such as cavernoma and dural arteriovenous fistula (DAVF) can also become symptomatic due to hemorrhage. Furthermore, children may develop balance disorders from cerebral ischemia or infarct related to vertebrobasilar insufficiency, embolic stroke, vasculitis, or hypercoagulable state. These conditions may lead to cerebellar infarct and an array of symptoms that includes vertigo and disequilibrium. For children with suspected vascular conditions, a computed tomography (CT) angiogram or MR angiogram is useful for initial assessment.

Brainstem

Lesions of neoplastic, vascular, or infectious pathologies may involve the brainstem. Most primary tumors of the brainstem are astrocytomas, although the pathologic grade varies widely by location. The most common are diffuse intrinsic pontine gliomas (DIPG), which are highly malignant and often subsume the entire pons on imaging. These lesions are characterized by a triad of cranial neuropathy, ataxia, and long tract findings. There is currently no indication for surgical biopsy or cytoreduction, and there are few long-term survivors despite aggressive chemoradiation treatment.

In contrast, the second most common brainstem tumors are tectal gliomas, which are benign and indolent. Most of these children present with obstructive hydrocephalus from occlusion of the cerebral aqueduct, and the usual treatment consists of an endoscopic third ventriculostomy to treat the hydrocephalus, without biopsy of the lesion.

Astrocytomas can also develop in other areas of the brainstem and upper cervical spinal cord. These are more likely to present with focal neurologic deficits and balance disorders rather than hydrocephalus. They vary in the degree of aggressiveness, and some exophytic brainstem tumors may be amenable to surgical excision. Brainstem vascular malformations, namely, cavernomas, may also lead to deficits from either mass effect or hemorrhage. Due to its proximity to critical structures, surgical management of brainstem cavernomas is limited to those with repeated hemorrhages and presentation to the pial surface.

Last, lesions of infection or inflammatory lesions may also lead to balance disorders and can be seen on MR imaging as an area of T2 and FLAIR signal change and possible gadolinium enhancement. Potential etiologies include demyelination, cerebellitis, vasculitis, and metabolic abnormalities.

Cerebellopontine Angle

The primary structures within the CPA are the cranial nerves exiting through their respective foramina. The most common tumors of the cranial nerves are nerve sheath tumors, especially schwannomas of the vestibulocochlear nerve. While vestibular schwannomas are common in adults, they are rare in children and mostly limited to those with neurofibromatosis (NF) II, where bilateral vestibular schwannomas are pathognomonic of the condition. Schwannomas can form on other cranial nerves but are quite rare in children.

Other CPA lesions include glomus jugulare tumors, meningiomas, and dermoid and epidermoid cysts. While unusual in adults, epidermoid cysts are the most common CPA tumor in children, often with minimal impact on the surrounding cranial nerves. The classic vestibular finding in patients with CPA tumors is Bruns nystagmus, which consists of slow, large-amplitude nystagmus when looking toward the lesion and smaller-amplitude nystagmus when looking away from the lesion. This is more common in larger tumors and is rarely seen in children.

The imaging modality of choice is MR imaging, with newer imaging techniques adding considerable information to the pathological diagnosis and proximity to important structures in the brain.[6] MR spectroscopy can help assess the degree of cellularity and necrosis within the lesion, and can help differentiate tumors from nonneoplastic lesions such as abscesses, stroke, or multiple sclerosis. Diffusion tensor imaging (DTI) sequences can be used to demonstrate specific pathways through the brain, making surgical approaches to lesions within the brainstem and CPA safer.

Craniocervical Junction

Structural abnormalities and lesions of the craniocervical junction can lead to brainstem, cerebellar, and upper cervical spine findings. Although most craniocervical junction lesions and abnormalities are congenital and developmental, lesions of neoplastic, vascular, infectious, and inflammatory etiology can also result in mass effect and compression of the neural elements, leading to vestibular symptoms.

Chiari Malformation

Chiari malformation is a condition of cerebellar tonsillar descent through the foramen magnum. This imaging finding is found incidentally in roughly 0.3% of the general population and is most commonly asymptomatic. Chiari I malformation symptoms include occipital headaches, nystagmus, and ataxia, as well as bulbar symptoms (ie, central sleep apnea, speech, and swallowing abnormalities). The balance and vestibular manifestations can be subtle, and it may be useful to obtain objective testing.[7]

Of note, Chiari I malformations are rarely noted on prenatal imaging; in fact, the position of the tonsils can change markedly in the preschool years. The conformation of the posterior fossa and cerebellar tonsils appears to stabilize around age 6, although older children can develop a secondary Chiari from focal increased ICP related to obstructive hydrocephalus or a space-occupying lesion, whereby the cerebellar tonsils herniate through the foramen magnum. Asymptomatic children do not require treatment; however, those with persistent symptoms or signs (including syringomyelia) related to the Chiari malformation usually benefit from a variety of decompressive approaches. These range from a bony suboccipital decompression with or without C1 laminectomy, to expansile duraplasty and potentially tonsillectomy or tonsil coagulation, in order to provide greater space in the posterior fossa. The vestibular symptoms associated with a symptomatic Chiari improve in nearly all children after a decompression.[8]

Like Chiari I malformations, Chiari II malformations also involve tonsillar and brainstem descent through the foramen magnum but are associated with open neural tube defects. Chiari II malformations may involve caudal descent of the entire hindbrain, with resultant changes in the shape of the fourth ventricle and kinking of the cervicomedullary junction, a large massa intermedia, interdigitation of the cerebral hemispheres with an incompetent falx, and heterotopias within the cerebrum. Symptoms associated with Chiari II malformations can result in lower cranial nerve dysfunction. Patients with a Chiari II malformation without necessarily subjective symptoms will often have significant vestibular findings with loss of smooth pursuit and horizontal nystagmus. This is thought to result from the congenital cerebellar and brainstem malformations rather than an acquired finding that is preventable.[9]

Basilar Invagination

The upper cervical spine and its connection to the skull is a complex mechanism of unique bony and ligamentous structures that allow remarkable freedom of motion while maintaining patency of the neural canal and mechanical integrity. When these structures fail slowly over time, the upper cervical spine, most particularly the tip of the odontoid, can ascend into the intracranial space causing distortion and compression on the brainstem.

In the pediatric population, basilar invagination is most commonly associated with bony and connective tissue disorders including osteogenesis imperfecta, spondyloepiphyseal dysplasia, Marfan syndrome, and Ehlers-Danlos syndrome. With cranial settling, the tip of the odontoid may cause direct compression of the midline medulla or lower pons. Potential brainstem dysfunction includes balance and vestibular symptoms, particularly vertical down-beating nystagmus. Hearing loss and vestibular dysfunction occur in the majority of patients with osteogenesis imperfecta, although this can usually be attributed to otosclerosis rather than basilar invagination.[13]

Most children do not have dynamic instability, and basilar invagination tends to progress slowly, so intervention is indicated when the pathology becomes symptomatic. Symptoms mostly consist of headaches, lower cranial nerve dysfunction, and changes in corticospinal function.[14] Surgical intervention in children can be quite complex and requires the expertise of orthopedic and neurosurgeons. It typically involves cervical traction to attempt reduction of the basilar invagination with a posterior decompression and occipital-cervical fusion. If the anterior compression is not significantly improved with traction, a transoral resection of the odontoid may also be required.[14]

Foramen Magnum Stenosis

Children with skeletal dysplasia, particularly achondroplasia, can develop congenital narrowing of the foramen magnum, resulting in compression of the upper cervical spine. While the majority of these children present with central sleep apnea and/or upper motor neuron dysfunction, a small number will have more profound brainstem symptoms. Vestibular dysfunction is uncommon, but older children who are ambulatory will often present with a change in gait and balance. On MR imaging, T2 and FLAIR hyperintensity in the craniospinal junction are thought to represent gliosis from repeated neural injury. Treatment of foramen magnum stenosis is similar to the treatment of a Chiari I malformation, with a suboccipital craniectomy to enlarge the posterior fossa, and removal of the C1 lamina when indicated by imaging. Most surgeons perform a bony decompression without a duraplasty.[15] Radiographic T2 hyperintensity and clinical signs of myelopathy may persist, but many of these patients clinically improve in regard to their gait and balance.

Spinal Cord

Lesions of the spinal cord may lead to gait imbalance and ataxia in children, due to poor proprioception from dorsal column injury and weakness from corticospinal tract injury. Although lesions of neoplastic etiology are most common, vascular, inflammatory and infectious pathologies should also be considered.

Lesions of the spinal column are classified by compartment: extradural, intradural, extramedullary, and intramedullary lesions. All of these may result in compressive symptoms. In the pediatric population, developmental neoplasms (ie, dermoid and epidermoid cysts, teratomas), astrocytomas, ependymomas, and lesions associated with leukemia or neuroblastoma are the most common. Additionally, for children with NF II or von Hippel-Lindau disease, schwannomas and hemangioblastomas should be considered. In addition to imbalance, children with spinal cord compressive or intrinsic lesions may also display back or radicular pain, weakness, sensory loss, scoliosis, or sphincter dysfunction. Diagnosis can be made with MR imaging of the spine.

Conclusion

Balance and vestibular dysfunction in children can be secondary to structural lesions in the CNS. Balance is controlled by multiple neural pathways and can be altered by supratentorial, infratentorial, or spinal cord lesions, which cause dysfunction in the vestibular, visual, cerebellar, basal ganglia, or proprioceptive systems. True vestibular dysfunction is primarily associated with either lesions in the CPA that cause dysfunction of the vestibular nerve or other posterior fossa locations that impact the vestibular nuclei in the brainstem. MR imaging is the primary diagnostic modality to identify these structural lesions. Formalized objective balance and vestibular testing is often helpful to understand which neural pathways are playing a role in a symptomatic child, and allows correlation with anatomic findings on imaging to help determine if a surgical intervention is indicated.

Self-Assessment Questions

1. What percentage of tumors in children is found in the posterior fossa?
   a. 20%
   b. 50%
   c. 70%
   d. 95%

2. Treatment of cerebellar tumors may result in:
   a. Ataxia
   b. Cerebellar mutism
   c. Anosmia
   d. a and b
   e. All of the above

3. Medulloblastomas can cause abducens palsies by:
   a. Directly invading the nerve
   b. Causing intraventricular hemorrhage
   c. Blocking CSF flow through the fourth ventricle.

4. The primary management of posterior fossa tumors is:
   a. Radiation therapy
   b. Proton beam therapy
   c. Surgical resection

5. Chiari Type 1 malformation is defined as descent of the cerebellar tonsil through the foramen magnum by at least:
   a. 1 mm
   b. 5 mm
   c. 10 mm

6. Symptoms of Chiari 1 malformation include:
   a. Central sleep apnea
   b. Vertical nystagmus
   c. Swallowing dysfunction
   d. All of the above

7. Chiari malformation is found in 0.3% of the population and is most commonly:
   a. Associated with severe headaches
   b. A harbinger of progressive ataxia
   c. Asymptomatic

8. Symptoms of Chiari 2 malformation are almost always a result of:
   a. Demyelination
   b. Infection
   c. Hydrocephalus

9. CPA arachnoid cysts can produce symptoms of:
   a. Ménière's disease
   b. Multiple sclerosis
   c. Stroke

10. Foramen magnum stenosis can be seen in children with:
    a. Hyperthroidism
    b. Waardenburg's syndrome
    c. Achondroplasia

References

1. Stiller C, Nectoux J. International incidence of childhood brain and spinal tumors. *Int J Epidemiol.* 1994;23:458–464.
2. Packer R, Macdonald R, Vezina G, Keating R, Santi M. Medulloblastoma and primitive neuroectodermal tumors. *Handb Clin Neurol.* 2012;105:529–548.
3. Daszkiewicz P, Maryniak A, Roszkowski M, Barszcz S. Long-term functional outcome of surgical treatment of juvenile pilocytic astrocytoma of the cerebellum in children. *Childs Nerv Syst.* 2009;25(7):855–860.
4. Zacharoulis S, Moreno L. Ependymoma: An update. *J Child Neurol.* 2009;24(11):1431–1438.
5. Gudrunardottir T, Sehested A, Juhler M, Schmiegelow K. Cerebellar mutism—Review of the literature. *Childs Nerv Syst.* 2011;27: 355–363.
6. Poretti A, Meoded A, Huisman TA. Neuroimaging of pediatric posterior fossa tumors including review of the literature. *J Magn Reson Imaging.* 2012;35:32–47.
7. O'Reilly RC, Greywoode J, Morlet T, et al. Comprehensive vestibular and balance testing in the dizzy pediatric population. *Otolaryngol Head Neck Surg.* 2011;144(2):142–148.
8. Liebenberg WA, Georges H, Demetriades AK, Hardwidge C. Does posterior fossa decompression improve oculomotor and vestibulo-ocular manifestations in Chiari 1 malformation. *Acta Neurochir (Wien).* 2005;147:1239–1240.
9. Salman MS, Sharpe JA, Lillakas L, Steinbach MJ, Dennis M. Smooth ocular pursuit in Chiari II malformation. *Dev Med Child Neurol.* 2007;49:289–293.
10. Ibrahim GM, Alotaibi NM, Lipsman N, Nassiri F, da Costa L. De novo formation of a symptomatic arachnoid cyst in an adult. *Neurology.* 2017;88:331–332.
11. O'Reilly RC, Hallinan E. Posterior fossa arachnoid cysts can mimic Meniere's disease. *Am J Otolaryngol.* 2003;24(6):420–425.
12. Olaya JE, Ghostibe M, Rowe M, Zouros A. Endoscopic fenestration of a cerebellopontine angle arachnoid cyst resulting in complete recovery from sensorineural hearing loss and facial nerve palsy. *J Neurosurg Pediatr*, 2011;7: 157–160.
13. Kuurila K, Kentala E, Karjalainen S, et al. Vestibular dysfunction in adult patients with osteogenesis imperfecta. *Am J Med Genet.* 2003;120A:350–358.

14. Sawin PD, Menezes AH. Basilar invagination in osteogenesis imperfecta and related osteochondrodysplasias: medical and surgical management. *J Neurosurg.* 1997;86:950–960.

15. King JA, Vachhrajani S, Drake JM, Rutka JT. Neurosurgical implications of achondroplasia. *J Neurosurg Pediatr.* 2009;4:297–306.

CHAPTER 19

Neurodegenerative Diseases

David R. Lynch, Abigail Lynch, and Kim Schadt

Introduction

Balance disorders in children may have many causes, including neurodegenerative diseases. This chapter focuses on the prototypic neurodegenerative illnesses that are selectively associated with balance dysfunction, namely, ataxia. In this brief chapter, we cannot discuss those many diseases in which balance is only a modest part of the clinical picture. For example, although ataxia can be a symptom of degenerative peripheral neuropathies, the clinical approach to diagnosis and therapy reflects not only the ataxia but the associated issues of weakness and sensory loss. In addition, this chapter concentrates on genetic disorders more than acquired, as the balance dysfunction in acquired disorders is rarely seen in isolation.

Genetic Disorders of Balance: Inherited Ataxias

The most important aspect of diagnosing and understanding balance disorders (ataxias) in genetic terms is the inheritance pattern. In general, recessive disorders more commonly appear in children, while dominant disorders primarily have onset in adulthood. Apart from diseases of white matter (leukodystrophies such as Pelizius-Merzbacher disease, which are beyond the scope of this chapter), X-linked ataxias are rare. Maternal inheritance of balance disorders is observed; however, it typically reflects a component of a larger mitochondrial cytopathy.[1]

Autosomal-Recessive Disorders

Friedreich Ataxia

Friedreich ataxia (FRDA) is the most common hereditary ataxia, affecting 1 in 50,000 Caucasian individuals.[2] All individuals with FRDA have a mutation in both alleles of the frataxin (*FXN*) gene, resulting in an abnormally low functional level of the protein called frataxin. Frataxin is a small, nuclear-encoded mitochondrial protein that mediates the chaperoning of iron sulfur clusters to the enzymes of oxidative phosphorylation; thus, its absence leads to decreased adenosine triphosphate (ATP) production, reactive oxygen species production in model systems, and accumulation of iron within the mitochondria. Most individuals have a trinucleotide GAA repeat expansion in intron 1 of the *FXN* gene on both alleles, causing reduced transcription of frataxin mRNA and decreased expression of frataxin protein. A minority of cases are caused by a repeat expansion on one allele with a point mutation in the other. Such point mutations usually disrupt frataxin RNA splicing, or lead to a nonfunctional protein, and thus produce severe phenotypes. However, selected missense mutations can produce disease that is more slowly progressive.

Disease Characteristics. While presentation is variable, onset occurs typically in childhood or adolescence.[3] Symptomatology includes ataxia, generalized areflexia, early loss of position and vibratory sense, dysarthria, cardiomyopathy, and scoliosis. Additional manifestations may include hearing loss, optic atrophy, swallowing dysfunction, urinary urgency, and decreased insulin sensitivity with a higher tendency toward developing diabetes mellitus over time. The cardiomyopathy seen in FRDA can be severe. The initial presentation is usually hypertrophic; however, fibrosis and loss of systolic function occur over time. When present, cardiac dysfunction can lead to premature death.

With genetic diagnosis, it has become clear that there is substantial phenotypic variability in FRDA.[3] Patients may present later (occasionally as late as the mid-sixties) and a few patients develop prominent spasticity or rapidly progressive visual loss. Such variants are more likely to be present in persons with GAA repeat lengths at the shorter end of the pathologic range, or in those who carry a point mutation on one allele.

Diagnosis and Testing. The diagnosis is typically based on clinical findings confirmed with genetic analysis.[3] Molecular genetic testing is commercially available and is based on detection and sizing of the GAA repeat length. Direct deoxyribonucleic acid (DNA) sequencing can be used to identify point mutations, if necessary. Anatomically, early in the disease, FRDA primarily leads to loss of the dorsal columns with a resultant sensory ataxia; thus, brain magnetic resonance imaging (MRI) scans are normal at presentation, although sensory potentials are lost on nerve conduction testing. Additionally, MRI of the cervical spine shows atrophy (from loss of dorsal columns) in many people. Electrocardiograms (ECGs) and echocardiographs are also abnormal early in the disorder and throughout the clinical course.

As all sensory systems are affected, visual-evoked potentials, brainstem auditory-evoked responses (BAERs), and optical coherences tomography of the retina can be abnormal[4]; however, such testing is rarely clinically useful, as the specific diagnosis is made genetically. Detailed visual or audiological evaluation may be useful in select research situations.

Management. Antioxidants, such as idebenone or coenzyme Q10, may decrease oxidative injury and improve mitochondrial function, although clinical trials have provided equivocal results.[3] Annual surveillance by neurology, cardiology, orthopedics, and endocrinology is helpful for preventing secondary complications. Physical and occupational therapy should be initiated early to address progressive balance dysfunction and fine motor difficulties. Prognosis varies based on age at onset and GAA repeat length, with mean age of death in the mid-thirties due to the cardiomyopathy in many patients.

Ataxia Telangiectasia

Ataxia telangiectasia (AT) is an autosomal-recessive disorder, affecting both the central and peripheral nervous systems, which also causes major complications outside the nervous system. The mutated gene is called *ATM*, an acronym for ataxia telangiectasia mutated. Mutations in *ATM* are usually point mutations on both alleles. The gene product appears to be involved in double-stranded DNA repair. Clinically, AT is associated with manifestations suggestive of defective DNA repair; however, it is unclear how exactly these mutations are linked to neurodegeneration. The central nervous system abnormalities include progressive cerebellar atrophy with early loss of Purkinje cells; a variety of other abnormalities may develop over time.[5] Though its exact prevalence is unknown, estimates range from 1 in 20,000 to 100,000 live births.[6]

Disease Characteristics. Clinical manifestations include progressive ataxia, oculocutaneous telangiectasias, abnormal eye movements, and immune deficiencies.[5] In addition, patients have insulin resistance, radiation sensitivity, pulmonary dysfunction, and an increased incidence of malignancy, of which a majority are lymphomas and acute leukemias. Most children with ataxia telangiectasia are initially developmentally appropriate and do not experience delayed milestones early in life. The fluidity of gait is typically slow to develop, and children may walk with a narrow base; thus, initial symptomatology occurs early (typically less than 5 years of age). Children with AT have difficulty standing still due to balance problems, as well as underlying movement disorders that become more prominent over time. Gross and fine motor skills deteriorate in parallel with the emergence of abnormal eye movements. Unlike FRDA, eye movement abnormalities are prominent. There is often a delay in initiating eye movements (impaired saccadic initiation) and a lack of smooth pursuits as eyes tend to move in a series of small jumps instead of a single motion.[7] Additional ocular symptoms include oculomotor apraxia (inability to coordinate head and eye movements) and hypometric (small) saccades.[7] These symptoms all reflect the prominent cerebellar and particularly Purkinje cell involvement.

More recently it has been discovered that alternative phenotypes exist, including paroxysmally mild individuals; however, many of the individuals reported before molecular diagnostic testing may represent other disorders, particularly ataxia oculomotor apraxia type 1 (AOA1) and ataxia oculomotor apraxia type 2 (AOA2).[1] The variability of AT is likely to increase as the disorder becomes easier to diagnose through the recent development of practical molecular testing approaches.

Diagnosis and Testing. Diagnosis of AT can readily be made through the combination of imaging and molecular studies in the context of a child with early onset of ataxia.[1] Imaging studies demonstrate cerebellar atrophy, as well as other abnormalities on computed tomography (CT) scanning, such as pulmonary telangiectasias. An elevated serum α-fetoprotein (AFP) is found in most subjects, and immunoglobulin A (IgA) levels are often low. Until recently, biochemical diagnosis was based on radiation sensitivity testing of lymphocytes; now both DNA sequencing and protein-based assessment of ATM protein levels are used. Molecular testing is commercially available.

In contrast to FRDA, there is modest direct involvement of sensory systems.[3] Although vestibular reflexes are highly abnormal in AT, this appears to reflect cerebellar control of vestibular reflexes rather than abnormal vestibular input.

Management. Management is supportive and presently based on systemic disease manifestations. Life expectancy is shortened due to the multisystem involvement; median age of death is approximately 25 years.[8]

Ataxia With Oculomotor Apraxias

Ataxia oculomotor apraxias, which are autosomal-recessive disorders, are characterized by oculomotor apraxia, ataxia, cerebellar atrophy; and sensorimotor neuropathy[5]; thus, they resemble AT in many ways. However, not every patient exhibits all features. At the molecular level, AOA1 is associated with mutations in the protein aprataxin (from the gene *APTX*),[9] while AOA2 is caused by mutations in the protein senetaxin (*STX* gene).[10] Both proteins are involved in DNA repair, suggesting a molecular overlap with AT, and abnormalities of DNA repair can be seen in fibroblasts from AOA2 patients.[11] Still, at this point, neither has been associated with increased risk of neoplasm as is seen in AT.

Ataxia With Oculomotor Apraxia Type 1

Disease Characteristics. Symptom onset of AOA1 is typically in childhood, usually before age 10 years, and is characterized by a slowly progressive ataxia.[12] Clinical manifestations include oculomotor apraxia with eventual ophthalmoplegia, progressive neuropathy (primarily motor), and cerebellar atrophy. Additional features can include choreoathetosis and dystonia.

Diagnosis and Treatment. Molecular genetic testing is commercially available to detect mutations in the *APTX* gene.[9] Although most reported cases have been in persons of Japanese, Portuguese, or Italian descent, it is likely a global disorder. Serum creatine kinase (CK) and total cholesterol levels may be elevated, while albumin levels may be decreased. MRI scans reveal cerebellar atrophy, and peripheral neuropathy is often found with electromyography (EMG). As of yet, no definitive genotype-phenotype correlations have been confirmed, as homozygosity for a complete deletion may not create a paroxysmally severe phenotype.[13]

Management. Management is supportive and symptomatically driven. A high-protein, low-cholesterol diet may be useful for controlling serum abnormalities of hypoalbuminemia and hypercholesterolemia.[14] Because this disorder is newly identified, no data on long-term prognosis are available at present.

Ataxia With Oculomotor Apraxia Type 2

Disease Characteristics. In AOA2 presenting symptoms often surface in the second decade of life.[10] Clinical features are similar to those of AOA1 and include cerebellar atrophy, oculomotor apraxia, as well as sensory and motor neuropathy. Based on the age at onset, AOA2 is most commonly confused with FRDA, while AOA1 is more commonly confused with AT.

Many individuals have elevated serum α-fetoprotein (AFP).[10] After using AFP as a screening test, molecular genetic testing is commercially available to detect mutations in the *SETX* gene. MRI demonstrates cerebellar atrophy, while EMG and nerve conduction velocity (NCV) testing show features of peripheral neuropathy. There are no specific features on BAER testing.

Management. At present, treatment is supportive and symptomatically driven. As for AOA1, a low-cholesterol diet may be useful.[15]

Ataxia With Vitamin E Deficiency

Ataxia with vitamin E deficiency (AVED) was initially identified among people diagnosed with FRDA without the same genetic markers.[3] Such individuals were shown to have low levels of vitamin E. The disease results from mutations in the α-tocopherol transfer proteins, which facilitate absorption of vitamin E in the intestine.

Disease Characteristics. Symptoms of AVED typically present before or around the age of puberty and include progressive ataxia, lack of hand dexterity, loss of proprioception and vibratory sensation, and areflexia. The phenotype is extraordinarily similar to FRDA.[3] Other features often observed are dysdiadochokinesia, a positive Romberg sign, head titubation, decreased visual acuity, and positive Babinski sign. Unlike FRDA, pigmentary retinopathy can be seen, and individuals have presented with dystonia.[16] The phenotype and disease severity vary widely among families with different mutations; age of onset and disease course are more uniform within a given family, but symptoms and disease severity can vary even among siblings.

Diagnosis and Testing. The principal criterion for diagnosis is an FRDA-like neurologic phenotype in association with markedly reduced plasma vitamin E (α-tocopherol) levels in the absence of known causes of malabsorption.[1] In most cases, molecular analysis of TTPA, the gene-encoding α-tocopherol transfer protein and the only gene known to be associated with AVED, allows confirmation of the diagnosis.

Management. Treatment includes lifelong high-dose oral vitamin E supplementation to maintain plasma vitamin E concentrations in the high-normal range.[17] Early treatment may reverse or halt ataxia progression, and many subjects recover significantly.

Ataxia With Coenzyme Q10 Deficiency

Ataxia with coenzyme Q10 (CoQ) deficiency was identified as a syndrome in which patients with relatively selective ataxia were identified to have low levels of CoQ in muscle and responded to therapy with oral CoQ, albeit incompletely.[18] Primary deficiency responds more readily than secondary deficiency.[19] Since that time, it has been associated with several different genes and syndromes; these include AOA1, ADCK3 kinase, and ANO10.[20] In general, MRI reveals cerebellar atrophy. Because some forms are treatable or reversible, it demands that all patients presenting with autosomal-recessive ataxia receive a therapeutic trial of CoQ or a muscle biopsy to rule out this syndrome. Plasma and skin fibroblast can be used, but their exact sensitivity and specificity are unclear.

Marinesco-Sjögren Syndrome

Marinesco-Sjögren syndrome (MSS) is a less common syndrome than other inherited ataxias.

Disease Characteristics. Symptoms of MSS typically present in childhood and may include cerebellar ataxia, early cataracts, distal and proximal muscular weakness, hypotonia, and intellectual disability. Additional features may include short stature and scoliosis.[14]

Diagnosis and Testing. Diagnosis is typically based on clinical and imaging studies that show cerebellar hypoplasia and a small posterior fossa.[21] Molecular genetic testing for the one known gene, *SIL1*, is available clinically, and detects mutations in about 60% of patients.[22] In addition, many patients with similar clinical presentations may represent phenocopies with mutations in *SIL1*-associated pathways, creating a common mechanism behind all patients with this clinical presentation.[23]

Management. Treatment is largely supportive and aimed at managing symptomatic manifestations as they arise.[14] Lifelong physical therapy as well as ophthalmologic and neurologic care should be initiated in infancy. Life span appears to be near normal.

Autosomal-Dominant Disorders

Spinocerebellar Ataxias

Most autosomal-dominant disorders can be grouped under the auspice of the disorders called spinocerebellar ataxias (SCAs). These disorders, by definition, are dominant, and the pathology is generally associated with cerebellar atrophy[3]; however, in some of these disorders, other features are equally prominent and phenotypic variability is great. The SCAs are numbered, with at least 32 different genetic loci. The most common are SCA2 and SCA3, with SCAs carrying numbers above 18 being rare. They can also be grouped by the type of mutation, primarily into those for which the mutation is or is not a CAG repeat.

CAG Trinucleotide Expansion Disorders

SCA1, 2, 3, 6, 7, 12, 17, and dentato-rubral-pallido-luysian atrophy (DRPLA) are caused by CAG trinucleotide repeat expansions within the coding sequences of their respective genes.[1] Two disorders not associated with balance dysfunction, Huntington disease and spinobulbar muscular atrophy, are also caused by CAG repeat expansions. As the CAG tract codes for glutamine, repeats in this coding region give rise to extended sequences of glutamine. For this reason, such disorders have also been referred to as polyglutamine disorders.

Molecular genetic testing for CAG repeat length is highly specialized. The location of the CAG repeat expansion is within a different specific gene for each disorder.[1] The length of the repeat that gives rise to disease also differs between disorders. Sensitive and specific testing is therefore required to determine the difference in sizes among the normal and disease-causing CAG repeat allele. Each test is disease specific; however, the tests are typically sent as a panel due to similarities in clinical phenomenology among all SCAs. CAG repeat disorders are not readily detected by whole exome sequencing, which is rapidly becoming the technique of choice for diagnosing ataxia in the absence of information directing one to specific diagnoses. Thus, care must be exercised in interpretation of negative results of CAG repeat testing.[24]

In general, CAG repeat disorders share clinical genetic phenomenology. All are exclusively neuronal with rare exceptions. In addition, the length of the CAG repeats correlates with disease severity.[1] Longer repeats typically give rise to an earlier age of onset. Furthermore, the CAG repeat is unstable and expands over generations. This leads to the phenomenon of anticipation, in which earlier onset and increasing severity of disease manifest in subsequent generations of a family. This is least prominent in SCA6, in which the repeat remains stable from generation to generation, although it nevertheless correlates with disease severity.

Non-CAG and Repeat SCAs

The other SCAs are not caused by CAG expansion repeats, yet they share unusual genetic features. SCA 10 is caused by a pentanucleotide repeat and SCA 8 by a CTG repeat.[1] The other SCAs each have unique mutations, most frequently point mutations rather than repeat expansions.

Clinical Features of the Spinocerebellar Ataxias

The 31 autosomal-dominant types of SCA share many characteristic features including cerebellar atrophy as well as progressive neuronal dysfunction with eventual loss of cerebellar and brainstem neurons.[3] SCA7 is distinguished by macular degeneration, the only feature among SCAs that is sufficiently specific and routinely used to clinically determine a diagnosis. SCA2 is associated with slow saccades. SCA3 and SCA2 may be associated with L-dopa-responsive parkinsonism in some patients. SCA10 is associated with epilepsy and is most common among individuals of Mexican descent. SCA6 is normally a "pure" cerebellar degeneration with subclinical neuropathy and few other features; however, none of these features are sufficiently unique to confirm a diagnosis in the absence of genetic testing.

Although SCAs are typically adult disorders, they can occur in childhood.[3] This occurs when anticipation leads to an earlier age of onset, with eventual childhood presentation. In such situations where the anticipation is sufficient to lead to childhood onset, the expanded allele is usually transmitted from the father; however, maternal transmission can occur, particularly in SCA7. In addition, the earliest features of these disorders begin in childhood. Thus, as treatments develop, particularly those that are most effective early in disease, the understanding of the course of SCAs in childhood will become particularly important.[25]

Dentato-Rubro-Pallido-Luysian Atrophy

A particular form of SCA is dentato-rubro-pallido-luysian atrophy (DRPLA), an autosomal-dominant progressive ataxic disorder caused by CAG repeat expansions on chromosome 12p.[1] This is another disorder that may present with anticipation, particularly with paternal transmission. DRPLA can cause ataxia, involuntary movements, myoclonic epilepsy, emotional instability, and cognitive dysfunction. Imaging studies may reveal basal ganglia calcification as well as atrophy of the cerebellum and brainstem.[26] This condition can appear anytime from infancy to mid-adulthood with symptoms differing by age.

Childhood onset (before age 20 years) often involves myoclonus, seizures, behavioral changes, intellectual disability, and problems with balance and coordination. In some individuals, the disorder is essentially congenital and presents with autism and seizures.[27] When symptoms emerge in adulthood, ataxia is frequently the presenting symptom; patients may also experience choreoathetosis, psychiatric symptoms, and deterioration in cognitive functioning. A variant of DRPLA without the characteristic myoclonic epilepsy has been described in African American descendants from North Carolina and is referred to as Haw River syndrome.[28]

With regard to clinical testing in SCA and DRPLA, confirmation of a specific SCA diagnosis requires genetic testing.[3] Although it is presently available on only half of the SCAs, those are the most common disorders; therefore, a genetic diagnosis can be confirmed in more than 80% of cases. Adjunctive testing that is useful for ruling out nongenetic disorders includes MRI (which usually reveals cerebellar atrophy in SCAs) and occasionally other blood tests including examination of paraneoplastic antibodies. Interestingly, there are usually few audiological features of SCAs and DRPLA, distinguishing them from some of the recessive ataxias and mitochondrial disorders.

Episodic Ataxia

There are presently seven types of episodic ataxia, an autosomal-dominant disorder, which is typically diagnosed based on history and clinical manifestations. In forms where it is known, the genetic mutation is in various voltage-gated potassium (episodic ataxia type 1 [EA1]), calcium (episodic ataxia type 2 [EA2]), or less commonly, sodium channels.[29,30]

Disease Characteristics

Symptoms typically present during childhood or adolescence and include episodes of transient ataxia lasting from minutes to days, vertigo, tinnitus, nausea, and vomiting.[30] Individuals with EA1 experience episodes of ataxia with nystagmus that last for minutes. Episodes of ataxia in EA2 can last hours to days. Ocular manifestations may include gaze-evoked nystagmus or broken pursuits.[31] Between episodes, neurologic functioning is normal. Triggers can include sudden changes in posture, being startled, stress, exercise, and caffeine.

Diagnosis and Testing

Regarding diagnosis and testing, molecular genetic testing is not yet uniformly available.

Management

Acetazolamide or anticonvulsant therapy may be therapeutic.[30] The medication 4-aminopyridine is now also used in individuals unresponsive to other medications.

Maternal Mitochondrial Disorders

Mitochondrial diseases are caused by a dysfunction in the mitochondrial respiratory chain that impairs oxidative phosphorylation.[3] While many of these disorders are maternally inherited, some can be inherited as recessive or dominant disorders, reflecting the fact that most mitochondrial enzymes are coded by the nuclear genome. There is wide phenotypic variation among these disorders. Mitochondrial disorders can be further classified by the exact clinical syndrome or mutation. Progressive ataxias may also be associated with mitochondrial disorders, where clinical symptomatology may include seizures, auditory impairment, retinopathy, cardiomyopathy, diabetes, or short stature.[32] These disorders may also present with intermittent or progressive ataxia. The hallmark of mitochondrial disease is involvement of multiple organ systems including the heart, brain, retina, and skeletal muscle. Diagnosis begins with a clear and detailed extended family history. While there is no consensus on the diagnostic evaluation of a suspected primary mitochondrial disorder, laboratory studies commonly include a complete blood count, renal and liver function testing, electrolytes, fasting blood glucose, creatine kinase, lactate pyruvate, plasma amino acids, carnitine, acylcarnitine, organic acids, electrocardiogram, neuroimaging, and muscle biopsy as warranted. Additional evaluations may include audiological testing, ophthalmologic evaluation, cardiac assessment, thyroid function testing, electroencephalogram, and lumbar puncture. Management of these disorders is largely supportive and symptomatically driven.

Leigh Syndrome

Phenotypic variation is due to abnormalities of the pyruvate dehydrogenase complex or respiratory chain dysfunction. Individuals with Leigh syndrome (subacute necrotizing encephalomyelopathy) typically present in infancy or early childhood.[3] Clinical manifestations may include developmental delay or regression (loss of acquired skills), ataxia, dystonia, vomiting, hypotonia, respiratory insufficiency, seizures, lactic acidosis, ophthalmoplegia, peripheral neuropathy, and myopathy.

Neuroimaging demonstrates symmetric abnormal white matter signals in the brainstem, thalamus, and basal ganglia.[1] Genetically, Leigh syndrome is associated with a variety of mutations. The most common mutations are pyruvate dehydrogenase (PDHC) deficiency and respiratory chain enzyme defects including mutations in the *SURF1* gene. Other cases result from *LRPPRC*[33] and *NARS2* mutations.[34] Modes of transmission largely depend on the defect; inheritance may be autosomal recessive, X-linked, or spontaneously acquired and without a genetic cause. There is no cure, and the prognosis is typically poor with a median age at death of 2.4 years.[35]

Myoclonic Epilepsy With Ragged Red Fibers

Myoclonic epilepsy with ragged red fibers (MERRF), as the name indicates, is characterized by myoclonus, generalized epilepsy, ataxia, and myopathy.[1] Symptoms are progressive and tend to develop in childhood following previously typical development. Additional symptomatology may include cognitive dysfunction, bilateral deafness, peripheral neuropathy, cardiomyopathy with Wolff-Parkinson-White syndrome, lipomatosis, and spasticity. Genetically, MERRF is characterized by mtDNA point mutations, with A8344G and T8356C being most common. Prognosis varies widely and is associated with variations in age of onset, symptom type, and severity.

Mitochondrial Encephalopathy With Lactic Acidosis and Stroke-Like Episodes

Mitochondrial encephalopathy with lactic acidosis and stroke-like episodes (MELAS) is a progressive neurodegenerative disorder that typically develops in childhood[1]; however, it can be found in adults, sometimes presenting in a parent after the onset of disease in a child. Clinical manifestations result from transfer RNA mutations in mtDNA and consist of stroke-like episodes causing hemiparesis, cortical blindness, seizures, migraine headaches, recurrent vomiting, muscle weakness, and hearing loss. The most common mtDNA point mutation is A3243G. Prognosis is typically poor.

Neuropathy, Ataxia, and Retinitis Pigmentosa

Neuropathy, ataxia, and retinitis pigmentosa present most commonly in late childhood or adulthood.[3] There is a broad range and combination of features that may include developmental delay, ataxia, pigmentary retinopathy, muscular weakness, dementia, sensory polyneuropathy, and epilepsy. It most commonly results from T8993G mutations but at a lower overall mutation level than is seen in individuals with Leigh syndrome. There are exceptions to this generalization,[36] and individuals can even present in adulthood with myoclonus and ataxia.[37]

Kearns-Sayre Syndrome

Kearns-Sayre (KS) syndrome is a progressive, multiorgan system disorder with a characteristic triad of clinical features known to include (1) onset before 20 years of age, (2) pigmentary retinopathy, and (3) progressive external ophthalmoplegia. In addition, one or more of the following features are present: complete heart block, elevated cerebrospinal fluid (CSF) protein >1 g/L (100 mg/dL), or cerebellar ataxia.[38] Additional manifestations can include cognitive deficits, cardiac conduction abnormalities, and endocrine abnormalities including short stature, diabetes, or parathyroid dysfunction. Fatigability and progressive limb weakness are also common. The diagnostic finding is the presence of multiple mtDNA deletions. KS syndrome is sporadic and usually reflects recessive inheritance of mutations in the proteins controlling mitochondrial DNA replication. Serum CK levels, lactate, and pyruvate may be normal or slightly elevated. EMG reveals myopathy. Muscle biopsy reveals characteristic ragged red fibers with defects in cytochrome oxidase. Prognosis varies widely depending on disease severity.

Audiology in Mitochondrial Disease

In contrast to other inherited balance disorders, primary auditory function is frequently abnormal in mitochondrial diseases, and it is subclinically involved in many others[3]; thus, evaluation with BAERs, auditory nerve testing, and other approaches are important for directing evaluation to the mitochondrial genome or to other symptomatic disorders (eg, storage diseases, leukodystrophies).

Nongenetic Causes of Pediatric Balance Dysfunction

Paraneoplastic: Opsoclonus Myoclonus and Cerebellar Degeneration

Paraneoplastic cerebellar degeneration may occur as an effect of a systemic cancer.[39] In the general population, associated malignancies are most commonly ovarian, lung, and breast cancer, though other cancers, including Hodgkin lymphoma, are implicated in children. Symptoms including ataxia (both gait and limb), dysarthria, and dysphagia are a result of tumor cell–directed immune response that cross-reacts with cerebellar Purkinje cells. Symptoms typically develop over days to months and may precede the diagnosis of cancer. The disorder typically progresses rapidly but may plateau; however, progression may be halted with treatment of the underlying cancer or occasional immunotherapy.[39] The frequent occurrence of dysphasia and dysarthria assists in distinguishing this condition from other cerebellar syndromes.[39] Although tests for the paraneoplastic antibodies are available, they are frequently negative; thus, the diagnosis of paraneoplastic processes is a clinical diagnosis aided by laboratory testing.

Opsoclonus Myoclonus

Opsoclonus myoclonus (OM) is a specific form of paraneoplastic ataxia. Patients have balance dysfunction but also myoclonus of their limbs and uncontrollable random eye movements.[40] The associated tumor in children is usually neuroblastoma. Occasionally, like all paraneoplastic processes, no tumor is identified, and the process reflects another underlying autoimmune process. Selected antibodies can be identified in some subjects.[41] In OM, immune modulatory therapies are more likely to be efficacious than in other paraneoplastic disorders.

Conclusion

This review has presented only a few of the many degenerative disorders associated with balance dysfunction. Evaluation with MRI, NCV, immune, and most importantly genetic testing can lead to the diagnosis in most individuals.

Self-Assessment Questions

1. In general, which inheritance pattern is most common for childhood-onset ataxias?
2. What is the most commonly inherited ataxia?
3. Opsoclonus myoclonus is associated most commonly with which tumor in children?

4. Which cellular organelle is dysfunctional in Friedreich ataxia?
5. What are the systemic features of ataxia telangiectasia?
6. What is the major treatment method for ataxia with vitamin E deficiency?
7. What is meant by the phenomenon of anticipation as seen in autosomal-dominant ataxias?
8. What is the inheritance pattern of most CAG repeat diseases?
9. What is the inheritance pattern of disorders of the mitochondrial genome?
10. What tumors most commonly cause paraneoplastic cerebellar degeneration?

References

1. Vu TH, Hirano M, DiMauro S. Mitochondrial diseases. *Neurol Clin North Am.* 2002;20:809–839.
2. Filla A, De Michele G, Marconi R, et al. Prevalence of hereditary ataxias and spastic paraplegias in Molise, a region of Italy. *J Neurol.* 1992;239:351–353.
3. David R. Lynch, ed. *Neurogenetics: Scientific and Clinical Advances.* Vol 75. New York, NY: Taylor and Francis Group; 2006.
4. Noval S, Contreras I, Sanz-Gallego I, Manrique RK, Arpa J. Ophthalmic features of Friedreich ataxia. *Eye (Lond)*; 2012;26(2):315–320.
5. Sedgwick R, Boder E. Ataxia-telangiectasia. In: de Jong JMBV, ed. *Handbook of Clinical Neurology.* New York, NY: Elsevier; 1991:347.
6. Swift M, Morrell D, Cromartie E, Chamberlin AR, Skolnick MH, Bishop DT. The incidence and gene frequency of ataxia-telangiectasia in the United States. *Am J Hum Genet.* 1986;39:573–583.
7. Lewis RF, Lederman HM, Crawford TO. Ocular motor abnormalities in ataxia telangiectasia. *Ann Neurol.* 1999;46:287–295.
8. Crawford TO, Skolasky RL, Fernandez R, Rosquist KJ, Lederman HM. Survival probability in ataxia telangiectasia. *Arch Dis Child.* 2006;91:610–611.
9. Coutinho P, Barbot C. Ataxia with oculomotor apraxia type 1. In: Pagon RA, Bird TD, Dolan CR, Stephens K, eds. *GeneReviews.* Seattle, WA: University of Washington, Seattle; 1993.
10. Moreira MC, Koenig M. Ataxia with oculomotor apraxia type 2. In: Pagon RA, Bird TD, Dolan CR, Stephens K, eds. *GeneReviews.* Seattle, WA: University of Washington, Seattle; 1993.
11. Roda RH, Rinaldi C, Singh R, et al. Ataxia with oculomotor apraxia type 2 fibroblasts exhibit increased susceptibility to oxidative DNA damage. *J Clin Neurosci.* 2014;21:1627–1631.
12. Le Ber I, Moreira MC, Rivaud-Pechoux S, et al. Cerebellar ataxia with oculomotor apraxia type 1: Clinical and genetic studies. *Brain.* 2003;126:2761–2772.
13. van Minkelen R, Guitart M, Escofet C, et al. Complete APTX deletion in a patient with ataxia with oculomotor apraxia type 1. *BMC Med Genet.* 2015;16:61.

14. Coutinho P, Barbot C. Ataxia with oculomotor apraxia type 1. 2002 Jun 11 [updated 2015 Mar 19]. In: Adam MP, Ardinger HH, Pagon RA, Wallace SE, Bean LJH, Stephens K, Amemiya A, eds. *GeneReviews*. Seattle, WA: University of Washington, Seattle; 1993–2018.
15. Moreira MC, Koenig M. Ataxia with oculomotor apraxia type 2. 2004 Nov 15 [updated 2018 Jul 12]. In: Adam MP, Ardinger HH, Pagon RA, Wallace SE, Bean LJH, Stephens K, Amemiya A, eds. *GeneReviews*. Seattle, WA: University of Washington, Seattle; 1993–2018.
16. Becker AE, Vargas W, Pearson TS. Ataxia with vitamin E deficiency may present with cervical dystonia. *Tremor Other Hyperkinet Mov.* 2016; 6:374.
17. Schuelke M, Mayatepek E, Inter M, et al. Treatment of ataxia in isolated vitamin E deficiency caused by α-tocopherol transfer protein deficiency. *J Pediatr.* 1999;134:240–244.
18. Quinzii CM, Lopez LC, Naini A, DiMauro S, Hirano M. Human CoQ10 deficiencies. *Biofactors*. 2008;32:113–118.
19. Desbats MA, Lunardi G, Doimo M, Trevisson E, Salviati L. Genetic bases and clinical manifestations of coenzyme Q10 (CoQ 10) deficiency. *J Inherit Metab Dis.* 2015;38:145–156.
20. Balreira A, Boczonadi V, Barca E, et al. ANO10 mutations cause ataxia and coenzyme Q_{10} deficiency. *J Neurol.* 2014;261:2192–2198.
21. Anttonen AK, Lehesjoki AE. Marinesco-Sjögren syndrome. In: Pagon RA, Bird TD, Dolan CR, Stephens K, eds. *GeneReviews*. Seattle, WA: University of Washington, Seattle; 1993.
22. Krieger M, Roos A, Stendel C, et al. SIL1 mutations and clinical spectrum in patients with Marinesco-Sjögren syndrome. *Brain.* 2013;136(Pt 12):3634–3644.
23. Ezgu F, Krejci P, Li S, et al. Phenotype-genotype correlations in patients with Marinesco-Sjögren syndrome. *Clin Genet.* 2014;86:74–84.
24. Fogel BL, Lee H, Deignan JL, et al. Exome sequencing in the clinical diagnosis of sporadic or familial cerebellar ataxia. *JAMA Neurol.* 2014;71:1237–1246.
25. Maas RP, van Gaalen J, Klockgether T, van de Warrenburg BP. The preclinical stage of spinocerebellar ataxias. *Neurology.* 2015;85:96–103.
26. Koide R, Onodera O, Ikeuchi T, et al. Atrophy of the cerebellum and brainstem in dentatorubral pallidoluysian atrophy: Influence of CAG repeat size on MRI findings. *Neurology.* 1997;49:1605–1612.
27. Licht DJ, Lynch DR. Juvenile dentatorubral-pallidoluysian atrophy: New clinical features. *Pediatr Neurol.* 2002;26:51–54.
28. Burke JR, Ikeuchi T, Koide R, et al. Dentatorubral-pallidoluysian atrophy and Haw River syndrome. *Lancet.* 1994;344:1711–1712.
29. Leach EL, van Karnebeek CD, Townsend KN, et al. Episodic ataxia associated with a de novo SCN2A mutation. *Eur J Paediatr Neurol.* 2016;20:772–776.
30. Jen JC, Wan J. Episodic ataxias. *Handb Clin Neurol.* 2018;148:521–529.
31. Damji KF, Allingham RR, Pollock SC, et al. Periodic vestibulocerebellar ataxia, an autosomal dominant ataxia with defective smooth pursuit, is genetically distinct from other autosomal dominant ataxias. *Arch Neurol.* 1996; 53:338–344.
32. Da Pozzo P, Cardaioli E, Malfatti E, et al. A novel mutation in the mitochondrial tRNA(pro) gene associated with late-onset ataxia, retinitis pigmentosa, deafness, leukoencephalopathy and complex I deficiency. *Eur J Hum Genet.* 2009;17:1092–1096.
33. Thompson Legault J, Strittmatter L, Tardif J, et al. A metabolic signature of mitochondrial dysfunction revealed through a monogenic form of Leigh syndrome. *Cell Rep.* 2015;13:981–989.
34. Simon M, Richard EM, Wang X, et al. Mutations of human NARS2, encoding the mitochondrial asparaginyl-tRNA synthetase, cause nonsyndromic deafness and Leigh syndrome. *PLOS Genet.* 2015;11:e1005097.
35. Sofou K, De Coo IF, Isohanni P, et al. A multicenter study on Leigh syndrome: Disease course and predictors of survival. *Orphanet J Rare Dis.* 2014;9:52.
36. Claeys KG, Abicht A, Häusler M, et al. Novel genetic and neuropathological insights in neurogenic muscle weakness, ataxia, and retinitis pigmentosa (NARP). *Muscle Nerve.* 2016;54: 328–333.
37. Martikainen MH, Gorman GS, Goldsmith P, et al. Adult-onset myoclonus ataxia associated

with the mitochondrial m.8993T>C "NARP" mutation. *Mov Disord.* 2015;30:1432–1433.

38. Rowland L, Hays A, DiMauro S, De Vivo D, Behrens M. Diverse clinical disorders associated with morphological abnormalities of mitochondria. In: Scarlato G, Cerri C, eds. *Mitochondrial Pathology in Muscle Diseases.* Padua, Italy: Piccin Medical Books; 1983: 141–158.
39. Dalmau J, Rosenfeld RM. Overview of paraneoplastic syndromes of the nervous system. In: Rose BD, ed. *UpToDate.* Wellesley, MA: UpToDate; 2012.
40. Dalmau J, Rosenfeld RM. Opsoclonus myoclonus ataxia. In: Rose BD, ed. *UpToDate.* Wellesley, MA: UpToDate; 2012.
41. Panzer JA, Anand R, Dalmau J, Lynch DR. Antibodies to dendritic neuronal surface antigens in opsoclonus myoclonus ataxia syndrome. *J Neuroimmunol.* 2015;286:86–92.

CHAPTER 20

Seizure Disorders

Cristina Y. Go

Introduction

Neurologic complaints of vertigo and dizziness are common in the general population, with a lifetime prevalence of 20% to 30%.[1] Dizziness was recognized by Jackson and Gowers as a manifestation of epilepsy more than 100 years ago.[2] However, the possibility of epilepsy as a cause of transient episodes of dizziness continues to be underrecognized by most physicians. This is even more so in the pediatric population. The reason for this may be due to the young patient's inability to fully describe what he or she is experiencing. Dizziness is defined as a sensation of disturbed or impaired spatial orientation without a false or distorted sense of motion.[3] Vertigo is the sensation of self-motion when no self-motion is occurring, or the sensation of distorted self-motion during an otherwise normal head movement.[3] It is usually a result of a disturbance in the vestibular system. Isolated epileptic vertigo is a rare type of focal seizure due to epileptic activity arising from parts of the brain that represent the vestibular system, including the frontal, temporal, parietal, and occipital cortex. In this chapter, one illustrative case is presented to discuss the phenomenon of epileptic vertigo, the different brain structures involved, and the role of electroencephalography (EEG) in the evaluation of the dizzy child.

Case

A 7-year-old, right-handed girl presented at the age of 5 years with a fall followed by unresponsiveness for a few minutes. A few months later, she started experiencing clusters of events where she would complain of "dizziness" for less than 10 seconds without alteration of level of consciousness. Eventually, she has episodes of screaming, "I'm falling," at times associated with a scared look on her face and eye deviation or limb stiffening. She also described a funny feeling in her legs as if she was being pulled backward. Because of these symptoms, she was referred to a neurologist. She had a normal neurologic examination, and her initial workup included normal 1.5-tesla cranial magnetic resonance imaging (MRI) and a normal routine EEG study. She presented to a tertiary pediatric epilepsy center for further evaluation after failing multiple anticonvulsants. An initial 24-hour video EEG did not capture her typical events; however, the interictal EEG was abnormal, showing occasional focal discharges over the left frontoparietal and temporal head regions. A repeat longer video EEG recording with medication taper captured multiple typical episodes of dizziness not associated with nystagmus. Some of these events were followed by stiffening of the limbs. Most of the isolated episodes of dizziness were not associated with clear changes on scalp EEG, but the episodes of dizziness followed by limb stiffening showed ictal changes arising from the left frontal, central, and parietal head regions (Figure 20–1). A 3-tesla cranial MRI showed thickening of the cortex with blurring of the gray-white matter interface in the left frontal region, suspicious for cortical dysplasia (Figure 20–2). Positron emission tomography (PET) scan showed subtle asymmetric reduction of fluorodeoxyglucose (FDG) activity on the left superior to middle frontal region. She underwent invasive EEG monitoring with subdural grid and depth electrodes covering the left frontal, temporal, and parietal regions. Episodes of dizziness with or without limb stiffening were captured and associated with EEG changes originating from the depth electrode in the MRI lesion with rapid propagation. Based on the invasive EEG data, the patient had cortical excision of the left superior and middle frontal gyri, including the left frontal MRI abnormality and supplementary motor area. Pathology showed oligodendroglial-like cells and heterotropic neurons in the subcortical white matter. Postoperative, she has rare, transient episodes of dizziness and no longer had motor manifestations of seizures.

Mechanism

More than a century ago, vertigo and epilepsy were felt to be closely related. Bladin[4] wrote

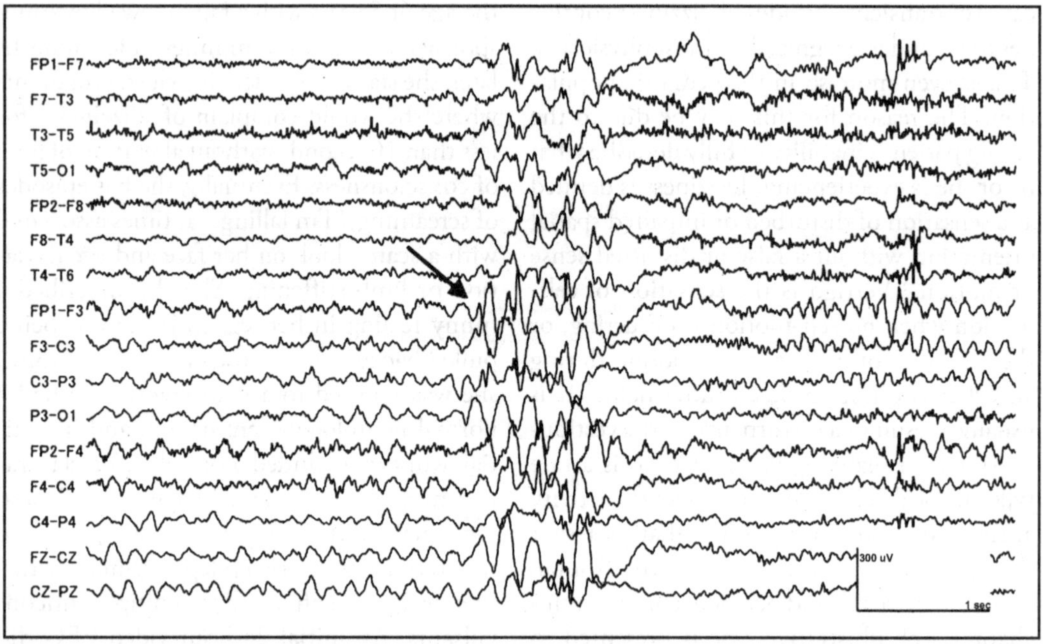

Figure 20–1. Scalp electroencephalography (EEG). During an ictal event, EEG shows burst of spike-wave discharges followed by attenuation with superimposed fast activity and buildup of rhythmic activity over the left frontocentral and parietal head regions (*arrow*).

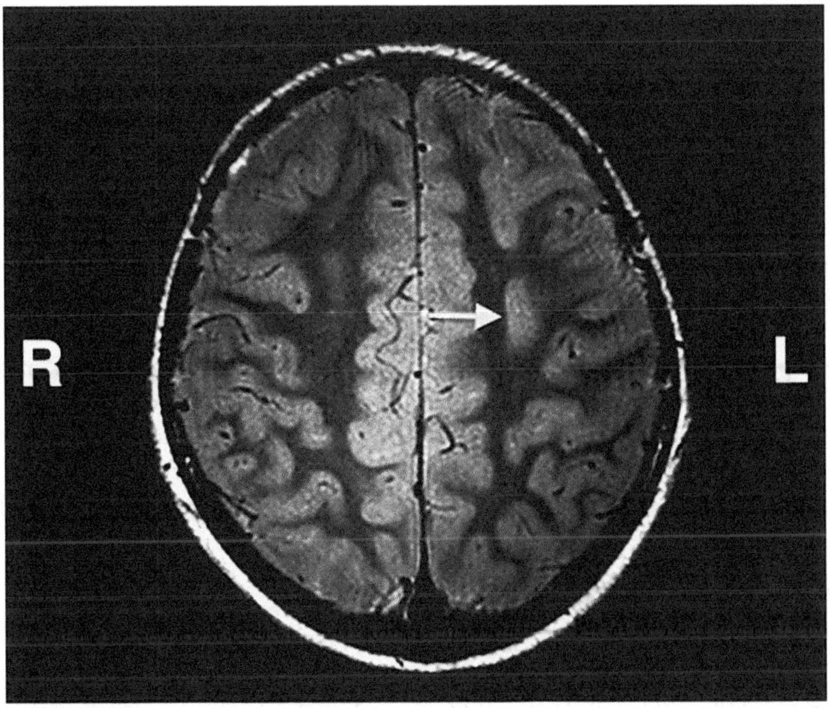

Figure 20–2. Brain magnetic resonance image. Axial proton density shows blurring of gray–white matter junction in the left superior frontal gyrus (*arrow*).

eloquently on the history of epileptic vertigo and how in ancient times, it "was recognized that persistent attacks of vertigo might develop into epilepsy." The term, "epileptic vertigo" was loosely used to define a paroxysmal cerebral disorder. In 1861, Ménière described the inner ear as being involved most often in vertigo. However, Gowers mentioned that in some cases, distinguishing vertigo caused by inner ear and epilepsy could be difficult. Seizures causing vertigo have traditionally been thought to arise mostly from the temporal regions. Cortical stimulation studies in the conscious human brain by Penfield[5] showed that stimulation of the posterior region of Brodmann area 22 produced the sensation of vertigo. In a study of 30 patients with epilepsy presenting predominantly with episodes of dizziness who had normal ontological assessment including clinical, audiometric, and caloric testing, 47% complained of a feeling of rotation, often followed by nausea.[2] All patients had an abnormal EEG with 93% showing temporal or bitemporal sharp or slow waves.

Other areas of the brain are also involved in producing the symptom of vertigo. The stimulation of the occipital lobe was reported to induce a vertiginous seizure.[6] Kinetopsia, or illusions of visual motion, has been reported in epileptic dysfunction involving the junction of the parietal, temporal, and occipital cortices, also known as V5.[7] Cerebral perfusion patterns by PET studies in response to cold caloric stimulation demonstrated activation in the contralateral temporoparietal junction, posterior insular cortex, putamen, anterior cingulate cortex, and primary sensory cortex.[8] Based on animal studies,[9] the posterior insula is thought to be the core of the vestibular cortex, integrating visual and somesthetic signals, and has strong interconnections with other numerous vestibular regions of the brain, including the premotor cortex, frontal eye fields, inferior frontal gyrus, precentral gyrus, anterior cingulate cortex, supramarginal and angular gyri, superior lip of the intraparietal sulcus, temporoparietal junction, and V5 area.[7,10] Epileptic activity in the different parts of the brain involved in vestibular processing can cause symptoms of vertigo. In a study involving 40 patients with partial seizures who underwent video EEG monitoring for aura presenting as vertigo or dizziness, the ictal-onset areas were seen in the mesial temporal (8 cases), lateral temporal (20 cases), frontal (4 cases), parietal (1 case), and occipital lobes (7 cases).[11]

Differential Diagnosis

When vertigo is followed by clinically evident seizure activity (confusion, focal sensory or motor symptoms, or a convulsion), the epileptic etiology is easier to diagnose. Most neurologists would call this symptom an "aura," which is defined as "a subjective ictal phenomenon that, in a given patient, may precede an observable seizure; if alone, constitutes a sensory seizure."[12] A systematic review of 84 studies describing 11,354 patients presenting with vertigo/dizziness and seizures showed that vestibular symptoms accompanied by other seizure-related symptoms or signs (epileptic vertigo or dizziness [EVD]) were seen in 9.3%, and those presenting mainly with isolated vertigo or dizziness as their seizure semiology (i-EVD) comprised only 0.8% of the total cohort.[13] Therefore, when episodic or recurrent vertigo occurs in isolation, it is important to rule out other etiology for the symptom.

Vertigo is due to a dysfunction of the vestibular system and can be due to problems arising from the peripheral (labyrinth, vestibular nerve) or central (brainstem, various areas in the cortex where cortical projections from the peripheral system terminates) system.

Common peripheral causes include infections (ie, vestibular neuronitis, otitis media), Ménière's disease, benign paroxysmal positional vertigo (BPPV), benign paroxysmal vertigo in children, acoustic neuromas, trauma (ie, vestibular concussion), perilymph fistula, Tullio's phenomenon, drugs and toxins (ie, streptomycin, aminoglycosides, minocycline), and motion sickness due to information mismatch from the visual and vestibular systems. A full discussion of the peripheral vestibular causes of vertigo can be found in Chapters 14 and 15.

Some of the central causes of vertigo to be considered aside from epilepsy include migraine (especially basilar-type migraine) (Chapter 16), transient ischemic attack (TIA) and stroke, multiple sclerosis, tumors, neurovascular cross-compression at the root entry zone of the eighth cranial nerve (vestibular paroxysmia), and other lesions affecting the vestibular cortical regions (Chapter 18).

Other causes include psychogenic (ie, panic attacks) and hyperventilation syndrome (Chapter 24).

The presence of hearing loss and tinnitus usually points to a more peripheral etiology of vertigo. However, normal hearing does not rule out a peripheral disease.

The duration of symptoms can provide a very important clue to the diagnosis of vertigo. Vertigo in BPPV typically lasts 30 to 60 seconds. In benign paroxysmal vertigo of children, the attacks can last seconds to minutes and are not associated with alteration of level of consciousness; the child is neurologically intact with the exception of abnormal vestibular function (Chapter 15). The same duration of vertigo is also seen in epileptic vertigo, although usually less than 30 seconds, and is often associated with lateralizing sensory or motor manifestations with or without alteration of level of consciousness. Isolated vertigo as sole manifestation of a seizure is very rare.[13] Vestibular paroxysmia lasts seconds to minutes and can occur at rest or with certain head position changes.[14] Most TIA symptoms last less than 20 to 30 minutes, and those affecting the posterior circulation usually produce vertigo. Vertiginous attacks due to Ménière's disease last minutes to 24 hours and patients usually have a history of tinnitus or some hearing loss. For attacks lasting for more than 24 hours, the diagnoses to consider include vestibular neuritis, multiple sclerosis, and stroke; and for those lasting weeks and months, consider psychogenic etiology.

Diagnostic Workup

Key information in the patient's history can point to the possibility of epilepsy as a cause of vertigo: a personal or family history of epileptic seizures, duration of symptom, absence of positional triggers, presence of visual or complex auditory hallucinations, and episodes associated with alteration of level of consciousness. All patients who have recurrent episodes of vertigo should have a complete neurologic examination to look for any focal abnormalities as well as an otologic examination as outlined in Chapter 4.

When neuro-otologic examinations are normal and epileptic seizure as the cause of vertigo is suspected, EEG becomes an indispensable diagnostic tool. In a study of 50 children presenting with vertigo, 50% were diagnosed with vertiginous seizures based on their EEG findings, with over half showing temporal paroxysmal discharges and the rest showing diffuse paroxysmal discharges.[15] In most neurophysiology laboratories, routine outpatient EEGs are short, about 25 to 30 minutes of recording, and studies are performed using 19 scalp electrodes based on the 10 to 20 system of electrode placement and include activation procedures such as photic stimulation and hyperventilation.[16] However, it is important to remember that a single normal EEG study does not rule out the possibility of seizures. Interictal epileptiform discharges (IEDs) tend to increase during sleep,[17] and sleep deprivation can increased the yield of recorded IEDs by up to 30% to 70%.[18] Therefore, if the initial baseline EEG is negative, a sleep-deprived EEG recording is recommended. A longer recording, using ambulatory EEG systems but ideally with video EEG monitoring, is warranted to capture the events and correlate the clinical and electrographic findings.

Any destructive or infiltrative lesion affecting the vestibular cortex can cause vertigo. Neuroimaging studies are indicated especially when the neurologic examination and/or EEG show focal findings. Among the different modalities available, MRI is more helpful than computed tomography (CT), especially in the investigation of the posterior fossa and also more sensitive in visualizing subtle signal changes in the gray-white matter junction that might point to possible cortical malformations. Other structural and functional imaging modalities such as PET, single-photon emission computed tomography (SPECT) scans, and magnetoencephalography (MEG) may also be performed as part of the workup, especially if surgery is being considered.[19]

Treatment

When seizures are determined to be the cause of episodic vertigo, treatment with antiepileptic drugs (AEDs) can be discussed with the patient and the family. Most physicians would start treatment after two unprovoked seizures because of the increased risk of subsequent seizures. The choice of AED is mainly based on the EEG findings. However, since there are a wide variety of AEDs to choose from, other factors that might influence the choice of AED also include side-effect profile, frequency of taking the medication, and cost, all of which could affect medication compliance.[20] When the patient continues to have seizures despite optimal medical management, a referral to an epilepsy center for presurgical evaluation is necessary.[21]

Conclusion

Vertigo as a sole manifestation of seizure is rare. The diagnosis is easier when the symptom occurs as an aura followed by motor involvement or alteration of level of consciousness. However, when the episodes of vertigo are short and lack positional triggers, and there is a personal or a family history of epilepsy, then the patient should have a complete neuro-otologic assessment and EEG as part of his or her diagnostic evaluation.

Self-Assessment Questions

1. Which statement is true regarding epileptic vertigo?
   a. It is a frequent manifestation of seizure.
   b. The term can be used interchangeably with dizziness.
   c. It is associated mainly with lesions in the temporal lobe.
   d. It is a type of nonepileptic seizure.
   e. None of the above.

2. Which is not a common peripheral cause of vertigo?
   a. Drugs
   b. Tullio's phenomenon
   c. Migraine
   d. Acoustic neuroma
   e. Ménière's disease

3. Which statement regarding duration of symptoms of vertigo is correct?
   a. Benign paroxysmal vertigo of children lasts seconds to minutes.
   b. Vertigo from stroke usually lasts 20 to 30 minutes.
   c. Epileptic vertigo lasts less than a minute.
   d. Both a and c.
   e. All of the above.

4. Workup and management for recurrent episodes of vertigo includes:
   a. Complete neuro-otologic examination
   b. Normal awake EEG, which can rule out epilepsy as a cause of vertigo

c. Cranial CT scan, which is sufficient
d. Trial of anticonvulsants before diagnostic tests are performed
e. A normal hearing test, which essentially rules out a peripheral disease

5. Cerebral perfusion PET studies in response to cold caloric stimulation demonstrated activation of:
   a. Ipsilateral temporoparietal junction
   b. Contralateral posterior cingulate cortex
   c. Ipsilateral primary sensory cortex
   d. Ipsilateral anterior cingulate cortex
   e. Contralateral posterior insular cortex

References

1. Neuhauser HK, Radtke A, von Brevern M. Burden of dizziness and vertigo in the community. *Arch Intern Med.* 2008;168:2118–2124.
2. Kogeorgos J, Scott DF, Swash M. Epileptic dizziness. *Br Med J.* 1981;282:687–689.
3. Bisdorff A, von Brevern M, Lempert T, Newman-Toker DE. Classification of vestibular symptoms: Towards an international classification of vestibular disorders. *J Vestib Res.* 2009;19:1–13.
4. Bladin PF. History of epileptic vertigo: Its medical, social, and forensic problems. *Epilepsia.* 1998;39:442–447.
5. Penfield WG, Boldrey E. Somatic motor and sensory representation in the cerebral cortex of man as studied by electrical stimulation. *Brain.* 1937;60:389–443.
6. Penfield WG, Jasper H. Epilepsy and functional anatomy of the human brain. Boston, MA: Little, Brown; 1954.
7. Laff R, Mesad S, Devinsky O. Epileptic kinetopsia: Ictal illusory motion perception. *Neurology.* 2003;61:1262–1264.
8. Bottini G, Sterzi R, Paulesu E, et al. Identification of the central vestibular projections in man: A positron emission tomography activation study. *Exper Brain Res.* 1994;99:164–169.
9. Guldin WO, Grusser O-J. Is there a vestibular cortex? *Trends Neurosci.* 1998;21:254–259.
10. Lopez C, Heydrich L, Seeck M, Blanke O. Abnormal self-localization and vestibular vertigo in a patient with right frontal lobe epilepsy. *Epilepsy Behav.* 2010;17:289–292.
11. Kim DW, Sunwoo J-S, Lee SK. Incidence and localizing value of vertigo and dizziness in patients with epilepsy: Video-EEG monitoring study. *Epilepsy Res.* 2016;126:102–105.
12. Blume WT, Luders HO, Mizrahi E, Tassinari C, van Emde Boas W, Engel J. ILAE Commision Report: Glossary of descriptive terminology for ictal semiology: Report of the ILAE Task Force on classification and terminology. *Epilepsia.* 2001;42:1212–1218.
13. Tarnutzer AA, Lee S-H, Robinson KA, Kaplan PW, Newman-Toker DE. Clinical and electrographic findings in epileptic vertigo and dizziness: A systematic review. *Neurology.* 2015;84:1595–1604.
14. Lehnen N, Langhagen T, Heinen F, Huppert D, Brant T, Jahn K. Vestibular paroxysmia in children: A treatable cause of short vertigo attacks. *Dev Med Child Neurol.* 2015;57:393–396.
15. Eviatar L, Eviatar A. Vertigo in children: Differential diagnosis and treatment. *Pediatrics.* 1977;59:833–838.
16. Mendez OE, Brenner RP. Increasing the yield of EEG. *J Clin Neurophysiol.* 2006;23:282–293.
17. Niedermeyer E, Rocca U. The diagnostic significance of sleep electroencephalograms in temporal lobe epilepsy. A comparison of scalp

and depth tracings. *Eur J Neurol.* 1972;7: 119–129.
18. Ellingson RJ, Wilken K, Bennett DR. Efficacy of sleep deprivation as an activation procedure in epilepsy patients. *J Clin Neurophysiol.* 1984; 1:83–101.
19. Widjaja E, Raybaud C. Advances in neuroimaging in patients with epilepsy. *Neurosurg Focus.* 2008;25:E3.
20. Raspall-Chaure M, Neville BG, Scott RC. The medical management of the epilepsies in children: Conceptual and practical considerations. *Lancet Neurol.* 2008;7:57–69.
21. Go C, Snead III OC. Pharmacologically intractable epilepsy in children: Diagnosis and preoperative evaluation. *Neurosurg Focus.* 2008;25:E2.

CHAPTER 21

Pediatric Movement Disorders

Teesta Soman and Ana Marissa Lagman-Bartolome

Introduction

Movement disorders are conditions characterized by involuntary motor movements that are abnormal in velocity, frequency, initiation, implementation, or posture. These disorders are rare in children; hence, diagnosis and treatment may be challenging.

These disorders are classified into hyperkinetic (dystonia, myoclonus, chorea, dyskinesia, tremor, tics) and hypokinetic (parkinsonism) disorders. Diagnosis involves pattern recognition. Description of the phenomenology of the movements is required for accurate classification.

There are neurologic conditions that may manifest in childhood with abnormal movements and balance abnormalities but are not classified as movement disorder, such as hypotonia, global developmental delay, and cerebral palsy.

Hypotonia is described as reduced resistance to passive range of motion in joints. It is an impairment of the ability to sustain postural control and movement against gravity.[1] Infants with hypotonia may present with poor control of movements, delayed motor skills, and hypotonic movement patterns, which include alterations in postural control, increased range of motion of joints, and abnormal stability and movement mechanics. Global developmental delay (GDD) is defined as a significant delay in two or more of the following developmental domains: gross/fine motor, speech/language, cognition, social/personal, and activities of daily living.[2] Cerebral palsy is a nonspecific, descriptive term pertaining to nonprogressive disordered motor function that is evident in early infancy and is characterized by changes in muscle tone (typically spasticity or rigidity), muscle weakness, involuntary movements, ataxia, or a combination of these abnormalities.[3]

Hyperkinetic Disorders

Dystonia

Clinical Diagnosis

Dystonia is defined as a syndrome of sustained muscle contraction affecting any part of the body, which frequently causes twisting and repetitive movements or abnormal postures as well as balance problems. Classification of dystonia is based on age of onset, etiology, or somatic distribution. Etiology of dystonia is described in Table 21–1. Primary dystonia refers to dystonia as the only clinical

Table 21–1. Classification of Dystonia

Classification	*Types*	*Description*
Primary	Genetic dystonias	DYT 1-20
Secondary	Infectious	Encephalitis
	Vascular	Stroke
	Toxic	
	Autoimmune	Vasculitis
	Others	Multiple sclerosis
Neurodegenerative	Lysosomal storage disorders	Niemann-Pick type C, Krabbe, GM gangliosidosis, neuronal ceroid lipofuscinosis, Pelizaeus Merzbacher, metachromatic leukodystrophy, Sandhoff disease
	Mitochondrial disorders	Leigh's disease, Mohr- Tranenbrug syndrome, MELAS NARP (neuropathy, ataxia, retinitis pigmentosa) LHON-dystonia syndrome Pyruvate dehydrogenase complex deficiency
	Amino acid and organic acidurias	Glutaric aciduria type I, propionic aciduria, isovaleric acidemia, methylmalonic acidemia, homocystinuria, maple syrup urine disease, d-2-hydroxyglutaric aciduria, tetrahydrobiopterin metabolism disorders
	Other metabolic disorders	Molybdenum cofactor deficiency, GLUT1 deficiency, Wilson's disease, CSF neurotransmitter disorders, Pantothenate kinase associated neurodegeneration (PKAN), Lesch-Nyhan disease
	Trinucleotide repeat disorders	Spinocerebellar ataxia type 3 (Machado-Joseph), dentato-rubro-pallido-luysian atrophy (DRPLA)

Source: [19]

feature, while secondary dystonia, also called symptomatic dystonia, occurs in the context of a precipitant such as brain injury or toxic drug exposure. Heredodegenerative dystonias consist of a heterogeneous group of inherited, progressive neurodegenerative conditions as listed in Table 21–1.

Primary Dystonia

Primary dystonia syndromes are genetic in nature. On examination, there are dystonia and sometimes other neurologic findings, but these are not associated with known neuropathologic findings. The most common forms include the following.

1. Primary Torsion Dystonia (DYT-1). This condition begins in early to late childhood with dystonia in the lower extremities and is progressive. It is an autosomal-dominant disorder caused by a mutation in *TOR1A* gene, with incomplete penetrance. Cognition is largely intact, although executive function may be impaired.[4] This condition responds to some medications, and remarkable response has been noted with deep brain stimulation.[5]

2. Dopa-Responsive Dystonia (DRD, DYT5, Segawa Disease). This is also known as hereditary progressive dystonia with diurnal fluctuations[6] presenting in children with previously normal motor and cognitive development. It typically begins with foot dystonia, gait abnormalities, and hyperreflexia, progressing to generalized dystonia.

It is an autosomal-dominant disorder caused by a point mutation in the gene for guanosine triphosphate cyclohydrolase 1, which is the gene involved in the synthesis of tetrahydrobiopterin, a cofactor in dopamine synthesis. Autosomal-recessive forms of *DYT5* also occur due to mutation in the tyrosine hydroxylase gene. Dopa-responsive dystonia responds well with treatment of levodopa.

3. Myoclonus-Dystonia (DYT11). Myoclonus-dystonia presents with dystonia of arms, trunk, and oromandibular regions associated with brief myoclonic jerks in childhood or adolescence. Myoclonic jerks may cause a loss in balance and precipitate falls. It improves with alcohol. It is a rare autosomal-dominant disorder involving mutations or deletions in the ε-sarcoglycan gene on chromosome 7 (*SGCE*).

Over the course of the past few years, over 20 genes have been identified in association with primary dystonias. Some of the other genetic dystonia that may present in childhood include DYT-6 (*THAP1*), DYT 12 (*ATP 1A13*), DYT 24 (*ANO3*), DYT 25 (*GNAL*), and DYT 28 (*KMT2B*).[7]

Secondary Dystonias

Pantothenate Kinase-Associated Neurodegeneration (PKAN, Hallervorden-Spatz Disease). PKAN is a complex neurodegenerative disorder with clinical features including extrapyramidal features (dystonia, dysarthria, and rigidity), choreoathetosis, ataxia, corticospinal tract involvement (spasticity, hyperreflexia, extensor plantar response), and 66% may present with pigmentary retinopathy. PKAN classically presents with early onset (3–4 years old) of movement abnormalities, most commonly dystonic symptoms in younger children followed by rapid disease progression with loss of ability to ambulate within 10 to 15 years of onset. Other clinical features include global developmental delay and seizures. Atypical PKAN presents with mean age of onset at 13 to 14 years with more prominent behavioral and speech problems followed by pyramidal and extrapyramidal signs that occur later.

Diagnosis includes genetic testing for mutations in pantothenate kinase 2 (*PANK2*), which regulated synthesis of acetyl coenzyme A resulting in iron accumulation in the globus pallidus. Cranial magnetic resonance imaging (MRI) shows the typical "eye of the tiger" appearance consisting of hypointensity of the globus pallidus with central area of increased signal on T2 images. Management remains symptomatic. Deferiprone and vitamin B5 have been used to alter the disease course, with limited benefit.

Wilson's Disease (WD). Wilson's disease is a disease of copper metabolism involving systemic manifestations including liver (acute liver failure, liver cirrhosis), cornea (Kayser-Fleischer rings), and brain (degeneration and necrosis of lenticular nuclei, brainstem, thalamus, cerebellum, and cerebral cortex) involvement.

Clinical onset is late childhood, early adolescence, or the third to fourth decade of adulthood. It initially presents with bulbar symptoms (dysphagia, drooling, and dystonia of bulbar muscles); speech difficulties (dysarthria, ataxic speech, hypophonia, scanning speech, and rarely anarthria and mutism); limb dystonia that impairs writing and walking; dystonic posturing of trunk, neck, jaw, and face ("vacuous smile"); cerebellar features (tremor, unsteady gait, and limb ataxia); and psychiatric or behavioral disturbances (hyperactivity, inattention, impulsivity, or psychosis). Patients with WD may present with other movement disorders as well. Biochemical markers including low serum ceruloplasmin, high 24-hour urinary copper excretion, and high serum free copper estimation are not confirmatory but are suggestive of WD. Liver biopsy is recommended to document increased copper metabolism. MRI shows diffuse volume loss (75%) and hypointensity (T1 images) of basal ganglia (66%) due to iron deposition in exchange for copper.

First lines of therapy include copper chelating agents (D-penicillamine, trientine, ammonium tetrathiomolybdate) to control toxic levels of copper. Zinc salts (zinc sulfate, zinc gluconate, and zinc acetate) are also used as well as dietary control (decreasing consumption of copper-rich foods like chocolate, nuts, shellfish, and liver) and symptomatic treatment of movement and psychiatric disorders.

Management of Dystonia

Children or adolescents who present with dystonia should be given a trial of levodopa (L-dopa/carbidopa combination at 50/12.5 mg to 100/25 mg administered for 5–7 days). Anticholinergic medication, which includes trihexyphenidyl (Artane: initial 1 mg/day to 40–80 mg/day or occasionally higher), can be given as well. The next line of treatment includes baclofen, clonazepam, muscle relaxants (tizanidine, cyclobenzaprine), and anticonvulsant medications (carbamazepine, gabapentin).[8] Oral baclofen (started at 5–10 mg/day and gradually titrated as tolerated) is useful in children with spasticity or as an adjunct to trihexyphenidyl. Botulinum toxin injection is the treatment of choice for most forms of focal dystonia (blepharospasm, jaw dystonia, spasmodic dystonia, cervical dystonia, and focal dystonia of hand) and in generalized dystonia in children to target specific group of muscles, with benefit lasting for 3 to 4 months.

Surgical Treatment of Dystonia

Intrathecal Baclofen. Intrathecal baclofen (ITB) administered through an implanted intrathecal catheter is considered for patients with intractable generalized secondary dystonia. Complications of ITB include infections at the catheter or pump site, decreased head and neck control, drowsiness, cerebrospinal leaks, and catheter or pump malfunction. Two of the most serious potential complications include baclofen withdrawal, which occurs with pump depletion or malfunction (severe exacerbation of dystonia, itchiness, hyperthermia, agitation, seizures, and psychosis), and overdose, which occurs during programming (hypotension and respiratory depression).

Deep Brain Stimulation. Deep brain stimulation (DBS) of the globus pallidus interna is an important therapy for treatment of patients with refractory dystonia (DYT-1 or non-DYT-1 primary generalized dystonia) but is less effective for secondary dystonia, such as in cerebral palsy.[9] There is a delay of several months between implantation of stimulators and benefit; however, improvement continues over 6 months to a year. Complications of DBS include brain hemorrhage; stroke; infection at local site, on chest, or overlying the area of the leads; lead breakage (fracture of wire) or migration; battery failure; and death. A few cases of depression and suicide have also been reported in adults.

Paroxysmal Dyskinesia

Paroxysmal Nonkinesiogenic Dyskinesia/DYT 8

Paroxysmal nonkinesiogenic dyskinesia is also known as paroxysmal dystonic choreoathetosis or paroxysmal dyskinesia of Mount and Reback. This disorder has been linked to a gene on chromosome 2q34, which is the myofibrillogenesis regulator 1 (MR-1) gene. Clinical features include transient episodes of abnormal involuntary movement or dyskinesias (chorea, ballismus, dystonia, and dysphagia) precipitated by exposure to alcohol, coffee, tea, chocolate, fatigue, hunger, and stress. Attacks last for 10 to 15 minutes or even longer, up to several hours. Neurologic examination is normal in between the attacks.

This condition is resistant to treatment. Medications that have been tried include benzodiazepines, acetazolamide, neuroleptics (haloperidol), and antiepileptics (valproic acid, carbamazepine, and gabapentin), and they had variable effect. Clonazepam is usually the most effective treatment.

Paroxysmal Kinesiogenic Dyskinesia/DYT 10

Paroxysmal kinesiogenic dyskinesia (PKD) is also known as paroxysmal kinesiogenic choreoathetosis with age onset at 6 to 16 years. Attack onset may coincide with puberty, although an adult onset idiopathic form also exists. Attacks can be unilateral or bilateral and occur multiple times a day, lasting a few seconds to minutes. Precipitating factors include sudden movements like standing up, walking, running, or jumping, or even focal movements like stretching of the arms. Other triggers are caffeine, marijuana, cold, humidity, hunger, external motion, and startle (rare). Anxiety can lower the threshold for paroxysms. Neurologic examination is normal in between events. This is an autosomal-dominant disorder; hence, family history is often positive with the proline-rich transmembrane protein 2 (PRRT2) gene. The patient may outgrow symptoms in adulthood.

PKD responds well to treatment with antiepileptics, and carbamazepine is usually the drug of choice.

Paroxysmal Exercise-Induced Dyskinesia

Movements usually involve lower extremities but both upper and lower extremities can be affected. Attacks usually last 5 to 30 minutes and are precipitated by continuous walking, running, or exercise, as well as cold and stress. Paroxysmal exercise-induced dyskinesia can be familial or sporadic. Autosomal-dominant paroxysmal exercise-induced dyskinesia combined with primary generalized epilepsy has been associated with mutations in the *SLC2A1* gene that codes for the glucose transported GLUT1, which responds to the ketogenic diet.

Myoclonus

Clinical Diagnosis

Myoclonus is defined as a brief, shock-like, jerky involuntary movement involving one or more muscle groups. Myoclonus may result in disturbance of balance and cause falls. Classification of myoclonus can be based on distribution (focal, multifocal, segmental, or generalized) or origin of the myoclonus generator—cortical, subcortical, brainstem, spinal, or segmental. Myoclonus is associated with several epileptic neurodegenerative conditions including mitochondrial disorders (mitochondrial encephalopathy with ragged red fibers or MERRF, Lafora body disease, neuronal ceroid lipofuscinosis [NCL]) and other neurometabolic disorders such as nonketotic hyperglycinemia, GLUT1 deficiency, biotinidase and cobalamin deficiency, Wilson's disease, sialidosis type 1, and lipid storage disorders (GM gangliosidoses, Gaucher disease type III, juvenile galactosialidosis).[10]

Hyperekplexia

Hyperekplexia is defined as a pathological exaggeration of normal startle response. It is described as a reflex jerk to auditory, somatic, or visual stimuli producing sudden grimace or abduction of arms and flexion of neck, trunk, elbows, hips, and knees. Hereditary hyperekplexia is due to mutation in the α-subunit of glycine receptor leading to disruption in the chloride ion channel. It manifests in neonates as repeated episodes of stiffness ("stiff-baby syndrome"), occasionally with apnea. A classic feature includes a prominent startle response to nose taps that does not suppress with repeated testing. In older children or adults, there is hyperekplexia, wide-based gait (compensatory to repeated falls secondary to startle), tonic spasm, and paroxysmal jerks that may respond to clonazepam. These patients may also present with seizures, and some are at risk of respiratory arrest as tonic laryngeal spasm may occur. This condition is also known as idiopathic hyperekplexia in the absence of family history, and glycine receptor mutation has not been identified in these patients.

Chorea

Clinical Diagnosis

Chorea is described as an involuntary movement that is brief, irregular, nonrhythmic, and nonpurposeful and that flows from one body part to another, occurring randomly without any pattern. The movements last longer than myoclonus but are briefer than dystonia. Chorea is usually present at rest and may increase with distracting maneuvers. It is partially suppressible or incorporated into voluntary movement to mask the impairment and disappears with sleep. The term *ballismus* is used when there are large-amplitude, intense, and flinging movements involving proximal muscle groups. Common etiologies of chorea in children are listed in Table 21–2.[11]

Sydenham's Chorea

Sydenham's chorea (SC) is the most common cause of secondary chorea in children, which is autoimmune in origin. Chorea usually begins within 2 to 6 months following infection with group A β-hemolytic streptococcal pharyngitis. The movements are usually generalized, although 20% to 30% of patients have hemichorea. Other movements include a "piano playing" pattern of repetitive hand movements, motor impersistence (unable to maintain firm grasp or "milkmaid's grip"), and Adder's tongue or darting tongue (unable to maintain tongue protrusion). Other clinical features include emotional lability and behavioral changes including obsessive-compulsive behavior. About 30% of patients may have recurrent symptoms months or years after cessation of initial illness. Female patients may have recurrence of symptoms years later when exposed to oral contraceptives or estrogen therapy or during pregnancy (chorea gravidarum).

Diagnosis of Sydenham's chorea is by history and is supported by the presence of elevated antistreptolysin O (ASO) titer, elevated anti-DNA-ase B titer, and a positive streptozyme test or positive throat culture for streptococcus pyogenes.

SC is usually self-limited and resolves within 6 months. Valproic acid or tetrabenazine are useful in severe or prolonged cases. Other treatments given are prednisone at 2 mg/kg/day for 4 weeks and intravenous immunoglobulin for severe and protracted cases. Treatment with oral penicillin for 10 days is also given to prevent rheumatic fever as well as penicillin prophylaxis for dental or surgical interventions if indicated in the presence of carditis.

Tremor

Clinical Diagnosis

Tremor is described as a rhythmic, involuntary, oscillatory movement around a central point involving one or more body parts. Tremor can be broadly classified into rest

Table 21–2. Etiology of Chorea in Childhood

Classification	*Etiology*	
Primary	Benign hereditary chorea	TTIF-1 gene on chromosome 14
Secondary	Infection	Bacterial, viral, and tuberculous meningoencephalitis
	Endocrine or nutritional derangement	Hypo-/hypernatremia, hypocalcemia, hyperthyroidism, hypo-/hyperglycemia, hypomagnesemia, vitamin B12 deficiency in infancy, hyperthyroidism, hypoparathyroidism
	Vascular	Stroke, moyamoya disease, antiphospholipid antibody syndrome, hypoxic ischemic injury, post-pump chorea (after cardiac surgery)
	Autoimmune	Systemic lupus erythematosus, demyelinating disorders, Sydenham's chorea, vasculitis, NMDA-receptor encephalitis, central nervous system vasculitis, Rasmussen's encephalitis, Behçet's disease, systemic lupus erythematosus[11]
	Toxins	Manganese, methanol, carbon monoxide, bilirubin (kernicterus)
	Drugs	Neuroleptics, oral contraceptives, phenytoin, gabapentin, ethosuximide, valproic acid, amphetamine, lithium, anticholinergics, antihistamines, opioid agonists, calcium channel blockers
	Neurodegenerative	Huntington's disease (akinetic-rigid syndrome in childhood); Huntington's-disease-like illness 3; spinocerebellar ataxia 1, 2, 3, 6, and 17; ataxia-telangiectasia; Pelizaeus-Merzbacher disease type 1
	Neurometabolic disorders	Organic acidemia (propionic acidemia, methylmalonic acidemia, cobalamin C disease, glutaric aciduria type 1), aminoaciduria (nonketotic hyperglycinemia, homocystinuria, phenylketonuria), mitochondrial disorders (Leigh syndrome, POL-G related disorders, pyruvate carboxylase deficiency, pyruvate dehydrogenase complex deficiency), Lesh-Nyhan disease, Wilson's disease, neurodegeneration with brain iron accumulation, lipid storage disorders (GM gangliosidosis, Sandhoff disease, metachromatic leukodystrophy, Gaucher type 2, Niemann-Pick disease type C), GLUT1 deficiency, and neurotransmitter diseases
	Pregnancy	Chorea gravidarum
	Psychogenic	
	Paroxysmal disorders	Exercise-induced dyskinesia Paroxysmal kinesigenic or nonkinesigenic dyskinesia

tremor and action tremor. Rest tremor is present when the limb is fully at rest, supported by gravity without any voluntary contraction of involved muscles. Tremor occurring during voluntary contraction of muscles is known as action tremor. Action tremor can be postural (when the limb is held in a certain posture), kinetic (when performing a certain movement), or intentional (when exacerbated toward the end of a goal directed movement). Table 21–3 lists some common etiologies of tremor in children.

Essential Tremor

Clinical Diagnosis. Essential tremor is a familial, autosomal-dominant condition, with onset in childhood or early or late adulthood. Tremor is postural involving the arms, but the face, neck, legs, and voice may also be affected with frequency ranging from 4 Hz (adults) to 10 Hz (younger children). It is typically absent at rest. The remaining neurologic examination and cognition are normal, although tandem gait may become abnormal later in the course.

Management. Management for mild tremor may only require modification of activities, such as larger pencil grip. Propranolol is used at doses of 40 to 80 mg/day in children. Adverse effects include hypotension and limited exercise tolerance. Primidone at a dose of 50 to 100 mg/day in children is also effective.

Table 21–3. Etiology of Tremor in Childhood

Classification	*Etiology*	
Physiologic	Metabolic	Hyperthyroidism, hyperparathyroidism, hypoglycemia
	Neurometabolic disorders	Wilson's disease, cystinosis, Hartnup's disease, neurodegeneration with brain iron accumulation, biotinidase deficiency, MELAS, Kearns-Sayre syndrome, Niemann-Pick disease type C, fucosidosis, GLUT1 deficiency, neurotransmitter diseases
	Drugs	Caffeine, theophylline, caffeine-containing drinks, amphetamines, valproic acid, ß-agonists, etc
	Withdrawal of drugs	Benzodiazepines
	Systemic	Fever, sepsis, anxiety, stress, fatigue
Primary or idiopathic		Essential tremor, task-specific, orthostatic, idiopathic palatal tremor
Associated with neurological disorders		Parkinsonism, Wilson's, multiple sclerosis, stroke, AV malformation, head trauma, midbrain tremor
Peripheral neuropathies		Commonly associated with mild or moderate weakness and associated with sustained posture, or in the context of muscle fatigue
Other rhythmical movement disorders		Head bobbing, hereditary chin quivering, spasmus nutans, and psychogenic

Source: [20]

The most significant side effect is sedation, but this can be minimized by initiation of therapy at low doses with slow titration. Other drugs that have provided benefit include benzodiazepines (alprazolam or clonazepam), gabapentin, and topiramate. Deep brain stimulation of the thalamus has been found very effective in disabled adult patients. Tremors may respond to alcohol, hence the risk for alcoholism in patients with severe essential tremor.

Ataxia

Clinical Diagnosis

Ataxia refers to a disturbance in the smooth performance of voluntary motor acts leading to poor coordination and balance problems. It includes unsteadiness of stance (abasia), decomposition of complex movements into isolated, successive parts (asynergia), abnormal excursions in movement (dysmetria), impaired performance of rapid alternating movements (dysdiadochokinesis), and impaired check/excessive rebound responses.[12] Lesions in the vermis result in truncal ataxia and head bobbing (titubation), while cerebellar hemispheric lesions cause limb ataxia. Common etiologies of ataxia in children are listed in Table 21–4.

Acute Cerebellar Ataxia

Clinical Diagnosis. Acute cerebellar ataxia is characterized by rapid onset of ataxia, fine motor incoordination, and headache, initially preceded by prodromal febrile or viral illness (75%) or following immunizations (varicella, rabies, hepatitis B).

Etiology of acute cerebellar ataxia is uncertain, but it is considered to be a post-viral inflammatory disease. Initial evaluation should include neuroimaging to exclude mass lesion or cerebellar malformation and lumbar puncture to rule out central nervous system infection. Metabolic workup to exclude glutaric aciduria, which presents with episodic ataxia, should be considered as well.

Management. There is no specific treatment for acute cerebellar ataxia. Spontaneous complete recovery occurs in 90% of patients. Steroids and intravenous immunoglobulin have been used for treatment as well as acyclovir because of association with varicella. The mainstay of treatment is physical and occupational therapy, but treatment is often not successful and children with even static forms of ataxia usually fail to improve despite intervention.

Tic Disorders and Tourette Syndrome

Tics

Tics are defined as intermittent, sudden, repetitive, nonrhythmic, and discrete movements.

Clinical Diagnosis

When the movements involve the skeletal muscles alone, they are known as motor tics. When the laryngeal and/or pharyngeal musculature is also involved, leading to the production of sound, they are known as phonic or vocal tics. *Motor tics* can be simple like eye blinking, grimacing, nose twitching, or shoulder jerking. Complex motor tics appear to be more purposeful like kicking, jumping, tapping, hitting oneself, head shaking, or body flexion. Motor tics might also occasionally cause balance problems. *Simple vocal tics* include sniffing, grunting, squeaking, throat clearing, humming, or coughing. *Complex vocal tics* include repetitive spoken words or syllables, shouting, echolalia, palilalia, and at times, coprolalia. This is less common. Simple motor or vocal tics such as eye blinking and sniffing are often mistaken for allergy symptoms, and children are subjected to repeated visits to the doctor as well as administered anti-allergic medications.

Table 21–4. Etiology of Ataxia in Childhood

Classification	*Etiology*	
Primary	Spinocerebellar ataxias (Machado-Joseph disease), ataxia-telangiectasia, ataxia-oculomotor apraxia, Friedrich's ataxia, dentato-rubro-pallido-luysian atrophy (DRPLA), olivopontocerebellar atrophy (OPCA), Marinesco-Sjögren syndrome, Pelizaeus-Merzbacher disease, childhood ataxia with central hypomyelination (CACH) syndrome	
Secondary	Static injury or structural	Cerebral palsy, stroke, trauma, hypoxic injury, Joubert's syndrome, Dandy-Walker malformation, Chiari malformation, cerebellar malformations
	Metabolic disorders	Hartnup's disease, lipidoses, mitochondrial disorders, glutaric aciduria, Refsum's disease, lysosomal storage disorders, propionic acidemia, maple syrup urine disease, urea cycle disorders, porphyria, congenital disorders of glycosylation (CDG), abetalipoproteinemia, electrolyte or glucose disturbances
	Vitamin deficiency	B12, E, thiamine
	Neoplastic or paraneoplastic	Tumors of cerebellum or brainstem, neuroblastoma of chest or abdomen
	Neurodegenerative disorders	Ceroid lipofuscinosis
	Niemann-Pick type C	
	Hypothyroidism	
	Drugs/toxins	Antiepileptic medications; antihistamines; barbiturates; lithium; alcohol; chemotherapy; heavy metal poisoning like lead, mercury, thallium, and bromide
	Immune mediated, demyelinating	Acute postinfectious cerebellitis, Millet-Fischer variant of Guillain Barré syndrome, multiple sclerosis
	Paroxysmal	Dominant familial episodic ataxias (EA1, EA2)
	Calcium channel disorders	
	Basilar migraine	

Source: [19]

Tics occur more frequently in boys and usually start around the age of 7 years. However, it can start as early as 3 to 5 years of age. Tics can occur throughout the day and even occasionally in sleep. Tics wax and wane in frequency and intensity over weeks to months. They can migrate from one location to another. One unique feature of tics that distinguishes them from other movement disorders is that a sensory (premonitory) urge is present, often described as a feeling of pain, burning, or restlessness. The performance of the movement/tic provides transient relief from the sensation. This premonitory urge is often reported even by children, particularly those over the age of 10 years. Tics can be voluntarily suppressed by the individual for short periods of time. Family history is often positive. In many children, tics spontaneously subside as they grow into adults.

Etiology

Primary or hereditary tic disorders are the most common. Tics may also occur secondary to infections, drugs, toxins, stroke, head trauma, and metabolic or degenerative disorders. Table 21–5 shows the classification and diagnosis of tics in children.

Tourette Syndrome (also known as Gilles de la Tourette Syndrome)

Tourette syndrome (TS) is a condition associated with motor and vocal tics, present for over 1 year with no tic-free interval of more than 3 months. Comorbidities associated with TS include attention deficit hyperactivity disorder (ADHD), obsessive-compulsive disorder (OCD), rage attacks, conduct disorder, oppositional defiant disorder, learning disability, and sleep disorders. Often, these symptoms are more disabling to the patients than the tics themselves. Table 21–6 shows the *Diagnostic and Statistical Manual of Mental Disorders,* fifth edition (*DSM-5*) diagnostic criteria for Tourette syndrome.

Table 21–6. Clinical Criteria for Diagnosis of Tourette Syndrome (*DSM-5*)

- Two or more motor tics, one or more vocal tics
- Duration more than 1 year
- Age of onset—before 18 years
- Not a symptom of any other or medical condition or physiological effects of a substance

Table 21–5. Classification and Diagnosis of Tic Disorders

Provisional tic disorder	Single or multiple motor or vocal tics, for at least 4 weeks, but not longer than 12 months
Persistent (chronic) motor tic disorder or chronic vocal tic disorder	Single or multiple motor or vocal tics, but not both present at some time during the illness throughout a period of more than 1 year, without a tic-free period of more than three consecutive months
Tourette syndrome	See Table 21-6
Tic disorder not otherwise specified	Cases that do not meet the criteria for a specific tic disorder

Management

Not all tics require medical treatment. Often, reassurance alone is sufficient. Indications for treatment include the following:

1. The tics are extremely severe in intensity or frequency, causing functional impairment.
2. Tics are causing social impairment, eg, poor self-esteem, bullying.
3. Tics are causing pain or a likelihood that the child may hurt himself or herself or others.

Medical suppression is only partial, and often additional educational, psychological, or social support is needed. Teachers and other community members should be educated, and parents, teachers, and the child should be accepting of these impairments.

Medications. Typical neuroleptics (pimozide, haloperidol, fluphenazine) and atypical neuroleptics (risperidone, Seroquel, Abilify [aripiprazole]) have been the mainstay of treatment for tics and TS. Some commonly used medications are listed in Table 21–7. Children with tics and ADHD can be treated with stimulants, and this was demonstrated in the TACT study (Treatment of ADHD in Children with Tics). In this 16-week study, for tics, all treated groups improved (not placebo) with a 25% reduction in tic rating scales. Thus, tics were not exacerbated with a stimulant (methylphenidate) and showed a reduction, even in the group treated with Methylphenidate alone.

Botulinum Toxin. Botulinum toxin injections can be used if a particular tic is very disabling. Botulinum toxin injections have been reported to abolish the sensory urge as well as the motor movement themselves. However, this is not usually used in children.

Deep Brain Stimulation. Deep brain stimulation (DBS) is the newest and most exciting option for severe tics, and a few anecdotal cases have been reported. It is not a clinically approved (U.S. Food and Drug Administration) therapy for tics. The TSA medical and scientific advisory groups have issued a statement regarding DBS. A comprehensive review of treatment by the Medical Advisory Board of the Tourette Syndrome Association is available (https://tourette.org).

Hypokinetic/Akinetic Rigid Movement Disorders

Akinetic rigid disorders (also known as parkinsonism) are characterized by bradykinesia and

Table 21–7. Medications for Management of Tics

Name	*Dose*	*Side Effects*
Risperidone	0.5 to 2 mg/day	Extrapyramidal effects (eg, rigidity), weight gain, hypertension
Clonidine	0.05 to 0.1 mg three times a day	Sedation
Guanfacine	0.5 to 2 mg twice a day	Sedation
Tetrabenazine	25 to 100 mg/day	Depression

rigidity. Postural instability causing balance problems is often associated with this condition.

Clinical Diagnosis

Juvenile Parkinson's Disease

Juvenile Parkinson's disease is defined as parkinsonism with onset at age 20 years or less. Tremors, bradykinesia, rigidity, and postural instability occur, often symmetrically.[13] Dystonia and autonomic dysfunction may be more common than in adult Parkinson disease.[14]

The cause of juvenile parkinsonism is often not found. Most common etiologies of parkinsonism in childhood are listed in Table 21–8. Japanese studies were first to identify an autosomal-recessive form of juvenile parkinsonism (AR-JP), now known to harbor the *parkin gene mutation* (*PARK2*, 6q25.2-27).[15] This genetic form may account for more than 50% of juvenile parkinsonism and young-onset Parkinson disease. Patients with *PARK2* usually progress slowly and respond well to levodopa, but experience motor fluctuations and levodopa-induced dyskinesias early in the course of treatment.

Table 21–8. Etiology of Parkinsonism in Childhood

Primary Conditions	
	Juvenile parkinsonism
	Juvenile Huntington's disease
Secondary Conditions	
Infection	Viral—Epstein-Barr virus, HIV
	Spirochete—Neurosyphillis
	Mycoplasma
Metabolic/endocrine	Hypoparathyroidism
	Pseudoparathyroidism
	Wilson's disease
Neurodegenerative	Mitochondrial disease
	Niemann-Pick C disease
	GM2 gangliosidosis
	PKAN
Structural lesions	Sphenoid wing meningioma
Drug induced	Neuroleptics
	Calcium channel blockers (Flunarizine)
	Valproic acid
Trauma	Repetitive head injury ("pugilist's encephalopathy")
	Direct trauma to substantia nigra

Autosomal-dominant juvenile parkinsonism (AD-JP) was found to have mutations in α-*synuclein* (*SNCA*, 4q21). The age at onset varies, with some patients developing symptoms before age 20 years. AD-JP carries a mean age to death of 9.2 years (range 2–20 years) but is otherwise phenomenologically similar to adult Parkinson's disease.[16]

Juvenile Huntington's Disease (Westphal Variant)

About 5% to 10% of all Huntington's disease cases have onset before age 20 years. Patients with juvenile Huntington's disease may have a more rapid progression of symptoms, and disease duration is shorter than in adults, with age at death usually in the second or third decade. In contrast to the adult form of Huntington's disease, which has predominant choreic movements, personality changes, and dementia, juvenile Huntington's disease typically presents with bradykinesia, rigidity, dystonia, and epilepsy, and is often associated with paternal transmission.

Huntington's disease is due to an unstable triplet repeat expansion (>39 CAG repeats) in the *ITI 5* gene (4p16.3) encoding huntingtin. MRI shows atrophy of the cortex and striatum (particularly caudate) and has been demonstrated by volumetric imaging studies as well. There is no clear correlation with the number of triplet repeats and severity of the disease, but there is an inverse correlation the number of CAG repeats and age at onset.[17] *Genetic anticipation* with earlier age at onset in subsequent generations is often observed in families with Huntington disease.

Management

Dopaminergic agents improve motor function.[18] Levodopa is used as the first line of treatment. Motor fluctuation may frequently occur. Dopaminergic agents also include Amantadine, MAO-B inhibitor (eg, entacapone, tolcapone), COMT inhibitor (eg, selegiline, rasagiline), or dopamine agonist (ropinirole). Psychiatric problems like depression and anxiety must be treated symptomatically. Cognitive decline, autonomic disturbances, and gait problems are unfortunately not amenable to treatment. Physical therapy and supportive care for other medical issues should be considered.

Self-Assessment Questions

Case Histories

Case 1

A 10-year-old girl presented with a 2-week history of abnormal movements. The movements were involuntary and consisted of constant movement of her hands. They started in her hands and then progressed to involve her arms. Her parents described her as clumsy, frequently dropping things, restless, and irritable. Her speech was occasionally slurred. She was reported to have strep throat infection 2 months prior to onset of symptoms but has been otherwise healthy. On neurologic examination, she appeared anxious and fidgety with rapid, purposeless, jerky movements in her arms. She was occasionally dysarthric. She had difficulty holding her arms up and difficulty maintaining a continuous grip; however, on motor examination she had normal power, tone, and reflexes. The rest of the examination was normal.

A proper diagnostic test for this child would be which of the following?

a. MRI
b. Examination of cerebrospinal fluid
c. Antistreptolysin O titer
d. None of the above

Case 2

A 15-year-old boy noticed that his leg would stiffen and freeze when changing from seated to standing position. Stiffness improved after a few seconds. Three months later, he noticed that his arms and face would also be occasionally involved, lasting less than 20 seconds. These episodes would occur if he was thinking about a movement. He occasionally reported a sensation of chills down his spine before movements. Born 4 weeks premature but otherwise healthy, he was diagnosed with ADHD but was not on medication. There is no family history of any similar episodes. His neurologic examination was normal. MRI of the head was normal. Routine EEG was normal.

What is the likely diagnosis?

a. Paroxysmal dyskinesia
b. Myoclonus
c. Seizures
d. Tics

Case 3

A 10-year-old boy begins to get into trouble at school for making faces and acting out. The teacher is worried about his behavior. The movements consist of repetitive eye blinking and grimacing. His physical examination was normal.

In order to diagnose this child with tic disorder, which investigation is required?

a. Serum ceruloplasmin
b. Brain MRI
c. α-Fetoprotein level
d. History and physical examination alone

Case 4

A 5-year-old girl, right handed, presented with very gradually progressive symptoms since the age of 2 years consisting of curling of her right-foot toes when walking and jerking of objects from her hand. Later, when writing, it was noticed that she would grip a pen with the fist with contraction of the forearm muscles. She also has frequent falls when walking. Her half-sister had similar problems from 9 years of age and currently is 23 years of age. The neurologic examination was normal except for the involuntary twisting movements in her feet.

What would the best medication to consider for her be?

a. Levodopa
b. Trihexyphenidyl
c. Baclofen
d. Botulinum toxin injections

Additional Questions

1. The factor that best differentiates Tourette syndrome from other chronic tic disorders is the presence of:
   a. A familial inheritance pattern
   b. Both motor and vocal tics
   c. Complex motor tics
   d. Coprolalia
   e. Male gender

2. Ataxia telangiectasia can be diagnosed by measuring levels of which of the following?
   a. Lactic acid
   b. α-Fetoprotein
   c. Long-chain fatty acids
   d. Serum albumin

3. Friedreich ataxia is inherited as which of the following?
   a. Autosomal dominant
   b. Autosomal recessive
   c. Sporadic mutation
   d. None of the above

4. Which of the following statements regarding tic disorders is true?
   a. Girls are more affected than boys.

b. Magnetic resonance imaging frequently demonstrates the etiologic abnormality.
c. Movements are exaggerated with anxiety.
d. Voluntary activities requiring concentration worsen abnormal movements.

5. Which of the following is associated with Gilles de la Tourette syndrome?
   a. Brief periods of loss of consciousness
   b. Gastroesophageal reflux
   c. Seizures
   d. Laboratory evidence of prior streptococcal infection
   e. Obsessive-compulsive behavior

6. Of the following, the most common cause of chorea in childhood is:
   a. Acute rheumatic fever
   b. Pantothenate kinase-associated neurodegeneration
   c. Hyperthyroidism
   d. Juvenile Huntington disease
   e. Systemic lupus erythematosus

References

1. Peredo D, Hannibal M. The floppy infant: Evaluation of hypotonia. *Pediatr Rev*. 2009;30: e66-e76.
2. Shevell M, Ashwal S, Donley D, et al. Practice parameter: Evaluation of the child with global developmental delay: Report of the Quality Standards Subcommittee of the American Academy of Neurology and the Practice Committee of Child Neurology Society. *Neurology*. 2003;60:367–380.
3. Swaiman K, Ashwal S, Ferriero D. Cerebral palsy. In: Swaiman K, Ashwal S, Ferriero D, eds. *Pediatric Neurology Principles and Practice*. 4th ed. Philadelphia, PA: Mosby Elsevier; 2006:491–504.
4. Jahanshahi M, Torkamani M. The cognitive features of idiopathic and DYT1 dystonia. *Mov Disord.* 2017;32(10):1348–1355. doi:10.1002/mds.27048
5. Dupre D, Nangunoori R, Koduri S, Angle C, Cantella D, Whiting D. Disease stabilization of DYT1-positive primary generalized dystonia with deep brain stimulation of the globus pallidus interna: A 15-year follow-up. *Oper Neurosurg*. 2018;14(5):E53–E57.
6. Segawa M, Hosaka A, Miyagawa F, Nomura Y, Imai H. Hereditary progressive dystonia with marked diurnal fluctuation. *Adv Neurol.* 1976;14:215–233.
7. Meijer IA, Pearson TS. The twists of pediatric dystonia: Phenomenology, classification, and genetics. *Semin Pediatr Neurol.* 2018;25:65–74.
8. Swaiman K, Ashwal S, Ferriero D. Disorders of balance and movement. In: Swaiman K, Ashwal S, Ferriero D, eds. *Pediatric Neurology Principles and Practice*. 4th ed. Philadelphia, PA: Mosby Elsevier; 2006:1271–1311.
9. Elia AE, Bagella CF, Ferré F, Zorzi G, Calandrella D, Romito LM. Deep brain stimulation for dystonia due to cerebral palsy: A review. *Eur J Paediatr Neurol.* 2018;22(2):308–315.

10. Christensen CK, Walsh L. Movement disorders and neurometabolic diseases. *Semin Pediatr Neurol.* 2018;25:82–91.
11. deGusmao CM, Waugh JL. Inherited and acquired choreas. *Semin Pediatr Neurol.* 2018; 25:42–53.
12. Swaiman K, Ashwal S, Ferriero D. Cerebellum and the hereditary ataxias. In: Swaiman K, Ashwal S, Ferriero D, eds. *Pediatric Neurology Principles and Practice*. 4th ed. Philadelphia, PA: Mosby Elsevier; 2006:1241–1269.
13. Muthane UB, Swamy HS, Satishchandra P, Subhash MN, Rao S, Subbakrishna D. Early onset Parkinson's disease: Are juvenile- and young-onset different? *Mov Disord.* 1994; 9(5):539–544.
14. Cardoso F, Camargos ST, Silva Junior GA. Etiology of parkinsonism in a Brazilian movement disorders clinic. *Arquivos de Neuro-Psiquiatria.* 1998;56(2):171–175.
15. Bertoli-Avella AM, Giroud-Benitez JL, Akyol A, et al. Novel parkin mutations detected in patients with early-onset Parkinson's disease. *Mov Disord.* 2005;20(4):424–431.
16. Golbe LI, Di Iorio G, Sanges G, et al. Clinical genetic analysis of Parkinson's disease in the Contursi kindred. *Ann Neurol.* 1996;40(5): 767–775.
17. Foroud T, Gray J, Ivashina J, Conneally PM. Differences in duration of Huntington's disease based on age at onset. *J Neurol Neurosurg Psychiatry.* 1999;66(1):52–56.
18. Miyasaki JM, Martin W, Suchowersky O, Weiner WJ, Lang AE. Practice parameter: Initiation of treatment for Parkinson's disease: An evidence-based review: Report of the Quality Standards Subcommittee of the American Academy of Neurology. *Neurology.* 2002;58(1):11–17.
19. Soman T, Lang AE. Movement disorders. *Continuum Lifelong Learning Neurol.* 2009;15(6): 167–190.
20. Lang A. Other Movement Disorders. In: Goldman L, Bennett JC, eds. *Cecil Textbook of Medicine.* 24th ed. Philadelphia, PA: Saunders; 2011.

CHAPTER 22

Ocular and Oculomotility Abnormalities in Children

Y. Arun Reginald

Introduction

An individual's balance is dependent on the integration of accurate afferent vestibular, visual, and proprioceptive information and the calibration and coordination of efferent posture and movement.

During critical periods of visual system plasticity in infancy, sensorimotor "cross talk" between the developing afferent and efferent system is important for mutual calibration.[1–2] Thus, degradation of visual information due to ocular abnormalities present in early development may impact balance directly and indirectly through induction of efferent oculomotility deficits such as nystagmus and strabismus. Conversely, nystagmus, strabismus, and other efferent deficits may affect balance directly or indirectly through additional afferent visual deficits (Figure 22–1).

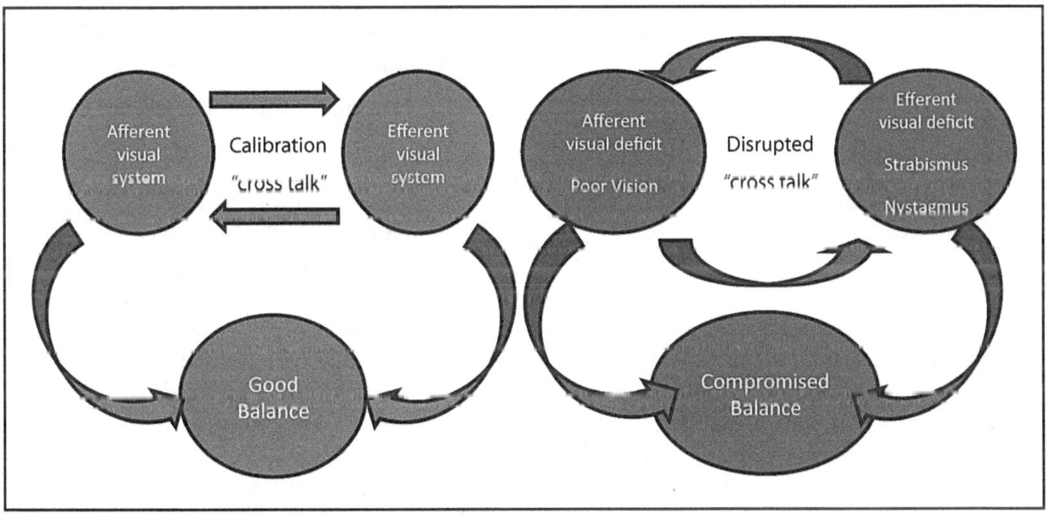

Figure 22–1. Relationship between afferent and efferent visual input and balance. Causes and impact of disrupted "cross talk" on balance.

In adults and adolescents, acute ocular and oculomotility disorders may cause intrusive imbalance symptomology and rapid presentation (Table 22–1). In infants and young children, sensory adaptive mechanisms exist to suppress subjective awareness of image blur (in poor vision), image jump (in nystagmus), or image doubling (in strabismus). In this age group, ocular and oculomotility disorders have transient, well-tolerated, or no symptoms but may result in long-term visual compromise (amblyopia, strabismus, reduced fusion, loss of stereopsis, eccentric viewing, and limited visual acuity) and abnormal postural adaption (torticollis).

Ocular and oculomotility assessment in balance disorder allows for the following:

- Identification of cases where visual system deficits are causative
- Identification of untreated visual impairments that compound balance issues due to other causes, posing limits on function and rehabilitation
- Detection of noncontributory ocular stigmata of systemic and/or inherited causes of imbalance

Visual assessment in imbalance should include the following[3]:

- Age-appropriate assessment of near and distance visual acuity, visual field, and stereopsis
- Oculomotility assessment to detect:
  - Nystagmus and saccadic intrusions
  - Incomitant strabismus and supranuclear/internuclear gaze paresis
  - Ocular torticollis (eye-related abnormal head posture)

Table 22–1. Impact of Ocular and Oculomotility Disorders in Adults and Children

Disorder	*Adults and Adolescents*	*Infants and Young Children*
Afferent defect, reduced acuity, reduced field	Blurring, visual-field defect (scotoma)	Suppression leading to amblyopia[a] Abnormal head posture
Strabismus	Diplopia	Suppression with associated loss of fusion/stereopsis Abnormal retinal correspondence[b] Abnormal head posture
Nystagmus and saccadic intrusions	Oscillopsia[c]	Suppression with associated reduced vision Abnormal head posture toward null point

[a]Ambylopia: central suppression of visual information from a structurally normal eye(s) within the critical developmental period results in a persistent visual deficit (often termed "lazy eye").

[b]Abnormal retinal correspondence: a binocular sensory adaptation to compensate for a long-standing strabismus. The fovea of the straight (nondeviated) eye and a nonfoveal retinal area of the deviated eye are paired, sometimes permitting single binocular vision.

[c]Oscillopsia: subjective perception of blurring or jumping associated with involuntary repetitive eye movements.

Abnormal Head Posture

Abnormal head postures (AHP) may arise from nonocular causes (muscular, skeletal, neurologic, and otolaryngologic) or ocular causes. Abnormal head posture due to eye-related conditions (ocular torticollis) may be adopted for the reasons outlined in Table 22–2. The ocular tilt reaction (OTR) is covered later in this chapter.

Table 22–2. Eye-Related Conditions Leading to Abnormal Head Posture (AHP)[a]

Optimize visual acuity	Nystagmus	AHP to view in null point of nystagmus, that is, eccentric viewing in position of least nystagmus intensity (null point) gives highest visual acuity as the image is at the fovea for longer.
	Ptosis	AHP may clear visual axis of lid or lashes.
	Refractive error	AHP may counter significant astigmatism.
		AHP may create pinhole effect on pupil (smaller aperture improves vision in the presence of mild refractive error).
Maintain binocularity	Strabismus	AHP moves eyes out of the field of unmatched extraocular muscle action in incomitant[b] strabismus reducing diplopia and improving vision.
Center the field of binocular vision	Visual field defects	Children with homonymous hemianopia or altitudinal scotomas[c] may adopt AHP to centralize intact visual field in relation to their body.
Center field of conjugate gaze	Supranuclear-gaze paresis Ocular apraxia	AHP, with face turned toward the paretic side to center range of limited eye movement to the body.
Paradoxical AHP	Strabismus	AHP to *maximize* separation of images as binocularity is not possible. The paradoxical AHP allows the peripherally displaced, false image from the strabismic eye to be more easily ignored.
	Ocular tilt reaction	Inappropriate righting reflex in the context of erroneous graviception due to otolith–ocular pathway lesion.
Cosmesis	Deformity/scar	AHP to hide orbital deformity, asymmetry, or scar.

[a]Adapted from SP Kraft.[6]

[b]Incomitant strabismus: present only in some fields of gaze (eg, lateral gaze in sixth nerve paresis).

[c]Altitudinal scotoma: vertical visual-field defect.

In childhood torticollis without a clear nonocular cause, eye examination is indicated due to the following:

- Prolonged, untreated ocular torticollis can lead to musculoskeletal adaptive changes that may persist as musculoskeletal torticollis even if the underlying ocular deficit is rectified. Ocular torticollis in early childhood can result in facial bone deformities such as plagiocephaly. Recognition and treatment of the ocular cause allow potential prevention of this condition.
- Initial ocular torticollis in childhood incomitant strabismus may allow binocular fusion. However, resolution of torticollis results in more normal posture but may signify loss of fusion and asymptomatic suppression of the deviating eye, placing the child at risk of amblyopia. Amblyopia untreated within the critical period results in permanent visual loss ("lazy eye").
- Surgical intervention for ocular torticollis due to nystagmus aims to centralize the null point to the primary gaze.[4–5] However, surgery may reduce nystagmus intensity, increasing foveation time, and give additional improvement in binocular vision.[5]

Ocular Tilt Reaction

A lesion of the otolith-ocular (gravioceptive) pathway leads to an abnormal internal estimate of gravito-inertial acceleration causing an inaccurate perception of earth vertical (Table 22–3). This inappropriately triggers the righting reflex normally seen in response to head tilting. This results in torticollis, vertical ocular (skew) deviation, and ocular torsion, termed the ocular tilt reaction (OTR).

The OTR results from a synergistic but inappropriate righting reflex in the context of erroneous gravioception. Clinically, the OTR consists of the triad of

1. Abnormal head tilt—toward lesion and away from true earth vertical
2. Skew deviation—eye ipsilateral to the lesion is lower, contralateral eye is higher
3. Ocular torsion—both eyes tort in roll axis toward the lower eye

Skew deviation and OTR may follow lesions along the otolith-ocular pathway (Table 22–4).

Other ocular signs along with ipsilesional OTR include spontaneous nystagmus (mixed horizontal and torsional) in primary position, lid nystagmus, head nystagmus, ipsipulsion of eyes at saccades (hypermetric ipsilesional saccades, hypometric contralesional saccades) and in dark or at blink (ipsilesional), and impaired contralesional smooth pursuit (Table 22–5).

Nystagmus and Saccadic Intrusions

Involuntary eye movements are classified by the speed of the initial phase that drives the eyes away from fixation (Table 22–6).

By convention, jerk nystagmus is described as beating in the direction of the fast phase that is clinically easier to appreciate. Actually this is the corrective phase, the pathological phase is the slow initial drift from fixation. Thus, the conjugate slow up-drift of the eyes followed by a fast downward corrective phase that is seen in cerebellar pontine lesions such as Chiari malformations is described as downbeat or downbeating nystagmus.

Clinically, nystagmus is documented in the nine positions of gaze (Figure 22–2A). The arrows (Figure 22–2B) denote the direction of beating (direction of fast corrective phase). Pendular nystagmus has arrows at each end.

Table 22–3. The Ocular Tilt Reaction: Lesions of the Otolith–Ocular (Gravioceptive) Pathway

	Normal		*Ocular Tilt Reaction*	
Imbalance in vestibular input triggers righting reflex.	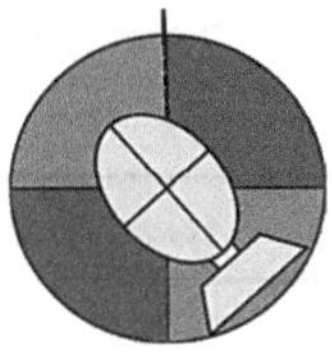	Whole body is tilted to the right. True earth vertical is to the left.	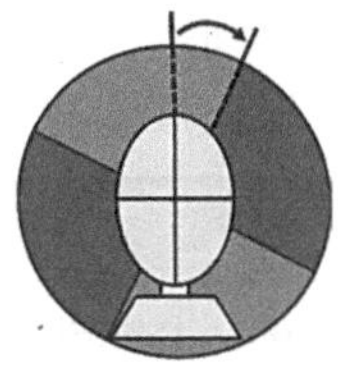	Body upright. Otolith–ocular pathway lesion is on the left. **Vertical is erroneously perceived to the left.**
Compensatory head posture.	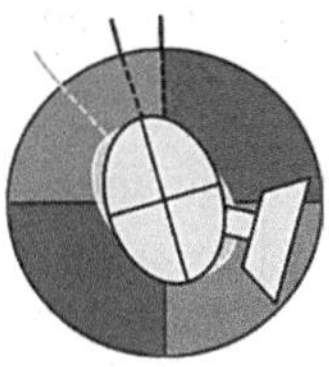	Normal head tilt toward true earth vertical. Head tilt to left reducing deviation.	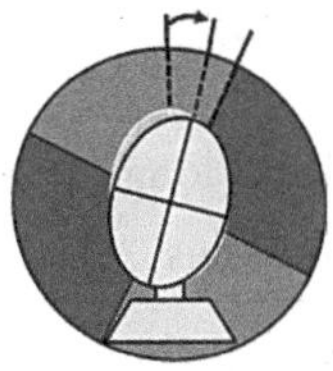	Inappropriate head tilt toward erroneous vertical plane. **Head tilt to left causing deviation.**
Head posture influences eye position in relation to horizon.	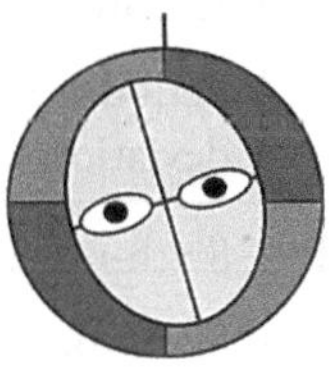	Head tilt reduces vertical deviation of eyes at true horizontal plane.	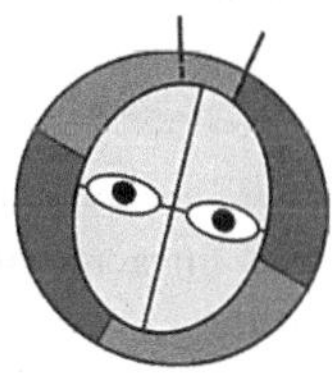	Abnormal head tilt causes vertical deviation of eyes at true horizontal plane. **Abnormal head tilt.**
Compensatory vertical eye movement (pitch axis).	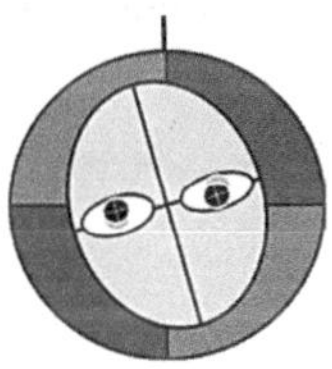	Eyes move vertically, aligning to earth horizontal, reducing vertical disparity.	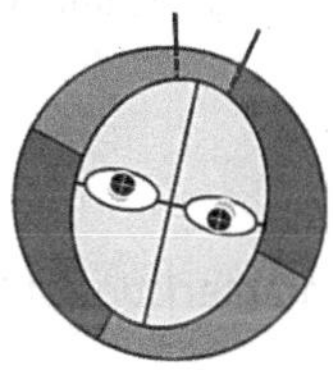	Eyes move further vertically, aligning to erroneous horizontal, increasing vertical disparity further. **Skew deviation.**
Compensatory torsional eye movement (roll axis).	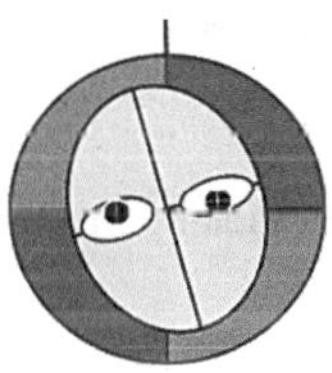	Both eyes roll, aligning to true earth vertical. Counter roll toward the lower eye aligns eyes.	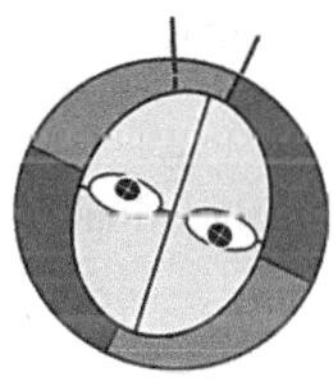	Both eyes roll, aligning to erroneous vertical. Inappropriate torsion toward the lower eye. **Ocular torsion.**
Resultant ocular fundal alignment.	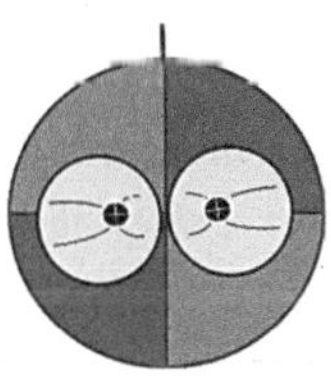	Ocular fundi, and therefore image perception, is better aligned with earth vertical.	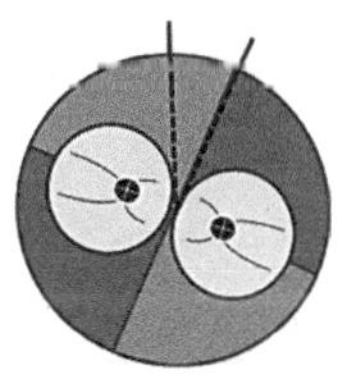	Ocular fundi, and therefore image perception, is misaligned. **(1) Vertically** **(2) Torted.**

Table 22–4. Otolith–Ocular Pathway Lesions and Their Associated Skew Deviation and Ocular Tilt Reactions (OTR). *ICP* intracranial pressure

Location		***Ocular Signs***	***Associated Features***
Peripheral	Peripheral vestibular	Ipsilesional OTR	Tullio phenomenon (irritative cause)
Brainstem	Vestibular nucleus	Ipsilesional OTR	Wallenberg syndrome[a]
	Cerebellum	Sustained ipsilesional alternating OTR	Ataxia and other cerebellar signs
Midbrain	Medial longitudinal Fasciculus	Contralesional OTR	Internuclear ophthalmoplegia
	Interstitial nucleus of Cajal	Contralesional OTR	Paroxysmal skew/OTR Ipsilateral OTR (irritative cause) Periodic alternating skew deviation
Nonlocalizing	Raised intracranial pressure	Skew deviation OTR	Sixth-nerve paresis Symptoms of raised intracranial pressure

[a]Wallenberg syndrome (lateral medullary syndrome) results from vascular (ipsilateral vertebral artery, posterior inferior cerebellar artery occlusion/dissection), or demyelination.

Table 22–5. Characteristics of Wallenberg Syndrome

Location	***Laterality***	***Clinical Sign***
Inferior cerebellar peduncle	Ipsilesional	Lateropulsion
	Ipsilesional	Limb ataxia
Spinal nucleus of trigeminal nerve	Ipsilesional	Impaired facial pain/temperature sensation
Nucleus ambiguus	Ipsilesional	Dysarthria, dysphagia, loss of gag reflex
Descending sympathetic fibers	Ipsilesional	Horner's syndrome
Spinothalamic tract	Contralesional	Impaired trunk limb pain/temperature sensation
Vestibular nucleus		Vertigo

Table 22–6. Classification of Involuntary Eye Movements

Slow initial phase	Slow corrective phase	Pendular nystagmus
	Fast corrective phase	Jerk nystagmus (beating in direction of fast phase)
Fast initial phase	Fast corrective phase, intermittent	Saccadic intrusions
	Fast corrective phase, sustained	Saccadic oscillation

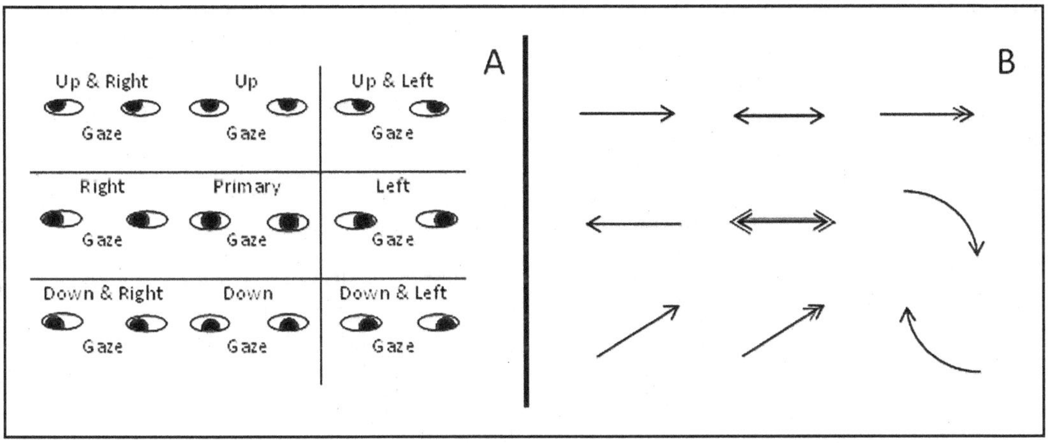

Figure 22–2. A. Nine positions of gaze. **B.** Arrows denote the direction of beating (direction of fast corrective phase), for example, pendular nystagmus has arrows at each end. Increasing numbers of arrows denotes increasing frequency, while additional lines denote increased amplitude. Direction of torsional nystagmus is indicated with curved lines.

Increasing numbers of arrows denotes increasing frequency, while additional lines denote increase amplitude. Direction of torsional nystagmus is indicated with curved lines (see Figure 22–2B).

Nonvestibular Nystagmus: Infantile Nystagmus Syndrome

Infantile nystagmus syndrome (INS) describes a spectrum of involuntary eye movements of early onset (<4 months). The exact mechanism has not been elucidated, but visual maladaptation due to early disruption of sensorimotor integration is implicated.[7–8] INS may be seen without an identifiable precipitating visual disorder, as idiopathic INS, or associated with sensory visual loss due to an identifiable anterior pathway (retina to lateral geniculate body) pathology (Table 22–7).

Initial signs of precipitating visual system disorders may be subtle or absent in early infancy. Specialized ocular investigations such as electrodiagnostic testing (electroretinogram [ERG]), visual-evoked potential, and magnetic resonance imaging (MRI) are useful in some cases. Early eye examination (Table 22–8) may allow optimization of visual potential and

Table 22–7. Anterior Pathway Pathology Leading to Infantile Nystagmus Syndrome

Etiology		*Dysfunction*
Refractive amblyopia	High bilateral myopia/hyperopia Anisometropia (intereye difference)	In marked refractive error, no clear image forms on the retina.
Ocular-media opacity	Congenital corneal dystrophies Anterior segment dysgenesis Congenital glaucoma Congenital cataract Persistent fetal vasculature Vitreous hemorrhage	Media opacity of the cornea, anterior segment, lens, and vitreous blocks the pathway of light to the retina, degrading visual information.
Retinal	Leber's congenital amarosis Cone dystrophy Acromotopsia Congenital stationary night blindness Peroxisomal disorders Isolated foveal hypoplasia	Retinal disease disrupts the architecture and function of the photoreceptors, glial cells, and ganglion cells responsible for visual-information transduction and conduction.
Optic nerve	Optic nerve hypoplasia Optic atrophy	Optic neuropathy results in poor conduction of visual information.
Chiasmal	Ocular albinism Oculocutaneous albinism Achiasmia Chiasmal glioma	Chiasmal misrouting, maldevelopment, or compression result in degradation of visual information to the posterior pathway.

treatment of refractive error, amblyopia, head posture, and strabismus. Systemic associations of these conditions can be significant (for example, albinism-associated immune and hematological deficiency; endocrine dysfunction associated with optic nerve hypoplasia), and early recognition allows appropriate referral and management. The inherited nature of some of these conditions also has implications on risk to siblings and future children.

Table 22–8. Clinical Characteristics of Infantile Nystagmus Syndrome

Direction	Usually horizontal, may have vertical element (elliptical) Uniplanar: Direction of nystagmus the same in all positions of gaze Increased intensity on lateral gaze Right beating on right gaze, left beating on left gaze
Symmetry between eyes	Conjugate: Both eyes move in same direction in phase Amplitude and frequency usually equal between eyes
Waveform	Jerk nystagmus (increasing-velocity slow phase at ENG) Pendular
Onset	Before 4 months of age
Intensity	Increases with fixation Decreases in darkness Decreases with convergence (convergence-blocking syndrome)
Associated features	Null zone where nystagmus intensity is minimal and vision optimal Abnormal head posture at null zone Head oscillation
Other ocular features	Reversed optokinetic nystagmus (OKN drum quick phase beat in same direction as the stripes/drum rotates) Inverted smooth pursuit Latent nystagmus Strabismus
Management	Cycloplegic refraction and treatment of refractive error (astigmatism common) Inclusion of base out prisms into glasses (stimulate convergence blocking syndrome) Extraocular muscle surgery to place null zone in primary position Extraocular muscle surgery without moving the muscles (resection and reattachment) has been reported to reduce the intensity of nystagmus

Nystagmus that displays features that are atypical for idiopathic INS, warrants further investigation (MRI/ERG) to rule out chiasmal gliomas or occult retinal diseases, for example (Table 22–9).

Latent Nystagmus: Latent Fixation Nystagmus, Fusional Maldevelopmental Nystagmus Syndrome, and Manifest Latent Nystagmus

Latent nystagmus occurs due to early disruption of binocular fusion by strabismus or media opacity. Monocular fixation, induced by covering one eye, evokes latent nystagmus. In children who develop amblyopia due to suppression of strabismus or poor vision due to ocular media opacity, this latent nystagmus becomes manifest (manifest-latent nystagmus), as they now monofixate without occlusion. The clinical presentation, features, and management of latent nystagmus are outlined in Table 22–10.

Spasmus Nutans

Spasmus nutans is a disorder characterized by the triad of nystagmus, head nodding and abnormal head posture. Although this condition resolves spontaneously in some children, perhaps reflecting delayed motor calibration or maturation. Spasmus nutans-like presentation has been recognized to occur in infantile suprasellar tumors, most commonly optic pathway glioma, and therefore MRI is indicated.[9] The clinical presentation, features and management of spamus nutans are outlined in Table 22–11.

Table 22–9. Characteristics of Nystagmus Associated with Chiasmal Glioma or Occult Retinal Disease

Signs associated with chiasmal glioma	Onset after 4 months
	Monocular or asymmetric nystagmus amplitude
	Dysconjugate/disjunctive (eyes dissociated in direction or phase of nystagmus)
	Multiplanar nystagmus
Signs associated with retinal dystrophy[2]	Severe photophobia
	High myopia
	Paradoxical (pupillary constriction rather than dilation when lights turned off)
	Oculodigital sign (self-stimulatory behavior—repetitive pushing on eye by thumb)

Table 22–10. Clinical Characteristics, Features, and Management of Latent Nystagmus

Direction	Latent nystagmus is only clinically obvious on occlusion. The fast phase of both eyes beats toward the fixating (uncovered) eye. Therefore, switching fixation (moving cover to other eye) instantaneously reverses the direction of the fast phase of nystagmus in both eyes.
Symmetry between eyes	Conjugate: both eyes in phase beating in same direction dependent on fixation
Waveform	Small-amplitude horizontal jerk nystagmus Decreasing-velocity waveform at ENG ENG subclinical (manifest-latent) nystagmus is seen without occlusion
Onset	Latent nystagmus early infancy Conversion to manifest-latent nystagmus (ie, nystagmus without occlusion) indicates development of suppression and amblyopia
Intensity	Increases in abduction of the eye (ie, direction of fixating eye obeys Alexander's law) Decreases in adduction
Associated features	Head turn to fixate with preferred eye in adduction (dampening nystagmus, null zone)
Other ocular features	Infantile esotropia (most common) and other infantile strabismus Monocular media opacity (corneal, lens, vitreous) Nasotemporal asymmetry at optokinetic testing Normal nasally directed OKN response when target moves toward nose Impaired temporally directed OKN response when target moves toward the temple Dissociated vertical deviation (DVD), on occlusion the covered eye is vertically deviated upward. The vertical deviation is considered *dissociated*, because upon uncovering the deviated eye, this eye takes up fixation without the paired (*associated*) corrective vertical movement in the fellow eye normally seen in most forms of strabismus.
Management	Early treatment cause of disruption of binocular function (strabismus, media opacity) Occlusion therapy of associated amblyopia Extraocular muscle surgery/botulinum toxin injection to move null position into primary position.

ENG electronystagmography; *OKN* optokinetic nystagmus.

Table 22–11. Clinical Characteristics, Features, and Management of Spasmus Nutans

Direction	Mutiplanar, direction changing in direction of gaze
Symmetry between eyes	Marked asymmetry, may appear clinically monocular but found to be bilateral and asymmetric at slit-lamp microscopy or electronystagmography Dissociated between eyes in relation to phase (disjunctive) and direction (dysconjugate)
Waveform	Small-amplitude high-frequency dissociated pendular "shimmering" nystagmus. Head nodding may change waveform to a slower waveform more symmetric between the eyes. Subclinical nystagmus at ENG may persist after clinical resolution.
Onset	6 months (within first year) Resolution within months to years
Intensity	Intermittent and asymmetric, reduced by head nodding
Associated features	Compensatory head nodding, though head nodding is at lower frequency than nystagmus Variable head tilt which does not have a clear ocular cause
Other ocular features	Usually no other ocular or systemic features Optic atrophy, afferent pupillary defects, visual loss, and strabismus raise suspicion of infantile suprasellar mass Concurrent neurofibromatosis type 1 and diencephalic syndrome (emaciation, hyperactivity, and euphoria) similarly are associated with optic-pathway glioma
Management	Magnetic resonance imaging to exclude suprasellar mass Electroretinography to exclude occult retinal disease Exclusion of neurodegenerative disorders, Pelizaeus-Merzbacher disease, and Leigh's disease

Summary

The visual system provides critical input for the maintenance of balance. In addition, eye movements provide a window into the function of the peripheral vestibular system. As outlined in summary Table 22–12, the differential diagnosis of involuntary eye movements is, however, extensive. It is the specific features and characteristics of these eye movements that allow for localization of the deficit. Recognizing the subtleties of these eye movements often requires the expertise of a subspecialist ophthalmologist. However, the ability to recognize eye movements associated with activation of the vestibular end organs and to distinguish them from those of primary ocular or oculomotility deficits is crucial for the clinician looking after children with vestibular and balance disorders.

Table 22–12. Summary of the Characteristics and Localization of Involuntary Eye Movements

Involuntary Eye Movement	***Downbeat Nystagmus***	***Upbeat Nystagmus***	***Torsional Nystagmus***	***Periodic Alternating Nystagmus***	***Seesaw (+ Hemi-Seesaw) Nystagmus***	***Opsiclonus Saccadic Intrusions***
Direction	Fast phase beats down in primary position Increases in lateral gaze	Fast phase beats up in primary position	Upper pole beats away from lesion	Alternates: beats 90 seconds to one side, then 90 seconds to other	Alternates: 1. Depression and excyclotorsion of one eye 2. Elevation and incyclotorsion of other eye	Erratic, multidirectional bursts
Waveform	Jerk	Jerk	Jerk	Jerk Obeys Alexander's law		Initiated by fast movement (ie, saccadic)
Symmetry	Conjugate	Conjugate	Conjugate	Conjugate	Dissociated vertical movement and torsion	Conjugate or monocular
Location of lesion	Pontomedullary junction Cerebellar flocculus	Superior cerebellar peduncle Bilateral midline pontomesencephalic or pontomedullary junctions	Pontomedullary junction Cerebellar Midbrain	Cerebellum (nodulus and uvula)	Seesaw diencephalic (chiasmal) Jerk (hemi-seesaw) lateral medullary or midbrain	Cerebellum (fastigial nucleus) Pons (damage to omnipause cells)
Etiology	• Arnold Chiari • Cerebellar degeneration • Vertebrobasilar infarct • Demyelination • Drugs • Idiopathic	• Cerebellar degeneration • Infarct (cerebellar) • Demyelination • Tumors	• Infarction • Demyelination • Vascular angioma • Arnold Chiari • Tumor • Seizure • Idiopathic	• Congenital • Albinism • Cerebellar degeneration • Demyelination • Tumor • Visual loss	• Parasellar tumor • Craniopharyngioma • Chiasmal glioma • Achiasmia • Infarct/hemmoraghe • Trauma • Visual loss	• Paraneoplastic Neuroblastoma • Idiopathic • Encephalopathic • Parainfectious • Toxic-metabolic

Source: Adapted with permission from AM Wong.[10]

Self-Assessment Questions

1. Does strabismus cause imbalance in children?
2. Does nystagmus cause imbalance in children?
3. Abnormal head posture related to ocular disease (ocular torticollis)
   may be adopted for:
   a. Cosmesis
   b. To center restricted visual field
   c. To center field of binocularity
   d. Reduce nystagmus intensity
   e. All of the above
4. What is the ocular tilt reaction (OTR), and what is the cause?
5. Is the skew deviation in the OTR always ipsilesional?
6. How are nystagmus and saccadic intrusions differentiated?
7. How is nystagmus described clinically?
8. What are the ocular causes of infantile nystagmus?
9. Is opsoclonus a form of nystagmus?
10. Where does downbeat nystagmus localize?

References

1. Harris C, Berry D, A developmental model of infantile nystagmus. *Semin Ophthalmol.* 2006; 21:63–69.
2. Brodsky MC. *Pediatric Neuro-Ophthalmology.* 2nd ed. New York, NY: Springer; 2010.
3. Buncic JR. Wobbly eyes in infancy. In: Taylor D, Hoyt C. *Pediatric Ophthalmology and Strabismus.* 3rd ed, Philadelphia, PA: Elsevier; 2008.
4. Kraft SP, O'Donoghue EP, Roarty JD. Improvement of compensatory head postures after strabismus surgery. *Ophthalmology.* 1992; 99:1301–1308.
5. Von Noorden GK, Sprunger DT. Large muscle recessions for the treatment of congenital nystagmus. *Arch Ophthalmol.* 1991;109:221–224.
6. Kraft SP. Abnormal head posture in children. In: Taylor D, Hoyt C. *Pediatric Ophthalmology and Strabismus.* 3rd ed. Philadelphia, PA: Elsevier; 2008.

7. Hertle RW, Dell'Osso LF. Clinical and ocular motor analysis of congenital nystagmus in infancy. *J AAPOS.* 1999;3:70–79.
8. Tychesen L, Hurtig RR, Scott WE. Pursuit is impaired but the vestibule-ocular reflex is normal in infantile strabismus. *Arch Ophthalmol.* 1985;103:536.
9. Gottlob I, Wizov SS, Reinecke RD. Spasmus nutans: A long term follow-up. *Invest Ophthalmol Vis Sci.* 1995;36:2736–2771.
10. Wong, AM. *Eye Movement Disorders.* New York, NY: Oxford University Press; 2008.

CHAPTER 23

Postural Orthostatic Tachycardia Syndrome

Stephanie A. Moody Antonio

Introduction

Dizziness is a word applied to a vast and varied number of symptoms. In contrast to true vertigo, which can be clearly described as the sensation of movement or spinning, other forms of dizziness, including lightheadedness, can be very difficult to describe, especially for children. Whereas vertigo most likely suggests a peripheral or central vestibular disorder, and disequilibrium or gait disturbances suggest neurologic, musculoskeletal, or multifactorial disorders, nonspecific lightheadedness has a varied differential diagnosis and requires a thoughtful approach.

In this chapter, we consider disorders that result in the sensation of lightheadedness that must be differentiated from vestibular disorders, particularly postural orthostatic tachycardia syndrome (POTS). Lightheaded dizziness can be described as wooziness, internal spinning, spaciness, or foggy-headedness. It may be associated with syncope, the sudden but brief loss of consciousness or presyncope, the sense of impending loss of consciousness. Transient lightheadedness on standing is a common and most often nonpathologic phenomenon, but lightheadedness that persists for longer than 1 minute is considered abnormal.[1]

Orthostatic Intolerance

Orthostatic intolerance is defined as the inability to or discomfort with standing upright due to dizziness, headache, fatigue, or other symptoms that are relieved by sitting or lying down. Orthostatic intolerance (OI) is caused by a disruption in autonomic and cardiovascular compensatory mechanisms that allow for an upright posture when 70% of the human blood volume is below the level of the heart.[2] On assuming an upright posture, blood pools in venous reservoirs below the heart, including the splanchnic circulation and legs. The gravitational shift in blood volume reduces venous return to the heart, hydrostatic blood pressure, and cerebral perfusion. The normal physiologic response to gravitational pull of blood volume on standing is increased heart rate and blood pressure, which supports return of blood to the heart and adequate circulation to the brain. The primary mechanisms to defend against orthostatic stress include adequate blood volume, skeletal muscle compression, and autonomic-mediated adjustments to vascular tone, heart rate, and cardiac contractility. When venous pooling results in a sudden drop in blood pressure, baroreceptors in the carotid sinus and aortic arch detect a reduction in stretch. As a result, a reflex arc through the baroreceptors, glossopharyngeal and vagus nerves, and nucleus tractus solitaries increases sympathetic outflow resulting in vasoconstriction, tachycardia, and increased cardiac contractility. Additional defenses to postural challenge include local and humoral effects. The renin-angiotensin-aldosterone system releases epinephrine and vasopressin, which influence local and central control of vascular tone.[1]

OI occurs when compensatory responses to postural change are inadequate, either due to overwhelming environmental stressors or to dysfunction of compensatory mechanisms. Environmental or physical factors, such as heat exposure, prolonged standing, emotional trigger, intense exercise, fasting, lack of sleep, or rapid weight loss contribute to physiologic stress.[3]

These factors may overwhelm an otherwise healthy regulatory system and result in symptomatic orthostatic intolerance. OI can be defined by timing as acute (less than 1 week), subacute (<3 months) or chronic (>3 months).[2] Disorders of postural tolerance can be classified by the pattern of physiologic response into 3 basic patterns: neurally mediated syncope, orthostatic hypotension, and postural tachycardia syndrome.[1,4]

Neurally Mediated Syncope

Syncope is the sudden and transient loss of consciousness and postural tone due to an abrupt fall in blood pressure with spontaneous recovery.[5] Syncope induced by exercise or with cardiac symptoms, such as arrhythmia or chest pain, may indicate cardiogenic syncope, which is rare in children but may be life-threatening.[1] Neurally mediated syncope (also called simple faint, vasovagal syncope, reflex syncope, and cardiogenic syncope) refers to a heterogeneous group of events in which there is bradycardia, vasodilation, decreased blood pressure, and cerebral hypoxia.[1,5] This paradoxical response to orthostatic stress may be caused by abnormal activation of the parasympathetic nervous system.[1]

Neurally mediated syncope (NMS) is not unusual and has been reported in 15% to 20% of children, with approximately 0.5 to 3 cases per 1,000, peaking at age 15 years.[1,3] Neurally mediated syncope is the most common type of syncope in children. It is more common in adolescent girls than boys.[2] Young people typically experience a sudden but brief sense of dizziness or lightheadedness, pallor, warmth, diaphoresis, nausea, abdominal discomfort, auditory and visual disturbances, and cognitive slowing prior to loss of consciousness.[4] Common scenarios include opportunities for excess pooling of blood, such as standing motionless (limited muscle pumping and vascular compression), straining against a closed glottis, and warm environments (vasodilation). NMS may also be triggered by emotions or pain, due to disrupted autonomic activity. In toddlers, syncopal spells commonly called "breath-holding" can occur as a result of crying combined with the Valsalva effects of a prolonged silent cry, which leads to reduced venous return and hypotension. The incidence of breath-holding has been reported to occur in up to 5% of children between 6 months and 2 years and generally resolves by age 3 to 4 years.[3]

Orthostatic Hypotension

Initial orthostatic hypotension is a transient sensation of lightheadedness that occurs due to delayed activation of sympathetic compensatory mechanisms to the effects of gravity when a person stands upright. It is defined by a decrease in systolic blood pressure (BP) of >40 mm Hg or decrease in diastolic BP of >20 mm Hg that occurs within 10 to 15 seconds of standing and is typically restored within 30 seconds. Heart rate increases very briefly. Prolonged supine position is a risk factor.[2]

In contrast to initial orthostatic hypotension, true orthostatic hypotension develops over several minutes and persists while the patient is upright. In adults, orthostatic hypotension (OH) is defined as sustained reduction in systolic blood pressure of 20 mm Hg or diastolic pressure of 10 mm Hg within 3 minutes of standing or head-up tilt, with or without tachycardia. There are no universally accepted criteria specific for children, although the same BP parameters are usually employed. While adults may not show tachycardia due to cardiac denervation, children may demonstrate supine tachycardia which increases when upright.[2] Orthostatic hypotension is caused primarily by failure of vasoconstriction of the peripheral vasculature and inadequate adjustments to heart rate and cardiac contractility.[4] Other mechanisms may contribute, such as decreased baroreflex sensitivity, impaired left ventricular compliance, or primary hypertension. OH can be classified as nonneurogenic or neurogenic, which may be further subtyped into primary or secondary disorders of the autonomic nervous system. Non-neurogenic causes include reduced intravascular volume (dehydration, anemia, adrenal insufficiency, diabetes insipidus), disorders of cardiac output, excessive vasodilation (fever), and medications that interfere with autonomic function.[6] Neurologic diseases associated with OH include primary autonomic neuropathies, multiple system atrophy, Parkinson disease, diabetic neuropathy, multiple sclerosis, and Guillain-Barré syndrome.[6] The frequency of orthostatic hypotension increases with age and is uncommon in children.

Postural Orthostatic Tachycardia Syndrome

Postural orthostatic tachycardia syndrome (POTS) is a disorder characterized by multiple complaints including nonspecific dizziness or lightheadedness, exercise intolerance, headache, fatigue, nausea, palpitations, diaphoresis, tachypnea, abdominal discomfort, and weakness triggered on standing upright and relieved by sitting or lying down. Symptoms range in severity from fairly mild to disabling. POTS is differentiated from orthostatic hypotension by maintenance of normal blood pressure. The symptomatology is typically more complex than either orthostatic hypotension or neurally mediated syncope, and the diagnosis is complicated by the enormous number of symptoms and comorbid complaints, which likely contribute to delay in diagnosis and treatment. The syndrome is a result of failure to maintain normal vascular tone while upright.

POTS has been increasingly recognized since it was first described in 1993 and is thought to affect millions of teens.[7] In one study, 30% of children who presented to a pediatric clinic complaining of dizziness had symptoms and postural tachycardia consistent with POTS.[8] POTS is most common in adolescent girls.[9] It is associated with lower body mass index (BMI), Caucasian race, high achievers, athletes, and psychiatric comorbidities.[2] In adolescence, POTS typically occurs within a few years of pubertal growth spurt.

Pathophysiology

The pathophysiology of POTS is likely heterogeneous and includes dysfunction or dysregulation of the autonomic nervous system, resulting in excessive upright sympathetic activation or excessive parasympathetic inhibition.[2] Several authors have described subtypes based on clinical characteristics and pathologic findings.[10,11] These subtypes may have different pathophysiologic mechanisms and as a result may manifest with varied signs and symptoms. Relative hypovolemia is one of the most consistent findings and likely a common endpoint for the various etiologies.[7,11] Peripheral or splanchnic vasodilation, hyperadrenergic state on response to orthostatic challenge, distal sudomotor denervation, low cardiac stroke volume, and high arterial resistance may each play a role in the development of relative thoracic hypovolemia.[7,11] A reduced renin-aldosterone ratio during standing has been demonstrated in POTS patients, which led Fu et al[12] to propose that some of the deconditioning effect of POTS is due in part to blunted adrenal function.

Clinical Presentation

The most common orthostatic symptoms associated with POTS are lightheadedness, palpitations, presyncope and syncope, weakness, tremulousness, nausea, and shortness of breath. These symptoms indicate sympathetic activation, versus the parasympathetic cardioinhibitory response thought to occur in cases of orthostatic hypotension.[11] In some cases, heat, exercise, eating, or menstruation exacerbates symptoms.[11] Fatigue, headache, chronic pain, sleep disturbance, and reduced quality of life are also common.[11,13] Most patients have multiple symptoms.[9] In a series of pediatric patients with autonomic dysfunction, chronic pain (headache or abdominal pain) was present in 88%, dizziness in 74%, fatigue in 65%, and altered-temperature sensation in 34%.[7,14] The combination of orthostatic intolerance with fatigue and other general symptoms typically leads to deconditioning, as patients accommodate to uncomfortable symptoms by reducing activity. In severe cases, limited tolerance to upright posture is debilitating, restricting ability to attend school, participate in social activities, or independently perform activities of daily life.

Predisposing Factors and Comorbidities

Disorders that cause secondary OI include diabetes, systemic lupus erythematous, paraneoplastic syndrome, eating disorders, medications (vasodilators, anxiolytics, diuretics), heavy-metal poisoning, Addison's disease, hyperthyroidism, autonomic neuropathies, anemia, and dehydration.[2,7]

In many cases, a significant viral illness or injury with prolonged recovery precedes the development of POTS. Cases have been linked to infectious mononucleosis, Lyme disease, and vigorous physical activity in competitive athletes.[10] Joint hypermobility and specifically, Ehlers-Danlos syndrome have been identified in 57% and 22%, respectively.[9] POTS may be associated with or overlap with chronic fatigue syndrome, migraine, functional gastrointestinal disorders, sleep disturbances, fibromyalgia, and cyclic vomiting syndrome.[2,9,15]

Whether fatigue is a primary symptom or merely a secondary effect of postural intolerance, avoidance of or inability to tolerate upright activity leads to deconditioning, which very likely further exacerbates the symptoms. Prolonged avoidance of exercise and chronic bedrest induce a distinct form of deconditioning with reduced blood volume, redistribution of blood volume, cardiac atrophy, baroreflex changes, and reduction in skeletal muscle pump, which further aggravates all forms of OI, including POTS.[2]

POTS has several features characteristic of an immune-mediated syndrome, including female predominance, preceding viral syndrome, and evidence of autonomic denervation.[2] Up to 15% of adults with POTS have antibodies to ganglionic acetylcholine receptor, which is also present in patients with autoimmune autonomic ganglionopathy.[7,16]

The number of children with this antibody is unknown, but one case was presented in which an 11-year-old with orthostatic intolerance responded to immunoglobulin.[7] Other studies have demonstrated thyroid-specific autoantibodies and autoantibodies that cross-react with cardiac proteins and adrenergic receptors. Disorders of mast cell activation have been found in some patients with POTS, with some symptoms overlapping and others distinctive.[2] Patients with mast cell activation disorder have episodic fatigue, syncope/pre-syncope, nausea, headache, and tachycardia, but also present with flushing, dermographism, pain, and urticaria.

Evaluation of Orthostatic Intolerance

The tests and consultations that may be indicated to evaluate OI are summarized in Table 23–1. A cardiologist may be involved early to rule out cardiogenic syncope. Consultations with neurology and gastroenterology may also be indicated. The tilt table test with continuous recording of blood pressure and heart rate for up to 10 minutes forms the basis for the diagnosis and can differentiate IOH, OH, and POTS. Tilt angles of 60° to 70° are typically utilized. A standing orthostatic test is a validated means of diagnosis of IOH and OH but is not yet validated for POTS in children.[2]

While there is no absolute consensus on the diagnostic criteria, Singer et al proposed the following for symptomatic children based on Tilt test: POTS can be defined by an increase in heart rate of ≥40 bpm or absolute orthostatic HR of ≥130 beats/min in children age 13 years or younger and ≥120 beats/min in children older than 14 years within 5 minutes of head-up tilt.[17] Typically, there is no variation in blood pressure over the first 5 to 10 minutes. However, in the case of hypovolemia or severe vasodilation, the blood pressure may drop. In hyperadrenergic POTS, the blood pressure may increase or fluctuate. A drop in blood pressure after 10 minutes may occur as a result of a normal adrenergic response.[11] In contrast, patients with OH will show a sustained monotonic decrease in BP and progressive elevation of heart rate in the

Table 23–1. Evaluation of Suspected Postural Orthostatic Tachycardia Syndrome

Consultations	*Basic Workup*
Cardiology to rule out arrhythmia, cardiogenic syncope, cardiac dysfunction	Complete blood count, electrolytes, fasting serum blood glucose, thyroid stimulating hormone, Lyme titer, Epstein-Barr virus titer
Neurology to evaluate dizziness, headaches, fatigue, screen for autonomic neuropathy	Head-up tilt table
Gastroenterology to evaluate nausea, vomiting, abdominal pain	24-hour urine sodium
	Plasma catecholamines—supine and standing
	Electrocardiogram
	24-hour Holter monitor to assess baseline heart rate, heart rate during activity, and correlate symptoms to heart rate

first 3 minutes.[2] Alternatively, a typical tilt test for IOH will demonstrate a sudden elevation of heart rate and drop in BP with rapid recovery of BP and stabilization of heart rate to a baseline upright value that may be slightly elevated compared to supine values.[2]

Serum electrolytes, complete blood count, liver function tests, thyroid function tests, and infectious serologies may be helpful to rule out other causes of dizziness and fatigue.[7] A 24-hour urine sodium is useful to rule out dehydration and electrolyte imbalance. Plasma catecholamines can be measured supine and after standing. High norepinephrine levels after standing indicate a hyperadrenergic state. Additional tests include electrocardiography, cardiac echo, Holter monitor, autonomic reflex screening, thermoregulatory sweat test, ganglionic antibody, and exercise tolerance test.[11]

Management

Management strategies of OI and POTS are tailored to the clinical situation, depending on the severity and chronicity of the symptoms. Patients with mild symptoms may not need a complete evaluation and may respond to increased fluid and salt intake. Patients with prolonged orthostatic intolerance, chronic fatigue, and deconditioning require a multitiered approach (Table 23–2). Sleep, stress management, and avoidance of triggers should be encouraged.[9] Salt and water loading is the first-line therapy for OH and POTS. Claydon et al demonstrated improved cardiovascular and cerebrovascular stability during an orthostatic challenge in patients with neurogenic syncope or OH after drinking 500 mL of water.[18] Ideal salt and water intake for adolescent girls is 5000 to 8000 mg and 2.5 to 3 liters daily. Boys may require an additional 0.5 to 1 liter. Sports drinks are appropriate in place of or in addition to water. Intravenous hydration is sometimes necessary but should not be required long term.[2]

A monitored graded increase in endurance exercise has been proposed as the most effective means of management.[12] Exercise improves exercise tolerance, increases cardiac output, improves venous return, increases blood volume and total hemoglobin, and normalizes heart rate response to standing. Weight training for lower extremities can improve muscle pump and prevent venous pooling. Exercise can be targeted to heart rate (60% to 70% of maximal heart rate) and may include recumbent bike, swimming, Pilates, and resistance training. Upright exercise and walking can be added as exercise tolerance improves over 2 to 3 months.

Propranolol has been suggested as the first-line treatment in pharmacologic therapy and was reported effective in controlling heart rate and postural symptoms in adults and children[7]; however, propranolol may reduce cardiac output and contribute to fatigue.[7,12] A double-blinded controlled trial comparing propranolol to placebo, followed by exercise training in adults with POTS, demonstrated that both propranolol and exercise reduced standing heart rate, but exercise was more effective in restoring orthostatic tolerance. Fu et al reported that exercise training was superior to propranolol in improving adrenal function and patient quality of life for adult patients with POTS.[12] Additional pharmacologic therapies are proposed to increase blood volume, support cardiovascular function, modulate autonomic function, or address comorbidities such as gastrointestinal dysregulation, fatigue, anxiety, depression, and pain.[2,19] A comprehensive review of the pharmacological treatment of POTS was published by Miller and Raj in 2018. Most patients require multiple medications. Over time, the majority of patients with childhood-onset POTS improve, but unfortunately, symptoms can persist into adulthood.[9]

Table 23–2. Management Goals in Postural Orthostatic Tachycardia Syndrome

Goal	*Technique*
Increase fluid intake	Daily intake of noncaffeinated fluid to maintain urination >4 times daily (Girls 2.5 to 3 L; Boys 3 to 3.5 L)
	24-hour sodium excretion should be >170 mEq if adequate plasma volume to combat hypovolemia
	16 ounces of water can be taken prior to activity for an effect that may last 1 to 2 hours.
	IV saline
Increase salt intake	At least 2 to 4 grams of sodium daily
Exercise	Slow escalation of aerobic exercise, starting recumbent if necessary
Increase peripheral resistance	Support stockings and abdominal binder
Psychological support	Patient and family education, evaluation, and management of comorbid sleep disorders, migraine, depression
Control heart rate	β-Blocker pharmacotherapy decreases heart rate, blocks peripheral vasodilation
Other medications and role	α-Agonist (midodrine)—vasoconstrictor
	Mineralocorticoid (fludrocortisone)—increases blood volume
	Erythropoietin—increases production of red blood cells
	Serotonin reuptake inhibitors (citalopram, fluoxetine)—relieves depression and anxiety
	Clonidine—lowers heart rate and blood pressure
	Modafinil—stimulant that can improve mental alertness
	Pyridostigmine—increases vagal tone
	Desmopressin—antidiuretic

Conclusion

Lightheadedness should be differentiated from vertigo and disequilibrium, which are more likely to be associated with central or peripheral vestibular disorders. Neurally mediated syncope, orthostatic hypotension, and POTS often present with lightheadedness, presyncope, and syncope and can be differentiated from one another by timing, precipitating factors, and chronicity. POTS is a potentially debilitating condition in children and adolescents that presents with intolerance to upright posture often after a significant medical illness. It can be diagnosed by identifying tachycardia, dizziness, headache, and other symptoms, in the absence of hypotension on orthostatic challenge. After ruling out cardiogenic etiologies, POTS can be effectively managed with adequate fluid intake, salt loading, graded exercise rehabilitation, and medications such as β-blockers.

Self-Assessment Questions

1. Orthostatic intolerance is defined as:
   a. Decreased blood pressure when exercising
   b. Development of dizziness, headache, and fatigue when standing upright relieved when sitting down
   c. Dizziness when standing upright that resolves after 1 minute
   d. All of the above

2. The primary mechanisms to combat the gravitational shift in blood pressure when standing upright include:
   a. Adequate blood volume
   b. Increased cardiac contractility
   c. Skeletal muscle contraction
   d. Activation of sympathetic nervous system
   e. All of the above

3. Syncope associated with tachycardia or chest pain is suggestive of:
   a. Reflex syncope
   b. Simple faint
   c. Vasovagal syncope
   d. Cardiogenic syncope

4. Paradoxical activation of the parasympathetic nervous system in response to orthostatic stress may be manifested by:
   a. Bradycardia and vasodilation
   b. Tachycardia and cerebral hypoxia
   c. Vasoconstriction and diaphoresis
   d. Tachycardia and syncope

5. Orthostatic hypotension is defined as:
   a. The sustained reduction in systolic blood pressure of 20 mm Hg or diastolic pressure of 10 mm Hg within 3 minutes of standing
   b. The sustained reduction in systolic blood pressure of 20 mm Hg and increase in heart rate of 20 beats per minute within 3 minutes of standing
   c. A reduction in systolic blood pressure of 30 mm Hg and syncope within 3 minutes of standing

d. A reduction in systolic blood pressure of 20 mm Hg or diastolic pressure of 10 mm Hg immediately on standing that resolves within 3 minutes

6. POTS is characterized by:
    a. Orthostatic intolerance
    b. Sustained tachycardia on standing
    c. Fatigue
    d. All of the above

7. POTS is defined as:
    a. An increase in heart rate that occurs immediately on standing lasting less than 1 minute
    b. An increase in heart rate of greater than 30 beats per minute that occurs within 10 minutes of standing with or without a change in blood pressure
    c. A drop in blood pressure 10 minutes after standing
    d. A paradoxical response to standing caused by abnormal activation of the parasympathetic nervous system

8. Which one of these statements is true?
    a. Neurally mediated syncope is common in older people, especially with comorbid factors such as diabetes.
    b. "Breath-holding" is a type of neurally mediated syncope common in young children.
    c. POTS is most common in boys and young men.
    d. The frequency of orthostatic hypotension decreases with age.

9. Which one of these statements is false?
    a. Relative thoracic hypovolemia is one of the most consistent findings in POTS.
    b. Peripheral and splanchnic vasodilation may play a role in the development of symptoms in patients with POTS.
    c. Adrenal function may play a role in the pathophysiology of POTS in some patients.
    d. POTS is more common than reflex syncope in children younger than 12 years.

10. Management of POTS includes:
    a. Glucocorticoids
    b. Graduated exercise training
    c. Increased salt and fluid intake
    d. Support stockings

References

1. Stewart JM, Medow MS. Orthostatic intolerance: Introduction and importance. emedicine .com. http://www.emedicine.medscape.com/article/902155-overview. January 6, 2011
2. Stewart JM, Boris JR, Chelimsky G, et al. Pediatric disorders of orthostatic intolerance by the Pediatric Writing Group of the American Autonomic Society. *Pediatrics.* 2018; 141(1):e20171673.
3. Wieling W, Ganzeboom KS, Saul JP. Reflex syncope in children and adolescents. *Heart.* 2004;90(9):1094–1100.
4. Freeman R, Wieling W, Axelrod B, Benditt D, Benarroch E, Biaggioni I. Consensus statement on the definition of orthostatic hypotension, neurally mediated syncope and the postural tachycardia syndrome. *Clin Auton Res.* 2011;21:69–72.
5. Sealy B, Lui K. Diagnosis and management of vasovagal syncope and dysautonomia. *AACN Clin Issues.* 2004;15(3):462–477.
6. Maule S, Papotti G, Naso D, Magnino C, Testa E, Veglio F. Orthostatic hypotension: Evaluation and treatment. *Cadiovasc Haematol Disord Drug Targets.* 2007;7:63–70.
7. Johnson JN, Mack KJ, Kuntz NL, Brands CK, Porter CJ, Fischer PR. Postural orthostatic tachycardia syndrome: A clinical review. *Pediatr Neurol.* 2010;42:77–85.
8. Marsh AM, Fischer PR, Brands CK. *Dizziness in a pediatric and adolescent referral population.* Paper presented at Pediatric Academic Societies, 2005.
9. Boris JR. Postural orthostatic tachycardia syndrome in children. *Auton Neurosci.* 2018; 215:97–101. https://doi-org.evms.idm.oclc .org/10.1016/j.autneu.2018.05.004
10. Stewart JM, Gewitz M, Weldon A, Munoz J. Patterns of orthostatic intolerance: The orthostatic tachycardia syndrome and adolescent chronic fatigue. *J Pediatr.* 1999;135:218–225.
11. Low PA, Sandroni P, Joyner M, Shen WK. Postural tachycardia syndrome (POTS). *J Cardiovasc Electrophysiol.* 2009;20:352–358.
12. Fu Q, VanGundy TB, Shibata S, Auchus RJ, Williams GH, Levine BD. Exercise training versus propranolol in the treatment of the postural orthostatic tachycardia syndrome. *Hypertension.* 2011;58:167–175.
13. Bagai K, Song Y, Ling JF, et al. Sleep disturbances and diminished quality of life in postural tachycardia syndrome. *J Clin Sleep Med.* 2011;7(2):204–210.
14. Staud R. Autonomic dysfunction in fibromyalgia syndrome: Postural orthostatic tachycardia. *Curr Rheumatol Rep.* 2008;10(6):463–466.
15. Ojha A, Chelimsky TC, Chelimsky G. Comorbidities in pediatric patients with postural orthostatic tachycardia syndrome. *J Pediatr.* 2011;158:20–23.
16. Thieben MA, Sandroni P, Sletten DM. Postural orthostatic tachycardia syndrome: The Mayo Clinic experience. *Mayo Clin Proc.* 2007;82:308–313.
17. Singer W, Sletten DM, Opfer-Gehrking TL, et al. Postural tachycardia in children and adolescents: What is abnormal? *J Pediatr.* 2012; 160(2):222–226.
18. Claydon VE, Schroeder C, Norcliffe LJ, et al. Water drinking improves orthostatic tolerance in patients with posturally related syncope. *Clin Sci.* 2006;110:343–352.
19. Miller AJ, Raj SR. Pharmacotherapy for postural tachycardia syndrome. *Auton Neurosci.* 2018;215:28–36. doi:10.1016/j.autneu.2018 .04.008

CHAPTER 24

Vertigo, Dizziness, and Mental Health

Gillian Liberman, Wanda A. Dillon, Philip Gerretsen, and Sharon L. Cushing

Introduction

The prevalence of mental illness among children and adolescents worldwide is estimated to be 10% to 20%, making it one of the leading causes of disability in the pediatric population.[1] Vertigo, among other otologic symptoms, can present as a physical reaction to psychological stress in children.[2] In a large series of pediatric patients presenting with vertigo, dizziness, or imbalance, a variety of diagnoses related to mental health (ie, anxiety, psychogenic vertigo, etc) accounted for a significant proportion (6%–13%) of the disease, and this is likely an underestimate of prevalence.[3–6] As such, an assessment of mental health symptoms should be part of the workup in children presenting with vertigo or dizziness.

The nomenclature used to describe physical manifestations of mental health can be confusing, contradictory, and misleading. In many cases, often without meaning to, an unnatural separation of the body and mind occurs in our description and classification of such disorders. Many such descriptors essentially pit the body against the mind, for example, somatic versus nonsomatic complaints, medically explained versus medically unexplained disorders, and functional versus organic disorders. This often has the effect of leaving the patient in question feeling that his or her symptoms are not real given that there is no "objective physical basis" for their complaints. It also creates an assumption that disorders of the mind versus the body are mutually exclusive of each other whereas, in fact, they often coexist in a continuum.

Over the years, a number of clinical entities have been defined in an effort to describe the physical symptoms that this patient population is experiencing. These include conversion disorder as well as disorders related to abnormal percepts in response to physiologic stimuli such as space motion discomfort, phobic postural vertigo, visual vertigo, and chronic subjective dizziness, all of which are defined later in this chapter. Most recently, the diagnostic criteria for persistent postural-perceptual dizziness (PPPD) have been defined. Some may argue that the diagnosis of PPPD does not belong in this chapter given its definition as a functional disorder, defined as "arising from a change in the mode of action of an organ,"[7] unrelated to structure or cellular deficits, which distinguishes them from psychiatric conditions[8] as stated by the International Classification of Vestibular Disorders (ICVD). There is, however, significant overlap in the presentation, treatment, and outcomes across these disorders; therefore, we have included PPPD in this chapter.

The labeling of such disorders, even in the absence of a perfect understanding of the underlying pathophysiology, is important to clinicians, to patients, and to their families, as well as to medical systems and funders. A disorder that carries a label and a set of diagnostic criteria can be diagnosed, treated, communicated, and funded in a way that is not possible of a disorder without a label. This is relevant despite the fact that the label itself has no impact on the functional consequences of the symptoms or on patients' and their families' lives.

As clinicians who care for children presenting with dizziness, vertigo, and disequilibrium, we may benefit from changing how we think about, discuss, and view these disorders, as well as how we treat the individuals who present with them. In an ideal world, all multidisciplinary teams that look after children presenting with dizziness and vertigo would include individuals with expertise in the assessment, presentation, and management of mental health symptoms. In fact, one could argue that a screening assessment for mental health conditions is as important as an audiogram in the evaluation of this population. This type of framework would shift the focus to actively looking for, identifying, and treating indications of mental health concerns, as opposed to passively assuming them when everything else has been ruled out.

Defined Disorders

In the next section, we review the diagnostic characteristics for both conversion disorder and PPPD. This is followed by an examination of the clinical presentation of such patients, their characteristics as well as those of their families, which is particularly important in the pediatric populations, as well as external factors that may contribute to their manifestation of symptoms.

Conversion Disorder

Vertigo can present as a function of a conversion disorder that is defined as a physical reaction to psychological stress.[2] In fact, there is a long-standing history of vertiginous symptoms as a symptoms of conversion disorder.[9]

The specific diagnostic criteria for conversion disorder, according to the *Diagnostic and Statistical Manual of Mental Disorders*, fifth edition (*DSM-5*),[10,11] that describe it as a functional neurologic symptom disorder are as follows:

1. One or more symptoms involving sensory function or voluntary motor control suggestive of a neurologic or medical condition.
2. Symptoms cannot be explained by medical or neurologic cause after thorough investigation, and it is often considered a diagnosis of exclusion.
3. Symptoms cause significant distress or problems in social, work, school, or other areas, or they are significant enough that medical evaluation is recommended.[12]

Conversion disorders in children can be complex in their presentation, with many conversion symptoms being the norm.[13–15] Conversion reaction in children often represents a need for emotional help or support in a child who does not have any other way of communicating his or her distress. It is important to note and communicate to the patient and his or her family that conversion reaction and the physical symptoms it creates are real in the way they are experienced by the child. Vertigo as a symptom of conversion disorder can be long lived and have a significant impact on functioning and quality of life. These symptoms can keep the patient from school, extracurricular activities, peers, and activities of daily living. It is important to note the patient is not "faking," making them up, or malingering; they do not have control over these symptoms.

Persistent Postural-Perceptual Dizziness

PPPD represents a new diagnostic label applicable to some patients presenting with physical manifestations of mental health related to dizziness and vertigo. It has been defined in the form of diagnostic criteria by the International Classification of Vestibular Disorders of the Bárány Society.[16] Through expert consensus and review of the literature, the criteria for diagnosis of this disorder were defined (Table 24–1).

The ICVD divides vestibular diseases and disorders into structural, functional, and psychiatric conditions based on either proven or presumed pathophysiologic mechanisms.[17] Where functional deficits are defined as "arising from a change in the mode of action of an organ,"[7] unrelated to structure or cellular deficits, this distinguishes them from psychiatric

Table 24–1. Criteria for the Diagnosis of Persistent Postural Perceptual Dizziness (PPPD)[16]

A. One or more symptoms of dizziness, unsteadiness, or nonspinning vertigo are present on most days for 3 months or more.	1. Symptoms last for prolonged (hours-long) periods of time, but may wax and wane in severity. 2. Symptoms need not be present continuously throughout the entire day.
B. Persistent symptoms occur without specific provocation but are exacerbated by three factors.	1. Upright posture 2. Active or passive motion without regard to direction or position 3. Exposure to moving visual stimuli or complex visual patterns
C. The disorder is precipitated by conditions that cause vertigo, unsteadiness, dizziness, or problems with balance including acute, episodic, or chronic vestibular syndromes, other neurologic or medical illnesses, or psychological distress.	1. When the precipitant is an acute or episodic condition, symptoms settle into the pattern of criterion A as the precipitant resolves, but they may occur intermittently at first, and then consolidate into a persistent course. 2. When the precipitant is a chronic syndrome, symptoms may develop slowly at first and worsen gradually.
D. Symptoms cause significant distress or functional impairment.	
E. Symptoms are not better accounted for by another disease or disorder.	

conditions.[8] By this definition, functional is not a synonym for psychogenic or psychosomatic disorders, which is how it is often used, for example, in the conversion disorder, which is also known as a functional neurologic disorder.[17] The conceptualization and pathophysiology of functional disorders, including PPPD, are not well understood. There is a suggestion that PPPD may arise from functional changes in postural control mechanisms, multisensory information processing, or cortical integration of spatial orientation and threat assessment. As a result, PPPD is classified as a chronic functional vestibular disorder, which may last months to years, and is not thought to be a structural or psychiatric condition.[16] There are multiple other disorders that have been provided with distinct labels over the years that describe many entities that may now be considered within the domain of PPPD. These include phobic postural vertigo,[18] which was felt to arise from anxiety-related conscious awareness of discrepancies between anticipated and actual movement that occur transiently in the course of normal voluntary motion.[18] Other groups defined space motion discomfort (SMD), which is felt to be a combination of uneasiness about spatial orientation and increased awareness of motion stimuli.[19,20] Similarly, visual vertigo (VV) is described as sensations or unsteadiness or dizziness on exposure to complex or moving visual stimuli, identified in patients following acute peripheral or central vestibular losses.[21] The final entity is chronic subjective dizziness (CSD), the clinical diagnosis of which is very similar to PPV, but with a focus on physical as opposed to psychological symptoms.[12]

In addition to the diagnostic criteria for PPPD outlined in Table 24–1, there are many modifiers and descriptors[16] of which the current chapter aims only to provide a summary thereof.

A diagnosis of PPPD is made on clinical history as defined in Table 24–1, criteria A to D.[16] Specifically, the primary symptoms include dizziness, a nonmotion symptom, unsteadiness, a sensation of instability, wobbling, or veering when upright or walking, and certain types of nonspinning vertigo, such as swaying, rocking, bouncing, or bobbing. There are no findings on physical exam, laboratory testing, or diagnostic imaging that are specific for a diagnosis of PPPD. Despite this, these modalities of investigation remain important as they serve to distinguish PPPD from other disorders as well as identify when a concurrent vestibular disorder exists. In most cases, symptoms of PPPD develop as the acute symptoms of the precipitating condition (where one has been identified) remit. These patients are generally not symptom free, meaning that the symptoms they report are always being experienced. In other cases, the symptoms may be stuttering in onset, initially lasting days to weeks prior to becoming persistent. Rarely, the onset of PPPD is gradual. Precipitants can include disorders causing episodic attacks of vertigo (ie, benign paroxysmal positional vertigo [BPPV], Ménière's, vestibular migraine), trauma (ie, concussion), autonomic dysfunction (ie, postural orthostatic tachycardia syndrome [POTS]), chronic anxiety and depressive disorders, as well as neurologic conditions (ie, poststroke), among others. A precipitant condition may not be identified in all cases, although patients will often be able to clearly identify the onset of their symptoms of PPPD.[16]

Given the recency of its formal definition, the incidence and prevalence of PPPD can only be estimated. Approximately 25% of individuals presenting with neuro-otologic disorders (ie, BPPV, Ménière's) subsequently evolve into conditions that would now likely be defined as PPPD.[22–25] Studies prior to the advent of the formal definition of PPPD suggest that of all patients presenting to a tertiary care center for evaluation of vestibular symptoms, 15% to 20% were diagnosed as having PPV[25] or CSD.[12] Regardless of the exact number, suffice it to say that this diagnosis is common in clinics that evaluate, assess, and treat patients presenting with vertigo and dizziness.

There is a certain degree of heterogeneity to the time course and precipitating factors that lead to PPPD that bring into question whether these are individual disorders or a single pathophysiologic entity. It is more likely at this stage of our understanding that separate mechanisms, in the presence of susceptible characteristics, lead to one recognizable and definable set of clinical features.[16] Despite its formal classification, it remains debated as to the degree it is distinct from conversion or some other somatic symptom disorder. A recent systematic review of PPPD highlights that this is a useful diagnostic label defining a series of, at times, vague and difficult to characterize, but functionally impactful symptoms, allowing for a structured management plan.[26]

Presentation

Clinical Characteristics

On history, there is often a long-standing pattern of symptoms leading to significant dysfunction and disruption of the daily routine. Symptoms are much more likely to be constant, which is counter to the episodic nature of peripheral vertiginous complaints. In general, patients' complaints persist longer and have greater impact on daily functioning than might be expected, for example, in comparison with a peripheral vestibular disorder. With this in mind, there will often be associated school absence and inability to participate in extracurricular activities. They will often display hypersensitivity across a variety of sensory stimuli including motion. They will also report and appear to have a significant fear of falling in the absence of a history of fall or fall-related injury. There may be associated symptoms that fall outside the domain of otolaryngology and, therefore, a thorough and broad history is required. Families may fail to readily offer up details of other types of physical complaints, particularly if a clinician has previously suggested that their basis may be in the mental health domain. There is often a detectable level of hypervigilance for symptoms, and families will often come in with elaborate symptom logs. Given the diagnostic challenge of these disorders coupled with the clinical concern of not missing a significant finding, these children often have a history of a significant number of tests and consultations.[2]

On physical examination, there are often extreme fluctuations of stance and gait. Many of these children will arrive in the clinic requiring significant assistance from their parents or require a mobility aid or even a wheelchair. These types of assistive devices are not generally necessary even in the child with congenital bilateral vestibular loss. These individuals will demonstrate uneconomic postures where there is wastage of muscular energy, anxious movements that are slow and variably hesitating, inconsistent with what one observes in neurologic disorders. Furthermore, the knees will be held in abnormal position, and the individual may be seen as though he or she is walking on ice (ie, walking on fixed ankles). They will often touch and hold onto surrounding objects, but not in all conditions. For example, they will hold onto the wall with simple walking, but not while walking on tiptoes (ie, ice walking). These patterns of gait and stance are often very different than what is seen in individuals with bilateral vestibular loss, for example. These individuals will also demonstrate significant sway in the upper body while the base remains stable. Their movements will have increased amplitude, which decreases with distraction.

Patient Characteristics

There are a distinct set of characteristics that are common and potentially predispose to the development of a conversion disorder. These include (1) have performance excellence in at least one area of their life, such as school, sports, or music; (2) experience a great deal of self-induced or family imposed performance pressure; (3) do not have the opportunity to develop adaptive coping strategies to cope with the stress; and (4) have difficulty identifying and talking about difficult emotions.[27,28] Most pediatric patients diagnosed with physical manifestations of mental health have not experienced behavioral problems. They tend to be children and adolescents who have little-to-no conflict with authority figures; they are often approval and perfection seeking.[18,29,30] The child or adolescent may present as a parentified child; meaning the child acts in a parenting role to their own parent. Children and adolescents can present with co-occurring depression or anxiety.

Family and Caregiver Characteristics

When a child or adolescent presents with vertigo as a function of mental health symptoms, management should include assessment of the family system, including a full family and caregiver mental health history. Unlike adult patients, we need to consider the family structure and the impact that it is having on the development of the child presenting with symptoms. To understand the developmental impact of the caregiver-child relationship, there are a few basic principles that need to be defined and reviewed.

Attachment

Attachment refers to the bond between parent/caregiver and child. When a child is securely attached to his or her parent or caregiver, the child believes that the parent is capable of consistently meeting the child's physical and emotional needs in a calm and predictable manner.[31] Practically, this means that parents respond to their children's distress in consistent and predictable ways. When an attachment crisis occurs as a result of trauma, illness, or death, for example, parents may become less able to respond to their child's distress and emotional needs.

Emotional Expression

In some families, expressing different emotions is not a role that is well modeled for the child. The family environment is structured in such a way that the child feels unsafe to express sadness, anger, or worry.

Illness Within the Family

In other families, a parent's or sibling's mental or physical health may take up the majority of the space within the family, making it difficult for the patient to feel he or she can express his or her own emotional needs. It is not uncommon for a conversion disorder diagnosis to follow some sort of trauma or attachment crisis within the family. The child or adolescent may present as a parentified child; meaning he or she acts in a parenting role. For these reasons, a full assessment of past and current family functioning is essential when considering a conversion disorder diagnosis and treatment interventions.

Impact on Functioning

When a child or adolescent first experiences dizziness or vertigo symptoms, it is quite distressing for both the patient and the family system. It is not uncommon for families to seek multiple medical opinions. The patient often begins to limit his or her activities due to symptoms. It is of particular concern when a patient's school attendance becomes inconsistent or stops all together. The vertigo symptoms begin to take up more space as patients and families spend more time focused on the symptoms. As one would expect, when a child's daily routine changes due to illness, the family's daily routine changes as well. Parents often feel the need to take time off work. Rather than one of natural progression toward individual and familial milestones, an illness narrative becomes the family's story. Anxiety, frustration, isolation, and low mood may follow if vertigo symptoms persist and go untreated.

Presentation of Diagnosis to the Patient and Family

The presentation of a diagnosis related to physical manifestations of mental health to patients and their family should be done in a thoughtful and supportive manner. Close attention should be paid to the language used in conveying the diagnosis, as this can greatly impact the acceptance of the diagnosis and the move toward appropriate treatment. It is essential that the patient and the family understand that the clinical team believes that the symptoms are real. Talking with patients and families about the continuum and intersection of the mind and body and providing psycho-education of the impact of psychological stress on the body is very important. It is also important to ensure that the patient and family do not feel blamed or responsible for the symptoms. When possible, including a mental health professional in the conversation with the family can be of benefit.

Treatment Interventions

Integrated care is required when children present with physical manifestations of mental health. This can include any or all of the following education, cognitive behavioral therapy, pharmacotherapy, physical therapy, etc, with a strong emphasis on helping the child regain confidence to conquer avoidance behaviors.

Individual and Family Therapy

The first step in any treatment intervention is the development of a safe, therapeutic relationship between the patient and health professionals providing treatment. Treatment goals should include a return to functionality, and coping skills to manage symptoms and lessen the impact they are having on the patient's life. Support should be provided to identify and express difficult emotions in adaptable ways for the patient and the family.

A combination of individual and family therapy is often indicated. Individual therapy may include cognitive behavioral therapy,[32] mindfulness, and psychotherapy to support the development of skills to manage anxiety related to the vertigo symptoms as well co-occurring symptoms of depression and anxiety. Family therapy may be of benefit to reduce the family's illness narrative created by the vertigo symptoms; increase distress tolerance; and support the family's gradual return to regular routines (eg, regular mealtimes, return to school, work, etc).

Pharmacotherapy

Drugs labeled "antidepressants" are valuable, safe interventions for the treatment of psychosomatic illness, which can include dizziness and/or imbalance. Unfortunately, individuals often have stigmatized fears of the adverse effects associated with antidepressants (eg, "It will turn me into a zombie"). The goal of antidepressant medication is to ease symptoms to help the individual better cope with his or her disorder(s). Recommendations with documented efficacy include selective serotonin reuptake inhibitors (SSRIs) or serotonin and norepinephrine reuptake inhibitors (SNRIs). These antidepressants improve mental, emotional, and physical symptoms by regulating nerve signaling throughout the nervous system. SSRIs and SNRIs are not habit forming (ie, not addictive), and patience is required to achieve optimal outcomes.[33] Patients and their families should routinely be informed of the common adverse effects of these antidepressants, which can include a transient worsening of dizziness or nausea at the outset of treatment or with each dose increase. If not informed of these expected adverse effects, many individuals may discontinue the treatment prematurely, passing up the opportunity for subsequent beneficial effects. For this reason, it is important to provide patients and their families with detailed information about the recommended medication, including an outline of the dosing schedule and a list of the common and rare side effects. Encouraging patients and their families to ask questions and to discuss possible fears related to this form of intervention will help foster trust and an adaptive attitude toward medication, and ultimately any other recommended treatments.[34]

The goal of antidepressant treatment is full remission of the patient's symptoms. Similar to guidelines used for the treatment of anxiety and depression, individuals should be informed that treatments should progress in a stepwise, algorithmic way until the treatment goal of full remission is achieved.[35,36] The emphasis on the goal of full remission fosters hope and maximizes the expectation of full recovery. Patients and families experience greater despair and a higher risk of relapse if patients are partially treated.[35,36] Medication discontinuation is recommended after a period of at least 6 months to 2 years of the individual being symptom free.[35] Individuals will be more willing to trial an antidepressant if aware that the goal is eventual medication discontinuation once a satisfactory period of remission has occurred. To achieve the best possible outcome with an antidepressant or any other recommended treatment, ie, mindfulness, psychotherapy, cognitive behavioral therapy, etc, interventions should be started when individuals are motivated and feel that it is the right treatment option for them.[34] Patient motivation or acceptance of treatment is important to readdress if an individual expresses any ambivalence or resistance to starting or continuing with an intervention. This will maximize the chance of an optimal outcome, relieve any unnecessary pressures associated with the interventions, and ultimately lead to a greater readiness by the individual to try the recommended treatments.[34]

Case Study 1

A 15-year-old female was referred to Otolaryngology for episodic and debilitating vertigo. Symptoms are worse in the mornings often keeping her home from school. Neurootologic and ancillary testing are normal. The patient reports a history of school avoidance and anxiety and was therefore referred to social work for further assessment and treatment. Biopsychosocial assessment reveals that the patient lives with her mother and younger siblings. There is a history of maternal depression and anxiety. The patient often acts in a caregiving role with her siblings and her mother when her mother's mental health symptoms are severe. The assessment reveals evidence of an insecure attachment as the patient's mother has been physically and emotionally absent at times due to her own mental health symptoms. The patient excels at school and was playing elite soccer until the vertigo episodes started. She reports that she is currently experiencing periods of low mood and irritability. She reports anxiety related to school performance, peer relationships, and recurrent vertigo symptoms. She is currently not attending school on a consistent basis. She reveals that when she stays home from school due to feeling unwell, her mother takes care of her and relieves her of taking care of her siblings as is otherwise the routine.[37]

A conversion disorder diagnosis was provided following full assessment. The language used in talking with the patient and her family is extremely important. Treatment interventions included psychoeducation regarding the mind-body connection. Individual therapy, including CBT to support the development of strategies to manage anxiety and mood, is provided. Family therapy is provided to support the shifting of roles, boundaries, and communication patterns within the family. A functional approach was used to support a gradual return to regular routines.[38] At the conclusion of the treatment intervention, the patient had attended school for 5 days, two consecutive weeks in a row. She was reporting using CBT strategies to manage vertigo and anxiety symptoms. The family's communication style became more responsive and emotionally supportive. A recommendation to continue with family therapy was made.

Case Study 2

A 15-year-old male athlete was referred to the Multi-Disciplinary Neurotology Clinic for sudden-onset dizziness approximately 3 days after hitting his head on a snowmobile approximately a year and half ago. He reported constant dizziness with episodic worsening, particularly on awakening or in anticipation of an event, such as a hockey game, which "disappears" once playing. He would also experience an increase in symptoms when preparing for tests and exams. Additional symptom complaints included occasional headaches, periods of chest tightness, muscle tension, and shortness of breath. The patient reported missing 1 to 3 days of high school per week over the past 1.5 years due to the inability to cope and manage with the chronic symptoms. Following a thorough psychiatric assessment, a diagnosis of chronic dizziness with agoraphobia and possible panic disorder was given. A trial of sertraline was recommended. Dosing instructions and side effects were discussed. The patient and his parents were also given the opportunity to discuss any concerns they may have had regarding the medication treatment recommendation. He was also recommended individual CBT. With gradual increases in the medication and bimonthly therapy sessions, he reported near complete resolution in his chronic dizziness approximately 6 months later. He also reported coping better with stressful events. Continued optimization of his medication was recommended to help him with the residual symptoms. He has now returned to school full-time and feels he is the same as he was before the head injury.

Self-Assessment Questions

1. Define a conversion disorder.
2. List specific diagnostic criteria for conversion disorder according to the *DSM-5*.
3. List typical patient characteristics in a patient diagnosed with vertigo as a function of a conversion diagnosis.

4. List typical family/caregiver characteristics of a family in which their child has been diagnosed with a vertigo as a function of a conversion diagnosis.

5. An integrated approach to treatment of a conversion disorder is of most benefit to the patient and family. What treatment interventions are included in this approach?

6. Define PPPD.

7. List medications that have documented efficacy in the treatment of vertigo as a function of a conversion disorder.

References

1. Child and adolescent mental health. In: WHO, ed 2015.
2. Caulley L, Kohlert S, Gandy H, Olds J, Bromwich M. When symptoms don't fit: A case series of conversion disorder in the pediatric otolaryngology practice. *J Otolaryngol Head Neck Surg.* 2018;47(1):39.
3. O'Reilly RC, Greywoode J, Morlet T, et al. Comprehensive vestibular and balance testing in the dizzy pediatric population. *Otolaryngol Head Neck Surg.* 2011;144(2):142–148.
4. Ravid S, Bienkowski R, Eviatar L. A simplified diagnostic approach to dizziness in children. *Pediatr Neurol.* 2003;29(4):317–320.
5. Riina N, Ilmari P, Kentala E. Vertigo and imbalance in children: A retrospective study in a Helsinki University otorhinolaryngology clinic. *Arch Otolaryngol Head Neck Surg.* 2005; 131(11):996–1000.
6. Erbek SH, Erbek SS, Yilmaz I, et al. Vertigo in childhood: A clinical experience. *Int J Pediatr Otorhinolaryngol.* 2006;70(9):1547–1554.
7. Combe A. Observations on mental derangement: Being an application of the principles of phresnology to elucidation of the causes, symptoms, nature and treatment of insanity. In: Anderson J, ed. Edingurgh1831.
8. In: Drossman DA, ed. *The Functional Gastrointestinal Disorders.* 3rd. ed. Mclean, VA: Degnon Associates Inc.; 2006.
9. Baijens LW, Verdonschot R, Vanbelle S, et al. Medically unexplained otorhinolaryngological symptoms: Towards integrated psychiatric care. *Laryngoscope.* 2015;125(7):1583–1587.
10. American Psychiatric Association. DSM 5 development. Highlights of changes from DSM-IV-TR to DSM 5. http://www.dsm5.org/Documents/changes%20from%20dsm-iv-tr%20to%20dsm-5.pdf
11. American Psychiatric Association. DSM-5 Task Force. *Diagnostic and Statistical Manual of Mental Disorders.* Arlington, VA: Author; 2013.
12. Staab JP, Ruckenstein MJ. Expanding the differential diagnosis of chronic dizziness. *Arch Otolaryngol Head Neck Surg.* 2007;133(2):170–176.
13. Ani C, Reading R, Lynn R, Forlee S, Garralda E. Incidence and 12-month outcome of non-transient childhood conversion disorder in the U.K. and Ireland. *Br J Psychiatry.* 2013;202: 413–418.
14. Kozlowska K, Nunn KP, Rose D, Morris A, Ouvrier RA, Varghese J. Conversion disorder in Australian pediatric practice. *J Am Acad Child Adolesc Psychiatry.* 2007;46(1):68–75.
15. Kozlowska K, Palmer DM, Brown KJ, et al. Conversion disorder in children and adoles-

cents: A disorder of cognitive control. *J Neuropsychol.* 2015;9(1):87–108.
16. Staab JP, Eckhardt-Henn A, Horii A, et al. Diagnostic criteria for persistent postural-perceptual dizziness (PPPD): Consensus document of the committee for the Classification of Vestibular Disorders of the Barany Society. *J Vestib Res.* 2017;27(4):191–208.
17. Bisdorff AR, Staab JP, Newman-Toker DE. Overview of the International Classification of Vestibular Disorders. *Neurol Clin.* 2015; 33(3):541–550, vii.
18. Brandt T. Phobic postural vertigo. *Neurology.* 1996;46(6):1515–1519.
19. Lilienfeld SO, Jacob RG, Furman JM. Vestibular dysfunction followed by panic disorder with agoraphobia. *J Nerv Ment Dis.* 1989; 177(11):700–701.
20. Jacob RG, Redfern MS, Furman JM. Space and motion discomfort and abnormal balance control in patients with anxiety disorders. *J Neurol Neurosurg Psychiatry.* 2009;80(1):74–78.
21. Bronstein AM, Guerraz M. Visual-vestibular control of posture and gait: Physiological mechanisms and disorders. *Curr Opin Neurol.* 1999; 12(1):5–11.
22. Best C, Tschan R, Eckhardt-Henn A, Dieterich M. Who is at risk for ongoing dizziness and psychological strain after a vestibular disorder? *Neuroscience.* 2009;164(4):1579–1587.
23. Cousins S, Kaski D, Cutfield N, et al. Predictors of clinical recovery from vestibular neuritis: A prospective study. *Ann Clin Transl Neurol.* 2017;4(5):340–346.
24. Godemann F, Siefert K, Hantschke-Bruggemann M, Neu P, Seidl R, Strohle A. What accounts for vertigo one year after neuritis vestibularis—Anxiety or a dysfunctional vestibular organ? *J Psychiatr Res.* 2005;39(5):529–534.
25. Heinrichs N, Edler C, Eskens S, Mielczarek MM, Moschner C. Predicting continued dizziness after an acute peripheral vestibular disorder. *Psychosom Med.* 2007;69(7):700–707.
26. Trinidade A, Goebel JA. Persistent postural-perceptual dizziness—A systematic review of the literature for the balance specialist. *Otol Neurotol.* 2018;39(10):1291–1303.
27. Ali S, Jabeen S, Pate RJ, et al. Conversion disorder—Mind versus body: A review. *Innov Clin Neurosci.* 2015;12(5–6):27–33.
28. Grattan-Smith P, Fairley M, Procopis P. Clinical features of conversion disorder. *Arch Dis Child.* 1988;63(4):408–414.
29. Staab JP, Rohe DE, Eggers SD, Shepard NT. Anxious, introverted personality traits in patients with chronic subjective dizziness. *J Psychosom Res.* 2014;76(1):80–83.
30. Yan Z, Cui L, Yu T, Liang H, Wang Y, Chen C. Analysis of the characteristics of persistent postural-perceptual dizziness: A clinical-based study in China. *Int J Audiol.* 2017;56(1): 33–37.
31. Bowlby J. *Attachment and Loss. Vol 1: Attachment.* 2nd ed. New York, NY: Basic Books; 1982.
32. Yu YC, Xue H, Zhang YX, Zhou J. Cognitive behavior therapy as augmentation for sertraline in treating patients with persistent postural-perceptual dizziness. *Biomed Res Int.* 2018;2018:8518631.
33. Staab JP. Assessment and management of psychological problems in the dizzy patient. *Continuum.* 2006;12(4):189–213.
34. Miller WR, Rose GS. Toward a theory of motivational interviewing. *Am Psychol.* 2009; 64(6):527–537.
35. Gelenberg AJ, Freeman MP, Markowitz JC, et al. Practice guideline for the treatment of patients with major depressive disorder. American Psychiatric Association. *Am J Psychiatry.* 2010:1–152.
36. Canadian Psychiatric Association. Clinical practice guidelines. Management of anxiety disorders. *Can J Psychiatry.* 2006;51(8 suppl 2): 9S–91S.
37. Kozlowska K, Williams LM. Self-protective organization in children with conversion and somatoform disorders. *J Psychosom Res.* 2009; 67(3):223–233.
38. Maisami M, Freeman JM. Conversion reactions in children as body language: A combined child psychiatry/neurology team approach to the management of functional neurologic disorders in children. *Pediatrics.* 1987;80(1):46–52.

SECTION IV

Treatment

CHAPTER 25

Multisensory Deficits

Joan Vertes

At 8 years of age, Alex seemed bright, active, and verbal. However, his teachers were concerned. He was unable to keep up in gym class; he could run across the balance beam but could not walk without falling off. He was slow to change out of his winter clothes, especially his snow pants. When required to line up, he leaned against the wall or other students. At times he seemed lazy, lying across his desk, or holding his head up with one hand while writing with the other. At other times, he seemed restless or "fidgety," wiggling in his chair. His written work was messy. He needed frequent reminders to sit up, sit still, and pay attention.

Multisensory Deficits and Balance in Occupational Therapy

The need for occupational therapy (OT) intervention for children described as having poor balance has been well documented. Balance issues often exist along with other coordination difficulties, including gross motor, fine motor, and/or visual motor. When balance is poorly developed, it may interfere with the development of motor skills and affect children's ability to socialize with peers or to perform daily tasks, such as dressing.[1,2]

In the past, children with poor balance sometimes received the label of Clumsy Child Syndrome. Currently the term sensory processing disorder (SPD), also known as sensory integration dysfunction (SID), is utilized.[3,4] The prevalence of SPD in children has been estimated to be 5% to 13% in those entering kindergarten; and 56% to 70% in those with other disabilities including autism spectrum disorders.[5,6]

The evolving theory of sensory integration (SI), originally developed by Dr. A. Jean Ayres, in the 1960s, has contributed to our understanding of SPD. Occupational therapists (OTs) use and study SI more than any other approach.[6] The clinical term *sensory integration* as used by OTs should be differentiated from the cellular one used by neuroscientists, which refers to "converging information in the brain from one or more sensory domains."[4(p1)]

SI refers to "the organization of sensations for use."[2(p5)] Based on her study of OT, neuroscience (including brain plasticity), sensorimotor development (based on the work of Piaget), and education, Ayres theorized that sensations form a foundation from which normal development can occur, through interaction with the body in the environment, enabling children to modulate behavior, learn and participate at home, in school, or on the playground, just like their peers. Information is taken in from any of the 8 senses: vestibular (balance and posture), proprioception (information from muscles and joints), tactile, visual, auditory, olfactory, taste, and interoception (sensations from inside the body as hunger or thirst). It is organized in the central nervous system. Through adaptive and purposeful responses, normal learning and behavior are achieved. If the sensory information is not efficiently organized in the brain, motor responses may be disorganized or not appropriate.

Knowledge of SI theory helps us to appreciate how multiple sensory systems contribute to the development of normal balance as well as the importance of using multisensory modalities in therapy, rather than single modalities. Effective processing and integration of vestibular, proprioceptive, and visual information are required for balance and postural control. Children with SPD may rely on different combinations of sensory information than typically developing peers.[4] They have also been found to rely more heavily on vision to compensate for difficulties in performing motor tasks.[7]

Low self-esteem and immature social skills are often seen in children with SPD. They may be picked for teams last or behave differently than peers. They may ultimately exhibit anxiety, frustration, anger, or depression.[8]

Alex in Occupational Therapy

Subsequent to ruling out medical causes, Alex's (example described above) doctor referred him to OT. Based on sensory motor assessment, the OT hypothesized that poor processing of basic sensory input, including vestibular, proprioceptive, tactile, and visual information may have resulted in Alex's lack of adaptive motor responses, and poor posture; he seemed to lack awareness of the displacement of his center of gravity; he did not shift his weight or use equilibrium reactions to balance. He leaned against the wall to compensate and to help himself feel where his body was in space. He was required to sit down to put on his snow pants since standing on one foot was difficult. Maintaining balance for long periods in his seat at his desk was challenging and tiring. Alex craved movement (wiggling) to remain upright against gravity. Holding his head up with one hand helped him remain seated and keep his eyes on his page but prevented him from stabilizing his paper which moved as he wrote. This, along with his use of overlapping thumb (immature grip) to stabilize the pencil in his hand (however, reduces mobility) contributed to messy written work.

Principles of Therapy

Ayres outlined several principles, which differentiated her frame of reference from others. She stressed that following the child's lead while he experienced sensorimotor development was important for change. Rather than pre-plan, structure, or direct sessions, therapists must collaborate with children. The treatment space (OT gym) is set up with sensory-rich opportunities based on the needs of the individual. Children are enticed to participate actively through play and rely on inner drive to choose activities to help them learn. An adaptive response and the just right challenge are sought (gear for success, not too hard or easy), as well as repetition. "Research suggests that learning is enhanced by emotion, spontaneity, and play, which are the essential ingredients in a SI approach used within OT. Physiological data shows increased cortical blood volume during performance of novel integration activities in a spontaneous, playful manner."[9(p817)]

OT interventions may be guided by Ayres theory either in its pure form, Ayres SI, or as part of a sensorimotor approach, where not all of the principles delineated previously are followed, eg, suspended equipment (swings) unavailable, or group treatment (more adult directed). Some other frames of reference used to work with children with coordination difficulties may include neurodevelopment, psychosocial, or cognitive. Occupational therapists use their clinical judgment and expertise to choose and combine these as appropriate.

A family centered approach is important. Collaboration is ongoing between parents, children, and therapists, to set goals and provide education. Parents are especially concerned about social participation, self-regulation, and perceived competence for their children.[10] They are helped to reframe their expectations and to advocate for their children with teachers and family members. In Alex's case, it is important for teachers and parents to understand that rather than being lazy, he may be working harder than others to attend and to accomplish similar tasks.

Therapy may be administered in hospitals or private clinics, schools, or homes. Originally developed for the learning-disabled population, OT using an SI frame of reference has also been used with various other populations, including developmental delay, autism spectrum disorder, fragile-X syndrome, CP, visual or hearing impairment, premature birth, and prenatal drug exposure.[11]

Sensory Modulation/Regulation

Initially in therapy, sensory modulation, or the manner in which children regulate or grade responses,[4] must be addressed. Some children cannot get enough vestibular input (hyporesponsive to, or overwhelmed by[4] vestibular input). They may become a danger to themselves or others in seeking it; eg, jumping prone (on tummy) onto a therapy ball of their own size with no one nearby to catch them.

Children with hyporesponsivity to proprioceptive input, such as Alex (previous example), may not notice the input to the same degree as others[4]; eg, they sometimes press too hard with their pencils to obtain sufficient feedback, breaking them or becoming tired quickly. They may "fix" or compensate with proximal muscles when required to use distal muscles, eg, hiking shoulders during wheelbarrow walk, locking knees during balance tasks, or using an immature quadruped grasp to provide stability for distal finger muscles.[12] These immature stabilizing patterns may interfere with mobility and performance.

Children receiving weak proprioceptive feedback from their muscles and joints may compensate with vision. If they are watching their fingers move to hold the pencil and to form letters, they are not free to look at the teacher or the blackboard. When playing catch, they may throw the ball with too much force, alienating possible friends.

Other children may be hyperresponsive; they may become anxious or overreact to vestibular input such as swinging or car rides with fear, nausea, headache, and/or loss of balance.

Example/Hyperresponsive

Jaclyn presented as a quiet-spoken 4-year-old girl, who held herself stiffly, barely moving her head. Parents described her as fearful and somewhat rigid in personality. She played games only when she was allowed to make the rules. She did not alternate feet on the stairs. She held the class back when they went upstairs or downstairs for recess or library periods. In OT she sat down on the 3-inch-high mat first in order to "climb" on or off of it. She refused to sit in the swing, clinging to the OT. She was desperate to keep her feet on the ground. She refused to put her head back or try a somersault.

Changes in relationship to gravity frightened Jaclyn. Ayres referred to this as gravitational insecurity.[2]

Developmental Components of Balance

Various developmental components of balance are addressed on an ongoing basis: muscle tone, equilibrium and righting reactions, gravitational insecurity, ocular pursuits, and/or reflex integration.[2,12]

Children with SPD who have low/normal muscle tone may present as "floppy" with poor posture, sometimes slouching over their desks, as Alex did in the previous example, or resting their head on one hand so that it is not free to stabilize the paper while they write. They tend to tire easily. Muscle tone cannot be changed. Rather the child is helped to gain stability, strength, and endurance.

Consequences of immature equilibrium reactions can be demonstrated to parents by asking them to stand on one leg. Ideally following shifting of weight, one experiences shortening of the muscles on the non-weight-bearing side or lengthening on the weight-bearing side along with rotation between shoulders and hips.

Children with immature equilibrium reactions appear stiff when required to balance. They seem to move their body as a block and do not adequately shift their weight or use trunk rotation to master changes in gravitational demands. Running can look awkward.

Primitive reflex integration underlies development of more mature postural reactions, righting, and equilibrium reactions. Initially, babies explore their environment and move using innate reflexes, eventually developing more mature motor skills. Some do not adequately integrate these reflexes, eg, children sitting in class turn to watch the teacher on the right side of the room and experience increased extensor tone in the right arm, accidentally brushing their notes off the desk (asymmetrical tonic neck reflex or fencing position). They may benefit from being placed in the center of the class close to the teacher, who has been made aware of the issue. Some children lean over their desk with their whole bodies (influence of poor integration of the symmetrical tonic neck reflex, low muscle tone).

Intervention Example

Gregg runs into the OT gym and begins to jump up and down on the large mat (vestibular and proprioceptive input). His therapist folds one end of the mat so that he is enticed to jump from one height to another. When he does not jump with both feet together (fear, bilateral issues), she places an inner tube on the lowest level, to provide a visual cue and added security. He jumps with both feet together. After five repetitions, the OT adds a ramp to the edge of the mat and hands Gregg a scooter board. He lies on his tummy (extension against gravity) and rides down, crashing into a large body pillow. A few minutes later, she hangs the hammock swing and he approaches with curiosity. The therapist guides him to lie on his tummy in the swing, which is a completely new experience for him (motor planning). She hands him a rope ladder, which is attached to a hook in the ceiling. He pulls himself forward slightly and lets go, slapping his hands down on the mat in fear, providing himself with proprioceptive input. He is encouraged to try to climb "Gregg Mountain" again. He alternates hands, counts two rungs, and then lets go (vestibular). With the therapist's encouragement and grading of the activity, he masters the just right challenge, gradually climbing to the sixth rung. He smiles with glee and pride in his success. He reaches for the ladder again and again, learning through active participation and repetition. Vestibular and proprioception input are provided as he uses cocontraction of his muscles to alternate hands (bilateral motor coordination) and counts (cognitive) the rungs.

Intervention

A heavy emphasis on vestibular (swings, trampoline, scooter boards), proprioceptive, and tactile input combined with vision and auditory information is provided in therapy. Children learn to feel where their bodies are in space, and to use adaptive responses. They are facilitated to work more efficiently against gravity (see Gregg, as discussed previously). Often they begin to take more risks, and to expose themselves to more and more activities requiring balance and holding their heads upside down, such as using the monkey bars.

As postural adjustments become more automatic, SPD children become freer to follow teacher directions and to attend to other motor and social tasks.

Proprioceptive input is thought to facilitate regulation over other systems such as vestibular and tactile, in addition to modulating arousal overall.[13] Jaclyn (example of gravitational insecurity) would benefit from heavy proprioceptive input, such as tug of war, jumping on a mini trampoline (rebounder) with hands held, helping to move the mats.

"Hot dog in a bun" is a favorite activity in OT and at home to calm the children: the child is rolled in a blanket and mustard- or chocolate-covered frogs' legs are firmly rolled over him (therapy ball). This provides deep pressure/touch. As he pulls himself out of the bun, he receives proprioceptive input.

The visual and vestibular systems work closely together. When our head moves, our eyes move. Occupational therapists may work on log rolling down an incline (vestibular, whole body), later adding in a game of Eye Spy (vision). The child may advance to rolling using vision and targeting, eg, the child slides down a ramp while lying on his tummy on a scooter board, picks up beanbags from the floor, and aims at a target.

Strategies are developed with parents and children to optimize behavior and performance. They can now understand why wiggling in their chairs helps them to maintain balance and to attend. Sitting on a gym ball or on a core disc (similar to a hot water bottle slightly filled with air) is sometimes recommended for home and school use. Blocks may be needed to help keep their feet grounded. Seat push-ups where the child sits in his chair and pushes his body up, holding it for a count of 5, can be a fun sensory-input break; wall-stands, in which children walk up the wall with their feet while holding their weight through their arms, help to prepare muscles for work and children to attend.

Frequent breaks (every 20 to 30 minutes) in school with opportunities to run errands for the teacher or carry heavy books are often recommended. Recess is important. Children are encouraged to walk or jump part way to school (similar to adults having coffee before beginning their day).

Chewing gum or crushed ice and sucking from a straw in a water bottle are useful strategies (oral-motor, proprioception). Toys such as small koosh balls, or thin wiry rings to fidget with often reduce distractibility.

Weighted vests or heavy-pressure clothing may aid in regulation or calming and with attention. Weights worn around their wrist while writing can help children feel where their arms are in space and encourage resting of their arm on the desk rather than up in space (poor proprioceptive awareness).

Conclusion

In conclusion, occupational therapists consider various sensory and motor components that impact balance and posture. The theory of sensory integration guides assessment and treatment practices as the processing and organization of multisensory input are critical for the development of balance. Multiple sensory modalities are used in treatment to improve the child's ability to produce adaptive responses and to learn new skills, thus allowing performance and behavior to match their peers.

Self-Assessment Questions

1. Occupational therapists receive many referrals for children with poor balance. What theory have they studied and used most often to address sensorimotor development of balance? Please define it.
2. List possible presenting complaints of children with sensory processing disorder (SPD) who experience poor balance.
3. List some important principles used by occupational therapists in an SI approach.
4. OT using an SI approach has been used with which populations?
5. What help do parents seek for their children? Describe the benefits of incorporating family-centered care.
6. What multisensory input may have contributed to Alex's (see case study) difficulties with balance and posture?
7. What is meant by sensory modulation, and what are the 2 subtypes?
8. How can immature reflex patterns interfere with children's performance?
9. How can gravitational insecurity affect performance?
10. What is involved in therapy sessions to address balance and posture?

References

1. Richardson PK, Atwater SW, Crowe TK, Dietz, JC. Performance of preschoolers on the pediatric clinical test of sensory integration for balance. *Am J Occup Ther.* 1992;46:793–800.
2. Doumas M, McKenna R, Murphy B. Postural control deficits in autism spectrum disorder: The role of sensory integration. *J Autism Dev Dis.* 2016;46(3):853–861.
3. Ayres AJ. *Sensory Integration and the Child.* Torrance, CA: Western Psychological Services; 1979.
4. Miller LJ, Nielsen DM, Schoen SA, Brett-Green BA. Perspectives on sensory processing disorder: A call for translational research. *Front Integr Neurosci.* 2009;3:22. https://doi.org/10.3389/neuro.07.022.2009
5. Ahn R, Miller LJ, McIntosh D. Prevalence of parent's perceptions of sensory processing disorders among kindergarten children. *Am J Occup Ther.* 2004;56:287–302.
6. Schaaf RC, Dumont RL, Arbesman M, May-Benson TA. Efficacy of occupational therapy using Ayres Sensory Integration: A systematic review. *Am J Occup Ther.* 2018;72:7201190010p1–7201190010p10. https://doi.org/10.5014/ajot.2018.028431
7. Su C-T, Wu M-Y, Yang AL, Chen-Sea M-J, Hwang I-S. Impairment of stance control in children with sensory modulation disorder. *Am J Occup Ther.* 2011;64:443–452. https://doi.org/10.5014/ajot.2010.09074
8. Schaaf R, Nightlinger K. Occupational therapy using a sensory integrative approach: A case study of effectiveness. *Am J Occup Ther.* 2007;61:239–246.
9. Peyton JL, Bass WT, Burked BL, Frank M. Novel motor and somatosensory activity is associated with increased cerebral cortical blood volume measured by near-infrared optical topography. *J Child Neurol.* 2005;20:817–821.
10. Cohn E, Miller LJ, Tickle-Degnen L. Parental hopes for therapy outcomes: Children with sensory modulation disorder. *Am J Occup Ther.* 2000;54:36–43.
11. Spitzer S, Smith Roley S. Sensory integration revisited: A philosophy of practice. In: Smith Roley S, Imperatore Blanche E, Schaaf RC, eds. *Understanding the Nature of Sensory Integration with Diverse Populations.* San Antonio, TX: Psychological Corporation; 2001:3–28.
12. Imperatore Blanche E, Schaaf RC. Proprioception: A cornerstone of sensory integrative intervention. In: Smith Roley S, Imperatore Blanche E, Schaaf RC, eds. *Understanding the Nature of Sensory Integration with Diverse Populations.* San Antonio, TX: Psychological Corporation; 2001:109–124.
13. Bundy AC, Lane SJ, Murray EA, eds. *Sensory Integration Theory and Practice.* 2nd ed. Philadelphia, PA: F.A. Davis; 2002.

CHAPTER 26

Vestibular Rehabilitation

Michael Karl

Introduction

Recent research indicates that vestibular dysfunction in children is more common than previously believed.[1] Based on a 2012 survey of parents in the United States, Li and colleagues reported that 18.6% of children were believed to have significant balance and dizziness concerns.[1] Central and peripheral vestibular impairments can lead to poor balance, increased fall risk, delays in gross motor development, decreased reading acuity, learning delays, gaze instability, and symptoms of dizziness or vertigo.[2] Despite the prevalence of vestibular problems in children, many children go untreated, which can lead to progressive delays in motor and reading function.[3–6] The low rate of treatment may be a result of a number of factors including some children's difficulty communicating symptoms and poor recognition by caregivers and medical providers of the signs of vestibular disorders in children. Additionally, there is a lack of pediatric specific examination equipment, facilities that provide this highly specialized care, and research on optimal treatment dosage and effectiveness. Some of the most common causes of vestibular dysfunction in the pediatric population include benign paroxysmal vertigo of childhood, vestibular migraine, recurrent otitis media, damage due to cytomegalovirus or other infections, and concussion/traumatic brain injury.[7,8] With early recognition and appropriate testing, vestibular rehabilitation can be effective in treating vertigo, balance and motor delays, and gaze instability in children.[2,9–14] Vestibular rehabilitation consists of specific interventions that are targeted to promote restoration and adaptation of functioning systems, substitution strategies for vestibular loss, and habituation for reduction of symptoms such as visual motion sensitivity.

Signs and Symptoms of Vestibular Dysfunction in Children

The vestibular system consists of the peripheral sensory apparatus (otoliths, semicircular canals, hair cells, vestibular nerve, and vascular supply), the central processing system (vestibular nuclear complex and cerebellum), and motor output resulting in eye movement and postural control (via the vestibulo-ocular, vestibulospinal, and vestibulocollic reflexes). Dysfunction in any one or more of the components of the vestibular system can result in impairments in functional mobility, gaze stability, and/or complaints of motion sickness, dizziness, or vertigo. Table 26–1 outlines common signs and symptoms of central and peripheral vestibular dysfunction.

Therapeutic Evaluation of a Child With Vestibular Dysfunction

The therapeutic evaluation and rehabilitation of vestibular dysfunction in children are typically performed by an occupational and/or physical therapist. The details related to inclusive medical evaluation and laboratory vestibular function testing of children have been outlined earlier within this textbook. These results and a detailed medical history should be reviewed by the rehabilitation professional before the physical examination. Prior to the assessment and treatment, the therapist should review specific precautions related to the child's pathology. Precautions that may require treatment/evaluation modifications include syncope, orthostatic hypotension, seizure disorders, low muscle tone, joint instability, spasticity, nausea, emesis, surgical

Table 26–1. Signs and Symptoms of Vestibular Dysfunction in Children

Signs and Symptoms of Central Vestibular Dysfunction
• Delayed acquisition of gross motor milestones • Impaired balance abilities • Delayed or below-age level performance on visuomotor and visual perception tests • Persistent tonic reflexes • Possible visual instability when moving (± Dynamic Visual Acuity Test) • Possible sensory integrative dysfunction • Incoordination • Laboratory vestibular function testing may be normal or abnormal • Associated diagnoses including migraine, attention deficit hyperactivity disorder, autism
Signs and Symptoms of Peripheral Vestibular Dysfunction
• Intermittent positional vertigo and/or nystagmus • Visual instability when moving (Positive Head Impulse Test and Dynamic Visual Acuity Test) • Impaired balance abilities • Complaints of spinning sensation or dizziness • Possible hearing loss or tinnitus • May avoid or be fearful of movement • Incoordination • Abnormal laboratory vestibular function testing

precautions, and poor balance. Additionally, the therapist should be aware that vestibular testing and treatment are likely to temporarily increase children's symptoms and may need to prioritize testing procedures.

Regardless of the source of dysfunction, signs and symptoms of vestibular impairment can generally be broken down into the following categories: postural, vertigo, vestibulovisual, and dizziness (Table 26–2).[15] A comprehensive evaluation requires a systematic assessment in all of these domains to determine the nature and type of lesion if possible, mechanism of recovery, and specific impairments that require intervention.[16]

Essential components of an assessment may include the following:

- Review of medical history, vestibular function testing, and other relevant previous testing and interventions
- Review of developmental history (age that child achieved independent sitting, crawling, walking, bike riding)
- Review of the nature, severity, and timing of symptoms including use of a validated symptom questionnaire completed by the parent/patient
- Examination of joint range of motion, muscle strength and tone, sensation and proprioception
- Clinical balance tests (Chapter 8), gait (Chapter 9), and mobility assessments
- Computerized dynamic posturography (Chapter 7)
- Developmental reflexes (Chapter 2)
- Standardized developmental assessments
- Vision and oculomotor tests
- Vestibulo-ocular reflex (VOR) tests
- Positional vertigo assessment
- Motion Sensitivity Quotient Test

Symptom questionnaires are important tools to not only quantify the severity of symptoms or functional impairments, but to also help direct treatment and assess the effectiveness of rehabilitation interventions. There are several questionnaires that have been validated for the pediatric population. The Pediatric Dizziness Handicap Inventory (DHI-PC) was adapted from the adult Dizziness Handicap Inventory and can be used to quantify the severity and impact of vestibular-related impairments in children.[17] The Pediatric Vestibular Symptom Questionnaire

Table 26–2. Vestibular Symptom Definitions[15]

Postural symptoms—balance symptoms related to maintenance of postural stability, occurring only while upright (seated, standing, or walking).
Vertigo—the sensation of self-motion (of head/body) when no self motion is occurring or the sensation of distorted self-motion during an otherwise normal head movement.
Vestibulovisual symptoms—visual symptoms that usually result from vestibular pathology or the interplay between visual and vestibular systems. These include false sensations of motion or tilting of the visual surround and visual distortion (blur) linked to vestibular (rather than optical) failure.
Dizziness—the sensation of disturbed or impaired spatial orientation without a false or distorted sense of motion.

(PVSQ) is validated to assess for the presence and severity of vestibular symptoms in children.[18] The Pediatric Visually Induced Dizziness Questionnaire (PVIDQ) can be used to assess for the presence and severity of symptoms of visual motion-related dizziness, ie, moving in a crowd or watching a movie on a large screen.[19] The Post-Concussion Symptom Inventory (PCSI) assesses for the presence and severity of concussion symptoms in children and has a number of versions that can be completed by parents or children as young as 5 years old.[20] Finally, the Sensory Profile (Pearson, Inc, San Antonio, TX, 1999) can be used to screen for sensory processing and integration deficits as reported by parents or caregivers of children.

The assessment of joint range of motion, sensation, muscle strength, and tone are standard tests used by occupational and physical therapists and are not covered in detail in this chapter. While such an assessment is not specific to children with suspected vestibular involvement, impairments in strength, sensation, coordination, range of motion, and tone can result in poor motor output leading to gross motor deficits and falls. Particular attention should be paid to the assessment of trunk and lower extremity strength/muscle tone as well as cervical spine, hip, and ankle range of motion. Assessment of gait is covered in detail elsewhere in this book. Developmental reflexes can be used to assess for reflex integration and the presence of protective and righting reactions for safety and are outlined in more detail in Chapter 2. Coordination and developmental assessments are included in pediatric standardized tests and should be completed if the child is able to participate. The standardized developmental assessments to evaluate these functions include the following:

- Peabody Developmental Motor Scale, second edition (PDMS-2) (Pro-Ed, Austin, TX, 2000) for ages birth through 83 months. The subtests of reflexes, stationary abilities, locomotion, and object manipulation are performed to obtain a composite gross motor score. The fine motor scale tests grasping and visual motor integration.
- Bruininks-Oseretsky Test of Motor Proficiency, second edition (BOT-2) (Pearson, Bloomington, MN, 2005) for ages 4 through 19 years. Subtests for balance and bilateral coordination (body coordination) and strength, running speed, and agility (strength and agility) can be used to assess balance and gross motor function. Additional subtests of upper limb coordination, dexterity, fine motor, and visual motor function can also be performed to obtain a total motor composite score.

Clinical balance tests are used to determine balance ability and assess for risk of falls. When utilized in combination with computerized dynamic posturography, these tests can help determine whether sensory information from the vestibular, visual, and somatosensory systems are appropriately coordinating to maintain postural stability. A detailed review of the visual system occurs elsewhere in this book. The somatosensory system provides information about body position and the movement of body segments relative to each other and the support surface. There are several reliable balance tests that have been validated within the pediatric population and/or have established normative pediatric values. These scales include the following:

- Modified Clinical Test of Sensory Interaction on Balance (mCTSIB), which assesses static balance on firm ground and foam with eyes open and then eyes closed for 30 seconds each for a total possible score of 120 seconds. A score of less than 111 seconds has been found to be sensitive (88%) and specific (85%) for hypofunction.[21]

- Functional Reach Test (5 years and older) measures a child's ability to reach forward from a stationary position without changing the original base of support and is correlated with anterior/posterior limits of stability testing.[22,23] The Pediatric Reach Test is a modification of the functional reach test that incorporates lateral reaching.[23]
- Single leg balance with eyes open and with eyes closed is an effective, quick screening test for ambulatory children to detect balance deficits.[24]
- Balance Error Scoring System (BESS, ages 5 and older) or modified-BESS (ages 5 to 14) can be used to assess static balance in different foot positions on firm and foam surfaces with eyes closed.[25]
- Pediatric Balance Scale (PBS) is a 14-item scale modified from the adult Berg Balance Scale that can be used to track balance function in young school-age and preschool-age children. Due to developmental and ceiling effects, the PBS is best for children between 3 and 6 years old.[26–28]

The pediatric norms for these scales are listed in Table 26–3.

Vision and oculomotor screening should be performed because impairments in binocular visual function can lead to deficits in reading or dynamic balance and can be associated with symptoms such as headache, dizziness, and diplopia. While the oculomotor and vestibulo-ocular examination and treatment techniques are similar to those used with adults, keeping a child motivated and on task when testing can be challenging. It is essential to keep children engaged in testing by using objects and interacting in a manner that attracts and maintains their attention. For both examination and treatment purposes, it is recommended that therapists have a variety of toys, stickers, balls, and other items that make noise, light up, or will motivate and keep a child's interest. Additionally, assessments should be performed in a quiet location without distractions and when the child is not overly fatigued to control for potential confounding factors in performing a thorough examination. See Table 26–4 and Figure 26–1.

Clinical vestibular screening should be performed to assess the function of the peripheral vestibular system. If laboratory vestibular function tests have been done, results between clinical and lab tests can be compared to guide medical and rehabilitative treatment. Since vestibular function is present at a very early age, testing can be performed on young children if they are cooperative and cognitively able to perform testing. Screening that can be performed without specialized equipment includes the Head Impulse Test, Dynamic Visual Acuity Test, and Dix-Hallpike and roll tests for positional vertigo. If infrared goggles or Frenzel lenses are available, then post-headshake nystagmus, post-rotary nystagmus, Dix-Hallpike and roll tests, and gaze-evoked nystagmus testing can also be performed. Tables 26–5 and 26–6 outline clinical vestibular tests.

Table 26–3. Pediatric Balance Norms

Modified Clinical Test of Sensory Interaction on Balance (mCTSIB)[21]

	Typically Developing	*SNHL (Sensory Neural Hearing Loss), Normal Vestibular Function*	*SNHL, Bilateral Vestibular Hypofunction*	*SNHL, Unilateral Vestibular Hypofunction*
mCTSIB Mean Total Score in seconds (Standard Deviation)	118.6 (4.3)	116.0 (6.3)	84.4 (23.3)	98.4 (20.4)

Functional Reach[22]

Age (years)	*Reach Distance (inches)*
5 to 6	6.7
7 to 8	8.2
9 to 10	10.2
11 to 12	11.9
13 to 15	11.8
Adults (20 to 39)	16.7

Single-Leg Balance[24]

Age in Years	*Eyes Open (Seconds)*	*Eyes Closed (Seconds)*
5	10	<5
7	15	5
9	30	15
11	30+	30

Modified BESS Normative Scores[25]

Age in Years	*Mean Errors*	*Median Errors*	*Standard Deviation*
5 to 7	8.55	8	4.44
8 to 10	6.18	5	4.20
11 to 14	4.57	4	3.04

BESS Normative Scores[25]

Age in Years	*Mean Errors*	*Median Errors*	*Standard Deviation*
5 to 7	23.07	23	8.23
8 to 10	18.99	18	8.53
11 to 14	15.94	16	15.94

Table 26–4. Visual/Oculomotor Assessment

Test	*Procedure*	*Normal Outcome*
Smooth pursuits	Head stabilized, child follows a slowly moving toy/sticker vertically and horizontally	Child able to keep eyes fixed on target and demonstrates full ocular range of motion
Saccades	Child quickly moves eyes vertically and horizontally between two stickers spaced roughly 18 inches apart	Movements should be accurate, fast, and equal between both eyes
Convergence	Child looks at a sticker as it moves slowly toward the child's nose (child reports when it appears to double)	Eyes adduct symmetrically; distance of 6 cm or less from child's forehead achieved before target appears to double
Cover/uncover test for ocular alignment	Child looks at object held in front of him or her as one eye is covered, then uncovered; repeat on other side	No corrective eye movement occurs when eye is covered/uncovered
Static visual acuity	Assess using age-appropriate chart (ie, LEA symbols, see Figure 26–1)	If impaired, refer to pediatric optometrist or neurologist

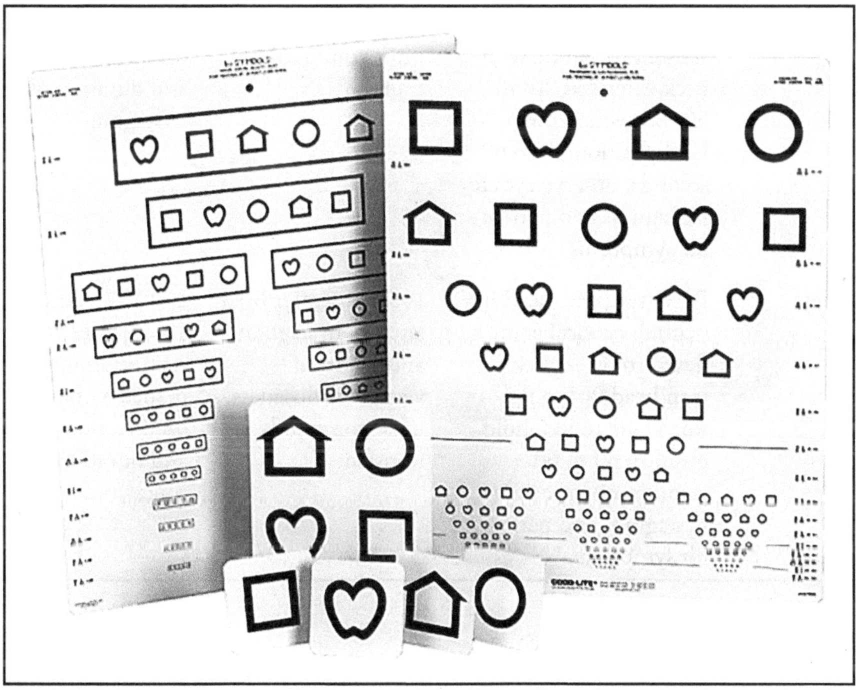

Figure 26–1. LEA Symbols Chart. (With permission, LEA Test Intl, LLC.)

Table 26–5. Clinical Vestibular Tests in Room Light

Test	*Procedure*	*Results*	*Implication*
Head impulse test	With child's eyes fixed on target, apply a rapid (>180°), unpredictable rotation of the head (<20°) in the plane of each canal	Positive—corrective saccade during movement	Hypofunction on side of corrective saccade Gaze stabilization exercises indicated
Dynamic visual acuity (DVA) test	Compare static visual acuity to visual acuity when examiner rotates child's head 20° to each side in horizontal plane at 2 Hz (120 bpm)	Positive—greater than 2 line difference between static and dynamic visual acuity	Impaired gaze stability Gaze stabilization exercises indicated
Dix-Hallpike	Patient in long sitting with head rotated 45° toward the side being tested; patient quickly assisted to supine with neck extended 20° to 30° below horizon; hold position 30 to 60 seconds, observe eyes for nystagmus and patient for symptoms	Positive—after brief latency, nystagmus, and report of vertigo or dizziness, most commonly transient	BPPV—perform appropriate repositioning maneuver based on direction and duration of nystagmus
Roll test	Patient supine, head in neutral, cervical spine flexed to 30°; quickly turn head 90° to the side being tested, hold position 30 to 60 seconds, observe eyes for nystagmus and patient for symptoms	Positive—after brief latency, nystagmus, and report of vertigo or dizziness, most commonly transient	BPPV—perform appropriate repositioning maneuver based on direction and duration of nystagmus

Table 26–6. Clinical Vestibular Tests With Fixation Removed (Frenzel lenses or infrared goggles required)

Test	*Procedure*	*Results*	*Implication*
Spontaneous and gaze-evoked nystagmus	Observe eyes at rest, then with gaze held left, right, up, and down at 20° to 30° from center resting position; be sure to avoid end range (physiologic nystagmus)	Positive—in cases of peripheral involvement, beating toward more active side	Acute, uncompensated hypo-/hyperfunction
Post headshake nystagmus	Examiner shakes child's head back and forth 20 times (at ~2 Hz) then observes eyes for nystagmus	Positive—nystagmus of short duration in one direction	Indicative of uncompensated unilateral vestibular hypofunction; nystagmus is away from side of hypofunction
Postrotatory nystagmus	Child sits in a rotating office chair and closes his or her eyes as the examiner rotates the chair to the right for 30 seconds at 0.5 Hz; examiner stops the chair and immediately puts the goggles on the child, then times the nystagmus until it stops; repeat in other direction	Positive—nystagmus of <29 seconds total between both directions	Indicative of hypofunction
Dix-Hallpike and roll tests	Same as in room light	Same as in room light, though nystagmus will typically be stronger and easier to observe without fixation	Same as in room light

Vestibular Rehabilitation

After completing a detailed interview, review of medical history, and physical examination, vestibular rehabilitation should be initiated, if appropriate. Treatment is individualized to the child's particular impairments, functional deficits, developmental level, and cognitive abilities. The child's and parents'/caregiver's goals, interests, and concerns should also be incorporated into treatment planning. Regardless of the underlying diagnosis, rehabilitation strategies can generally be broken down into the following four categories based on the intended mechanism of recovery:

- Restoration—impaired vestibular function is recovered using the original anatomy and function.[29]

- Adaptation—lost vestibular function is rehabilitated via long-term changes in the neuronal response to head movements with the goal of reducing symptoms and normalizing gaze and postural stability.[30]
- Habituation—the reduction in a behavioral response (ie, sensation of dizziness) by repeated exposure to a provocative stimulus, such as walking in a crowded hallway, with the goal of reducing symptoms. Exercises are chosen on the basis of movements or situations that provoke symptoms and are performed repetitively until a temporary and modest increase in symptoms occurs.[30]
- Substitution—the use of alternative strategies (eg, smooth pursuit eye movements, saccades, assistive devices, etc) to substitute for missing vestibular function.

As mentioned earlier in this chapter, vestibular impairments can generally be broken down into the following categories: postural, vertigo, vestibulovisual, and dizziness.[15] Rehabilitation strategies for each impairment type are reviewed separately with these categories in mind, but in most cases treatments will need to be directed to address multiple impairments. Vestibular rehabilitation is an exercise-based approach that typically includes supervised exercises in clinic and home-based activities to be performed with parents, caregivers, school staff, or independently for older children. These exercises should address the impairments and functional limitations identified during evaluation and are generally intended to promote gaze stability (gaze stability or ×1 and ×2 viewing exercises), reduce dizziness or vertigo, and improve balance, functional mobility, and gait (balance and gait training).[30]

Lacour and Bernard-Demanze (2014) wrote a review article describing some key principles for enhancing the success of vestibular rehabilitation.[29] They recommend emphasizing active rehabilitation to provide the central nervous system (CNS) with normal sensorimotor cues to regulate vestibular function and promote neural plasticity. They suggest initiating vestibular rehabilitation early to take advantage of the sensitive period after a vestibular insult as neural circuitry patterns use synaptic competition mechanisms (ie, use it or lose it). This is especially true in young children as delays in initiating rehabilitation are likely to lead to progressive motor deficits.[4,31,32] The authors also warn against using a stereotyped protocol as the sensory and behavioral strategies used for recovery are different among individuals. In some cases, it may be necessary to focus on the reduction of anxiety and stress first to promote compliance in vestibular rehabilitation, reduce fear of movement, and enhance vestibular adaptation. Use ecological situations and motivate patients by designing interventions that mimic daily life and that are fun, rewarding, and meaningful. Vestibular rehabilitation activities need to be interesting, motivating, challenging, and adaptable in order to allow for both successes and failures to promote motor learning and maximize participation in therapy. Finally, parents and caregivers should be involved in carrying out the treatment plan to promote compliance, as daily performance of home exercises is essential for rehabilitation to be successful.

Rehabilitation for Postural Impairments

Postural symptoms can include delayed acquisition of motor milestones such as independent sitting and walking, frequent falls, bumping into objects, avoiding movement, and body lean or head tilt. The ability to assume, maintain, and move in sitting, standing, and walking develops during childhood. Acquisition of these skills is dependent on the functioning and interaction of three sensory systems (vision, vestibular, and somatosensory systems). The CNS integrates information from these sensory systems to coordinate neuromotor output to maintain upright posture and control movement. Ideally, this integration occurs through experimentation and movement in a rich environment that allows use of all intact systems. Somatosensory system effectiveness for balance approaches adult norms by age 6 to 7 years, and use of vision for postural control continues to mature until around age 15 years.[33] Young children (under age 6 years) with absent or severely impaired vestibular function will develop progressive motor delay, even when their visual and somatosensory systems are intact, if intervention does not occur before this critical window of balance development.[4,31,32]

Impairments in muscle strength, tone, and joint range of motion may contribute to problems with gross mobility or postural stability and should be addressed based on findings from the examination. As these are findings not specific to vestibular dysfunction and are commonly treated by pediatric physical and occupation therapists, detailed intervention strategies are not discussed in this chapter.

Postural interventions to promote adaptation and restoration are indicated when some vestibular function is present on one or both sides. Exercises can be targeted to improve the use of remaining vestibular function, vision, somatosensation, and the integration of all 3 systems to maintain balance. For balance and postural control to improve, these systems must be challenged to create losses of balance in a safe and controlled manner. Variables that can be manipulated to progressively challenge balance at a level appropriate to the specific child's abilities and development include the following:

- *Base of support* (start large and progressively decrease): sitting, standing with feet apart, feet in tandem, stand on one foot
- *Surface* (firm to unstable): firm, exercise mat, physioball, balance disk, wobble board, or moving between surfaces
- *Add movement through environment:* popping bubbles, marching, kicking a ball, walking while bouncing a balloon or ball, walking on a balance beam, walking backward, skipping, moving up/down stairs, navigating through an obstacle course
- *Add head movement:* bouncing while sitting on ball, scanning for hidden objects or stickers while standing on a balance beam, nodding yes or no while reading (known as ×1 viewing)
- *Vision* (allow fixation then gradually remove): eyes open and fixed on stationary target such as picture of favorite cartoon character, then follow moving target such as bubbles, scan busy background to find hidden sticker, balance with eyes closed, or with moving background (optokinetic), modify challenge with speed and predictability of movement and by introducing complexity and/or changes in contrast
- *Dual task:* recite alphabet, complete memory task, complete problem-solving task, carry a cup of water, use flashcards

Postural interventions to promote substitution are indicated when vestibular function is absent or severely limited bilaterally, and should emphasize the use of vision and somatosensory information to maintain balance. The clinician can promote the use of the visual system to maintain balance by allowing patients to use visual fixation such as looking at a stationary sticker or toy. As with adaptation/restoration interventions, the clinician can then progressively increase the balance demands. This can be accomplished by narrowing the child's base of support, adding movement such as walking or bouncing on a ball while sitting, and changing the support surface. As a child's balance improves, the clinician can gradually challenge the use of visual fixation by having children perform eye movements between two or more targets, scan for a hidden object, or track a moving target.

In order to promote the use of somatosensory information for balance, rehabilitation should begin with the child maintaining both feet on firm ground while sitting (on a therapy ball or T-stool if appropriate) or standing. Initially, it may be necessary to allow children to use a hand on a wall, counter, or the therapist in order to provide additional stability. In these positions, children can play with toys, play board games, or watch a video. As static balance improves, the clinician can add movement by having the child kick a ball, play catch, reach for a toy, or dance to his or her favorite song. Challenge children by having them race through an obstacle course, walk over hurdles, crawl through a tunnel, or walk on a low balance beam. If appropriate, the clinician should try to decrease the use of visual input by having the child scan for a hidden object while walking around the gym, search for a sticker with the child's favorite cartoon character on a busy background, or by closing their eyes. Somatosensory input can also be augmented with the use of weights, compression, and increased impact during physical activities.

Even with timely and intense rehabilitation, children without a functional vestibular system will be at an increased risk for falling compared to typically developing children. Due to this increased fall risk, it is important to prepare children by promoting the use of protective reflexes and anticipatory reactions to reduce the risk of injury. This can be practiced by having a child sit on a ball or stand on a rocker board as the therapist moves the ball or board underneath the child to simulate a loss of balance. Another option is to have the child lean against the therapist, who then removes his or her support, requiring the child to use ankle, hip, or stepping strategy to recover in conditions that gradually become less predictable. Although vestibular input for protective reflexes may be absent, somatosensation and central preprogramming in predictable situations may be able to compensate and reduce the risk of falls in children with profound vestibular loss.

In patients with severe, bilateral vestibular hypofunction, the clinician should also educate caregivers on safety strategies and equipment to reduce the chance of injury. Such recommendations may include installing nightlights at home, having the child use a flashlight when walking in the dark, avoiding walking on very uneven ground, and using a helmet for a child with severe imbalance. Additionally, therapists should assess children for assistive equipment and bracing needs such as orthotics in children with hypotonia or a walker when vestibular hypofunction is present with other comorbidities that limit a child's ability to safely mobilize independently.

Rehabilitation for Vertigo

Vertigo is the sensation of self-motion when not moving or the sensation of distorted self-motion during an otherwise normal head movement.[15] This false sense of motion is not limited to spinning and needs to be differentiated from dizziness, the sensation of disturbed or impaired spatial orientation without a false of sense of motion.[15] The terms *vertigo* and *dizziness* are commonly interchanged by both laypeople and health care providers, but every effort should be made to clarify what a symptomatic child is experiencing to aid in the diagnostic and rehabilitation process. Conditions that may cause episodic vertigo include vestibular migraine, benign paroxysmal vertigo of childhood, Ménière's disease, acute vestibular neuronitis, perilymph fistula, traumatic brain injury, and benign paroxysmal positional vertigo (BPPV). Medical and surgical management of these conditions is outlined in detail in other chapters in this book.

While medical management is often indicated for other conditions causing vertigo, vestibular rehabilitation is the primary treatment for BPPV. Assessment for BPPV includes the Dix-Hallpike and roll tests, which are ideally performed without fixation but can be done in room light if infrared goggles or Frenzel lenses are not available. The underlying physiology of BPPV is discussed in Chapter 15. While less common in the pediatric population compared to older adults, BPPV has been reported and successfully treated in children who have had head trauma.[11,12,34] Interpretation of a positive Dix-Hallpike and roll test and the recommended repositioning maneuvers for the various forms of BPPV are outlined in Tables 26–7 and 26–8.[35] The canalith repositioning maneuver (Table 26–9) has been proven in numerous studies and a Cochrane review to be a very effective treatment for posterior canal BPPV, the most common form of BPPV.[35,36] For detailed descriptions of other less commonly used repositioning maneuvers, the reader is referred to the clinical practice guideline developed by Bhattacharyya et al (2017).[35]

These maneuvers can be modified for patient comfort and other specific precautions by positioning the child in a parent's lap, using bolsters, or using a tilt table if the clinician keeps in mind the position of the affected canal relative to gravity. Restricting movement or sleeping upright after repositioning, which has been recommended in earlier treatment guidelines, is no longer recommended. Treatment should be effective within one to a few sessions, otherwise, an alternative diagnosis or treatment should be considered (eg, different canal involved or repositioning maneuver; central positional vertigo).[35] Other symptoms (imbalance, dizziness/motion sensitivity, gaze instability) that may occur concurrently with vertigo may be treated with vestibular rehabilitation and are covered in the postural, dizziness, and vestibulovisual rehabilitation sections of this chapter.

Table 26–7. Dix-Hallpike Test Interpretation: Identification of Canal Involvement and Recommended Repositioning Maneuver With Anterior and/or Posterior Canal Involvement[35]

Canal	*Right Dix-Hallpike Test Results*	*Treatment*
Right posterior	Upbeating and right torsional nystagmus	Right canalith repositioning maneuver (CRM) or Semont liberatory maneuver (LM)
Right anterior	Downbeating and right torsional nystagmus	Right CRM or LM
Left anterior	Downbeating and left torsional nystagmus	Left CRM or LM
Left posterior	No nystagmus	Perform left Dix-Hallpike test

Table 26–8. Roll Test Interpretation: Identification of Canal Involvement and Recommended Repositioning Maneuver with Horizontal (Lateral) Canal Involvement[35]

Canal	*Right Roll Test*	*Left Roll Test*	*Treatment*
Right horizontal canalithiasis (geotropic form)	Transient right beating (geotropic or toward the earth) with more severe nystagmus and symptoms	Transient left beating (geotropic)	Right Lempert 360° roll maneuver (barbecue roll maneuver) or Gufoni maneuver
Left horizontal canalithiasis (geotropic form)	Transient right beating (geotropic)	Transient left beating (geotropic) with more severe nystagmus and symptoms	Left Lempert 360° roll maneuver (barbecue roll maneuver) or Gufoni maneuver
Right horizontal cupulolithiasis (apogeotropic form)	Persistent left beating (apogeotropic or away from the earth)	Persistent right beating (apogeotropic) with more severe nystagmus and symptoms	Right Lempert 360° roll maneuver (barbecue roll maneuver) or Gufoni maneuver
Left horizontal cupulolithiasis (apogeotropic form)	Persistent left beating (apogeotropic) with more severe nystagmus and symptoms	Persistent right beating (apogeotropic)	Left Lempert 360° roll maneuver (barbecue roll maneuver) or Gufoni maneuver

Table 26–9. Canalith Repositioning Maneuver

1. The patient is sitting in the upright position with the head turned 45° toward the affected ear (the ear that was positive on the Dix-Hallpike testing).
2. The patient is rapidly laid back to the supine head-hanging 20° position, which is then maintained for 20 to 30 seconds.
3. Next, the head is turned 90° toward the other (unaffected) side and held for about 20 seconds.
4. The head is turned a further 90° (usually by rolling from the supine position to sidelying on the unaffected side) such that the patient's head is nearly in the facedown position. This is also held for 20 to 30 seconds.
5. The patient is then brought into the sitting position.

Rehabilitation for Vestibulovisual Impairments

Children with unilateral or bilateral vestibular hypofunction, central vestibular dysfunction, or congenital nystagmus often demonstrate deficits in gaze stability, also known as vestibulovisual dysfunction. Vestibulovisual symptoms are visual symptoms that usually result from vestibular pathology or the interplay between the visual and vestibular systems. These symptoms include false sensations of motion or tilting of the visual surround and visual distortion (blur) of vestibular origin.[15] A number of different terms have been used to describe such symptoms, including external vertigo, oscillopsia, visual lag, visual tilt, and movement-induced blur. Dysfunctions of the visual system that may cause such symptoms include impaired visual fixation, convergence insufficiency or excess, and saccadic dysfunction. Ocular abnormalities are covered in detail elsewhere in this book. Smooth pursuits, saccades, and the cervical ocular reflex can be effective in maintaining visual stability at slower speeds of head movement. The only system that can maintain gaze stability with the rapid head and body movements that occur during activities such as running and vigorous play is the vestibular system. Assessment of the vestibular ocular reflex (VOR) has been outlined earlier and includes the clinical head impulse test, clinical or computerized dynamic visual acuity test, and video head impulse test (vHIT).

As with postural symptoms, treatment strategies for deficits in gaze stability can be broken down into restoration/adaptation (some vestibular function present on one or both sides) or substitution (bilateral vestibular areflexia). The mechanism of restoring gaze stability with restoration/adaptation exercise is challenging the VOR to stabilize images on the fovea of the retina. This generates a retinal image slip error signal and drives adaptive change in the VOR.[37] This can be done effectively by the therapist moving the child's head or by the child actively moving his or her own head and body while attempting to maintain a clear visual image of a target of interest[38] (Table 26–10). Optimal dosage

Table 26–10. Vestibulovisual Restoration/Adaptation Activities

General tips for vestibulovisual exercises: Use items with print or pictures of interest and age appropriate to child. This may include index, playing, or flash cards; popsicle sticks with stickers; books with large font/pictures; toys; electronic devices with games; pictures; and PowerPoint presentations. The target of interest should be small enough to challenge acuity but clear enough to identify.

Have child actively move his or her head, or alternatively the therapist or caregiver passively moves the child's head (vertically, horizontally, diagonally, or randomly), while the child identifies or points to the letter, number, picture, or character that he or she sees. The head movement must be fast enough to produce an error message (retinal slip) and challenging to see clearly (aka ×1 viewing). Perform for 30 seconds and eventually progress up to 2 minutes. Provocation of symptoms is expected but should settle within minutes. Activities should be fun, challenging, and followed with home exercises performed with parents/caregivers. Total duration of exercises should be 12 to 20 minutes per day and performed daily.

Progressions:

- Increase duration
- Increase speed
- Have multiple targets
- Apply more complex background: busy wallpaper, striped or checkered fabric, busy part of clinic
- Incorporate balance challenge: sitting, standing, tandem, unilateral stance, and progress from firm to compliant surface
- Add movement: moving target (opposite direction from head movement is known as ×2 viewing), body movement while walking, bouncing on ball, swinging in net, running, skipping, dancing, or jumping

of gaze stabilization exercises for vestibular hypofunction in children is not known, but a recent clinical practice guideline for adults suggests that exercises should be performed in the range of 12 to 20 minutes per day.[30] Rehabilitation is recommended to last for 2 to 6 weeks in patients with unilateral hypofunction and 8 to 12 weeks in patients with bilateral hypofunction.[30]

In contrast, substitution exercises (Table 26–11) are intended to compensate for absent vestibular function. This can be accomplished by performing activities to promote the use of the cervical-ocular reflex (COR), saccades, smooth pursuits, and central preprogramming to reduce oscillopsia and image blur with head and body movement.[39–44] With the development of the vHIT, it has been shown that covert saccades, which are detectible with the vHIT but not the clinical head impulse test, can be quite effective at compensating for vestibular loss and reducing or eliminating vestibulovisual symptoms.

Rehabilitation for Dizziness

In the Bárány Society consensus document on classification of vestibular disorders, dizziness is defined as "the sensation of disturbed or impaired spatial orientation without a false or distorted sense of motion."[15,45] This does not include vertiginous sensations, hallucinations, or light-headedness, but can coexist with vertigo, postural, or vestibulovisual symptoms. During the initial interview, the clinician should clarify what the child or parent means if he or she uses the term "dizziness." Additionally, the clinician should inquire about the

Table 26–11. Vestibulovisual Substitution Activities

Cervical-ocular reflex—same as restoration/adaption (×1 viewing) but will likely have to start with slower movements and will not be able to achieve same speed as when vestibular function is present
Smooth pursuits—have child track/identify target that is moving while keeping head/body still
Saccades—have child move eyes between different targets while keeping head/body still
Eye/head movement between targets—start with two or more targets spaced about 30° to 40° to each side of the child's midline. Have child perform saccade to one target, then quickly follow by moving head to the target. Repeat to other side.
Progressions: • Increase duration • Increase speed • Apply more complex background: busy wallpaper, striped or checkered fabric, busy part of clinic • Incorporate balance challenge: sitting, standing, tandem, unilateral stance, and progress from firm to compliant surface • Add movement: moving target or body movement while walking, bouncing on ball, swinging, running, skipping

duration of symptoms and aggravating factors such as head motion, position, visual surround or movement, sound, or exercise. If dizziness accompanies other symptom categories, the clinician should focus on addressing these other categories first with the restoration, adaptation, or substitution activities outlined earlier in this chapter. Once those impairments are adequately addressed, if dizziness is the only or predominant symptom remaining, habituation exercises may be indicated. Valid and reliable assessments to quantify degree of dizziness and aggravating movements include the Pediatric Visually Induced Dizziness Questionnaire (PVIDQ) and Motion Sensitivity Quotient Test, which consists of a series of 16 movements with assessment of duration and intensity of dizziness for each movement.[19,46–48]

Based on answers on the PVIDQ or provocative positions, movements, or situations found from the patient's history, physical examination, or the Motion Sensitivity Quotient Test, habituation activities can be designed and dosed so that the child's symptoms are temporarily and moderately increased. With repeated and gradually more demanding exposure to such activities, the sensation of dizziness should diminish. Initially, the child may use visual fixation on a target of interest to avoid excessive symptom production. The clinician should choose activities that produce a mild to moderate level of dizziness and gradually progress to more symptom-provoking movements or situations. Then, as with other rehabilitation strategies, the duration of exercise can be increased or movement, balance, or cognitive demand can be added. Immersive virtual reality environments, such as head-mounted systems, are one way to engage children in fun and challenging habituation activities.

An example of habituation treatment for a child who experiences dizziness when exposed to complex visual patterns or backgrounds is optokinetic habituation. A source of optokinetic stimulation such as a disco ball or large piece of fabric with stripes or patterns can be an effective treatment.[49,50] Initially, the child may start by sitting in a darkened room with moving lights from a disco ball while looking at a picture of a favorite cartoon character. Once symptoms are provoked to a moderate level, the disco ball is turned off, and the child can rest until symptoms have diminished. This exposure is then repeated, as tolerated. The child can then perform this while standing, walking, looking at multiple targets, playing catch, or kicking a ball. Optokinetic habituation exposure has shown some promise in treating the symptoms of motion sickness, but research in this area is limited.[51]

For any habituation treatment to be effective and to improve compliance with home exercise recommendations, it is essential that the clinician clearly communicate to children, if they can understand, and caregivers the rationale for activities and expectations for short-term increases in dizziness to promote long-term reduction of symptoms. To promote more rapid functional improvements, the clinician should design a daily home exercise program that mimics activities done in the clinic using available equipment and motivating activities.

Another condition that may result in both dizziness and postural symptoms is persistent perceptual postural dizziness (PPPD).[52] PPPD encompasses a number of overlapping conditions and historic terminology such as space and motion discomfort, visual vertigo, and chronic subjective dizziness, among others. It is a functional neurological disorder, characterized by nonspinning vertigo and perceived unsteadiness. The symptoms are exacerbated with upright postures and in situations with complex or moving visual stimuli, and the symptoms are not better accounted for by another condition.[53] PPPD develops in about 25% of patients seen for acute or episodic vestibular conditions such as BPPV, vestibular neuronitis, concussion, and vestibular migraine, and is the second most common condition seen in specialty dizziness centers.[53,54] Vestibular rehabilitation following habituation principles to address dizziness and postural symptoms, in combination with cognitive behavioral therapy and medication can be effective in treating this common and challenging diagnosis.[52]

Treatment Outcomes

The effectiveness of vestibular rehabilitation in adults with vestibular hypofunction, BPPV, concussion, and balance deficits is fairly well documented.[30,35,55–57] In contrast, there has been relatively little research on rehabilitation for vestibular dysfunction in children, but the results so far have been promising. Krebs and colleagues (1993) first demonstrated that vestibular rehabilitation could be effective in improving balance, gait speed, and dizziness symptoms in children with bilateral hypofunction in a study comparing weekly vestibular rehabilitation sessions and home exercises versus placebo exercises.[14] Rine and Braswell have done pioneering work in the assessment and treatment of children with vestibular deficits, demonstrating effectiveness and the importance of tailoring interventions to the child's level of development.[2,3,5,10,16] They reported that three weekly, 30-minute vestibular rehabilitation sessions over 12 weeks resulted in improved motor development and postural control outcomes compared to placebo treatment in children with bilateral sensory neural hearing loss and vestibular impairment.[10] Others have also shown that vestibular rehabilitation is effective in improving balance and mobility deficits in children with hearing loss and vestibular impairment.[9,13,58,59] Although the incidence of BPPV is much less in children than in adults, repositioning maneuvers have been effective in treating children with this diagnosis.[11,12,34] Vestibular rehabilitation, as part of a multimodal treatment program including graded aerobic exercise and treatment of cervical spine dysfunction, has proven to be effective in improving balance, decreasing postconcussion vestibulovisual symptoms, and allowing children and adults to return to school, sport, and work after concussion.[56,60–65]

Acknowledgment. Thank you to Gaye Cronin for her valuable contribution to the foundation of this chapter from the prior edition of this text.

Self-Assessment Questions

1. Which of these is the most common cause of vertigo in children?
   a. Ménière's disease
   b. Vestibular neuronitis
   c. Benign paroxysmal vertigo of childhood
   d. Benign paroxysmal positional vertigo

2. The best test of motor development for a 7-year-old child is:
   a. Peabody Developmental Motor Scales (PDMS-2)
   b. Pediatric Dizziness Handicap Inventory

c. Bruininks-Oseretsky Test (BOT-2)
d. Motion Sensitivity Quotient Test

3. The function(s) of the vestibulospinal reflex include:
   a. Head-trunk righting
   b. Postural adjustments
   c. Protective reflexes
   d. All of the above

4. Two clinical tests of vestibular ocular reflex (VOR) function are:
   a. Clinical Head Impulse Test and convergence
   b. Saccades and smooth pursuits
   c. Dix-Hallpike and Dynamic Visual Acuity
   d. Dynamic Visual Acuity and clinical Head Impulse Test

5. The primary vestibular rehabilitation strategy for unilateral vestibular hypofunction due to vestibular neuronitis is:
   a. Adaptation
   b. Substitution
   c. Habituation
   d. Repositioning maneuvers

6. The critical age for vestibular rehabilitation to be effective in stopping progressive motor delays in children with congenital or early onset of vestibular dysfunction is:
   a. 2 years old
   b. 6 years old
   c. 9 years old
   d. 12 years old

7. Which symptom(s) fall under the vestibulovisual category according to the Bárány Society Consensus Document for the Classification of Vestibular Disorders?
   a. Impaired balance
   b. Oscillopsia
   c. Vertigo and nystagmus due to BPPV
   d. Motion sickness with car rides

8. Which self/parent-reported outcome measure(s) is/are appropriate for the child with vestibular-related symptoms?
   a. Pediatric Dizziness Handicap Inventory
   b. Post-Concussion Symptom Inventory
   c. Pediatric Visually Induced Dizziness Questionnaire
   d. All of the above

9. What is the primary function of the vestibular ocular reflex?
   a. Maintain upright posture
   b. Saccadic eye movement control
   c. Maintain gaze stability
   d. Smooth pursuit eye movements

10. When performing the Head Impulse Test, a corrective saccade is observed with impulses to the child's right side. This is indicative of:
    a. Left vestibular hypofunction
    b. Right vestibular hypofunction
    c. Saccadic dysfunction
    d. Impaired smooth pursuit function

11. The first system in typically developing children to reach adult-like function for maintenance of postural stability is?
    a. Visual
    b. Vestibular
    c. Otolithic
    d. Somatosensory

12. Key elements for successful vestibular rehabilitation include all of the following except:
    a. Exercises that are fun and motivating
    b. Challenging, but allow for success
    c. Avoid reproduction of symptoms
    d. Activities that are individualized to age, development, and impairments

13. Vertigo due to which condition is most responsive to vestibular rehabilitation?
    a. Benign paroxysmal vertigo of childhood
    b. Perilymph fistula
    c. Benign paroxysmal positional vertigo
    d. Vestibular migraine

References

1. Li CM, Hoffman HJ, Ward BK, Cohen HS, Rine RM. Epidemiology of dizziness and balance problems in children in the United States: A population-based study. *J Pediatr.* 2016;171:240–247.e3.
2. Braswell J, Rine RM. Preliminary evidence of improved gaze stability following exercise in two children with vestibular hypofunction. *Int J Pediatr Otorhinolaryngol.* 2006;70(11):1967–1973.

3. Braswell J, Rine RM. Evidence that vestibular hypofunction affects reading acuity in children. *Int J Pediatr Otorhinolaryngol.* 2006; 70(11):1957–1965.
4. Rine RM, Cornwall G, Gan K, et al. Evidence of progressive delay of motor development in children with sensorineural hearing loss and concurrent vestibular dysfunction. *Percept Mot Skills.* 2000;90(3 Pt 2):1101–1112.
5. Rine RM, Braswell J. A clinical test of dynamic visual acuity for children. *Int J Pediatr Otorhinolaryngol.* 2003;67(11):1195–1201.
6. Franco ES, Panhoca I. Vestibular function in children underperforming at school. *Braz J Otorhinolaryngol.* 2008;74(6):815–825.
7. Gioacchini FM, Alicandri-Ciufelli M, Kaleci S, Magliulo G, Re M. Prevalence and diagnosis of vestibular disorders in children: A review. *Int J Pediatr Otorhinolaryngol.* 2014;78(5): 718–724.
8. Bernard S, Wiener-Vacher S, Van Den Abbeele T, Teissier N. Vestibular disorders in children with congenital cytomegalovirus infection. *Pediatrics.* 2015;136(4):e887–895.
9. Rajendran V, Roy FG, Jeevanantham D. A preliminary randomized controlled study on the effectiveness of vestibular-specific neuromuscular training in children with hearing impairment. *Clin Rehabil.* 2013;27(5):459–467.
10. Rine RM, Braswell J, Fisher D, Joyce K, Kalar K, Shaffer M. Improvement of motor development and postural control following intervention in children with sensorineural hearing loss and vestibular impairment. *Int J Pediatr Otorhinolaryngol.* 2004;68(9):1141–1148.
11. Brodsky JR, Lipson S, Wilber J, Zhou G. Benign paroxysmal positional vertigo (BPPV) in children and adolescents: Clinical features and response to therapy in 110 pediatric patients. *Otol Neurotol.* 2018;39(3):344–350.
12. Fay JL. Benign paroxysmal positional vertigo in 2 children: A case series. *Pediatr Phys Ther.* 2016;28(3):355–360.
13. Ebrahimi AA, Jamshidi AA, Movallali G, Rahgozar M, Haghgoo HA. The effect of vestibular rehabilitation therapy program on sensory organization of deaf children with bilateral vestibular dysfunction. *Acta Med Iran.* 2017; 55(11):683–689.
14. Krebs DE, Gill-Body KM, Riley PO, Parker SW. Double-blind, placebo-controlled trial of rehabilitation for bilateral vestibular hypofunction: Preliminary report. *Otolaryngol Head Neck Surg.* 1993;109(4):735–741.
15. Bisdorff A, Von Brevern M, Lempert T, Newman-Toker DE. Classification of vestibular symptoms: Towards an international classification of vestibular disorders. *J Vestib Res.* 2009;19(1–2):1–13.
16. Rine RM. Vestibular rehabilitation for children. *Semin Hear.* 2018;39(3):334–344.
17. McCaslin DL, Jacobson GP, Lambert W, English LN, Kemph AJ. The development of the Vanderbilt Pediatric Dizziness Handicap Inventory for Patient Caregivers (DHI-PC). *Int J Pediatr Otorhinolaryngol.* 2015;79(10): 1662–1666.
18. Pavlou M, Whitney S, Alkathiry AA, et al. The Pediatric Vestibular Symptom Questionnaire: A validation study. *J Pediatr.* 2016;168:171–177.e1.
19. Pavlou M, Whitney SL, Alkathiry AA, et al. Visually induced dizziness in children and validation of the Pediatric Visually Induced Dizziness Questionnaire. *Front Neurol.* 2017;8: 656.
20. Sady MD, Vaughan CG, Gioia GA. Psychometric characteristics of the postconcussion symptom inventory in children and adolescents. *Arch Clin Neuropsychol.* 2014;29(4): 348–363.
21. Christy JB, Payne J, Azuero A, Formby C. Reliability and diagnostic accuracy of clinical tests of vestibular function for children. *Pediatr Phys Ther.* 2014;26(2):180–189.
22. Donahoe B, Turner D, Worrell T. The use of functional reach as a measurement of balance in boys and girls without disabilities ages 5 to 15 years. *Pediatr Phys Ther.* 1994;6(4): 189–193.
23. Bartlett D, Birmingham T. Validity and reliability of a pediatric reach test. *Pediatr Phys Ther.* 2003;15(2):84–92.
24. Condon C, Cremin K. Static balance norms in children. *Physiother Res Int.* 2014;19(1):1–7.

25. Hansen C, Cushman D, Anderson N, et al. A normative dataset of the balance error scoring system in children aged between 5 and 14. *Clin J Sport Med.* 2016;26(6):497–501.
26. Darr N, Franjoine MR, Campbell SK, Smith E. Psychometric properties of the pediatric balance scale using Rasch analysis. *Pediatr Phys Ther.* 2015;27(4):337–348.
27. Franjoine MR, Darr N, Held SL, Kott K, Young BL. The performance of children developing typically on the pediatric balance scale. *Pediatr Phys Ther.* 2010;22(4):350–359.
28. Franjoine MR, Gunther JS, Taylor MJ. Pediatric balance scale: A modified version of the Berg balance scale for the school-age child with mild to moderate motor impairment. *Pediatr Phys Ther.* 2003;15(2):114–128.
29. Lacour M, Bernard-Demanze L. Interaction between vestibular compensation mechanisms and vestibular rehabilitation therapy: 10 recommendations for optimal functional recovery. *Front Neurol.* 2014;5:285.
30. Hall CD, Herdman SJ, Whitney SL, et al. Vestibular rehabilitation for peripheral vestibular hypofunction: An evidence-based clinical practice guideline: From the American Physical Therapy Association Neurology Section. *J Neurol Phys Ther.* 2016;40(2):124–155.
31. Wiener–Vacher SR, Obeid R, Abou-Elew M. Vestibular impairment after bacterial meningitis delays infant posturomotor development. *J Pediatr.* 2012;161(2):246–251. e241.
32. Woollacott M, Debu B, Mowatt M. Neuromuscular control of posture in the infant and child: Is vision dominant? *J Mot Behav.* 1987; 19(2):167–186.
33. Hirabayashi S, Iwasaki Y. Developmental perspective of sensory organization on postural control. *Brain Dev.* 1995;17(2):111–113.
34. Reimer K, Ellis V, Cordingley DM, Russell K, Ellis MJ. Benign paroxysmal positional vertigo after pediatric sports-related concussion [published online ahead of print, May 25, 2018]. *Clin J Sport Med.* doi: 10.1097/JSM.0000000000000617
35. Bhattacharyya N, Gubbels SP, Schwartz SR, et al. Clinical practice guideline: Benign paroxysmal positional vertigo (update). *Otolaryngol Head Neck Surg.* 2017;156(3 suppl):S1–S47.
36. Hilton MP, Pinder DK. The Epley (canalith repositioning) manoeuvre for benign paroxysmal positional vertigo. *Cochrane Database Syst Rev.* 2014(12):CD003162.
37. Gauthier GM, Robinson DA. Adaptation of the human vestibuloocular reflex to magnifying lenses. *Brain Res.* 1975;92(2):331–335.
38. Mahfuz MM, Schubert MC, Figtree WVC, Todd CJ, Khan SI, Migliaccio AA. Optimal human passive vestibulo-ocular reflex adaptation does not rely on passive training. *J Assoc Res Otolaryngol.* 2018;19(3):261–271.
39. Blodow A, Pannasch S, Walther LE. Detection of isolated covert saccades with the video head impulse test in peripheral vestibular disorders. *Auris Nasus Larynx.* 2013;40(4):348–351.
40. Macdougall HG, Curthoys IS. Plasticity during vestibular compensation: The role of saccades. *Front Neurol.* 2012;3:21.
41. Schubert MC, Migliaccio AA, Clendaniel RA, Allak A, Carey JP. Mechanism of dynamic visual acuity recovery with vestibular rehabilitation. *Arch Phys Med Rehabil.* 2008;89(3): 500–507.
42. Kasai T, Zee DS. Eye-head coordination in labyrinthine-defective human beings. *Brain Res.* 1978;144(1):123–141.
43. Schubert MC, Das V, Tusa RJ, Herdman SJ. Cervico-ocular reflex in normal subjects and patients with unilateral vestibular hypofunction. *Otol Neurotol.* 2004;25(1):65–71.
44. Bockisch CJ, Straumann D, Hess K, Haslwanter T. Enhanced smooth pursuit eye movements in patients with bilateral vestibular deficits. *Neuroreport.* 2004;15(17):2617–2620.
45. Bisdorff AR, Staab JP, Newman-Toker DE. Overview of the International Classification of Vestibular Disorders. *Neurol Clin.* 2015; 33(3):541–550, vii.
46. Smith-Wheelock M, Shepard NT, Telian SA. Physical therapy program for vestibular rehabilitation. *Am J Otol.* 1991;12(3):218–225.
47. Norre ME, Beckers AM. Vestibular habituation training. Specificity of adequate exercise. *Arch Otolaryngol Head Neck Surg.* 1988; 114(8):883–886.
48. Akin FW, Davenport MJ. Validity and reliability of the Motion Sensitivity Test. *J Rehabil Res Dev.* 2003;40(5):415–421.

49. Pavlou M, Bronstein AM, Davies RA. Randomized trial of supervised versus unsupervised optokinetic exercise in persons with peripheral vestibular disorders. *Neurorehabil Neural Repair.* 2013;27(3):208–218.
50. Pavlou M, Lingeswaran A, Davies RA, Gresty MA, Bronstein AM. Simulator based rehabilitation in refractory dizziness. *J Neurol.* 2004; 251(8):983–995.
51. Golding JF, Gresty MA. Pathophysiology and treatment of motion sickness. *Curr Opin Neurol.* 2015;28(1):83–88.
52. Popkirov S, Staab JP, Stone J. Persistent postural-perceptual dizziness (PPPD): A common, characteristic and treatable cause of chronic dizziness. *Pract Neurol.* 2018;18(1):5–13.
53. Staab JP, Eckhardt-Henn A, Horii A, et al. Diagnostic criteria for persistent postural-perceptual dizziness (PPPD): Consensus document of the Committee for the Classification of Vestibular Disorders of the Barany Society. *J Vestib Res.* 2017;27(4):191–208.
54. Dieterich M, Staab JP, Brandt T. Functional (psychogenic) dizziness. *Handb Clin Neurol.* 2016;139:447–468.
55. Hillier S, McDonnell M. Is vestibular rehabilitation effective in improving dizziness and function after unilateral peripheral vestibular hypofunction? An abridged version of a Cochrane Review. *Eur J Phys Rehabil Med.* 2016;52(4):541–556.
56. Murray DA, Meldrum D, Lennon O. Can vestibular rehabilitation exercises help patients with concussion? A systematic review of efficacy, prescription and progression patterns. *Br J Sports Med.* 2017;51(5):442–451.
57. Porciuncula F, Johnson CC, Glickman LB. The effect of vestibular rehabilitation on adults with bilateral vestibular hypofunction: A systematic review. *J Vestib Res.* 2012;22(5–6):283–298.
58. Shah J, Rao K, Malawade M, Khatri S. Effect of motor control program in improving gross motor function and postural control in children with sensorineural hearing loss—A pilot study. *Pediat Therapeut.* 2013;3(141). https://doi.org/2161–0665.1000141.
59. Medeiros IR, Bittar RS, Pedalini MF, Lorenzi MC, Formigoni LG, Bento RF. Vestibular rehabilitation therapy in children. *Otol Neurotol.* 2005;26(4):699–703.
60. Gagnon I, Galli C, Friedman D, Grilli L, Iverson GL. Active rehabilitation for children who are slow to recover following sport-related concussion. *Brain Inj.* 2009;23(12):956–964.
61. Chan C, Iverson GL, Purtzki J, et al. Safety of active rehabilitation for persistent symptoms after pediatric sport-related concussion: A randomized controlled trial. *Arch Phys Med Rehabil.* 2018;99(2):242–249.
62. Grabowski P, Wilson J, Walker A, Enz D, Wang S. Multimodal impairment-based physical therapy for the treatment of patients with post-concussion syndrome: A retrospective analysis on safety and feasibility. *Phys Ther Sport.* 2017;23:22–30.
63. Reneker JC, Hassen A, Phillips RS, Moughiman MC, Donaldson M, Moughiman J. Feasibility of early physical therapy for dizziness after a sports-related concussion: A randomized clinical trial. *Scand J Med Sci Sports.* 2017;27(12):2009–2018.
64. Schneider KJ, Meeuwisse WH, Nettel-Aguirre A, et al. Cervicovestibular rehabilitation in sport-related concussion: A randomised controlled trial. *Br J Sports Med.* 2014;48(17): 1294–1298.
65. Storey EP, Wiebe DJ, D'Alonzo BA, et al. Vestibular rehabilitation is associated with visuovestibular improvement in pediatric concussion. *J Neurol Phys Ther.* 2018;42(3):134–141.

CHAPTER 27

Environmental Adaptations

Moira Pena, Nicole Captain, and Janet Woodhouse

Introduction

Background

The incidence, prevalence, and etiology of falls in the adult population, as well as the utility of programs associated with falls prevention are well established in the current literature.[1] Research that examines the specific contribution of balance disorders to falls and the ways in which their risk can be mitigated remains focused on adults.[1,2] Pediatric-specific resources outline postural control and assessments and by way of example focus on modifications to existing balance scales (eg, Berg balance scale to the pediatric balance scale).[3] Discussions of vestibular disorders[4] and their specific impact on daily living[5] can also be found. However, there are no pediatric-specific balance disorder guidelines in current literature that address the broad spectrum of diagnoses, assessments, and interventions. These guidelines are required to establish best practice for overall engagement in home and community.

The gap in knowledge in the realm of pediatric balance disorders is most evident in the spectrum of intervention. The paucity and availability of currently published evidence demonstrates that clear guidelines and additional resources are needed. Such guidelines would not only serve to better inform clinicians but would also encourage contributions to evidence- based practice. With this in mind, this chapter focuses on identifying the population needs, as well as discussing current recommendations and strategies of modifying environments to enable clients' participation in meaningful roles, routines, and occupations. Case studies will be used as examples to highlight clinical decision-making and establish a foundation for intervention. The primary focus is on environmental adaptations and supports for engagement in home and community within the scope of occupational therapy (OT) and allied health.

Population Needs

In order to explain and discuss balance disorders, the *International Classification of Functioning, Disability, and Health* (*ICF*)[6] framework that classifies health and health-related domains, will be implemented. These domains are separated into body, individual, and societal perspectives and also account for environmental factors or context.

Pediatric balance disorders encompass a broad and varied group of diagnoses that are discussed in detail in Chapters 13 through 25.

Despite the availability of clinical expertise and numerous diagnostic tools, many individuals remain undiagnosed despite significant balance dysfunction.[4] This may be particularly true in pediatrics, as a child may have one or more primary or secondary diagnoses, may have no family history, and may be in progression toward a formal diagnosis for an extended period of time. Within pediatric practice, it is essential to complete a full assessment to inform interventions. These interventions should facilitate safety and function with individual occupational performance issues in mind, regardless of the specific diagnosis or lack thereof.

Current Recommendations: Occupational Therapy Practice

Current practice is directed by the adult literature, which outlines general principles and guidelines of assessment (eg, safety issues, education, environmental, and preventative strategies). Although it is necessary to use established and current principles, they must be modified to accurately reflect the needs of a child and the child's family and take into consideration stage of development, individual functional abilities, and environmental factors (ICF).

Pediatric clinicians must use general principles in addition to clinical judgment and experience-based knowledge to tailor interventions to specific pediatric needs. Due to availability and overlap of a wide variety of assessment and follow-up regimes, it is often beneficial to collaborate with physiotherapy (PT) colleagues to address balance, postural control, and mobility concerns as well as activities of daily living (ADLs). This type of collaboration between health disciplines to assess and treat the client is known as interprofessional practice and is commonly accepted as best practice in pediatric rehabilitation. The current chapter highlights the unique occupational therapy (OT) scope on adaptations, compensatory strategies, and environmental modifications.

An evidence-based practice clinical framework should be utilized for assessment.[7–9] For example, the Person Environment Occupation Model (PEO) considers each child as an individual with specific needs and abilities as well as specific goals. In terms of outcomes, the Canadian Occupational Performance Measure (COPM)[7] captures individual- and family-centered goal-setting as well as individual perception of performance.

Assessment

OT assessment for children with balance disorders is based on the following theoretical frameworks.

Family-Centered Care

Daily occupations occur in the context of a family system; therefore, shared decision-making in service delivery intervention and evaluation is required. The family's understanding of the child and their environment are essential to practice. Family-centered practice (FCP) refers to "the attitudes and behaviors of a therapist that facilitates the family's role as lead negotiator in assessment, treatment and discharge." Evidence suggests that FCP is linked to efficient attainment of meaningful goals, greater carryover of program recommendations, and increased consumer satisfaction.[10]

Person Environment Occupational Model

The PEO model describes the transactional relationship between a person, their environment, and occupations. The model represents the dynamic interactions and complexity of occupation within environment, and the basic assumptions of the model are that a person is continually developing and is intrinsically motivated. The Venn diagram in Figure 27–1 illustrates the components (person, environment, and occupation) in three overlapping circles. Occupational performance is represented by the overlap of the three circles.

International Classification of Function

The *ICF* is a classification of health and health-related domains; it is structured around the following broad components: (1) body functions and structure, (2) activities (related to tasks and actions by an individual) and participation (involvement in a life situation), and (3) additional information on severity and environmental factors. Function and disability are viewed as a complex interaction between the individual's health condition, personal factors, and the contextual factors of the environment as outlined in Figure 27–2.

Case Study 1

The following case study is used to provide a framework for the OT assessment of a child who presents with a balance disorder. All names are fictitious.

Selene is an 11-year-old girl who was diagnosed with a posterior fossa tumour with obstructive hydrocephalus. She underwent

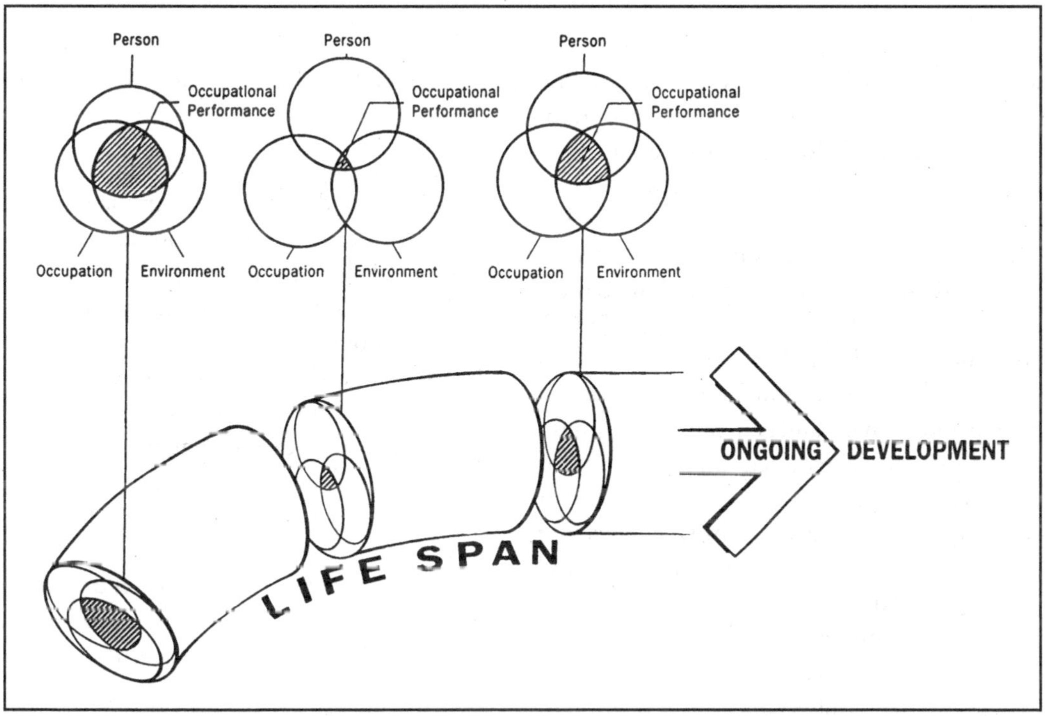

Figure 27–1. Person environment occupation model. (Reproduced with permission from Canadian Association of Occupational Therapists [CAOT] Publications ACE. From Law M, Cooper B, Strong S, Stewart D, Rigby P, Letts L. The person environment occupational model: A transactive approach to occupational performance. *Can J Occup Ther*. 1996;63(1):19–23.

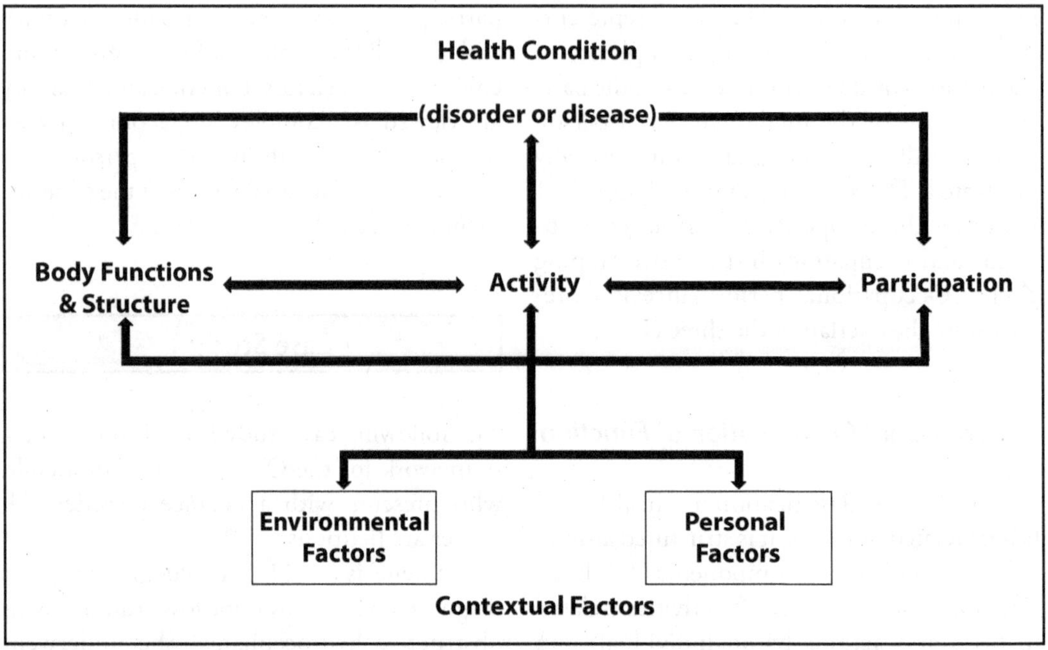

Figure 27–2. Diagram outlining the complex interaction between the individual's health condition, personal factors, and the contextual factors of the environment.

a surgical resection and was transferred to a pediatric inpatient rehabilitation program. She was referred for OT assessment and intervention as part of her interdisciplinary rehabilitation program. She resides with her mother and 2 older sisters in an apartment in a large urban center and was preparing to transition to a middle school to enter grade 6 at the time of diagnosis. Postoperatively, she was experiencing diplopia, impairments in coordination and balance, and generalized weakness. On admission, she required total assistance for self-care activities and used a wheelchair for mobility. Selene and her family have stated goals of returning to home and school and resuming her daily occupations.

Upon commencement, the OT utilized a family-centered practice approach to identify Selene and her family's concerns in relation to occupational performance (eg, how she manages the everyday activities that occupy her at home, school, and play). These included the following:

1. Current physical functional state of reduced endurance and stamina and impairments of vision, coordination, and balance limited her performance of feeding, dressing, grooming, transfers, and mobility.
2. Lack of participation in home, school, and community activities due to motor and communication challenges.
3. Recovery from surgery, including uncertainty of degree, amount, and rate of progress.
4. Environment, including issues of access for weekend visit home, return to school, and engaging in her community.

Based on the concerns and hopes of Selene and her family, the PEO model and *ICF* were used as a framework for her OT assessment.

PEO Assessment Components

In Selene's case, the PEO assessment comprised the components described in the following sections.

Person: Skills and Abilities, Intrinsic Motivation, Values, and Goals

1. Communication: Selene communicated using gestures. She presented with right-sided facial weakness and had poor lip and tongue control. Use of a writing device was compromised by evident physical-access challenges.
2. Assessment of Self-Care Activities: Selene was on a pureed diet and required assistance with finger feeding and utensil use. She drank thin liquids with assistance. Maximal assistance was required for dressing, grooming, and hygiene. She was continent of bowel and bladder and transferred with a standing pivot transfer with maximal assistance of one person.
3. Physical Function: Selene required assistance from lying to sitting and supervision to sit unsupported in bed. She presented with diplopia, generalized weakness, and static and dynamic balance impairment. On admission, she had poor head and trunk control and required a tilt wheelchair with a headrest. Sitting tolerance was approximately 10 minutes. Range of motion in her upper and lower extremities was full. Challenges with coordination of all limbs observed with greater left-sided involvement. Upper-extremity function was characterized by limited ability to reach, grasp, and release. In collaboration with PT, assessment measures including the Pediatric Balance Scale were utilized.[11]
4. Motivation: Selene was highly motivated to regain strength and function. She indicated preference through choice making and exerted positive efforts during all of her therapy.
5. Cognition: She demonstrated adequate attention to activities and appeared orientated to person and place.

Environment

The environment is defined as the context within which occupational performance takes place, and it is composed of cultural, socio-economic, institutional, physical, and social domains.

1. Physical: In her home environment, Selene lives in a two-bedroom apartment with elevator access. She shares a bedroom with her sister and a bathroom that is not wheelchair accessible.
2. Social: Selene's parents are separated, and her mother is experiencing financial challenges given her unpaid leave of absence from work during her daughter's hospitalization. Selene's family report that she is not comfortable or confident participating in social activities.
3. Cultural: Selene's family immigrated to Canada from South Asia 10 years ago and has no extended family living in the community. Selene's mother and sister are highly supportive and are actively involved in her rehabilitation program.
4. Institutional: Selene attends a large community school that is not accessible. The staff and students identified that they require support and education to provide assistance and accommodation for her return to school.

Occupation

Occupation is defined as self-directed meaningful tasks and activities engaged in throughout a life span.[7] Selene's occupations include the following:

1. Personal care activities of self-feeding, dressing, toileting, and showering
2. Functional mobility, including independent sitting, transfers, and walking
3. Student-/school-based occupation including reading, writing, and keyboarding
4. Home-based occupations such as meal preparation and leisure activities
5. Friendship and socialization

Assessment Components

Person/Occupation and Occupation/Environment Analysis

In collaboration with Selene and her family, the OT identified three occupational performance issues that were impacted by balance to be addressed during her rehabilitation program. These included dressing, showering, and writing. The assessment of these occupations was a dynamic process that occurred over time, and a balance between safety considerations (e.g., fall prevention) and the promotion of independence was achieved. During clinical observation of her occupation performance, Selene's balance control was assessed according to (1) her position, (2) the task being performed including gradation of complexity and demands of the occupation, (3) context of the activity and environment, and (4) her perception and awareness of stability and balance. Overall, postural control and adjustments are best learned in the context of task performance. Selene's performance was assessed on admission, and the tasks were graded as physical and functional gains were made.

Dressing. Person components included clinical observations of her physical ability to maintain a stable upright posture, and to adjust her posture and weight shift when reaching for articles of clothing, placing and positioning clothing on her body and adjusting her clothing. Cognitive and perceptual components included planning and organization of activities, spatial orientation of clothing, and attention to task.

The environment was structured to support her participation, safety, and success and included placement of clothing on bed, height of bed, family expectations, and availability of support personnel. Types of clothing (eg, elastic waistbands, shoes with hook and loop fasteners) are modifications that supported Selene's successful performance.

Bathing and Showering. Person components included postural control, transfer ability, safety awareness, endurance, planning, and sequencing. Environment components included hospital and home access, floor surface, lighting, assistive devices, time of day, family expectations, and availability of support personnel. In preparation for her discharge, a home safety assessment was completed with Selene and her family to provide recommendations on environmental accommodations to support her safety and independence. Recommendations included a bath seat with a back support to provide stabilization when showering, grab bars, and a handheld shower[12] in her bathroom and reorganization of closet and drawers to facilitate independence in clothing selection.

Writing. Writing assessment components included sitting posture, work surface and height, pencil grasp, fine motor skills, vision, as well as quality and quantity of written output. Certain other considerations such as motivation, past performance, values, and language were also assessed. Occupational therapists structure tasks and environments to assist patients in developing efficient motor strategies and motor problem-solving. They also provide meaningful practice that enables individuals to use their available motor function to its fullest potential in daily activity performance.

Over time, the OT grades the demands of the task to improve balance by altering (1) position of the person: size and shape of base of support, alignment; (2) object placement: position determines weight shift; (3) object characteristics (eg, weight and size); and (4) temporal demands (eg, stationary versus moving objects).

Interventions and Accommodations

The following case study illustrates a comprehensive intervention approach for a child who experiences balance issues and who also has a diagnosis of autism spectrum disorder (ASD).

Case Study 2

Tyson is an 8-year-old diagnosed with ASD and is having difficulties tolerating certain movement-related experiences. He becomes car sick easily and is intensely afraid of going up or down escalators and riding in elevators. He becomes anxious at the mall as he is not able to determine how quickly to move to avoid bumping into others. He is afraid of the sliding doors as he fears getting caught in them. He was often described as "clumsy" or "uncoordinated" and has not been able to learn to ride a bicycle despite frequent practice.

As previously highlighted, the OT's aim is to identify barriers to the client's ability to engage in activities that the client needs or wants to do at home and school (eg, their occupational performance). Using the PEO framework, a therapist will therefore assess person components (overall muscle tone, postural stability, equilibrium reactions, and Tyson's general ability to assume a variety of body positions), environmental components (where the challenges are taking place and whether environmental modifications can be made), and occupational performance components (the activities Tyson is motivated to engage in). The therapist will then work collaboratively with Tyson to come up with goals that are functional and validating to him.[13] It is important that he become actively engaged in the activity as motivation influences skill acquisition, performance, and the willingness to continue when a task becomes exceedingly challenging.[14–16] The occupational therapist's treatment plan can include both a remediation and a compensation approach.

Remediation Approach. Remediation approaches include engaging the child in activities that provide enhanced vestibular and proprioceptive sensation that simultaneously challenges posture with the aim of enabling Tyson to become more comfortable when in a car or when riding on an elevator. Intervention strategies relate to the five aspects of postural control, which include (1) tonic postural extension; (2) tonic flexion; (3) postural stability (balancing flexion and extension); (4) weight shifting, lateral flexion, and rotation; (5) righting and equilibrium reactions; and (6) oculomotor control. In addition, further exploring eye movements, such as convergence and eye teaming, can yield benefit as coordinated eye movements have a positive effect on balance.[13,17,18] Remediation strategies also include (1) targeting the vestibular-visual-auditory domains as they work in unison for balance, (2) working collaboratively with a behavioral optometrist, (3) engaging him in activities that require movement of the body through different planes (eg, horizontal [swinging side to side on a platform swing] and vertical [jumping on a trampoline]) as well as short obstacle courses to enhance input to the vestibular system; and (4) maximizing proprioceptive input prior to movement activities to enable Tyson to gain a better sense of his body in space (eg, playfully engaging him in activities that involve movement against resistance, such as tug-of-war, pushing hands together and apart, as well as weight-bearing activities such as animal walks and wheelbarrow walks).[17–19] Additional gains in the maintenance of balance can be achieved through the use of rhythm (eg, counting to help Tyson move his body through space in a coordinated manner).

Equilibrium reactions enable the child to maintain a desired body position through compensatory movements of the head, trunk, and limbs when there is need for the child to shift his or her balance.[19] Most equilibrium responses are very subtle and occur in response to relatively small changes in position. Occupational therapists develop activities that elicit subtle reactions in various positions (ie, prone, sitting, quadruped, kneeling, half-kneeling, and standing). This can be accomplished using any piece of equipment that moves or any activity that involves reaching.

The Cognitive Orientation to Daily Occupational Performance (CO-OP) is a cognitive behavioral approach that could also be a good fit for Tyson as it uses a variety of cognitive techniques such as the use of verbal scripts, verbal motor mnemonics, and guided discovery to enable him to successfully perform meaningful occupations while meeting his own chosen goals.[20]

Compensation Approach. The compensation approach is in direct opposition to remediation: instead of completing active rehabilitation to improve function, other strategies are used to help the child manage his or her environment more successfully. In Tyson's case, examples may include (1) going to the mall when it is less crowded so that the chances of bumping into others are fewer and (2) preparing ahead and studying a map of the mall together and determining if there are stairs that can be used instead so that he does not have to use the elevator or escalator if so desired. It is important to help children with ASD keep their anxiety in check to ensure successful participation in their daily activities.

Environmental Modifications. Other interventions may also be applicable depending on the particular client and needs identified during the assessment approach. As previously discussed, modifications to home, school, and community environments for safety and promotion of engagement in daily occupations are warranted to provide a safe environment for a child or teen with a balance disorder.

Summary

There is a paucity of current research to guide interventions for the pediatric population experiencing issues with balance. From a combination of existing evidence as well as clinical experience, it is possible to conclude that each child with a balance disorder will benefit from an individualized approach to assessment and treatment. This approach should focus on their unique presentation, associated needs, and individualized goals all while keeping safety and independence in mind. It is expected that through the publication of documented clinical experience as well as the previously discussed relevant case examples, best practice will continue to be established. It is intended that this publication will contribute to a solid foundation to guide clinical practice in assessments, interventions, as well as outcome measures. Continued research in the field is required for expansion of the knowledge base and continued refinement of clinical practice frameworks for our pediatric clients with balance disorders.

Self-Assessment Questions

1. What are two key considerations for completing an occupational therapy assessment with a child who presents with balance dysfunction?

2. List seven reasons that highlight the importance of collaborating with other health professionals when working with a child/youth with balance dysfunction?

3. List three advantages of using family-centered care in conducting assessment and treatment of children with balance dysfunction.

4. Define occupational performance and provide an example.

5. Using a person–environment–occupation framework, what are some components that would be considered in each of their respective areas during an occupational therapy assessment?

6. Interventions that address balance dysfunction can be graded to challenge the individual's performance. Describe methods of grading an activity.

7. Provide examples of environmental modifications for the case study of Selene (given in this chapter), and assess the types of environmental modifications you might consider in working with a child/youth with balance impairments to promote their participation in daily occupations.

8. Describe the process involved in setting valid and functional goals for children with balance impairments.

9. List three clinical considerations that should be taken into account before completing an assessment involving a child with a balance disorder.

10. List four clinical considerations regarding implementing interventions for a child with a balance disorder.

References

1. National Institute on Deafness and Other Communication Disorders: NIDCD Fact Sheet Balance Disorders. Bethesda, MD: U.S. Department of Health and Human Services, National Institutes of Health; 2011.
2. Stevens JA, Sogolow ED. Preventing falls: What works: A CDC Compendium of Effective Community-based Interventions from Around the World. Atlanta, GA: National Centre for Injury Prevention and Control; 2008.
3. Pope R. The common compensatory pattern: Its origin and relationship to the postural model. *AAO J.* 2003;13(4):19–40.
4. Mehta Z, Stakiw D. Childhood vestibular disorders: A tutorial. *Commun Disord Q.* 2004; 26(1):5–16, 55–58.
5. Cohen HS. Disability and rehabilitation in the dizzy patient. *Curr Opin Neurol.* 2006;19(1): 49–54.
6. *The International Classification of Occupational Functioning, Disability, and Health (ICF).* Geneva, Switzerland: World Health Organization; 2012.
7. Law M. *Canadian Occupational Performance Measure.* Ottawa, ON, Canada: CAOT Publications; 2005.
8. Law M, Cooper B, Strong S, Stewart D, Rigby P, Letts L. The person environment occupational model: A transactive approach to occupational performance. *Can J Occup Ther.* 1996;63(1):19–23.
9. Polatajko HJ, Mandich A. *Enabling occupation in children: The cognitive orientation to daily occupational performance (Co-op) approach.* Ottawa, ON, Canada: CAOT Publications; 2004:30–46.
10. Van Benthem K. Family-centered practice: Am I giving what it takes? *Occup Ther Now.* 2004;6:5–9.
11. Franjoine MR, Gunther JS, Taylor MJ. Pediatric balance scale: A modified version of the Berg balance scale for the school-age child with mild to moderate motor impairment. *Pediatr Phys Ther.* 2003;15:114–128. https://doi.org/10.1097/01.PEP.0000068117.48023.18
12. King EC, Novak AC. Effect of bathroom aids and age on balance control during bathing transfers. *Am J Occup Ther.* 2017;71(6):7106165030p1–7106165030p9.
13. Miller LJ, Wilbarger JJ, Stackhouse T, Trunne S. Appendix A: Use of clinical reasoning in occupation therapy: The Step SI model of intervention of sensory modulation dysfunction. In: Bundy A, Lane S, Murray E, eds. *Sensory Integration: Theory and Practice.* 2nd ed. Philadelphia, PA: F.A. Davis; 2002:435–451.
14. Anshel MH, Weinberg R, Jackson A. The effect of goal difficulty and task complexity on intrinsic motivation and motor performance. *J Sports Behav.* 1992;15(2):159–176.
15. Deci EL, Ryan RM. The initiation and regulation of intrinsically motivated learning and achievement. In: Boggiano AK, Pittman TS, eds. *Achievement and Motivation: A Social Development Perspective.* Cambridge, England: Cambridge University Press; 1992:3–36.
16. Dweck CS. Motivational processes affecting learning. *Am Psychol.* 1986;41:1040–1048e.
17. Lane SJ. Sensory modulation. In: Bundy A, Lane S, Murray E, eds. *Sensory Integration: Theory and Practice.* 2nd ed. Philadelphia, PA: F.A. Davis; 2002:101–122.
18. Lane SJ. Structure and function of the sensory systems. In: Bundy A, Lane SJ, Murray E, eds. *Sensory Integration: Theory and Practice.* 2nd ed. Philadelphia, PA: F.A. Davis; 2002: 35–70.
19. Weisz S. *Studies in Equilibrium Reaction.* Vol 88;1938:150–162.
20. Miller LJ. *Sensational Kids.* New York, NY: G.P. Putnam's Sons; 2007.

CHAPTER 28

Current and Future Research and Challenges

Sharon L. Cushing and Robert C. O'Reilly

Prevalence and Impact of Vestibular Dysfunction

Previous chapters outlined the prevalence of vestibular impairment in a number of populations and certainly our capacity to detect vestibular impairment continues to increase. Where the future lies is in further understanding the broader implication of a particular congenital and early acquired vestibular impairment in the setting of the child's developing brain. Future questions in this domain will no doubt include observation and exploration of structural changes that occur in children with congenital vestibular impairment as some work has already been undertaken in the adult world evaluating hippocampal volume.[1–3] In addition, better categorizing the functional impact of vestibular impairment beyond balance alone will be more feasible, with many of these methods outlined in Chapter 12. This is of particular importance as we examine both short- and longer-term outcomes, with an emphasis on children with sensorineural hearing loss in which we are aiming to explain variance in performance with hearing aids and cochlear implantation, particularly in experimental groups such as children with single-sided deafness.

Diagnostic Testing

We have seen diagnostic testing as well as its application to the pediatric population evolve significantly over the last several decades. In particular, the use of video head impulse test (vHIT) (Chapter 7) is particularly applicable to the pediatric population. The future will likely continue to see the evolution of diagnostic testing specifically with the pediatric population in mind, such as the use of different muscular targets for vestibular-evoked myogenic potentials,[4] which may reduce the effort of testing in children, increasing yield and reliability in younger children and even infants. Not only will techniques evolve but also the adaptation test equipment to include continued evolution of goggles that optimize their fit to the pediatric face. Such advances will go hand in hand with increased demands for diagnostics in the pediatric population.

Screening for Vestibular Impairments

Universal newborn hearing screening gained acceptance in many jurisdictions in the early 2000s. There are, however, still many places in the world and even throughout Canada and the United States where universal programs do not exist or programs still struggle with appropriate follow-up. The addition of hearing screening has greatly reduced the time to identification and intervention with hearing aids and cochlear implantation. Although likely a number of years away, it is feasible as, we look toward the future, to consider that one day we may also screen for vestibular impairment in newborns. In some places such as Ghent, Belgium, screening programs have already begun. The success, however, of screening programs lies not only in diagnosis but also in the ability to provide early intervention and effect a change the course of outcomes. Certainly, at this point in time, there is value in early identification as it may lead to the provision of early occupational and physical therapy. In this chapter, we focus on where such future therapeutics may lie as their capacity to apply to the pediatric population in a meaningful way would most certainly accelerate and drive the development of screening programs for vestibular impairment in children.

Future of Therapy for Vestibular Impairment

Vestibular dysfunction is a common problem, affecting up to 20% of the population. Some of these patients are able to centrally compensate for the dysfunction, alone or with the help of vestibular rehabilitation, and remain relatively functional; however, those who are unable to compensate often have debilitating oscillopsia and/or postural instability impairing their activities of daily living. Few proven treatment options for vestibular dysfunction exist, and the current mainstay of treatment is vestibular rehabilitation.

This chapter provides a thorough discussion of ongoing research that may underline the future of vestibular therapy. To date, the approaches to the treatment of vestibular dysfunction fall into three categories, which include the following:

1. *Sensory substitution*, whereby the stimuli that would typically excite the vestibular end organs (ie, head/postural movements) are translated into sensory stimuli targeted at one of the remaining intact sensory systems (ie, sound or vibration).
2. *Electrical stimulation* of the vestibular end organs using either transcranial (galvanic) or intracranial electrodes.
3. *Regeneration*, which includes the use of both hair cells and stem cells.

Sensory Substitution

Vibrotactile Feedback

Body Worn: Vestibular Vests

Over the past decade, vestibular vests have evolved and become an avenue for the rehabilitation of patients with chronic vestibular disorders. In essence, a sensor is fixed to a patient-worn vest, and it monitors inertial movements (both direction and angular acceleration are taken into account) as well as provides vibrotactile feedback. Over time, multiple modifications have been made to the vest. In one of the earliest renditions, two inertial sensors were used (one vibrating device placed on the shoulders and one placed on the right and left sides of the trunk).[3] Head tilt and center of pressure displacement were measured under different sensory conditions in six healthy participants with and without the vest, and overall the feedback provided by the shoulder and trunk sensors led to decreases in head tilt and sway in individuals with intact vestibular function. Given these promising initial results, vest therapy was applied to patients with vestibular end-organ dysfunction (unilateral and bilateral), where performance was measured using computerized dynamic posturography.[1] Anterior posterior sway was measured with a mounted gyroscope, and vibration was employed for tilt feedback. Vibrotactile feedback was found to significantly decrease anteroposterior tilt.[1] Subsequently, the effect of vibrotactile feedback on mediolateral tilt in addition to anteroposterior tilt was examined in 12 patients with vestibular hypofunction using posturography and during tandem walking.[2] Vibrotactile feedback led to decreased mediolateral body tilt during tandem walking and anteroposterior tilt during posturography.

Electrotactile Feedback

Tongue Worn

Tongue-worn electrotactile feedback aims to translate the information about head orientation, position, and motion, which is normally provided by the vestibular system, through electrotactile information on the tongue. Stimulation of the tongue occurs via pulses conducted through an electrode array. The tongue port (often in conjunction with a head-mounted accelerometer) allows "sensory substitution" and leads to functional compensation. In early reports, the tongue port was shown to enable a great degree of head and body postural coordination, and this persisted as a training effect for a period of time even after removing the vestibular substitution.[5]

Initial experiments were conducted in healthy adults (n = 8) under four conditions: firm-standing surface with and without electrotactile vestibular substitution system (EVSS), and foam-standing surface with and without EVSS.[6] Overall, there were more perturbations in center-of-foot pressure displacement with the foam surface than the firm surface, but EVSS decreased this destabilizing effect, suggesting that a sensory substitution system may help the central nervous system (CNS) compensate for postural instability induced by an altered support surface.

In patients with unilateral vestibular loss (n = 12), the use of EVSS led to less center-of-foot pressure displacement, suggesting its effectiveness in postural control for patients with unilateral vestibular weakness.[7] In a follow-up study, patients with unilateral vestibular loss performed better with respect to center-of-foot pressure displacement when using EVSS, and this stabilizing effect was most pronounced when standing on an "altered" foot-sensory condition (ie, foam).[8]

In a comparison (n = 19) of EVSS to standard-of-care vestibular rehabilitation (8 weeks) in patients with bilateral vestibulopathy, significant improvements in both the Dizziness Handicap Inventory as well as the Sensory Organization Test pre- and post-therapy were demonstrated in the EVSS, whereas little improvement occurred in the rehabilitation group.[9] Electrotactile tongue feedback has also been examined as a rescue therapy in patients with bilateral vestibular loss (n = 7) who do not respond to vestibular therapy.[10] On average, a statistically significant improvement in postural control evaluated by the Sensory Organization Test and a questionnaire was demonstrated.

Auditory Biofeedback

Auditory biofeedback has been investigated over the past few years and has been shown to lead to improvements in postural stability. This type of feedback works by translating center-of-pressure displacements and/or trunk and head accelerations into sounds that are modulated in frequency, level, intensity, and right/left balance.[11] A sound stimulus, therefore, substitutes partially for the lack of vestibular sensory information. Significant decreases in postural sway occur in patients with bilateral vestibular loss in the presence of auditory biofeedback in comparison with controls with intact vestibular function.[12] Specifically, patients with bilateral vestibular losses had decreased sway area (23%) and decreased trunk accelerations (46%) when standing on foam with the use of auditory biofeedback. Not surprisingly, auditory feedback leads to the largest gains in patients with the most severe dysfunction (bilateral vestibular loss) who are placed in the most challenging balance conditions (limited visual, eg, eyes closed; and somatosensory, eg, foam platform).[13] In keeping with this, auditory biofeedback had limited effect in vestibular patients in less challenging environments where full somatosensory information was present and accurate (eg, a flat, steady platform).[14]

Several variations on the characteristics of auditory biofeedback have been examined. In 2005, Hegeman et al[15] observed audio feedback that was triggered by either angular position or velocity changes. (Auditory feedback was via four speakers on each of the four walls of the room and was triggered when the patient deviated toward that wall at either a preset velocity or a position change.) Overall, an improvement in balance control with audio biofeedback in the vestibular patients was shown, in some cases, even reaching balance levels of the control subjects with intact vestibular function. In general, position-related information was found to be more useful than velocity-related information in reducing trunk sway.

Attempts have been made to understand the underlying physiologic mechanisms that lead to increased stability in the presence of auditory biofeedback. It has been suggested that it not only induces a mechanical increase in stiffness of the leg muscles but actually exerts a change in brain activity that likely aids in control of posture.[12]

Summary: Sensory Substitution

The understanding of the use and role of sensory substitution in the setting of bilateral vestibular impairment is evolving. As outlined, there are numerous options for the configuration and characteristics of the input stimulus and the sensory output of such systems. The miniaturization of such sensors is ongoing, making such devices more portable. The applications of such types of biofeedback have been shown to induce changes, specifically decreased movement amplitudes, in the activity patterns of muscles involved in postural control, in turn leading to a reduction in sway in individuals with bilateral vestibular loss.[16] The "real-world" utility of such approaches needs to take into consideration the cognitive demands that biofeedback places on the individual. This additional need for cognitive processing may detract from, or slow, their reactions to the world around them, which may be a detriment to overall function. The maintenance of balance is a complex task, and most of these devices simply use the vestibular inputs in four cardinal directions (anterior, posterior, medial, and lateral). There may be limitations and consequences to this oversimplification, particularly because these devices go from being tested using posturography to more challenging and realistic tasks. Despite these limitations, the utility of sensory biofeedback as a means of maintaining or training stability remains a relevant topic of research.

Electrical Stimulation of the Vestibular End Organs

Transcranial Vestibular Stimulation and Galvanic Vestibular Stimulation

Galvanic vestibular stimulation (GVS) is a form of transcranial direct stimulation whereby weak current is applied via electrodes attached to the mastoid bones. This current modulates the continuous firing levels of vestibular afferents. It may have a role in diagnosis as well as treatment of patients with vestibular loss. In the diagnostic setting, GVS is known to elicit different patterns of nystagmus pre-, during, and post-GVS in healthy volunteers compared with patients with complete unilateral vestibular loss.[17] It is postulated that these differences may be used to estimate the degree of vestibular function loss in patients. From a therapeutic standpoint, GVS has been shown to reduce sway amplitude and latency in patients with vestibular dysfunction, particularly when mechanical perturbations were introduced.[18] In addition to the effectiveness of this technique for vestibular symptoms in several studies, some authors have demonstrated neuroplastic changes following consistent use.[19] Although further study is required, GVS demonstrates potential for use as a prosthesis aimed at improving postural control.

Cochlear Implants

The auditory and vestibular systems are embryologically similar; they are also located in close proximity to one another. As outlined in Chapter 14, a large proportion of children with sensorineural hearing loss have an associated vestibular deficit. Across several studies, the prevalence of vestibular end-organ function in this population ranges from roughly 50% to 70%.[20–23] What is harder to understand is how cochlear implantation can improve vestibular function. Although this phenomenon is much less described in the literature, there are isolated reports and theories as to why it works.

Cochlear implants (CIs) have been shown to have a number of effects on vestibular and balance function. Initial concerns about the potential of eliciting a bilateral vestibular loss arose with the advent of bilateral cochlear implantation and as a result stimulated evaluation of vestibular and balance function in both pediatric and adult implant candidates. While some series have documented decrements in vestibular end-organ function following cochlear implantation,[24–27] others have demonstrated in some patients no change in function, or in some, even improvements in end-organ function following cochlear implantation.[27,28] A number of groups have documented improvements also in static and dynamic balance skills following cochlear implantation using tools such as computerized dynamic posturography and the Bruininks-Oseretsky test of motor proficiency, particularly when implants were on and activated.[20–22,24]

Similar improvements have also been documented on the Dizziness Handicap Inventory, particularly in the emotional subcategories at 4 months and 1 year post-op,[20] and parents also reported a marked improvement in their child's balance following surgery.[29] They further theorized that this effect was due to low-level current from the CI spreading beyond the cochlear nerve to stimulate the nearby vestibular nerve. Although this could lead to vestibular dysfunction, they postulated that it could also lead to improvement of vestibular function perhaps by providing vestibular cues. This hypothesis is feasible when one considers the literature regarding facial nerve stimulation from cochlear implantation. It has been demonstrated that 35% to 59% of children with CIs demonstrate electromyographic evidence of facial nerve stimulation, albeit subclinical. Indeed, the vestibular end organs and nerve are in much closer proximity to the electrode than is the facial nerve. Vestibular-evoked myogenic potential (VEMP) testing is an objective measure of vestibular stimulation with CIs. VEMP can be elicited with electrical stimulation in a proportion of children with CIs, demonstrating current spread from the cochlea to the vestibular system. The presence of electric VEMPs in acoustically nonresponsive ears, along with the shorter latencies of electrically driven VEMPs, suggests that electrical current can bypass the otoliths and directly stimulate vestibular neural elements.[30] Beyond the capacity to stimulate the end organ, we have demonstrated that stimulation from CI electrodes assists with recovery from asymmetric perceptual tilt as evidenced from the subjective visual vertical test.[31] Perception of visual vertical was assessed using the static Subjective Visual Vertical (SVV) test performed with and without stimulation in the participants with cochleovestibular loss. Trains of electrical pulses were delivered by an electrode in the left and/or right ear. Asymmetric spatial orientation deficits were found in nearly half of the participants with CIs (24/53 [45%]). The abnormal perception in this cohort was exacerbated by visual tilts in the direction of their deficit. Electric pulse trains delivered using the CI shifted this abnormal perception toward center (ie, normal; $p = 0.007$). Importantly, this benefit was realized regardless of which ear was stimulated. These results suggest a role for CI stimulation beyond the auditory system, in particular, for improving vestibular/balance function.[31] Attempts have been made to provide head-referenced stimulation of the cochlear implant, and this has been shown to improve stability in a small group.[32] These findings suggest that modifications to the cochlear implant in combination with developmental plasticity may prove useful in improving stability in patients with cochleovestibular dysfunction.

Vestibular Implants

Vestibular implants may hold the key to the treatment of individuals with bilateral vestibular impairment, and this section is not an exhaustive review of the current state of the art and the science that led us there but rather a summary of current approaches. There are several reviews on this topic in the literature which provide a more extensive description.[33,34] Vestibular implants generally are similar to cochlear implants in design and size.[35] They function via a miniature gyroscope, which detects three-dimensional head rotation, and a processor that manages inputs and decomposes them into vectors parallel to the planes of the semicircular canal. The processor then controls the stimulus output to a series of electrodes corresponding to the correct ampullary branch of the vestibular nerve.

Early reports of electrical stimulation of the vestibular system date back to 1964, when electrical stimulation of ampullary nerves was found to elicit eye movements.[36] More recently over the last decade, a number of groups across the globe have taken up the challenge of developing a vestibular prosthetic for human application. While the specific approach varies across the research groups in Geneva, Switzerland, Masstricht, the Netherlands, Baltimore, Maryland, and Seattle, Washington, the goal is the same, to provide baseline electrical activity to the vestibular end organs that would ultimately be modulated by head movement and have the capacity to restore or support vestibular reflexes such as the vestibulo-ocular reflex (VOR). To this end, a number of groups have examined the function of such implants in animal models. For example, the Johns Hopkins Multichannel Vestibular Prosthesis was found to partially restore the VOR for head rotations in any direction in rodents and rhesus monkeys with acquired bilateral vestibular deficits[37]; however, fine-tuning of the design, surgical approach, and stimulation paradigm remain a challenge. The three ampullary and two macular branches of the vestibular nerve lie in close proximity in vivo, making stimulus specificity difficult. Current spread to other afferent nerve fibers can distort the vestibular neural pattern leading to differences in the perceived versus true axis of head rotation, leading to spurious eye movements and visual blurring. Similarly, the University of Washington Group demonstrated that electrical stimulation delivered by a vestibular prosthetic implanted in rhesus monkeys demonstrated changes in eye velocity, which could ultimately be used to code head rotation.[38] A number of groups have proceeded to implant human subjects with either bilateral vestibular loss or other vestibular disorders such as Ménière's disease with such vestibular neural prosthetics and have demonstrated the capacity to restore vestibular reflexes such as the VOR.[39–41] It has, however, been demonstrated in adult models that the CNS can compensate for this differences seen in the animal models between the actual and perceived axis of rotation.[42] Furthermore, this discordance and the extent of disconjugate gaze improved significantly by the end of the first week of vestibular simulation. It has been suggested that humans may also be privy to similar adaptation over a similar timeline.

Physiologically, one of the main differences between the auditory and vestibular systems is the fact that in the vestibular system, there is a baseline neural firing rate that is challenging to replicate with and implant without eliciting uncontrolled eye movements and visual blurring. Ultimately, modulation of intensity and frequency of the restored baseline firing rate in the vestibular nerve generates controlled, smooth, conjugated eye movements; however, there is an adaptation phase that can be quite uncomfortable for patients. Typically, during the adaptation phase, the patient commonly experiences nystagmus and visual blurring; however, with training consisting of repetitive on–off periods of continuous electrical stimulation, the timeline of adaptation is decreased.[43,44]As a result, training is advocated and likely required in an effort to obtain controlled eye movements in response to neural firing. Similar features have been shown in animal models (guinea pigs) with adaptation occurring.[45] Ultimately, once the adaptation (nystagmus) phase has passed, VORs are elicited by head-motion stimulation in the presence of electrical stimulation, and therefore, it is believed that long-term replacement of vestibular function is possible.[46] Vestibular implants are also being tested for the treatment of vestibular disorders, such as Ménière;s disease, with the goal of activation being to abort an attack.[47–50]

Other considerations for vestibular implantation include hearing preservation, and optimization of electrode array is also important. Primate studies have demonstrated that the impact of vestibular implantation on hearing ranges from no significant change to small but measurable effects, with complete loss of hearing being possible but less common compared with the nonimplanted subjects, even following 5 months of chronic electrical stimulation.[51–53] In addition to preservation of hearing, it has been demonstrated that preservation of the rotational sensitivity of the semicircular canals can occur following implantation and chronic electrical stimulation.[52] Likewise, in chinchillas,[54] auditory brainstem thresholds obtained 3 to 9 weeks after implantation demonstrated in the majority of ears (4 of 6) a hearing loss of 5 to 10 standard deviations above the mean threshold for control ears across all frequencies with the thresholds of the remaining two ears being within one standard deviation of the control at nearly all frequencies compared with the non-implanted ear. It has been shown that hearing preservation is indeed possible even in the setting of cochlear implantation.[55] When hearing is lost following cochlear implantation, however, this can occur early or late; therefore, hearing thresholds should be followed in the long term.

Progress is being made in the development of a vestibular prosthetic, with new multichannel vestibular prostheses being smaller, more selective, easier to place, less power consuming, and appropriate for in vivo testing and measurement of impedances.[42] The vestibular prosthesis continues to hold much promise for the treatment of individuals with debilitating symptoms and safety concerns regarding bilateral vestibular loss and other peripheral vestibular disorders.

Regeneration

Molecular Genetics Gene Therapy and Viral Vectors

With the advent of powerful molecular genetic analysis on an individual and population basis, the genetic underpinnings of many peripheral and central disorders are being revealed. It is conceivable that in the not-too-distant future, the standard evaluation of individuals with vestibular disorders will include genetic analysis akin to the workup of patients with progressive ataxias.[56] In an excellent review, Frejo et al detail the molecular basis of vestibulopathies associated with hearing loss (DFNA9, DFNA11, DFNA15, DFNA28, DFNA102/103, EVAS, and both sporadic and familial Ménière's disease) as well the periodic vestibulopathies that heretofore were etiologically opaque (motion sickness, vestibular migraine, congenital vestibular hypofunction, and CANVAS syndrome).[57]

Information gained from studying gene function at the molecular level can be used to treat patients through gene therapy using viral vectors; however, such techniques are not currently U.S. Food and Drug Administration (FDA) approved. Over the past decade, much has been learned about the impact of genetic mutations on the development, anatomy, and function of the inner ear. Genes such as the H6 homeobox family 2 and 3 (*HMX2/3*) have been shown to play key roles in cell determination and development of the vestibular system, including the semicircular canals, utricle, saccule, sensory epithelia, as well as the endolymphatic duct and sac.[58] Knockout mice with no *HMX2/3* had an absence of vestibular end organs on computerized models despite the presence of a normal cochlea, and heterozygotes for this mutation were anatomically normal. *HMX2/3* may therefore be a worthy target for gene therapy in some individuals. Along those same lines, delivery of math using an adenovector resulted in recovery of the vestibular hair cells, neuroepithelium, and vestibular function in vitro and in vivo (in mice and rats) following aminoglycoside-mediated loss of hair cells.[59,60]

Given its accessibility via local rather than systemic approaches, the inner ear lends itself well to the introduction of novel genetic material via viral vectors. While most of the research has focused on viral transfection of the cochlea to restore hearing loss, there is an increasing amount of research into viral vectors for the purposes of ameliorating vestibular disorders. Applications of this therapy have focused mainly on hair cell regeneration and/or protection from ototoxicity. Many viral vectors have been tried, including herpes simplex type I virus, vaccinia virus, retroviruses, adenovirus, and adeno-associated virus, and a number of genes have also been examined.

Specifically, surgical techniques for gene transfer in which an adenoviral vector is administered through the posterior semicircular canal have been developed and described.[61] Such approaches have led to gene expression diffusely in the perilymphatic spaces with hearing preservation. Adenoviral vectors administered to the round window of mice were also found to lead to transgenic expression in vestibular and cochlear neurons,[62] whereas herpes viral vectors were much less concentrated in the vestibular structures and instead showed concentration mainly in the cochlea. It has also been demonstrated that not only can viral vectors concentrate within the inner ear, but that viral-mediated gene transfer leads to overexpression of glial cell line neurotrophic factor and is protective against ototoxicity.[63]

Hair cells within the inner ear are known to have the capacity to regenerate spontaneously in birds and lower vertebrates, but not in humans. Much work has been done in an attempt to uncover the mechanisms responsible for driving hair cell regeneration with the primary impetus of treating hearing loss. This interest has transferred over to the vestibular end organs, and adenoviral-mediated transfer of the *hath1* gene in sensory epithelium of cultured rat utricular maculae has been found to lead to new hair cell production, with hair cell regeneration occurring even after application of aminoglycoside to the cultures.[64] Likewise, delivery of atoh1 (a transcription factor and atonal homolog) to mice following damage to their vestibular end organs led to regeneration of vestibular hair cells with these mice recovering their balance function.[65,66] The atoh1 viral vector works by causing transdifferentiation of neighboring epithelial supporting cells and appears to lead to functional recovery of the vestibular system.[67] While it has been demonstrated that delivery, concentration, and restoration of function are possible using viral vectors to transfer genetic and transfection factors, one challenge that remains is how to obtain uniform distribution through the vestibular labyrinth without harming nearby structures such as the cochlea. Optimal amounts of viral vectors as well as toxicity, specificity, and serotype continue to be investigated. With this technology, functional restoration of the vestibular system with minimal toxicity may be on the horizon.

Stem Cells

In recent years, there has been increased interest in stem cells for many purposes, and their use in sensory restoration is only beginning to be elucidated. Damage to hair cells in the inner ear accounts for many balance disorders, and their inability to effectively regenerate explains why many vestibular insults are permanent. That being said, stem cells have been found in the vestibular sensory epithelium, but their limited ability to regenerate has not been adequate to restore function.[68,69] As early as 2003, cells with the capacity to differentiate into hair cells were isolated from the murine vestibular system and were found to have the capacity to differentiate into neurons.[70,71] It has been postulated that within the sensory epithelium, it is likely that the supporting cells are the progenitors of the new hair cells.[71] Embryonic stem cells, adult mouse inner ear stem cells, as well as cells within the CNS and vestibular end organs have all been reported to have the ability to differentiate into cells containing hair cell markers and proteins, and they demonstrate connections to spiral ganglion cells.[33,68]

Examination of stem cells within the vestibular system has been difficult, and several modes of doing so have been introduced.[72] Neural stem cells have been cultured with explants of rat inner ear. These cells were incorporated into the sensory epithelium of the vestibular organs, and this technique was recommended for further investigation of vestibular stem cells. Using similar techniques, mouse embryonic neural stem cells were cultured with mouse vestibular sensory epithelia in vitro, and the stem cells functioned like neurons, elongating their neurites toward, and attaching to, the vestibular hair cell at the typical locations.[73] In addition, patterns of synaptophysin, a marker for synaptic vesicles, were similar to those of developing sensory epithelia. Embryonic stem cells that responded to otic growth factors have also been generated.[69] Under these conditions, the cells organized into clusters exhibiting stereociliary bundles, and the cells responded to mechanical signals similar to those of normal hair cell transduction. In addition, the capacity for supporting cell division in mammalian vestibular organs can be enhanced by treatments with mitogenic growth factors, which are most effective in epithelia from neonates.[74]

From a therapeutic standpoint, one of the earliest challenges to stem cell use was the delivery method, such that there were adequate amounts delivered without disrupting normal cochlear function. Delivery methods for stem cells have included injection into the inner ear via utriculostomy which distributed the cells in the perilymph of the scala tympani and vestibuli.[75] Clearly, stem cells have the potential to pave the way for the treatment of both hearing and vestibular disorders through regeneration of the neural elements.

Summary Regeneration

The vestibular end organs are intricate structures composed of diverse cell types. Despite this complexity, the goal of regenerating their structure and function remains feasible on the basis of the cellular plasticity that exists even into adulthood within mammalian vestibular organs.[76] With that in mind, however, the morphology as well as the signal and response characteristics of vestibular cells are significantly more complex than the cochlea. However, the regeneration of different vestibular cell types in mammals with the goal of restoring sensory function is in evolution.

Conclusion

Vestibular dysfunction continues to be a common yet difficult problem to treat and carries with it an immense burden on health care systems, particularly given the morbidity and cost associated with falls in our aging population. Therapies have traditionally focused on central compensation and techniques to hasten or improve this process further. Future options for treatment include sensory substitution through a number of modalities, electrical stimulation and restoration of vestibular function, and finally, regeneration of the neural elements at the cellular level. While many challenges remain, it is an exciting time in this field, and clinicians treating individuals with vestibular and balance dysfunction will hopefully have a whole new set of tools in their armamentarium in the near future.

Self-Assessment Questions

1. The treatment of vestibular dysfunction can broadly be divided into three categories—what are they?

2. True or false: Vibrotactile feedback provided by use of a vestibular vest leads to decreased mediolateral and anteroposterior tilt.

3. True or false: Tongue-worn electrotactile feedback devices can aid recovery in unilateral but not bilateral vestibular losses.

4. In what scenario is auditory feedback most useful?

5. What is GVS?

6. Describe the possible effect of cochlear implantation on the vestibular function.

7. Explain how vestibular implants work.

8. Describe one of the obstacles facing vestibular implantation.

9. What are the H6 homeobox family 2 genes?

10. Describe one of the challenges of using viral vectors.

References

1. Kentala E, Vivas J, Wall C, 3rd. Reduction of postural sway by use of a vibrotactile balance prosthesis prototype in subjects with vestibular deficits. *Ann Otol Rhinol Laryngol.* 2003;112(5):404–409.
2. Wall C, 3rd. Application of vibrotactile feedback of body motion to improve rehabilitation in individuals with imbalance. *J Neurol Phys Ther.* 2010;34(2):98–104.
3. Wall C, 3rd, Weinberg MS, Schmidt PB, Krebs DE. Balance prosthesis based on micromechanical sensors using vibrotactile feedback of tilt. *IEEE Trans Biomed Eng.* 2001;48(10):1153–1161.
4. Camp AJ, Gu C, Cushing SL, Gordon KA, Corneil BD. Splenius capitis is a reliable target for measuring cervical vestibular evoked myogenic potentials in adults. *Eur J Neurosci.* 2017;45(9):1212–1223.
5. Tyler M, Danilov Y, Bach YRP. Closing an open-loop control system: Vestibular substitution through the tongue. *J Integr Neurosci.* 2003;2(2):159–164.
6. Vuillerme N, Cuisinier R. Sensory supplementation through tongue electrotactile stimulation to preserve head stabilization in space in the absence of vision. *Invest Ophthalmol Vis Sci.* 2009;50(1):476–481.
7. Vuillerme N, Pinsault N, Fleury A, et al. Effectiveness of an electro-tactile vestibular substitution system in improving upright postural

control in unilateral vestibular-defective patients. *Gait Posture.* 2008;28(4):711–715.

8. Vuillerme N, Hlavackova P, Franco C, Diot B, Demongeot J, Payan Y. Can an electro-tactile vestibular substitution system improve balance in patients with unilateral vestibular loss under altered somatosensory conditions from the foot and ankle? *Conf Proc IEEE Eng Med Biol Soc.* 2011;2011:1323–1326.
9. Polat S, Uneri A. Vestibular substitution: Comparative study. *J Laryngol Otol.* 2010;124(8): 852–858.
10. Barros CG, Bittar RS, Danilov Y. Effects of electrotactile vestibular substitution on rehabilitation of patients with bilateral vestibular loss. *Neurosci Lett.* 2010;476(3):123–126.
11. Chiari L, Dozza M, Cappello A, Horak FB, Macellari V, Giansanti D. Audio-biofeedback for balance improvement: An accelerometry-based system. *IEEE Trans Biomed Eng.* 2005; 52(12):2108–2111.
12. Dozza M, Chiari L, Horak FB. Audio-biofeedback improves balance in patients with bilateral vestibular loss. *Arch Phys Med Rehabil.* 2005;86(7):1401–1403.
13. Dozza M, Horak FB, Chiari L. Auditory biofeedback substitutes for loss of sensory information in maintaining stance. *Exp Brain Res.* 2007;178(1):37–48.
14. Horak FB. Postural compensation for vestibular loss and implications for rehabilitation. *Restor Neurol Neurosci.* 2010;28(1):57–68.
15. Hegeman J, Honegger F, Kupper M, Allum JH. The balance control of bilateral peripheral vestibular loss subjects and its improvement with auditory prosthetic feedback. *J Vestib Res.* 2005;15(2):109–117.
16. Allum JH, Honegger F. Vibro-tactile and auditory balance biofeedback changes muscle activity patterns: Possible implications for vestibular implants. *J Vestib Res.* 2017;27(1): 77–87.
17. Kim HJ, Choi JY, Son EJ, Lee WS. Response to galvanic vestibular stimulation in patients with unilateral vestibular loss. *Laryngoscope.* 2006;116(1):62–66.
18. Scinicariello AP, Eaton K, Inglis JT, Collins JJ. Enhancing human balance control with galvanic vestibular stimulation. *Biol Cybern.* 2001;84(6):475–480.
19. Utz KS, Dimova V, Oppenlander K, Kerkhoff G. Electrified minds: Transcranial direct current stimulation (tDCS) and galvanic vestibular stimulation (GVS) as methods of non-invasive brain stimulation in neuropsychology—A review of current data and future implications. *Neuropsychologia.* 2010;48(10): 2789–2810.
20. Buchman CA, Joy J, Hodges A, Telischi FF, Balkany TJ. Vestibular effects of cochlear implantation. *Laryngoscope.* 2004;114(10 pt 2 suppl 103):1–22.
21. Cushing SL, Gordon KA, Rutka JA, James AL, Papsin BC. Vestibular end-organ dysfunction in children with sensorineural hearing loss and cochlear implants: An expanded cohort and etiologic assessment. *Otol Neurotol.* 2013;34(3):422–428.
22. Cushing SL, Papsin BC, Rutka JA, James AL, Blaser SL, Gordon KA. Vestibular end-organ and balance deficits after meningitis and cochlear implantation in children correlate poorly with functional outcome. *Otol Neurotol.* 2009;30(4):488–495.
23. Licameli G, Zhou G, Kenna MA. Disturbance of vestibular function attributable to cochlear implantation in children. *Laryngoscope.* 2009;119(4):740–745.
24. Bonucci AS, Costa Filho OA, Mariotto LD, Amantini RC, Alvarenga Kde F. Vestibular function in cochlear implant users. *Braz J Otorhinolaryngol.* 2008;74(2):273–278.
25. Jacot E, Van Den Abbeele T, Debre HR, Wiener-Vacher SR. Vestibular impairments pre- and post-cochlear implant in children. *Int J Pediatr Otorhinolaryngol.* 2009;73(2): 209–217.
26. Wiener-Vacher SR, Obeid R, Abou-Elew M. Vestibular impairment after bacterial meningitis delays infant posturomotor development. *J Pediatr.* 2012;161(2):246–251. e241.
27. Szirmai A, Ribari O, Repassy G. Air caloric computer system application in monitoring vestibular function changes after cochlear implantation. *Otolaryngol Head Neck Surg.* 2001;125(6):631–634.

28. Ribari O, Kustel M, Szirmai A, Repassy G. Cochlear implantation influences contralateral hearing and vestibular responsiveness. *Acta Otolaryngol.* 1999;119(2):225–228.
29. Cushing SL, Chia R, James AL, Papsin BC, Gordon KA. A test of static and dynamic balance function in children with cochlear implants: The vestibular olympics. *Arch Otolaryngol Head Neck Surg.* 2008;134(1):34–38.
30. Parkes WJ, Gnanasegaram JJ, Cushing SL, McKnight CL, Papsin BC, Gordon KA. Vestibular evoked myogenic potential testing as an objective measure of vestibular stimulation with cochlear implants. *Laryngoscope.* 2017; 127(2):E75–E81.
31. Gnanasegaram JJ, Parkes WJ, Cushing SL, McKnight CL, Papsin BC, Gordon KA. Stimulation from cochlear implant electrodes assists with recovery from asymmetric perceptual tilt: Evidence from the subjective visual vertical test. *Front Integr Neurosci.* 2016;10:32.
32. Cushing SL, Pothier D, Hughes C, Hubbard BJ, Gordon KA, Papsin BC. Providing auditory cues to improve stability in children who are deaf. *Laryngoscope.* 2012;122(suppl 4): S101–S102.
33. Guyot JP, Perez Fornos A. Milestones in the development of a vestibular implant. *Curr Opin Neurol.* 2019;32(1):145–153.
34. Guyot JP, Perez Fornos A, Guinand N, van de Berg R, Stokroos R, Kingma H. Vestibular assistance systems: Promises and challenges. *J Neurol.* 2016;263 suppl 1:S30–35.
35. Valentin NS, Hageman KN, Dai C, Della Santina CC, Fridman GY. Development of a multichannel vestibular prosthesis prototype by modification of a commercially available cochlear implant. *IEEE Trans Neural Syst Rehabil Eng.* 2013;21(5):830–839.
36. Suzuki JI, Cohen B. Head, eye, body and limb movements from semicircular canal nerves. *Exp Neurol.* 1964;10:393–405.
37. Della Santina CC, Migliaccio AA, Hayden R, et al. Current and future management of bilateral loss of vestibular sensation—An update on the Johns Hopkins Multichannel Vestibular Prosthesis Project. *Cochlear Implants Int.* 2010;11(suppl 2):2–11.
38. Nie K, Ling L, Bierer SM, et al. An experimental vestibular neural prosthesis: Design and preliminary results with rhesus monkeys stimulated with modulated pulses. *IEEE Trans Biomed Eng.* 2013;60(6):1685–1692.
39. Golub JS, Ling L, Nie K, et al. Prosthetic implantation of the human vestibular system. *Otol Neurotol.* 2014;35(1):136–147.
40. Perez Fornos A, Guinand N, van de Berg R, et al. Artificial balance: Restoration of the vestibulo-ocular reflex in humans with a prototype vestibular neuroprosthesis. *Front Neurol.* 2014;5:66.
41. Guinand N, Van de Berg R, Cavuscens S, et al. Restoring visual acuity in dynamic conditions with a vestibular implant. *Front Neurosci.* 2016;10:577.
42. Chiang B, Fridman GY, Dai C, Rahman MA, Della Santina CC. Design and performance of a multichannel vestibular prosthesis that restores semicircular canal sensation in rhesus monkey. *IEEE Trans Neural Syst Rehabil Eng.* 2011;19(5):588–598.
43. Guinand N, Guyot JP, Kingma H, Kos I, Pelizzone M. Vestibular implants: The first steps in humans. *Conf Proc IEEE Eng Med Biol Soc.* 2011;2011:2262–2264.
44. Guyot JP, Sigrist A, Pelizzone M, Kos MI. Adaptation to steady-state electrical stimulation of the vestibular system in humans. *Ann Otol Rhinol Laryngol.* 2011;120(3):143–149.
45. Saginaw MA, Gong W, Haburcakova C, Merfeld DM. Attenuation of eye movements evoked by a vestibular implant at the frequency of the baseline pulse rate. *IEEE Trans Biomed Eng.* 2011;58(10):2732–2739.
46. Merfeld DM, Haburcakova C, Gong W, Lewis RF. Chronic vestibulo-ocular reflexes evoked by a vestibular prosthesis. *IEEE Trans Biomed Eng.* 2007;54(6 Pt 1):1005–1015.
47. Phillips JO, Bierer SM, Ling L, Nie K, Rubinstein JT. Real-time communication of head velocity and acceleration for an externally mounted vestibular prosthesis. *Conf Proc IEEE Eng Med Biol Soc.* 2011;2011:3537–3541.
48. Nie K, Bierer SM, Ling L, Oxford T, Rubinstein JT, Phillips JO. Characterization of the electrically evoked compound action potential

of the vestibular nerve. *Otol Neurotol.* 2011; 32(1):88–97.

49. Rubinstein JT, Nie K, Bierer S, Ling L, Phillips JO. Signal processing for a vestibular neurostimulator. *Conf Proc IEEE Eng Med Biol Soc.* 2010;2010:6247.
50. Rubinstein JT, Della Santina CC. Development of a biophysical model for vestibular prosthesis research. *J Vestib Res.* 2002;12(2–3):69–76.
51. Dai C, Fridman GY, Della Santina CC. Effects of vestibular prosthesis electrode implantation and stimulation on hearing in rhesus monkeys. *Hear Res.* 2011;277(1–2):204–210.
52. Rubinstein JT, Bierer S, Kaneko C, et al. Implantation of the semicircular canals with preservation of hearing and rotational sensitivity: A vestibular neurostimulator suitable for clinical research. *Otol Neurotol.* 2012;33(5): 789–796.
53. Bierer SM, Ling L, Nie K, et al. Auditory outcomes following implantation and electrical stimulation of the semicircular canals. *Hear Res.* 2012;287(1–2):51–56.
54. Tang S, Melvin TA, Della Santina CC. Effects of semicircular canal electrode implantation on hearing in chinchillas. *Acta Otolaryngol.* 2009;129(5):481–486.
55. Gantz BJ, Hansen MR, Turner CW, Oleson JJ, Reiss LA, Parkinson AJ. Hybrid 10 clinical trial: Preliminary results. *Audiol Neurootol.* 2009;14(suppl 1):32–38.
56. Choi KD, Choi JH. Episodic ataxias: Clinical and genetic features. *J Mov Disord.* 2016;9(3): 129–135.
57. Frejo L, Giegling I, Teggi R, Lopez-Escamez JA, Rujescu D. Genetics of vestibular disorders: Pathophysiological insights. *J Neurol.* 2016;263(suppl 1):S45–S53.
58. Wang X, Zhou J, Doyle ME, Egan JM. Glucagon-like peptide-1 causes pancreatic duodenal homeobox-1 protein translocation from the cytoplasm to the nucleus of pancreatic β-cells by a cyclic adenosine monophosphate/protein kinase A-dependent mechanism. *Endocrinology.* 2001;142(5):1820–1827.
59. Staecker H, Praetorius M, Baker K, Brough DE. Vestibular hair cell regeneration and restoration of balance function induced by Math1 gene transfer. *Otol Neurotol.* 2007;28(2):223–231.
60. Huang Y, Chi F, Han Z, Yang J, Gao W, Li Y. New ectopic vestibular hair cell-like cells induced by Math1 gene transfer in postnatal rats. *Brain Res.* 2009;1276:31–38.
61. Kawamoto K, Oh SH, Kanzaki S, Brown N, Raphael Y. The functional and structural outcome of inner ear gene transfer via the vestibular and cochlear fluids in mice. *Mol Ther.* 2001;4(6):575–585.
62. Staecker H, Li D, O'Malley BW, Jr, Van De Water TR. Gene expression in the mammalian cochlea: A study of multiple vector systems. *Acta Otolaryngol.* 2001;121(2):157–163.
63. Kanzaki S, Kawamoto K, Oh SH, et al. From gene identification to gene therapy. *Audiol Neurootol.* 2002;7(3):161–164.
64. Shou J, Zheng JL, Gao WQ. Robust generation of new hair cells in the mature mammalian inner ear by adenoviral expression of Hath1. *Mol Cell Neurosci.* 2003;23(2):169–179.
65. Baker K, Brough DE, Staecker H. Repair of the vestibular system via adenovector delivery of Atoh1: A potential treatment for balance disorders. *Adv Otorhinolaryngol.* 2009;66:52–63.
66. Schlecker C, Praetorius M, Brough DE, et al. Selective atonal gene delivery improves balance function in a mouse model of vestibular disease. *Gene Ther.* 2011;18(9):884–890.
67. Albu S, Muresanu DF. Vestibular regeneration —Experimental models and clinical implications. *J Cell Mol Med.* 2012;16(9):1970–1977.
68. Kesser BW, Lalwani AK. Gene therapy and stem cell transplantation: Strategies for hearing restoration. *Adv Otorhinolaryngol.* 2009; 66:64–86.
69. Oshima K, Shin K, Diensthuber M, Peng AW, Ricci AJ, Heller S. Mechanosensitive hair cell-like cells from embryonic and induced pluripotent stem cells. *Cell.* 2010;141(4):704–716.
70. Li H, Roblin G, Liu H, Heller S. Generation of hair cells by stepwise differentiation of embryonic stem cells. *Proc Natl Acad Sci USA.* 2003;100(23):13495–13500.
71. Li H, Liu H, Heller S. Pluripotent stem cells from the adult mouse inner ear. *Nat Med.* 2003;9(10):1293–1299.

72. Fujino K, Kim TS, Nishida AT, et al. Transplantation of neural stem cells into explants of rat inner ear. *Acta Otolaryngol Suppl.* 2004;(551):31–33.
73. Kim TS, Nakagawa T, Kita T, et al. Neural connections between embryonic stem cell-derived neurons and vestibular hair cells in vitro. *Brain Res.* 2005;1057(1–2):127–133.
74. Lambert PR. Inner ear hair cell regeneration in a mammal: Identification of a triggering factor. *Laryngoscope.* 1994;104(6 Pt 1):701–718.
75. Praetorius M, Vicario I, Schimmang T. Efficient transfer of embryonic stem cells into the cochlea via a non-invasive vestibular route. *Acta Otolaryngol.* 2008;128(7):720–723.
76. Li W, You D, Chen Y, Chai R, Li H. Regeneration of hair cells in the mammalian vestibular system. *Front Med.* 2016;10(2):143–151.

Self-Assessment Questions Answer Key

Chapter 1

1. c
2. e
3. d
4. d

Chapter 2

1. c
2. b
3. a
4. a
5. b
6. b
7. b
8. b
9. a

Chapter 3

1. a. Rotation of the top of the eye toward the lesioned ear
   b. Elevation of the eye on the side of the intact ear
   c. Tilt of the head toward the lesioned ear.
2. Patients with unilateral utricular lesions often fall, or feel pushed, toward the lesioned ear, reflecting the effect of descending vestibulospinal reflexes that maintain posture and balance.
3. Robust nystagmus with slow-phase eye movement toward the side of the lesion, as the vestibulo-ocular reflex (VOR) attempts to stabilize the eye in response to an inaccurately sensed head rotation.
4. Kinesthetic cues, tactile cues, and visual sensation
5. ■ Systematic changes in the weighting of various sources of sensory information
   ■ Reweighting of inputs to the neurons in the vestibular nucleus
   ■ Rebalancing the resting discharge of vestibular nuclear neurons
   ■ Progressive change in the response of vestibular nuclear neurons to motion stimuli
6. Patients who restrict head and body motion during the period of their recovery tend to have poorer outcomes than those who force themselves to safely and progressively experience destabilizing and challenging visual, vestibular, and support-surface environments.
7. a. Gaze-stabilization exercises
   b. Balance exercises

Chapter 4

1. Benign paroxysmal positional vertigo (BPPV) and benign paroxysmal vertigo of childhood (BPVC)
2. Vertigo resulting from a peripheral vestibular cause is always episodic. Episodes can be of a variety of durations, and the patient may feel unwell between acute episodes, particularly if they are clustered. Vertigo of a peripheral vestibular cause is never continuous. In addition, vertigo from a peripheral cause is always made worse with head movement.
3. Children with BPVC are at higher risk of developing true migraine later in life.
4. Fixation of the eyes can lead to suppression during both the static and dynamic assessment of eye and head movements.
5. Dynamic visual-acuity testing, head-thrust testing, pre- and post-rotatory nystagmus.
6. Head-thrust testing (abnormal when head is turned toward the affected ear), headshake testing (will have post-headshake nystagmus with the fast phase directed away from the affected ear), and Fukuda stepping test (deviation toward the side of unilateral weakness).
7. 5 years of age
8. Inability to suppress the VOR, dysmetric saccades, and saccadic smooth pursuit are all clinical findings that suggest central pathology.
9. Vertical nystagmus can indicate either a cranial cervical junction lesion, which will have downbeating nystagmus, or a pontine lesion with upbeating nystagmus.
10. Following an acute vestibular injury, there is the following progression: (a) third-degree nystagmus (nystagmus in the primary and both lateral positions of gaze), (b) second-degree nystagmus (nystagmus in the primary and one lateral position), (c) first-degree nystagmus (nystagmus is seen in only one position of lateral gaze), and (d) no spontaneous nystagmus.

Chapter 5

1. False
2. True
3. False
4. e
5. True
6. d
7. True
8. False
9. d
10. True

Chapter 6

1. a. Well tolerated
   b. Can use motorized or manual rotation
   c. Employs a physiologically relevant stimulus to access the VOR (ie, rotation)
   d. Can assess compensation and central adaptive changes
   e. Validity is unaffected by external or middle pathology (ie, cerumen or effusion)

2. a. Costly and space consuming
   b. Stimulus is delivered to both ears—no means of isolating one side
   c. At higher frequencies, additional stimuli (tactile and kinesthetic cues) occur
   d. Requires good head stabilization, which can be challenging
   e. Requires alerting
   f. Requires experience to interpret results
3. a. Off-vertical axis rotation (OVAR)
   b. Unilateral centrifugation test
4. a. Electronystagmography (ENG)
   b. Videonystagmography (VNG) (goggles, mask, chair-mounted or remote camera)
   c. Scleral coil
5. a. Gain
   b. Phase
   c. Symmetry
6. The gain of the response is the ratio of the slow-phase eye velocity to the chair velocity.
7. The symmetry of the response is the ratio of the rightward and leftward slow-phase eye velocities.
8. a. Gain
   b. Time constant
   c. Symmetry
9. In very young infants, the time constant is not always an effective measure of vestibular loss. In this age group, subjects with vestibular loss may have time constants close to the time constant of the normally functioning end organ, ≈6 seconds. The reason for this is that the neural networks that are responsible for the central storage of velocity information are relatively slow to develop. However, in older children, this test can be interpreted in the same manner as with adult patients.
10. Unilateral vestibular loss produces a reduction of the time constant for rotations toward the affected ear, which accompanies a reduction in the gain of the response in the same direction, producing an overall gain asymmetry.

Chapter 7

1. b
2. a
3. c
4. b
5. b
6. c

Chapter 8

1. a
2. a
3. c
4. b
5. a
6. b
7. a
8. c

Chapter 9

1. b
2. b and c

3. a
4. a and c
5. b
6. c
7. c
8. b
9. c
10. b

Chapter 10

Case 1

1. Yes, a gross motor assessment is indicated. As falls are impacting Jane's ability to participate in her community (school) via the performance of functional movements, it is necessary to know what functional movement and gross motor skills Jane is able to safely perform. It is necessary to investigate measures of impairment, but these will not translate into knowledge of movement skill performance and, therefore, balance, while these skills and movements are performed. More complex movement patterns and skills are required in a physical education class and general school play rather than isolated movements of muscles or joints. Assessment of age-appropriate functional tasks and gross motor skills provides robust and necessary information to determine if Jane requires help to safely participate in physical education classes.

2. a. Specific gross motor skills. The most important gross motor skills to include would be those that demand lower-extremity weight bearing, as Jane is having difficulty with falls when she is involved in games that demand standing. Running, hopping, and jumping skills should be a focus of the assessment and compared with typical performance of running, hopping, and jumping skills at age 6 years.
   b. Measures of lower-extremity impairment. As the falls are occurring while standing, it is necessary to assess for lower-extremity impairments such as tone, strength, range of movement, coordination, and sensation. Changes in any of these factors could significantly impact Jane's ability to perform gross motor functional tasks or skills. For example, a child who has mild trunk and lower-extremity hypotonia may have great difficulty in recruiting and producing muscle function at the speed and intensity required for movements in play or organized games. This may manifest in the inability to stand on one foot. When this task is required in the game of basketball while running or shooting, it may place Jane at risk for losing her balance and falling.
   c. Various types of gait. By systematically assessing various types of gait from basic to more demanding (gait on level surface, toe gait, heel gait, tandem gait), the physiotherapist will be able to determine at what point these gait tasks become more difficult to perform. If Jane has difficulty balancing when performing gait with a very narrow base of support (tandem gait), it would be useful to further assess the systems that are more heavily relied upon in this task, such as proprioception.

3. The use of an outcome measure can provide quantitative, and in this case, normative, data on dynamic balance in order to compare Jane's performance to that of children her age. In addition, observations/descriptions made with test performance could inform the assessor of the use of balance strategies and the quality of Jane's equilibrium reactions.
4. As Jane has not been described as having a specific health diagnosis, the use of the BOT2 or PDMS2 would provide useful information on Jane's gross motor performance. The GMFM has been researched primarily in the cerebral palsy population and would likely not provide information as useful, due to the potential ceiling effects with a child who appears to be performing at a relatively high level of function.
5. Yes. Assessment of stair ascent/descent is relatively easy to perform in a school setting and requires no additional equipment other than a staircase. Stair performance demands the use of concentric and eccentric muscle activity, graded movement, reciprocal stepping, and single-leg stance within function. These are all important factors to include within gross motor assessment, and difficulty with a component in stair ascent/descent may also be viewed when similar demands are made in functional skill performance. In addition, the need for railing use and adaptation of stepping patterns (eg, a step to pattern on descent) would indicate that further assessment of balance is required to ensure safe community mobility.

Case 2

1. Impairment measures, basic functional tasks, gross motor skills, and high-demand functional tasks should all be included in the gross motor assessment; however, due to the acuity of John's injury, his tolerance throughout the assessment, especially when performing the high-demand functional tasks, should be closely monitored.
2. Changes in the function of the vestibular system following brain injury could impact John's ability to maintain his balance and may need to be examined by a health care practitioner trained in vestibular assessment.
3. An assessment of motor coordination using tests such as the heel-to-shin test and rapid alternating movements, indicating dysmetria and dysdiadochokinesia, respectively, is indicated. In addition, a full somatosensory exam is indicated. A child with changes in the sensory system due to a sensory impairment can present with an ataxic gait pattern.
4. The BOT2 is a useful tool if it is to be used for discriminative purposes. It also has a specific balance component that is relatively short, allowing the physiotherapist to focus the assessment specifically on balance if patient tolerance is an issue. If a more evaluative measure for baseline performance is indicated, use of the Community Mobility and Balance Scale (CB&M) is suggested. Recent literature supports its use in a population of highly functioning children with acquired brain injuries.
5. If a specific outcome measure cannot be performed due to a child's tolerance or cognitive function, functional tasks that include level changes, narrowing of the base of support in sitting or standing position, a rotational component

of movement, and single-leg stance should be included in the assessment of dynamic balance.

Chapter 11

1. e
2. b
3. d
4. e
5. c

Chapter 12

1. They assess challenges faced during everyday behaviors and conditions rather than physiologic responses.
2. The otoliths and semicircular canals.
3. Subjective visual vertical.
4. The "continuous pointing task" involves participants being blindfolded and pointing to a previously viewed target while they are walking or being moved past it. Measuring the pointing direction of the arm provides a continuous indicator of how well the participant is able to perceive his or her location, and the location of objects around him or her in space, as well as their velocity and acceleration during passive or guided movement.
5. Path integration is the ability to keep internal track of one's position in space without using visual or auditory landmark cues. The primary sensory inputs used for path integration during walking include dynamic visual and acoustical flow, proprioceptive/efference copy, and vestibular inputs.
6. Spatial memory encoding.
7. The rotational elements of path integration tasks are misestimated to a greater degree than the translational element in the path for those with vestibular dysfunction.
8. Multisensory integration is the integration of redundant inputs from across the various sensory systems. It is advantageous, as integrating input from all the sensory systems leads to a more precise estimate of sensory percepts.
9. The "cue conflict approach" involves providing individual modalities with slightly incongruent information about a single perceptual event at the same time in an effort to dissociate individual sensory cues (ie, visual inputs from vestibular/proprioceptive inputs).
10. Decreasing cost; increasing accessibility and availability of VR hardware, software, and content; and the ability of VR to mimic everyday conditions and challenges. VR is able to simulate sensory information and introduce realistic sensory incongruencies and distracting stimuli that reflect real-world environments.
11. The time course (congenital versus acquired) and etiology of sensory deficits (eg, CMV versus stroke) are often different between children and adults.

Chapter 13

1. c
2. d

3. e
4. e
5. c
6. b

Chapter 14

1. Medical treatment:
   a. Lifestyle modifications
      1) A low-salt diet
      2) Avoidance of
         a) Caffeine and its derivatives
         b) Alcohol
   b. Medical therapies
      1) Diuretics
      2) Vasodilators
      3) Steroids
2. Surgical treatment:
   a. Nonablative
      1) Endolymphatic sac decompression/shunting
      2) Tympanostomy tube with Meniett Therapy
   b. Ablative
      1) Tympanostomy tube with intratympanic gentamycin
      2) Labyrinthectomy
      3) Vestibular nerve section
2. Up to 30%
3. In general, the vestibular end organs are more sensitive. This sensitivity is underestimated in the literature given that documentation of vestibular dysfunction is typically symptom based and not based on clinical exams or ancillary tests.
4. Head-thrust testing and dynamic visual acuity both examine high-frequency horizontal canal function. Head-thrust testing detects unilateral weaknesses, and dynamic visual acuity is abnormal in bilateral vestibular loss.
5. Vestibular function should be assessed in all children presenting with sensorineural hearing loss. Although vestibular dysfunction can occur with any etiology of hearing loss and there is large variability across any given etiologic group, severe vestibular dysfunction is most likely associated with the following etiologies:
   a. Meningitis (nearly 100%)
   b. Abnormal cochleovestibular anatomy (likelihood increases with the severity of the dysfunction and if it is associated with an underlying syndromic diagnosis)
   c. Usher syndrome. Vestibular function is typically severely and congenitally affected in type 1 Usher syndrome. With type 2 Usher syndrome, vestibular function is normally preserved, and it is variably, progressively, and more mildly affected in type 3 Usher syndrome.
   d. Ototoxicity
   e. Congenital cytomegalovirus

   This list is not exhaustive but includes the most common etiologic groups of sensorineural hearing loss associated with vestibular end-organ dysfunction.
6. a. Conductive hearing loss
   b. Autophony
   c. Aural fullness
   d. Pulsatile tinnitus
   e. Sound-/pressure-induced oscillopsia and vertigo (Tullio [sound] and Hennebert's [pressure] sign)
7. a. Latency
   b. Brief duration (usually <30 seconds)
   c. Fatigability
   d. Reversibility
   e. Geotropic rotatory

8. Ramsay Hunt syndrome occurs secondarily to reactivation of the latent varicella zoster virus in the geniculate ganglion. The presence of herpetic lesions distinguishes it from Bell's palsy.

9. a. Labyrinthine concussion
   b. Benign paroxysmal positional vertigo
   c. Perilymphatic fistula

10. a. Two or more definitive spontaneous episodes of vertigo 20 minutes or longer
    b. Audiometrically documented hearing loss on at least one occasion
    c. Tinnitus or aural fullness in the treated ear
    d. Other causes excluded

Chapter 15

1. False.

2. a. Posterior canal BPPV
   c. Anterior canal BPPV

3. A positive diagnostic maneuver is characterized by subjective vertigo and nystagmus, which typically demonstrate a latency of up to 20 seconds and fatigability after 30 to 60 seconds.

4. True.

5. b

6. d

7. Risk factors for BPPV in the pediatric population include vitamin D deficiency, migraine, vestibular migraine, and benign paroxysmal vertigo of childhood.

8. a and d

Chapter 16

1. d
2. b
3. f
4. d
5. d
6. c

Chapter 17

1. c
2. b
3. a
4. b
5. c

Chapter 18

1. c
2. d: a and b
3. c
4. c
5. b
6. d
7. c
8. c
9. a
10. c

Chapter 19

1. In general, recessive disorders more commonly appear in children, while dominant disorders have onset primarily in adulthood.
2. Friedreich ataxia is the most common form of hereditary ataxia, affecting 1 in 50,000 Caucasian individuals.
3. The associated tumor in children is usually neuroblastoma.
4. Mitochondria. All individuals with FRDA have a mutation in both alleles of the frataxin (*FXN*) gene, resulting in an abnormally low level of the protein called frataxin. Frataxin is a small, nuclear-encoded mitochondrial protein that mediates the chaperoning of iron sulfur clusters to the enzymes of oxidative phosphorylation; thus, its absence leads to decreased adenosine triphosphate production, reactive oxygen species production, and accumulation of iron within the mitochondria, resulting in injury caused by oxidative stress.
5. Systemic features include increased susceptibility to malignancies, conjunctival and cutaneous telangiectasia, insulin resistance, and recurrent pulmonary infections due to immunodeficiencies.
6. Lifelong high-dose oral vitamin E supplementation to maintain plasma vitamin E concentrations in the high-normal range.
7. Anticipation is a phenomenon whereby the symptoms of a genetic disorder appear earlier and with increasing severity as the disorder (most commonly seen in trinucleotide repeat disorders) is passed from one generation to the next.
8. Most CAG trinucleotide repeat disorders are characterized by an autosomal-dominant mode of inheritance.
9. Mitochondrial disease may be inherited from the mitochondrial DNA, or from the nuclear DNA, or may occur as a spontaneous mutation. Mitochondrial DNA diseases are transmitted maternally.
10. Associated malignancies are most commonly ovarian, lung, and breast cancer, although other cancers, including Hodgkin's lymphoma, are implicated in children.

Chapter 20

1. e
2. c
3. c
4. a
5. e

Chapter 21

Case 1

d

Case 2

a

Case 3

d

Case 4

a

Additional Questions

1. b
2. b
3. b
4. c
5. e
6. a

Chapter 22

1. In adults strabismus can cause significant diplopia resulting in balance disorder. Although children may suffer transient imbalance with acute strabismus secondary to diplopia, suppression of the deviated eye occurs quickly (days), resolving diplopia and imbalance; however, in this age group, suppression rapidly leads to amblyopia and loss of acuity and stereopsis (see Table 22–1).
2. Once again due to rapid suppression of image blur in children, transient oscillopsia is resolved centrally, resolving image jump and imbalance; however, reduced foveation time caused by nystagmus results in reduced vision, and an eccentric null position may result in marked abnormal head posture (see Table 22–1).
3. e
   Abnormal head posture may be adopted for all of these reasons. Patients may adopt an abnormal head posture and eccentric viewing as it centers a restricted field to the body (eg, hemianopia) or allows a patient to view binocularly straight ahead without diplopia or reduces the intensity of nystagmus, increasing image time at the retinal fovea (sharpest image) and improving vision. Other causes of ocular-related abnormal head posture are given in Table 22–2.
4. A lesion of the otolith-ocular (graviceptive) pathway leads to an abnormal internal estimate of gravitoinertial acceleration causing an inaccurate perception of earth-vertical axis. This inappropriately triggers the righting reflex normally seen in response to head tilting, resulting in (a) torticollis, (b) vertical ocular (skew) deviation, and (c) ocular torsion. This triad is termed the *OTR*.
5. No. Lesions of the spinothalamic tract can cause contralesional skew deviation (see Table 22–5).
6. Both conditions are involuntary eye movements. Nystagmus is initiated by a slow movement drifting from fixation; saccadic movements are initiated by a fast movement away from fixation (see Table 22–6).
7. The characteristics of nystagmus include the waveform (pendular versus jerk), amplitude (range of oscillation), direction of beating (fast corrective phase direction), conjugacy (whether the eyes move in phase in the same direction), plane (horizontal, vertical, rotary, symmetry, change on fixation), and presence of abnormal head posture and null position.
8. Nystagmus in infants may occur due to marked refractive error and media opacity (blurring image), congenital retinopathy (image degradation), as well as optic nerve and chiasmal pathology.
9. As opsoclonus is involuntary, erratic multidirectional bursts initiated by fast movements, this is a form of saccadic intrusion rather than nystagmus

(see Table 22–12). In children these multidirectional, often asymmetric, eye movements are associated with neuroblastoma requiring appropriate systemic workup.

10. Downbeat nystagmus is associated with lesions of the pontomedullary junction and cerebellar flocculus. This form of nystagmus may be seen in Chiari malformation, cerebellar degeneration, vertebrobasilar infarct, demyelination, and medication side effects.

Chapter 23

1. b
2. e
3. d
4. a
5. a
6. d
7. c
8. b
9. d
10. a

Chapter 24

1. Conversion disorder is defined as a physical reaction to psychological stress.
2. (1) One or more symptoms involving sensory function or voluntary motor control suggestive of a neurologic or medical condition. (2) Symptoms cannot be explained by medical or neurologic cause after thorough investigation; it is often considered a diagnosis of exclusion. (3) Symptoms cause significant distress or problems in social, work, school, or other areas, or they are significant enough that medical evaluation is recommended.[12]
3. (1) Performance excellence in at least one area of their life; school, sports, music. (2) Experience a great deal of self-induced or family imposed performance pressure. (3) Do not have the opportunity to develop adaptive coping strategies to cope with the stress. (4) Have difficulty identifying and talking about difficult emotions.[27,28]
4. Possibility of a recent trauma within family or for patient, possibility of recent attachment injury. Conversion disorder can develop in families where discussing difficult emotions is not role modeled. Possible development in families where a parent's mental or physical illness is the priority.
5. Individual therapy—cognitive behavioral therapy, mindfulness, skill building, supportive counseling, family therapy, pharmacotherapy
6. PPPD is classified as a chronic functional vestibular disorder, which may last months to years, and is not thought to be a structural or psychiatric condition.
7. Recommendations with documented efficacy include selective serotonin reuptake inhibitors (SSRIs) or serotonin and norepinephrine reuptake inhibitors (SNRIs).

Chapter 25

1. Occupational therapists use knowledge of Ayres' sensory integration (SI) theory

to appreciate how multiple sensory systems contribute to the development of normal balance and to the importance of using multisensory modalities in therapy. SI refers to organization of seven sensations in the brain, for use in an adaptive manner, enabling children to modulate behavior, learn, and participate in daily activities just like their friends.

2. Weak muscle tone; slouches in standing or when sitting at a desk; tires easily; immature equilibrium reactions; teachers report that the child slows the class down; does poorly in gym; does not alternate feet when taking the stairs; has low frustration tolerance; has poor handwriting; teacher must constantly remind child to sit up, sit still, and pay attention; may present as overly anxious.

3. Follow the child's lead; collaborate with the child; children must be active participants; set up the treatment space to be rich in sensory information and opportunities; encourage sensorimotor development; use repetition; therapists must use knowledge of play and should tap inner drive of the child; facilitate adaptive response; seek the right challenge for success.

4. Learning disability, attention deficit disorder with hyperactivity, developmental delay, autism spectrum disorder, fragile-X syndrome, cerebral palsy, visual or hearing impairment, premature birth, and prenatal drug exposure.

5. Parents seek social participation, self-regulation, and perceived competence for their children. Occupational therapists provide ongoing education to help parents reframe their expectations and collaborate with them to set goals for their children.

6. Vestibular, proprioceptive, and visual. Alex presented with immature equilibrium reactions (weight shift, elongation on weight-bearing side, trunk rotation) and weak muscle tone; the latter may have led to tiring easily and his slouched posture. The combination may explain his overall poor balance affecting participation in sports or simple tasks such as standing on one leg to put on his snow pants. Overly relying on vision to compensate for poor sensory feedback may have slowed performance as well. His writing was messy because he was not free to use one hand to stabilize his paper. He used an immature grasp to provide increased stability; however, this compensation interferes with mobility.

7. Sensory modulation refers to regulation and grading of sensory input. The two subtypes are hyperresponsiveness (oversensitivity to sensory input) and hyporesponsiveness (may not notice the input to the same degree as others).

8. Some children do not adequately integrate these reflexes, for example, children sitting in class turn to watch the teacher on the right side of the room and experience increased extensor tone in the right arm, accidentally brushing their notes off the desk (asymmetric tonic neck reflex or fencing position).

9. Changes in relationship to gravity yield extreme fear or hyperresponsivity. The child may not alternate feet on the stairs, may not jump with both feet together, may not use swings or park equipment, may be fearful of climbing and appear stiff, and may demonstrate rigid behavior.

10. Heavy use of a combination of vestibular (swings), proprioceptive (heavy work with muscles and joints), tactile

(deep-touch pressure, discrimination of touch), and visual (targeting, tracking, eye spy) sensory input in a playful and challenging manner; also, encouraging children to take more risks, to increase strength and endurance, and to be more able to feel where their bodies are in space and thus participate effectively with peers and in activities of daily living.

Chapter 26

1. c
2. c
3. d
4. d
5. a
6. b
7. b
8. d
9. c
10. b
11. d
12. c
13. c

Chapter 27

1. Safety and functional independence
2. a. Interprofessional practice is known to be best practice
   b. Provides a comprehensive assessment
   c. Allows for continuity of care
   d. Enhances communication
   e. Ensures no gaps in service
   f. Facilitates client/family centered care
   g. Allows for scope of practice
3. a. Link with attainment of meaningful goals
   b. Carryover of program recommendations
   c. Increased client satisfaction
4. Occupational performance is one's ability to engage/participate in a meaningful activity/occupation (ie, self-care, work, and leisure).
5. a. Person: physical, social and cognitive abilities, age, values, personality
   b. Environment: psychic, social, school
   c. Occupation: self-care activities, home management, school, and play
6. An activity can be graded by altering:
   a. Position of the person (ie, size and shape of base of support, alignment)
   b. Object placement (ie, position determines weight shift)
   c. Object characteristics (eg, weight and size)
   d. Temporal demands (eg, stationary versus moving objects)
7. Modifications to the environment should be targeted at the following levels/areas:
   a. *Physical.* Consider home and school. Consider all access points (ie, entrance into the building as well as interlevel access). If there were no elevator and the bathroom was not accessible, one would consider removal of barriers and universal design, for example, a roll in the shower could be useful to make the bathroom more accessible, as well as widening of doorways.
   b. *Social.* Consider psychosocial issues, socioeconomic status, and

the impact of finances. Additionally, consider intrinsic social factors as well as motivation. Selene did not feel comfortable or confident participating in social activities. Consulting a psychologist or social worker to help address this and formulate a plan to increase confidence may be useful; otherwise, grading activities and helping her to achieve success in OT activities would be appropriate.

c. *Cultural.* Take into consideration cultural background and be sensitive to differences and aware of your own beliefs in order to provide unbiased and supportive interventions. Another factor to consider is level of family support and type of involvement. In the case of Selene, act as a resource and educate the family on how to best support Selene in her rehabilitation.

d. *Institutional.* Consider community in terms of supports and resources as well as barriers. Selene's school is not accessible physically, and education about her situation is required for the staff and students. In a therapist's role, provide education, consultation, and advocate for the client in terms of what support she requires to be able to successfully reintegrate into school. For example, conduct training sessions for staff and/or an information session with students regarding safety or level of assistance required. Advocate for an educational assistant and be involved in school meetings regarding the level of assistance and accommodation for her return to school.

8. The process must start with a comprehensive assessment to inform goal setting and should include assessing overall muscle tone, postural stability, equilibrium reactions, and general ability of the child to assume a variety of positions. Next the therapist must work collaboratively with the child to come up with goals that are functional and validating to them. It is important that the child's priorities and level of importance of activities be considered first and foremost to ensure that the child is engaged in this rehabilitation process. To ensure that the child is functional, consider what the child must do every day, and if it was a previous activity that the child engaged in frequently, this is also a good indicator of functionality (or return to function). Moreover, it is important that the child be actively engaged in the activity (and want to participate and believes that it is important), because motivation influences skill acquisition, performance, and perseverance when difficulties are encountered.

9. a. Individual presentation and unique client characteristics
   b. Environmental barriers and facilitators
   c. Tasks and individual goals

10. a. Feasibility and time line of intervention
    b. Family goal and priorities
    c. Resources
    d. Relationship to safety and independence

Chapter 28

1. Sensory substitution, electrical stimulation, regeneration

2. True

3. False
4. Patients with the most severe dysfunction (bilateral vestibular loss) who are placed in the most challenging balance conditions (limited visual, eg, eyes closed; and somatosensory, eg, foam platform)
5. A form of transcranial direct stimulation whereby weak current is applied via electrodes attached to the mastoid bones. This current modulates the continuous firing levels of vestibular afferents.
6. While some series have documented decrements in vestibular end-organ function following cochlear implantation, 21 to 24 others have demonstrated in some patients no change in function, or in some, even improvements in end-organ function following cochlear implantation.
7. They function via a miniature gyroscope, which detects three-dimensional head rotation, and a processor, which manages inputs and decomposes them into vectors parallel to the planes of the semicircular canal. The processor then controls the stimulus output to a series of electrodes corresponding to the correct ampullary branch of the vestibular nerve.
8. The three ampullary and two macular branches of the vestibular nerve lie in close proximity in vivo, making stimulus specificity difficult. Current spread to other afferent nerve fibers can distort the vestibular neural pattern leading to differences in the perceived versus true axis of head rotation, leading to spurious eye movements and visual blurring. Thus a training period is often necessary. Placement can be quite difficult. There is also a possibility of worsening hearing.
9. Play key roles in cell determination and development of the vestibular system including the semicircular canals, utricle, saccule, sensory epithelia, as well as the endolymphatic duct and sac.
10. Obtaining uniform distribution through the vestibular labyrinth, not harming nearby structures such as the cochlea. Optimal amounts of viral vectors and toxicity, specific vector to be used.

Index

Note: Page numbers in **bold** reference non-text material

C

D

E

F

G

H

P

R

S

T

U

W

X

Y

Γ